T0181365

Register Now for Online Access to Your Book!

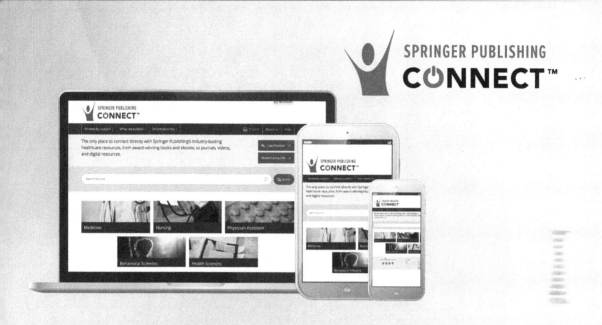

Your print purchase of *Neonatal Advanced Practice Nursing: A Case-Based Learning Approach* **includes online access to the contents of your book**— increasing accessibility, portability, and searchability!

Access today at:
http://connect.springerpub.com/content/book/978-0-8261-9415-2
or scan the QR code at the right with your smartphone. Log in or register, then click "Redeem a voucher" and use the code below.

PAFA1CY3

Scan here for quick access.

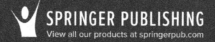

SPRINGER PUBLISHING
View all our products at springerpub.com

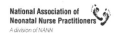

National Association of
Neonatal Nurse Practitioners
A division of NANN

Neonatal Advanced Practice Nursing: A Case-Based Learning Approach is a must have for your library. This case-based pathophysiology text is specifically designed for the neonatal advanced practice registered nurse (APRN) and provides both a pragmatic and clinical resource that the neonatal APRN has not had until now.

Each case is developed through the utilization of a system-based approach that is supported by current evidence, advanced physical assessment, and pathophysiology. This text closes the gap between didactic education and practice and promotes development of critical thinking through the use of realistic clinical cases.

Perfect for the new APRN or the most tenured among us! The Table of Contents alone reads as a veritable list of giants in the neonatal APRN world. Most contributors have served or currently serve in leadership positions at the national level.

Congratulations Sandy and Michele!

> —2016 Governing Council of the National Association of
> Neonatal Nurse Practitioners (NANNP)

Neonatal Advanced Practice Nursing

Sandra Bellini, DNP, APRN, NNP-BC, CNE, is an associate clinical professor who holds National Certification Corporation (NCC) certification as a neonatal nurse practitioner (NNP) and National League for Nursing certification as a nurse educator. Her current position is coordinator for the Neonatal Nurse Practitioner Program at the University of Connecticut School of Nursing. She has published and presented at the local, regional, national, and international levels. Dr. Bellini also serves as a reviewer for several journals and is a member of the editorial advisory board for *Nursing for Women's Health*, an Association of Women's Health, Obstetric and Neonatal Nurses journal. Dr. Bellini has 28 years of neonatal nursing experience at both the staff and advanced practice levels. Her current joint-appointment position incorporates 20% full-time equivalent (FTE) in clinical practice as an NNP at Connecticut Children's Medical Center, Neonatal Intensive Care Unit, Hartford, Connecticut. Dr. Bellini is also a certified regional trainer for the Neonatal Resuscitation Program (NRP) and a lead instructor for the STABLE Transport Program.

Michele J. Beaulieu, DNP, ARNP, NNP-BC, is a neonatal nurse practitioner at Johns Hopkins/All Children's Hospital. She is also an author and educator. Dr. Beaulieu graduated with her doctor of nursing (DNP) degree from the Frances Payne Bolton School of Nursing at Case Western Reserve University, Cleveland, Ohio. In addition to her full-time neonatal practice, Dr. Beaulieu has been the column editor for "Pointers in Practical Pharmacology" in *Neonatal Network: The Journal of Neonatal Nursing*, author and expert reviewer of various peer-reviewed manuscripts and books, and is the coinvestigator for several research studies. Her research interests include perinatal safety, extremely low-birth-weight infants, neonatal abstinence syndrome, and the management of high-risk newborns in the delivery room. Dr. Beaulieu has developed and taught clinical and online courses for undergraduate and graduate nursing programs, including those at the University of Connecticut. She is a member of Sigma Theta Tau (Delta Beta chapter) and is actively involved in several neonatal and women's health professional organizations, among them, the Florida Association of Neonatal Nurse Practitioners.

Neonatal Advanced Practice Nursing

A Case-Based Learning Approach

Sandra Bellini, DNP, APRN, NNP-BC, CNE

Michele J. Beaulieu, DNP, ARNP, NNP-BC

Editors

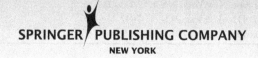

SPRINGER PUBLISHING COMPANY

NEW YORK

Springer Publishing Company, LLC
11 West 42nd Street
New York, NY 10036
www.springerpub.com

Acquisitions Editor: Elizabeth Nieginski
Composition: Westchester Book Publishing

ISBN: 978-0-8261-9415-2
e-book ISBN: 978-0-8261-9416-9
Instructor's Toolkit ISBN: 978-0-8261-9391-9
Image Bank ISBN: 978-0-8261-9395-7

Instructor's Materials: Qualified instructors may request supplements by e-mailing textbook@springerpub.com.

Printed by BnT

The author and the publisher of this Work have made every effort to use sources believed to be reliable to provide information that is accurate and compatible with the standards generally accepted at the time of publication. Because medical science is continually advancing, our knowledge base continues to expand. Therefore, as new information becomes available, changes in procedures become necessary. We recommend that the reader always consult current research and specific institutional policies before performing any clinical procedure. The author and publisher shall not be liable for any special, consequential, or exemplary damages resulting, in whole or in part, from the readers' use of, or reliance on, the information contained in this book. The publisher has no responsibility for the persistence or accuracy of URLs for external or third-party Internet websites referred to in this publication and does not guarantee that any content on such websites is, or will remain, accurate or appropriate.

Library of Congress Cataloging-in-Publication Data

Names: Bellini, Sandra, 1966– editor. | Beaulieu, Michele (Michele J.), editor.
Title: Neonatal advanced practice nursing : a case-based learning approach / [edited by] Sandra Bellini, Michele Beaulieu.
Description: New York, NY : Springer Publishing Company, LLC, [2017] | Includes bibliographical references and index.
Identifiers: LCCN 2016020388 | ISBN 9780826194152 (alk. paper) | ISBN 9780826194169 (e-book)
Subjects: | MESH: Neonatal Nursing—methods | Infant, Newborn, Diseases—nursing | Advanced Practice Nursing—methods | Problems and Exercises
Classification: LCC RJ245 | NLM WY 18.2 | DDC 618.92/00231—dc23
LC record available at https://lccn.loc.gov/2016020388

Printed in the United States of America.

I dedicate this book to my husband and favorite neonatologist, Joel Weiner, because although he's still clearly out of my league, I hope he never actually notices.

Our collective children, Travis, Eli, and Melanie, because they've emerged as intelligent, articulate, and sensitive adults we couldn't be more proud of.

. . . And to the sorority of breast cancer survivors in the world, I read this somewhere and wish I'd been clever enough to write it:

"Don't knock at Death's door and wait for him to answer. Ring the bell . . . and run.

He hates that!"

—sb

I dedicate this book to my late husband, Bob, without whom I would not be the person or professional I am today.

Through his love and support all things were possible.

—mjb

Contents

Contributors

Ana Arias-Oliveras, MSN, NNP-BC
Associate Program Director
Neonatal Nurse Practitioner Program
University of Pennsylvania
School of Nursing
Philadelphia, Pennsylvania

Bobby Bellflower, DNSc, NNP-BC
Associate Professor
University of Tennessee Health Science Center
College of Nursing
Memphis, Tennessee

Mary Beth Bodin, DNP, CRNP, NNP-BC
Neonatal Consultant
Tuscaloosa, Alabama

Elena Bosque, PhD, ARNP, NNP-BC
Neonatal Nurse Practitioner/Professional Development
Seattle Children's Hospital
Faculty, College of Nursing, Creighton University
Seattle, Washington

Terri A. Cavaliere, DNP, NNP-BC
Clinical Associate Professor
School of Nursing
Stony Brook University
Stony Brook, New York

Bresney Crowell, MSN, APRN, NNP-BC
Neonatal Nurse Practitioner
Medical University of South Carolina
Charleston, South Carolina

Regina M. Cusson, PhD, APRN, NNP-BC, FAAN

Professor
University of Connecticut School of Nursing
Storrs, Connecticut

Desiree A. Diaz, PhD, RN-BC, CNE, CHSE

Assistant Professor
University of Central Florida
Orlando, Florida

Donna Campbell Dunn, PhD, CRNP, CNM, FNP-BC

Assistant Professor
University of Alabama at Birmingham
School of Nursing
Birmingham, Alabama

Carolyn J. Herrington, PhD, RN, NNP-BC, CLC

Assistant Professor, Clinical
Wayne State University
Detroit, Michigan

Jacqui Hoffman, DNP, ARNP, NNP-BC

DNP-NNP Track Coordinator
University of Florida College of Nursing
Gainesville, Florida
Neonatal Nurse Practitioner
Pediatrix Medical Group
Tampa, Florida

Amy Jnah, DNP, NNP-BC

Clinical Assistant Professor
Director, Neonatal Nurse Practitioner Program
East Carolina University
Greenville, North Carolina

Patricia J. Johnson, DNP, MPH, APRN, NNP

Neonatal Nurse Practitioner
Maricopa Integrated Health System
Phoenix, Arizona

Kimberly Knoerlein, MSN, APRN

Children's Hospital at Dartmouth
Instructor of Pediatrics
Geisel School of Medicine at Dartmouth
Lebanon, New Hampshire

Joan Esper Kuhnly, DNP, APRN, NNP-BC, IBCLC, CNE

Associate Clinical Professor
University of Connecticut School of Nursing
Storrs, Connecticut

Maureen F. McCourt, MS, APRN, NNP-BC

Coordinator, Neonatal Nurse Practitioner Service
Women & Infants Hospital
Neonatal Nurse Practitioner Faculty Northeastern University
Providence, Rhode Island

Jacqueline M. McGrath, PhD, RN, FNAP, FAAN

Professor and Associate Dean for Scholarship and Research
University of Connecticut
School of Nursing
Storrs, Connecticut
Connecticut Children's Medical Center
Hartford, Connecticut

Kathryn R. McLean, MSN, RNC, NNP

Neonatal Nurse Practitioner
Women & Infants Hospital
Providence, Rhode Island

Leanne M. Nantais-Smith, PhD, RN, NNP-BC

Assistant Professor Clinical
Director of Advanced Practice and Graduate Certificate Programs
Coordinator Neonatal Nurse Practitioner Specialty
College of Nursing
Wayne State University
Detroit, Michigan

Desi Newberry, DNP, NNP-BC

Clinical Assistant Professor
East Carolina University
Greenville, North Carolina

Susan M. Quinn, MS, ARNP, NNP-BC

Maine Medical Center
Adjunct Faculty Neonatal Nurse Practitioner Program
University of Connecticut School of Nursing
Portland, Maine

Daphne A. Reavey, PhD, RN, NNP-BC

Coordinator, Neonatal Nurse Practitioner Program
University of Missouri-Kansas City
Neonatal Nurse Practitioner
Children's Mercy Hospital & Clinics
Kansas City, Missouri

Cheryl Riley, DNP, RN, NNP-BC

Coordinator, Neonatal Nurse Practitioner Program
Baylor University
Louise Herrington School of Nursing
Dallas, Texas

Tracey Bell Robertson, DNP, NNP-BC

Clinical Assistant Professor
East Carolina University
Greenville, North Carolina

Cheryl B. Robinson, DNS, MS, NNP-BC

Associate Professor
Neonatal Nurse Practitioner Specialty Track Coordinator
University of Alabama at Birmingham
School of Nursing
Birmingham, Alabama

Lori Baas Rubarth, PhD, APRN, NNP-BC

Associate Professor, Neonatal Nurse Practitioner Program Coordinator
Creighton University College of Nursing
Omaha, Nebraska

Suzanne Staebler, DNP, APRN, NNP-BC, FAANP

Associate Professor, Clinical Track
Specialty Program Coordinator, Neonatal Nurse Practitioner Program
Nell Hodgson Woodruff School of Nursing at Emory University
Atlanta, Georgia

Roxanne R. Stahl, APRN, MS, NNP-BC

Council Member, National Association of Neonatal Nurse Practitioners
Monroe Carell Jr. Children's at Vanderbilt
Vanderbilt University School of Nursing
Nashville, Tennessee

Lyn Vargo, PhD, RN, NNP-BC

Clinical Assistant Professor in Neonatal Nurse Practitioner Programs
University of Missouri–Kansas City (UMKC)
St. Louis, Missouri

Mary Beth Whalen, DNP, APRN, NNP-BC

UMass Memorial Healthcare
Adjunct Faculty Neonatal Nurse Practitioner Program
University of Connecticut School of Nursing
Worcester, Massachusetts

Catherine Witt, PhD, NNP-BC

Associate Professor, Coordinator, Neonatal Nurse Practitioner Program
Loretto Heights School of Nursing, Regis University
Denver, Colorado

Karen Wright, PhD, NNP-BC

Assistant Professor and Director
Neonatal Nurse Practitioner Program
Rush University
Chicago, Illinois

Foreword

I had the privilege of working with Dr. Patricia Benner at the University of California, San Francisco, during the 1980s. Benner's underlying philosophical approach was phenomenological, and she described how a nurse gains expertise through experience. The result of her early work was the book *From Novice to Expert: Excellence and Power in Clinical Nursing Practice* (1984).

In this book, she described how the novice must solve problems using theory and rules but, with actual practice, the nurse tests theory and the approach changes. Expert performance of skills and clinical judgments, or embodied intelligence, allows the nurse to see patterns within complex information. For Dr. Benner's research, she used nurses' exemplar cases to demonstrate levels of nursing expertise. Although these qualitative data have been valuable in education and practice, her work also has the rare ability to describe nursing practice and exalt the work of nurses.

In the mid-1980s, I was working as a neonatal clinical specialist at Children's Hospital of San Francisco (now California Pacific Medical Center) and had based the neonatal staff nurse orientation program on Benner's philosophical approach to how nurses gain expertise. I had been having trouble recruiting expert nurses to mentor new staff nurses because they told me that they could not always respond to the novices' questions about why they intervened with a sick infant, and it made them feel stupid. I had better success with recruitment when I quoted Dr. Benner and explained that it was because of expertise and intuitive and embodied knowledge that they had difficulty with rule-based explanations. After I organized an elegant, fun, memorable, sponsored evening for neonatal nurse mentors at the Fairmont Hotel, where Dr. Benner gave an inspirational talk about the power of expert nursing, I never again had any trouble with recruitment.

In Benner and colleagues' more recent book, *Educating Nurses: A Call for Radical Transformation* (2010), it is suggested that educators should transform the approaches to basic nursing training to incorporate experiential learning through case-based education, "to unify clinical and classroom teaching and teach from a stance of practice" (Benner, Sutphen, Leonard, & Day, 2010, p. 91). They recommended a "shift from a focus on covering decontextualized knowledge to an emphasis on teaching for a sense of salience, situated cognition, and action in particular situations" (Benner et al., 2010, p. 82).

I have had the opportunity to demonstrate that this approach can be implemented while teaching neonatal nurse practitioner (NNP) students in a course about common neonatal problems (Bosque, 2012). The benefits of closing the gap between didactics and practice through a case-based approach, with the promotion of critical thinking and role development in a supportive environment, were demonstrated by students' and lecturers' responses on a survey.

As educators, we know that we can provide information and receive perfect test answers without teaching the NNP student how to determine what stands out among so much detailed information in a busy neonatal intensive care unit (NICU). It is possible to prepare a new NNP graduate to pass the certification exam, and yet the novice NNP may have difficulty with critical thinking and nuanced decision making in the NICU. Expertise will develop with time, but educational efforts to "bring the NICU to the classroom" and have experts teach via paradigm cases should impart critical-reasoning knowledge to the student instead of only decontextualized information. This approach may not only improve the level of functioning of the novice NNP in training or practice, but also decrease stress and promote success and job satisfaction.

This book, which has been so well organized by the editors, Michele J. Beaulieu and Sandra Bellini, has been developed as a tool for educators to facilitate integrative learning for NNP students. It is the first of its kind. Common neonatal problems are included. Every chapter is presented in a similar manner. Pathophysiology is presented, but the focus is on the application of the background information to the cases. Questions are posed to support the critical-thinking and decision-making skills that are required of an effective NNP in the NICU.

During meetings with my fellow contributors, who are known as national leaders in neonatal advanced practice education and clinical practice, there were no controversies and no prolonged discussion. I believe that this approach to the education of the NNP is so natural and appealing that the goal was easily understandable to us all. This work captures the expertise of many seasoned neonatal educators and clinical providers and translates their experience into a useful, helpful product for others. The goal of our collective efforts is, as always, to benefit the family who has a sick or premature infant in the NICU. I am grateful to be a part of this work.

Elena Bosque, PhD, ARNP, NNP-BC
Neonatal Nurse Practitioner/Professional Development
Seattle Children's Hospital
Faculty, College of Nursing, Creighton University
Seattle, Washington

REFERENCES

Benner, P., Sutphen, S., Leonard, V., & Day, L. (2010). *Educating nurses: A call for radical transformation.* San Francisco, CA: Jossey-Bass.

Bosque, E. (2012). Toward salience: An application of integrative, case-based nursing education for neonatal advanced practice. *Advances in Neonatal Care, 12*(5), 292–302.

Preface

Educational materials written expressly for neonatal nurse practitioner (NNP) students are rare, indeed. More common, NNP programs and faculty rely on medical texts dedicated to neonatal medicine and designed for residents and neonatal fellows. Although these are invaluable resources for NNP students, this text is intended to begin where that didactic information leaves off.

The process of educating an advanced practice nurse requires, of course, that students gain significant *knowledge* during their studies focused on physiology, disease process, exam findings, appropriate evaluation, management strategies, and so on. Therefore, the purpose of this text is the next step in education for advanced clinical practice: Once the student has acquired substantive knowledge regarding the care of neonates, what does one *do* with that information? This book is intended to further develop the novice NNP into a safe and excellent clinician through *application* exercises designed to enhance critical-thinking skills. Similar to the way in which texts for neonatal medicine are useful in NNP programs, we believe this text will also be useful for the education of residents and fellows. Our practice in neonatal intensive care units (NICUs) is inherently interprofessional, so our educational journeys should be as well.

This book seeks to augment student learning through enhancement of *integration and application* of didactic knowledge. In other words, it is intended that students will have reviewed didactic material in other primary sources already in use. Following that, students should ask: "What does it all mean?" and "What do I do with this information?" The distinction between acquiring baseline knowledge and learning how to apply that knowledge requires strong critical-thinking skills. From an educational standpoint, critical-thinking skills and improved learning outcomes are enhanced when students are engaged in *active learning*, such as identifying problems and creating a list of differential diagnoses, for example, as opposed to *passive learning activities*, such as independent reading. The case-based learning format provides students with the opportunity to be *involved* in their learning process through active learning activities. Given that NNP education today is predominantly delivered in online formats, faculty can promote student interaction and team building in an online environment through collaborative group assignments. Conversely, students can also use the book for individual learning, such as review for the National Certification Corporation (NCC) certification exam.

This book comes to market at an opportune time in health professions education, and in nursing education, in particular. In their 2010 Carnegie Report, *Educating Nurses: A Call for Radical Transformation* (Benner, Sutphen, Leonard, & Day, 2010), Dr. Benner and colleagues clearly relay their recommendations that nursing students be educated differently going forward. In part, they argue that nurses graduating from undergraduate programs today are not prepared to function in the rapidly changing, complex health care environment. One area of education they select for improvement is related to building critical-thinking skills; yet another is for making learning environments more experiential to promote contextual learning. Although NNP students are, by definition, graduate students as opposed to undergraduate students, the reality is that they will still graduate as novices who will benefit from both improved critical-thinking skills and experiential learning, both of which can be promoted through case-based learning.

Developed through the collaborative efforts of experienced NNP faculty and NNPs from across the country, this book brings the didactic content of an NNP program to life. Each chapter provides a brief overview of the physiology/pathophysiology of disease processes in a systems format as a means of reinforcing content found in other texts. Following that review, real-life cases are provided for the student accompanied by critical-thinking/discussion questions. The many cases included will provide students with ample opportunity to build critical-thinking skills and emerge after graduation as confident and safe novice NNPs.

Sandra Bellini
Michele J. Beaulieu

REFERENCE

Benner, P., Sutphen, S., Leonard, V., & Day, L. (2010). *Educating nurses: A call for radical transformation.* San Francisco, CA: Jossey-Bass.

Acknowledgments

This book was a collaborative effort in the truest sense. From the outset, we wanted to use the creation of this case-based learning book as a means of bringing the national neonatal nurse practitioner (NNP) faculty and clinicians together to do something very creative and even "fun." Therefore, the contributing authors for this project represent a self-selected group of people who have much in common, including an odd definition of "fun" that only another NNP would understand!

We thank the long list of contributing authors who participated in this project. You are all excellent professionals whom we are honored to call friends and colleagues.

We thank our NNP students, past, present, and future, for sharing their passion for neonatal nursing. They continue to inspire us.

Last, but not least, we thank the many families who have allowed us the pleasure of caring for their newborns over many years. They have given us the privilege of intruding on what should otherwise be a very intimate and private event in their lives. In doing so, we have shared some of the greatest highs and lows that life has to offer. They will never know that they have had as much of an effect on us as we had on them.

An Overview of the Text

As an introduction to the book and the concept of case-based learning, the Foreword is written by Dr. Elena Bosque, who has published works on the integration of knowledge through a case-based approach to facilitate the neonatal nurse practitioner's (NNP's) learning in education and application in the clinical setting (Bosque, 2012). This book extends the work of Dr. Patricia Benner and supports the integrative educational approach outlined by Dr. Bosque.

The book is divided into three sections, each focusing on different aspects of neonatal care.

In Section I, case-based learning is approached through assessment of maternal risk factors and conditions that may place the fetus at risk, identifying factors that influence neonatal transition, and formulating a differential diagnosis based on maternal history and physical exam of the newborn.

In Section II, common diseases and disorders of the newborn are presented by body system. This section is rich in integration and application of critical thinking as it applies to various disease processes. Case studies in each of the chapters vary somewhat in their presentation to accommodate different teaching and learning styles and to allow for academic freedom on the part of the contributing authors. Some of the chapters include unfolding case studies, whereas others have case presentations with relevant questions. The number of case studies varies depending on the body system. The majority of chapters contain case studies related to the physiology/pathophysiology content review provided at the beginning of the chapter, followed by objective multiple-choice questions and discussion questions. The intent is to provide a review of content, followed by integration and application of concepts and reinforcement of learning. Content is based on material the NNP should know for safe practice and questions are in step with the types of questions that may appear on the National Certification Corporation (NCC) exam.

Section III focuses on a diverse presentation of topics, including discussion of health care maintenance of the newborn through the first year of life, as well as developmental outcomes of high-risk newborns. Two additional chapters in this section are unique to this book and to NNP educational materials in general, because they include the rare discussion of application of ethical principles, moral distress, and communication of sensitive information to families and the application of simulated best-practice methods in advanced practice nursing.

In the Afterwords, Dr. Regina Cusson and Dr. Jacqueline McGrath discuss the challenges of role transition and strategies for success in role development as an advanced practice nurse, as well as the importance of developing a purposeful plan for lifelong learning.

Finally, there is an Instructor's Toolkit containing additional discussion questions that can easily be incorporated into online class discussion and a Test Bank, as well as a primer on creating simulations for NNP programs as a means of providing experiential, case-based learning. A comprehensive Image Bank is also available. Qualified instructors can access both by e-mailing Springer Publishing Company at textbook@springerpub.com.

It is our hope that this book will appeal to neonatal nurses, novice NNPs, and students alike as they advance their learning about the care of neonates and their families. We believe that instructors will find this book a valuable resource in the education of NNPs.

Sandra Bellini
Michele J. Beaulieu

REFERENCES

Benner, P., Sutphen, S., Leonard, V., & Day, L. (2010). *Educating nurses: A call for radical transformation.* San Francisco, CA: Jossey-Bass.

Bosque, E. (2012). Toward salience: An application of integrative, case-based nursing education for neonatal advanced practice. *Advances in Neonatal Care, 12*(5), 292–302.

Assessing Maternal History and Neonatal Presentation Through Case-Based Learning

1

Identifying Maternal Risk Factors and Influence on Fetal Risk

Cheryl Riley and Lori Baas Rubarth

Chapter Objectives

1. Analyze and synthesize data on various placental perfusion disorders that can occur in pregnant women
2. Evaluate the clinical presentation and develop a plan of care for an infant born to a mother with abruption, placenta previa, or preeclampsia immediately after birth
3. Analyze the fetal risk factors associated with diabetes in the pregnant mother
4. Apply knowledge of maternal diabetes to develop an appropriate plan of care for the infant of a diabetic mother (IDM) immediately after birth
5. Analyze the fetal risk factors associated with bacterial and/or viral infections in the pregnant mother
6. Apply knowledge of maternal premature labor and/or premature rupture of membranes (PROM) to create an appropriate plan of care for a newborn infant
7. Analyze fetal risk factors associated with other maternal conditions, for example, systemic lupus erythematosus (SLE) and multiple gestation
8. Apply knowledge resulting from known maternal risk factors to create an appropriate plan of care for selected infant cases

This chapter focuses on maternal risk factors and their effect on the fetus. Placental physiology in the disease states of preeclampsia and hypertension, diabetes, and twin-to-twin transfusion syndrome (TTTS) and their effects on the fetus/infant are explored. Bacterial/viral infection, premature labor, PROM, SLE, and multiple gestation are also included. Finally, students will have the opportunity to engage in active learning through case studies provided.

COMMON MATERNAL COMPLICATIONS INFLUENCING FETAL RISK

HYPERTENSIVE DISORDERS

Hypertensive disorders are the most common obstetric complications in pregnancy world-wide, with an incidence of approximately 10% (McDonnold & Olson, 2013; Rugolo, Bentlin, & Trindade, 2012). These disorders are associated with adverse maternal outcomes and short- and long-term complications in the neonate. Hypertensive complications cover a broad spectrum of disorders, which are classified by the National High Blood Pressure Education Program Working Group on High Blood Pressure in Pregnancy (Gifford et al., 2000) into four categories: chronic hypertension (before or during the first 20 weeks of pregnancy), gestational hypertension (after 20 weeks of gestation without proteinuria), preeclampsia (hypertension developing after 20 weeks of gestation with proteinuria), and preeclampsia superimposed on chronic hypertension.

Preeclampsia

Preeclampsia is a multisystem disorder that is unique to pregnancy and can affect maternal brain, lungs, kidney, liver, coagulation cascade, and the fetus (McDonnold & Olson, 2013). Severity of the disease varies with the gestational age at onset and presenting symptoms. Mild disease is generally associated with good outcomes. Severe disease, especially if the onset is early in gestation, is associated with eclampsia, cerebral hemorrhage, renal failure, hepatic failure, HELLP (hemolysis, elevated liver enzymes, and low platelet) syndrome, prematurity, fetal growth restriction, oligohydramnios, placenta abruption, and intrauterine fetal demise (McDonnold & Olson, 2013). Signs and symptoms associated with the diagnosis of preeclampsia include blood pressure (BP) of at least 160 mmHg systolic or at least 110 mmHg diastolic, new proteinuria of at least 2 grams protein in a 24-hour urine collection or +2 to 3 on a urine dipstick, increased serum creatinine greater than 1.2 mg/dL, platelet count lower than 100×10^3/mcL, elevated hepatic enzymes, persistent headache or visual disturbances, and persistent epigastric pain (Lyell, 2004).

Pathophysiology

Although the pathophysiology is not completely understood, there are several theories, including decreased placenta perfusion resulting from either abnormal implantation or abnormal placental vasculature (Lyell, 2004; Moallem & Koenig, 2009). Lyell (2004) proposed that the maternal immune response to foreign paternal antigens of the fetoplacental unit is a cause of preeclampsia. This is supported by the increased incidence of preeclampsia in multiparous women pregnant by a new partner. Angiotension II sensitivity is also more common in women with preeclampsia, which is a potent vasoconstrictor.

Risk Factors

Risk factors for preeclampsia include nulliparity, type 1 diabetes, chronic hypertension, multiple gestation, prior preeclampsia, eclampsia, HELLP syndrome, prepregnancy obesity, extremes of age, and assisted reproduction (Lyell, 2004). Standard practice for the diagnosis of preeclampsia is to obtain baseline studies, including a 24-hour urine collection, to quantify protein and BPs at each visit. The diagnosis of preeclampsia is made when there is a new BP elevation of greater than or equal to 140 mmHg systolic or greater than or equal to 90 mmHg diastolic twice after 20 weeks gestation and greater than or equal to 300 mg protein in a 24-hour urine collection (McDonnold & Olson, 2013).

Management

Management of preeclampsia usually involves delivery, close observation, and seizure prophylaxis with magnesium sulfate. The only known treatment is delivery of the infant. In this case, the interests of the mother and infant are in direct conflict. Exceptions to this would be if there were severe uteroplacental insufficiency or intrauterine growth restriction (IUGR; Lyell, 2004). Timing of delivery is based on severity of disease. Criteria for immediate delivery are eclampsia, pulmonary edema, acute renal failure, neurologic deficits, abruption, nonreassuring fetal testing, and persistent severely elevated BP despite treatment with two hypertensive regimens. If there are less severe symptoms, delaying delivery until a complete course of antenatal steroids can be given is recommended. Delivery at 34 weeks is advised with severe preeclampsia without any contraindications, at 37 weeks for preeclampsia without severe findings and chronic hypertension that is difficult to control with medication, at 37 to 38 weeks for gestational hypertension and chronic hypertension controlled with medication, and at 39 weeks for well-controlled hypertension with no medication required (McDonnold & Olson, 2013).

Magnesium sulfate administration for prophylaxis of maternal seizures may cause muscle relaxation by competing with calcium (McDonnold & Olson, 2013; Rugolo et al., 2012). Magnesium crosses the placenta into fetal circulation and can cause neonatal respiratory depression requiring resuscitation. In addition, hypermagnesmia may decrease neonatal intestinal motility requiring slower-than-normal introduction of enteral feeding, especially in the preterm infant (McDonnold & Olson, 2013; Rugolo et al., 2012).

Early Neonatal Outcomes

Chronic stress to the fetus may be associated with accelerated fetal pulmonary maturity caused by the increase in cortisol production in the fetus (Rugolo et al., 2012). In this regard, preeclampsia may reduce the risk of respiratory distress, although there is controversy in the literature. Several large studies demonstrated that gestational age and preeclampsia were significant risk factors for respiratory distress syndrome (Langenveld et al., 2011; Rugolo et al., 2012).

Thrombocytopenia is a transient condition found in the first 72 hours after birth and usually resolves by day 10 of life. It is thought to occur as a result of "decreased platelet production associated with fetal hypoxia, microangiopathic sequestration, and destruction in the placental thrombi" (Rugolo et al., 2012, p. e534). Infants with IUGR are at higher risk for thrombocytopenia (Lyell, 2004; Rugolo et al., 2012).

Neonatal neutropenia occurs in approximately 50% of infants born to hypertensive mothers (McDonnold & Olson, 2013; Moallem & Koenig, 2009; Rugolo et al., 2012). Preeclampsia and neonatal neutropenia can be divided into two groups based on duration (Moallem & Koenig, 2009). The most common form usually resolves within the first 3 days of life and the more severe form may last up to 1 month (Moallem & Koenig, 2009). Increased duration and severity of neutropenia was associated with very-low-birth-weight infants and small-for-gestational-age infants secondary to placental inhibitors (McDonnold & Olson, 2013; Moallem & Koenig, 2009; Rugolo et al., 2012). Necrotizing enterocolitis (NEC) has been shown to occur in preterm infants with intrauterine distress and absent or reversed end-diastolic umbilical artery Doppler flow studies. As a result, preeclampsia should be considered a risk factor for NEC. Enteral feeds should be introduced cautiously in these infants. There is also an association with increased feeding problems such as gastric residuals, regurgitation, and gastroesophageal reflux (McDonnold & Olson, 2013; Moallem & Koenig, 2009; Rugolo et al., 2012). Close monitoring is required to identify feeding problems early.

Late Outcomes

It has been hypothesized that abnormal intrauterine environments may have long-term effects in adult life. The theory suggests that diseases, such as diabetes and cardiovascular disease, originate in utero from insults during critical periods of growth and development (McDonnold & Olson, 2013; Rugolo et al., 2012). There is a growing body of evidence that supports children born to preeclamptic mothers have higher systolic and diastolic BPs and higher levels of total cholesterol, triglycerides, insulin, and plasma epinephrine. A population-based study with more than a million children showed an increased risk of endocrine, nutritional, and metabolic derangements in adolescence and early adulthood among the cohort exposed to preeclampsia in utero (Wu et al., 2009).

Case 1.1

A 15-year-old gravida 1, para 0 (G1P0), Hispanic female presents to the labor and delivery (L&D) unit at 36 weeks of gestation by both her estimated date of delivery and ultrasound. She began prenatal care at 10 weeks of gestation and has had an uneventful pregnancy until 2 weeks ago when she began having severe headaches, increased weight gain, and pedal edema. Her vital signs on admission are stable with the exception of BP, which is 190/100 mmHg. She is noted to have +2 protein in her urine by dipstick. On exam, she complains of a pounding headache, epigastric pain, and has increased deep tendon reflexes. Her sister had preeclampsia with two of her pregnancies. She is started on magnesium sulfate, a 4-g loading dose given over 20 minutes and a 1-g maintenance dose. L&D unit calls the neonatal intensive care unit (NICU) and requests that the NICU team attend the delivery for preeclampsia.

1. *In reviewing Jennie's history, what are the risk factors that increase the chance of developing preeclampsia?*

   A. Nulliparity, family history of preeclampsia, and young age
   B. History of pounding headache, low socioeconomic status
   C. Low socioeconomic status (SES), history of pedal edema

   ANSWER: A. *Risk factors for preeclampsia include nulliparity, type 1 diabetes, chronic hypertension, multiple gestation, prior preeclampsia, eclampsia, HELLP (hemolysis, elevated liver enzymes, and low platelet) syndrome, prepregnancy obesity, extremes of age, family history, and assisted reproduction (Lyell, 2004).*

2. *Based on her presentation, what is your presumptive differential diagnosis? Include the data to support it.*

   A. Eclampsia
   B. Preeclampsia
   C. Chronic Hypertension
   D. Gestational Hypertension

(continued)

Case 1.1 (continued)

ANSWER: B. *Preeclampsia can be described as a blood pressure of at least 160 mmHg systolic or at least 110 mmHg diastolic, new proteinuria of at least 2 g protein in a 24-hour urine collection or +2 to 3 on a urine dipstick, increased serum creatinine greater than 1.2 mg/dL, platelet count lower than 100×10³/mcL, elevated hepatic enzymes, persistent headache or visual disturbances, and persistent epigastric pain (Lyell, 2004).*

PLACENTAL ABRUPTION AND PLACENTA PREVIA

Placental abruption is defined as premature separation of the placenta from the uterine wall prior to delivery; *placenta previa* is defined as a placenta located at or near the internal os. Both of these are serious complications that are responsible for up to one fourth of all perinatal deaths caused by third trimester bleeding (Matsuda et al., 2011).

Placental Abruption

The classic symptoms of placental abruption are bleeding and pain, but the clinical picture can vary from asymptomatic to massive bleeding leading to fetal death and severe maternal morbidity (Tikkanen, 2010). When the placenta separates from the uterus, hemorrhage into the decidua basalis occurs. Vaginal bleeding usually follows but can be hidden if it occurs behind the placenta. As a hematoma forms, this further separates the placenta from the uterine wall and can compromise the blood supply to the fetus (Tikkanen, 2010). Placental abruptions organized into four classes from 0 to 3. Class 0 is asymptomatic. Class 1 is mild and represents approximately 48% of all cases. There is no vaginal bleeding, slightly tender uterus, normal BP and heart rate (HR). There is no evidence of coagulopathy or fetal distress. Class 2 is moderate and represents approximately 27% of all cases. There is no vaginal bleeding to moderate vaginal bleeding, moderate to severe uterine tenderness with possible tetanic contractions, maternal tachycardia with orthostatic changes in BP and HR, fetal distress becomes evident, and hypofibrinogenemia (i.e., 50–250 mg/dL) is present. Class 3 is severe and represents 24% of all cases. Vaginal bleeding ranges from no bleeding to heavy vaginal bleeding, very painful tetanic uterus, maternal shock, hypofibrinogenemia (i.e., < 150 mg/dL), coagulopathy, and fetal death (Deering, 2015).

Although the primary cause of placental abruption is generally unknown, many risk factors have been identified. These are numerous and include maternal hypertension, maternal trauma, cigarette smoking, alcohol consumption, cocaine use, short umbilical cord, sudden depression of the uterus, chorioamnionitis, retroplacental fibromyoma with bleeding, previous abruption, advanced maternal age, maternal age younger than 20, male fetus, and low socioeconomic status (Deering, 2015; Matsuda et al., 2011; Tikkanen, 2010).

Management includes maternal fluid resuscitation and blood transfusion for hemodynamically unstable mothers. Perinatal morbidity and mortality associated with abruption ranges from 20% to 40% and accounts for 15% of perinatal deaths (Deering, 2015; Matsuda et al., 2011). The main causes of perinatal death include anoxia, exsanguination, stillbirth, and prematurity. Continuous fetal monitoring is indicated. Signs and symptoms of fetal compromise will include HR decelerations, decreased variability, tachycardia, sinusoidal heart rhythm, and death (Deering, 2015; Matsuda et al., 2011; Tikkanen, 2010). Resuscitation in the delivery room should be anticipated.

Placenta Previa

Placenta previa is fairly common within the first 20 weeks of pregnancy. In most cases, it resolves leaving approximately 10% that persist into later pregnancy. As the uterus grows, the placenta moves higher in the uterus. If this upward movement does not occur, then the risk of bleeding increases. The incidence of placenta previa is about one in 200 pregnancies. There are three types of placenta previa: a marginal placenta previa (low lying placenta) that is near the cervical os, which usually moves up during pregnancy; a partial placenta previa that covers part of the cervical os; and a complete placenta previa that blocks the cervical opening (Johnston, Paterson-Brown, & Paterson-Brown, 2011; Matsuda et al., 2011).

The cause of placenta previa is unknown but several risk factors have been identified. It is more common in women with an abnormally shaped uterus, with advanced maternal age, smoking, multiple births, previous cesarean sections (C-sections), or prior uterine surgery. If there is bleeding after 20 weeks of gestation, placenta previa should be suspected and confirmed with ultrasound imaging. This scan should be repeated at 32 weeks of gestation to assess the placenta position and plan for third trimester management. In the majority of cases, if the placenta remains low or is anteriorly placed at 32 weeks, it is unlikely that the placenta will migrate up in the uterus.

Mothers with a total placenta previa who have had previous bleeding should be admitted to the hospital from approximately 34 weeks of gestation to delivery. Those with partial placenta previa who are asymptomatic may be managed as outpatients. If this is the case, it is important to have an emergency plan. This includes having someone available to assist if the need arises and have ready access to the hospital. In preparing for delivery, it is critical to have discussed the plan of care with parents, including the possible need for blood transfusions and hysterectomy. A C-section may be recommended if the placental edge is less than 2 cm from the internal os in the third trimester.

Case 1.2

A 19-year-old gravida 1, para 0 (G1P0) woman is admitted to the labor and delivery (L&D) unit for abdominal pain and vaginal bleeding. She is 35 weeks gestation and received late prenatal care. The mother has a history of smoking and alcohol use, though she stopped both at 12 weeks of gestation when she discovered she was pregnant. You are called for a stat C-section for placenta abruption.

1. **What are your initial concerns for this infant?**
    A. Anemia and hypovolemia
    B. Cardiac arrhythmias and bounding pulses
    C. Low birth weight and late preterm birth
    D. Fetal alcohol syndrome and small for gestation

    ANSWER: A. *This infant is at risk for anemia, hypovolemia, shock, or birth depression due to blood loss, and also at risk for prematurity and its complications because of the need for early delivery due to bleeding (Deering, 2015).*

(continued)

Case 1.2 (continued)

You arrive in the operating room (OR) and receive report on the mother and baby. Both are tachycardic and the mother is hemorrhaging. You call for backup and have the crash cart brought into the OR.

2. *To prepare for this resuscitation, what equipment and supplies do you anticipate you will need?*

   A. Nothing until the infant is born

   B. Bag and mask (or T-piece resuscitator) only

   C. Bag and mask (or T-piece resuscitator), umbilical catheter or angiocatheter for IV insertion, and normal saline for volume replacement

   ANSWER: C. *After delivery, the neonatal nurse practitioner will follow Neonatal Resuscitation Provider guidelines: place on warmer, dry with warm towels, have bag and mask (or T-piece resuscitator) available as well as oxygen, suction, and intubation supplies. An umbilical venous catheter (UVC), emergency medication (saline), and supplies for intravenous (IV) catheter insertion will need to be available. Also, "O" negative, uncross-matched blood may be needed for emergency blood transfusion.*

A male infant is born with an HR of 50, no respiratory effort, very pale, and no tone. The estimated birthweight is 2.8 kg.

3. *What risk factors did the mother have for a placental abruption?*

   A. Appendicitis and bleeding

   B. Diabetes and short umbilical cord

   C. Alcohol consumption and maternal age younger than 20 years

   ANSWER: C. *There are numerous risk factors, including maternal hypertension, maternal trauma, cigarette smoking, alcohol consumption, cocaine use, short umbilical cord, sudden depression of the uterus, chorioamnionitis, retroplacental fibromyoma with bleeding, previous abruption, advanced maternal age, maternal age younger than 20 years, male fetus, and low socioeconomic status (Deering, 2015; Matsuda et al., 2011; Tikkanen, 2010).*

4. *A complete blood count (CBC) is drawn and the laboratory reports a hematocrit of 20%. What is your next step if the infant has stabilized?*

   A. Order a normal saline bolus of 28 mL to run over 30 minutes

   B. Order 28 mL packed red blood cells (PRBCs) to run over 2 hours

   C. Order 56 mL packed red blood cells to run over 3 hours

   ANSWER: C. *Acute blood loss has occurred so it is important to transfuse with 10 to 20 mL/kg of PRBCs IV over 2 to 3 hours or faster depending on infant's condition. In this case a bolus of saline or albumin for volume would have been given immediately, and followed up with uncross-matched blood if the infant had remained unstable. The PRBCs would be given over 2 to 3 hours to slowly resupply the infant's original blood supply (the timing and actual blood product depends on the stability of the infant at the time of transfusion) (Gomella, 2013).*

MATERNAL DIABETES

Maternal diabetes can cause multiple problems for the neonate. Early in gestation, the high maternal glucose levels are passed on through the placenta to the infant and can cause congenital anomalies. Glucose molecules cross the placenta, but the large molecules of insulin do not. About midgestation, the fetal pancreas begins to produce large amounts of insulin and fetal islet cells develop compensatory hyperplasia, resulting in fetal hyperinsulinemia (see Figure 1.1).

The most common problem that occurs in the IDM is an increase in the size or growth of the infant, in which the infant becomes large for gestational age (LGA). *LGA* is defined as greater than the 90th percentile for weight, and is considered a larger-than-normal infant. This often occurs more in the second and third trimesters with increases in fat and glycogen storage (Potter, 2013). Pregnancies with LGA infants lead to increased need for C-section and the risk of birth injuries. Prior to birth, it is important to assess pulmonary maturity because surfactant production appears to occur late in the fetal lungs of diabetic pregnancies, which can result in respiratory distress syndrome even at term gestation (Ramon & Moore, 2012).

Structural abnormalities can occur in infants whose mothers have poor glucose control during the period of rapid growth and development (3–8 weeks of gestation). Therefore, the infant born to a diabetic mother must be assessed for structural defects in the delivery room. These defects can include congenital heart defects (murmur), renal defects/renal vein thrombosis (observe for voiding and palpation size of kidneys), caudal/sacral agenesis (observation), neural tube defects (visualize infant's back), small left colon syndrome/meconium plug (failure to pass meconium in 24 hours and signs of obstruction), and skeletal dysplasia/hemivertebrae (observation/chest x-ray [CXR]). Episodes of maternal hyperglycemia promote fetal catabolism and hypoxia, which can cause the cardiac septal hypertrophy (cardiomyopathy), higher levels of erythropoietin with polycythemia, and possible sudden death in utero (Ramon & Moore, 2012).

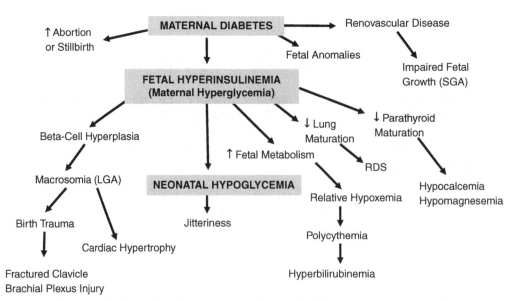

Figure 1.1 Algorithm of Infant Disorders With Infants of a Diabetic Mother

RDS, respiratory distress syndrome; SGA, small for gestational age.

After birth, hyperbilirubinemia and hyperviscosity can occur as a result of the polycythemia. Also, hypoglycemia occurs with the maternal glucose supply cutoff at the same time continued high levels of insulin are being produced by the neonate.

Neonates with hypocalcemia can develop neurologic symptoms such as being jittery, or lethargy, apnea or tachypnea, hypotonia, cyanosis, or seizures. Hypocalcemia and hypomagnesemia can occur in the IDM because of a delayed parathyroid gland response after birth (Rubarth, 2013). Some of these same symptoms can occur as a result of low calcium and low magnesium levels.

Maternal diabetes that is well controlled will have minimal symptoms and less risk for defects. There is a higher risk of congenital anomalies if glucose control is poor during the first trimester, but poor control later in pregnancy (as with gestational diabetes) can result in large infants with hypoglycemia. Maintenance of stable glucose levels is important in the insulin-dependent diabetic mother and the pregnant mother with gestational diabetes.

Case 1.3

A 32-year-old gravida 3, para 0 (G3P0) mother delivered a 4,200-g baby boy by C-section for failure to progress. Mother had a history of gestational diabetes with her previous pregnancies and both were delivered stillborn near term. In this pregnancy, mother has been on an insulin drip during labor, with uncontrolled glucose levels. Baby G was born with spontaneous cry and respirations, no murmur, Apgar score of 7/9 with a large caput succedaneum. Initial glucose level at 1 hour equals 32. Baby was put to breast and then nipple fed 15 mL of 20-cal. formula. Glucose level at 2 hours of age was 28.

The infant was admitted to the neonatal intensive care unit (NICU) and a peripheral IV was started with 10% dextrose water (D10W) at 80 mL/kg/d. A bolus of 8 mL of D10W (2 mL/kg) was provided over 15 minutes. Repeat glucose level equals 56. The infant's glucose dropped a second time to 27, so that the fluids were increased to 100 mL/kg/d. Further drops in the bedside monitoring of the glucose resulted in an increased glucose concentration of D12.5W and then placement of a UVC for glucose infusion of D15W at 120 mL/kg/d. Glucose stabilized at this glucose infusion rate (GIR).

1. *What is the most likely reason for this infant's hypoglycemia?*

   A. Maternal hypoglycemia
   B. Fetal hyperinsulinemia
   C. Increased catecholamine secretion
   D. Diminished glucagon storage

   ANSWER: B. *In diabetic pregnancies, maternal hyperglycemia results in fetal hyperglycemia, which "is accompanied by fetal pancreatic beta-cell hyperplasia and hyperinsulinemia" (Ramos & Moore, 2012, p. 77). At birth, the transplacental glucose is interrupted and hyperinsulinemia results in neonatal hypoglycemia and most commonly in macrosomic infants (Gomella, 2013).*

(continued)

Case 1.3 (continued)

2. **What is the GIR of this infant with the initial IV solution of D10W?**

   A. 4.5 mg/kg/min
   B. 5.5 mg/kg/min
   C. 6.9 mg/kg/min
   D. 8.7 mg/kg/min

   ANSWER: B. *For hypoglycemia, start IV glucose infusion of 6 mg/kg/min (Gomella, 2013). Refer to Zenk (2003, Appendix A) for details in calculation of GIR.*

3. **What is the GIR of this infant after the umbilical venous catheter (UVC) was inserted and the glucose stabilized?**

   A. 6.9 mg/kg/min
   B. 8.7 mg/kg/min
   C. 10.4 mg/kg/min
   D. 12.5 mg/kg/min

   ANSWER: D. *For hypoglycemia, start IV glucose infusion of 6 mg/kg/min (Gomella, 2013). Refer Zenk (2003, Appendix A) for details in calculation of GIR.*

4. **Which medication would you initially prescribe for this infant to inhibit insulin release from the pancreas?**

   A. Diazoxide
   B. Glucagon
   C. Hydrocortisone
   D. Octreotide

   ANSWER: A. *Diazoxide is used for treatment of persistent or severe hypoglycemia caused by hyperinsulinism. Glucagon is used for glucagon deficiency. Octreotide is for refractory hyperinsulinemia and hydrocortisone is for cortisol deficiency (Neofax, 2014).*

NEONATAL SEPSIS

Neonatal sepsis is a generalized bacterial or viral infection that occurs in neonates via many different routes. Infants are protected from bacterial infections in utero by the amniotic membranes and certain antibacterial factors present in the amniotic fluid. But some infants become infected in utero: (1) via the maternal bloodstream, (2) by ascending bacteria that either colonize or infect the mother's birth canal, (3) by these same bacteria as the infant descends through the birth canal at delivery, or (4) via nosocomial infection within the NICU environment. Infants can become infected through use of scalp electrodes to monitor fetal heart tones. The majority of bacterial infections occur by the ascending route with either ruptured or intact membranes leading to premature birth (Rubarth, 2011). PROM of greater than 24 hours can result in an increase in bacteria reaching the infant in utero (Anderson-Berry, Bellig, & Ohning, 2014). These bacterial infections can cause amnionitis and/or chorioamnionitis. The incidence of bacterial infections has declined as a result of administration of prophylactic antibiotics to pregnant women during labor and delivery.

Table 1.1 **Types and Function of White Blood Cells**

WBC	Subtype	Function of WBC
Neutrophils	Polymorphonuclear cells (polys, segs)	Phagocytosis—bacterial-fighting cells Mature type
	Bands	Immature type
	Metamyelocytes	Immature type
	Myelocytes	Very immature type
	Promyelocytes	Very immature type
	Blasts (stabs)	Most immature type
Lymphocytes	B-lymphocytes	Humoral, adaptive immunity (produce antibodies against infection)
	T-lymphocytes	Cell-mediated, adaptive immunity (mostly against viral infections; responds in inflammatory reactions)
	Natural killer cells	Against viral infections and tumor cells
Monocytes		Against fungal and viral infections
Eosinophils		Respond in allergic reactions and chlamydia infections
Basophils		Respond in hypersensitivity reactions

WBC, white blood cells.

Maternal signs of infection are a fever, foul-smelling or discolored amniotic fluid, or abdominal pain. Some predisposing factors that can lead to neonatal infection are as follows:

- Premature labor
- PROM
- Chorioamnionitis

- Maternal fever
- Prolonged or difficult labor
- Low-birth-weight or premature infant (with immature immune system)
- Maternal antibody status or vaginal flora

Most viral infections occur via the maternal bloodstream during early pregnancy (e.g., with TORCH [toxoplasmosis, other agents, rubella, cytomegalovirus [CMV], herpes simplex virus [HSV] infections) or can occur at delivery (e.g., with herpes virus). Other infants can also acquire infections from the environment during their prolonged stays in the NICU (e.g., pseudomonas, coagulase-negative staphylococcus; Anderson-Berry et al., 2014).

There are wide-ranging clinical manifestations of neonatal sepsis and no single set of criteria is reliable for diagnosing sepsis. Often the clinician states the infant "is not doing well" as a nonspecific sign of sepsis. Some of the signs can be subtle color changes or feeding difficulties. Temperature instability, increase in apnea, abdominal distension, and worsening respiratory distress are often early signs of neonatal sepsis. These signs can also be signs of other premature diagnoses such as respiratory distress syndrome, apnea of prematurity, feeding intolerance, and hypothermia. Many infants have feeding difficulties, but a combination of signs must lead the clinician to explore the possibility of sepsis. Signs of bloodstream infection lead to lethargy/hypotonia, mottling, cyanosis, pallor, hypotension, and shock. Meningitis occurs more frequently in late-onset infections, but signs of irritability or hypertonia must lead the clinician to do a lumbar puncture and send cerebral spinal fluid (CSF) for culture and sensitivities, Gram stain, glucose, protein, and cell count with differential. A CBC with differential, blood culture, urine bacterial antigen screen, CSF bacterial antigen screen, specific polymerase chain reaction (PCR) levels, and C-reactive protein (CRP) are well-accepted tests for neonatal sepsis (see Table 1.1 for types and functions of WBCs and Table 1.2 for measures of I:T ratio and total neutrophil count [TNC]).

Depending on the sensitivities of the blood cultures, treatment for bacterial sepsis always involves antibiotics. Treatment for viral infections can start with antivirals and can involve many variations of treatments, including antiretrovirals and protease inhibitors for human immunodeficiency virus (HIV), immunoglobulins specific for the virus (as with CMV), and granulocyte-colony stimulating factor (G-CSF).

Table 1.2 **Measures of Neutrophils (Bacterial-Fighting White Blood Cells)**

Test	Explanation of Test	Indicator of Infection
I:T ratio	Percentage of immature neutrophils (bands + other immature) ÷ Percentage of total number of neutrophils (segs + bands + other)	> 0.2
TNC	WBC (in thousands) × percentage of total neutrophils	< 2,000 infection < 1,000 critical level

I:T, immature:total; TNC, total neutrophil count; WBC, white blood cells.

Case 1.4

A mother was admitted to the labor and delivery (L&D) unit of a local, community hospital. The mother was at 36 6/7 weeks of gestation and was noted to be in active labor with ruptured membranes. She was A+ blood type, with negative antibody screen, rubella immune, Venereal Disease Research Laboratory (VDRL) test nonreactive, hepatitis B negative, and group B *Streptococcus* (GBS) was unknown. Because the mother was so close to 37 weeks and actively progressing, the attending obstetrician decided not start prophylactic antibiotics, but a GBS culture was sent. The mother delivered a 2,600-g infant about 5 hours after admission. The baby had a spontaneous cry and respirations, and appeared well with Apgar scores of 9 and 9 at 1 and 5 minutes, respectively. The infant stayed with the mother after the delivery with mother–baby care done by the couplet care nursing staff.

At about 12 hours of age, the mother called the nurse stating that the father was holding the infant and the baby appeared to be struggling and was making some grunting noises. The nurse enters the dimly lit room, turns on the overhead light, and sees that the baby is blue, pale, and grunting significantly. The baby is immediately brought to the Level II neonatal intensive care unit (NICU).

1. **What is your most likely diagnosis on admission to the NICU?**
   A. Coarctation of the aorta
   B. Bacterial sepsis
   C. Viral sepsis
   D. Congenital pulmonary airway malformation (CPAM)

   ANSWER: B. *Coarctation would not be a problem this early unless it was severe, but this is a common presentation for bacterial sepsis (Anderson-Berry, Bellig, & Ohning, 2014).*

2. **What is the most important part of your management plan to assist you in developing a diagnosis for this infant?**
   A. Complete blood count (CBC) with manual differential and blood culture
   B. Viral culture and polymerase chain reaction (PCR)
   C. Echocardiogram and oxygen
   D. Umbilical line placement

   ANSWER: A. *It is important to rule out infection as soon as possible, since a delay in treatment could result in significant mortality (Anderson-Berry, Bellig, & Ohning, 2014).*

   On admission to NICU:
   Vital signs: Heart rate (HR), 168; respiration rate (RR), 88 with occasional grunting; temperature, 36.4°C; blood pressure (BP), 32/18; mean BP, 23; saturation of 72% in room air. On physical examination, the infant presented with poor perfusion, gray/dusky color, no murmur noted, and continued with increased respiratory distress with significant retractions and nasal flaring. The infant is placed under a radiant warmer with nasal cannula placed at 100% oxygen with 0.5 L/min flow, which is increased to 1 L/min, and then 2 L/min to improve saturations to 85%. The baby was intubated and placed on a conventional ventilator with peak inspiratory pressure (PIP) = 26; rate = 30; positive end-expiratory pressure

(continued)

Case 1.4 *(continued)*

(PEEP) = 5; pressure support of 8 FiO$_2$ of 60% to 70%. Umbilical artery catheter (UAC) and umbilical venous catheter (UVC) were placed successfully and labs were drawn.

CBC with differential: white blood cell (WBC) = 2.1 thousands/mcL with 2% bands, 6% segmented neutrophils, 1% metamyelocytes, 1% promyelocytes, 83% lymphocytes, 5% monocytes, and 2% basophils.

CRP = 35 mg/L (3.5 mg/dL)

Blood culture is pending.

Antibiotics were started and the infant was transported to a Level III NICU for further care (see algorithms for GBS prophylaxis at the Centers for Disease Control [CDC] website: www.cdc.gov/groupbstrep/clinicians/neonatal-providers.html#algorithms).

1. *Which antibiotics would you start on this infant?*

   A. Acyclovir and vancomycin
   B. Ampicillin and gentamicin
   C. Zosyn and tobramycin with clindamycin

   ANSWER: B. *Ampicillin and gentamicin are broad-spectrum antibiotics used against the most common pathogens present in the NICU (Neofax, 2015). Ampicillin and gentamicin are the empiric antibiotics chosen for therapy for infants with early-onset sepsis (Embree & Alfattoh, 2016).*

2. *The mother's GBS was unknown and, according to the CDC guidelines for GBS prophylaxis, what should have been done?*

   A. Administer two (2) doses of penicillin G to the mother prior to delivery
   B. Admit the infant to the NICU at delivery for observation
   C. Admit the infant to the NICU at delivery for antibiotic treatment

   ANSWER: A. *See algorithms for intrapartum prophylaxis for GBS sepsis (CDC, 2016).*

3. *What is the infant's I:T ratio?*

   A. 0.25
   B. 0.33
   C. 0.40
   D. 0.47

   ANSWER: C. *The I : T ratio is figured based on the formula in Table 1.2. A ratio of bands to segs greater than 0.3 or ratio of immature neutrophils to total neutrophils greater than 0.1 can be predictive of sepsis in the neonate (Gomella, 2013), but most neonatal providers use the value of 0.2.*

4. *What is the infant's total neutrophil count?*

   A. 126
   B. 210
   C. 399

   ANSWER: B. *Total neutrophil calculations are based on the formula in Table 1.2. Total neutrophil counts less than 1,000 are critical. Additional information on WBC indices can be found in Gomella (2013).*

Systemic Lupus Erythematosus

SLE is a multisystem, autoimmune, connective tissue disorder that can affect almost all organ systems, including the joints, skin, heart, lungs, nervous system, and kidneys (Classen, Paulson, & Zacharias, 1998; Madazli, Yuksel, Oncul, Imamoglu, & Yilmaz, 2014). SLE mainly affects women in their childbearing years and is associated with increased maternal and fetal morbidity and mortality. Mothers with SLE have an increased risk of miscarriage, fetal growth restriction, death, preeclampsia, preterm birth, congenital heart block, and neonatal lupus erythematous (NLE; Classen et al., 1998; Madazli et al., 2014). The risk of acerbation of SLE during pregnancy is associated with the disease activity in the previous 6 to 12 months prior to pregnancy, so pregnancy should be planned during remission (Madazli et al., 2014). The American Rheumatism Association has established criteria for the diagnosis of SLE. If you have four of the following symptoms, and are a woman in your childbearing years, the following diagnoses can be made:

1. Rashes: a butterfly-shaped rash over the cheeks, or a red rash with raised round patches, or a rash on skin exposed to the sun

2. Mouth sores

3. Arthritis lasting for a few weeks in two or more joints

4. Lung or heart inflammation

5. Swelling of the tissue lining the lungs or the heart

6. Kidney problems

7. Blood or protein in the urine

8. Neurologic problems, including seizures, strokes, or psychosis

9. Abnormal blood tests: autoimmune hemolytic anemia, leucopenia, and thrombocytopenia; positive antinuclear antibody; anti–double-strand DNA (anti-dsDNA); antiphospholipid antibodies; or a false-positive blood test for syphilis (Hochberg, 1997).

Maternal treatments for flare-ups during pregnancy are anti-inflammatory, antimalarial, immunosuppressive, and anticoagulation drugs. Corticosteroids are also used to prevent flare-ups. Prednisone crosses the placenta and is therefore the drug of choice (Borchers, Naguwa, Keen, & Gershwin, 2010).

SLE patients frequently have the anti-Sjögren's-syndrome-related antigen A (SSA)/anti-Sjögren's syndrome type B (SSB) antibodies, which are associated with an increased risk of NLE that can result from transplacental passage of maternal autoantibodies causing fetal tissue damage and clinical symptoms of NLE (Borchers et al., 2010). This condition is rare, affects females more than males, and involves multiple organs. Infants with NLE may display cutaneous rashes and are at significant risk for heart block. The skin manifestations are typically found on the head, scalp, and chest. These skin lesions appear as erythematous flat patches that change to large scaly plaques. The skin lesions develop within the first few weeks after birth up to 1 month and usually resolve by 6 months of age, which correlates with the disappearance of maternal antibodies. Hydrocortisone cream may be helpful (Boh, 2004; Classen et al., 1998).

Cardiac involvement, including cardiac arrhythmias and conduction defects, is common in infants with NLE with an incidence of 65% (Femia, Callen, & Vleugels, 2014). The occurrence of congenital complete heart block occurs in approximately 15% to 30% of infants with NLE. Monitoring a fetal HR between 18 and 24 weeks of gestation will detect a large number of infants with heart block. Anti-SSA/Ro and anti-SSB-La antibodies bind to fetal cardiocytes and inhibit normal physiologic removal of apoptotic cells that result in an inflammatory reaction, which can lead to fibrosis of the cardiac conduction system (Yildirim, Tunaodlu, & Karaabac, 2013). Additionally, cross-reactivity of the SSA/SSB antibodies and downregulation of calcium channels may explain the cardiac rhythm disturbances that lead to decreased cardiac output and heart failure. These processes have the ability to cause myocarditis, hemorrhage, fibrosis, calcification, and necrosis in the conduction system, which leads to the development of various degrees of heart block (Yildirim et al., 2013). Morbidity and mortality depend on the degree of heart block and other organ systems involved. Some infants may require a pacemaker.

Thrombocytopenia, leukopenia, and anemia may be present at birth but these are transient. In addition, hepatomegaly occurs in 20% to 40% of patients and includes histologic changes such as cholestasis, fibrosis, and hepatitis (Boh, 2004). In many cases, hepatic symptoms are self-limiting though severe liver failure is possible (Femia et al., 2014).

Case 1.5

A baby girl was born at 36 weeks of gestation with Apgar scores of 9 and 9 at 1 and 5 minutes, respectively. She weighed 3.2 kg. Maternal history was unremarkable. Over the first week of life, the baby developed a rash over her face. Initial laboratory tests revealed a hemoglobin level of 11 g/dL and a platelet count of 24,000/mm^3. An electrocardiogram showed a normal sinus rhythm. Serologic testing reported a strongly positive anti-Sjögren's-syndrome-related antigen A (SSA) (Ro) and anti-Sjögren's syndrome type B (SSB), which confirmed the diagnosis of neonatal lupus erythematous (NLE).

1. *Based on the infant's complete blood count (CBC) results, your plan of care includes which of the following?*

   A. Transfuse with 10 mL/kg of packed red blood cells (PRBCs)
   B. Transfuse with 10 mL/kg of platelets
   C. Repeat CBC in the morning

   ANSWER: C. *Thrombocytopenia, leuckopenia, or anemia may be present at birth but is transient (Boh, 2004).*

2. *Initially, the rash on the infant's face covered her forehead, nose, and cheeks. The parents are very concerned with her appearance. Which of the following is your best response?*

   A. We will set up an appointment with a dermatologist as an outpatient
   B. We will send a viral culture to rule out any type of congenital virus
   C. We have ordered cortisone cream, which may help

   ANSWER: C. *Hydrocortisone cream may be helpful (Boh, 2004; Classen et al., 1998).*

(continued)

Case 1.5 (continued)

3. NLE is usually self-limiting because:
  A. Treatment with antibiotics cures it
  B. Maternal antibodies disappear at approximately 6 months
  C. The infant's immune system attacks maternal antibodies

ANSWER: B. *The skin lesions develop within the first few weeks after birth up to 1 month and usually resolve by 6 months of age, which correlates with the disappearance of maternal antibodies (Boh, 2004).*

The mother had not been diagnosed with systemic lupus erythematosus (SLE) prior to this pregnancy. She was referred to a rheumatologist and received the diagnosis of SLE though she had been asymptomatic.

MULTIPLE GESTATION

Multiple-gestation pregnancies with twins, triplets, or higher order multiples are considered high risk with a high incidence of premature births. The length of gestation is inversely related to the number of fetuses. Most women carrying multiples will deliver prior to 36 weeks, thereby contributing to the population of infants cared for in NICUs (Fletcher & Zach, 2015). There have been increased numbers of multiple births in the past few decades as a result of more widespread use of assisted reproductive technologies (ART) and women postponing pregnancy until their 30s or later. Women in the age group of 35 to 40 years have higher rates of multiple ovulation and, therefore, dizygotic (fraternal) twins. This is thought to occur because of higher levels of follicle-stimulating hormone (FSH) in older women (Fletcher & Zach, 2015). Women with higher parity also have higher rates of dizygotic twinning. The rate of dizygotic twinning is highest in the Black race, followed by Caucasian and Hispanic races, and lowest in the Asian race. There is also a familial tendency for dizygotic (fraternal) twins through the mother's lineage, and a probable genetic link for monozygotic (identical) twins (Genetics & Human Traits, 2016).

Understanding the terminology and pathophysiology of twinning is necessary to understand complications that can occur with multiple gestation pregnancies. With dizygotic twins, there are two eggs and two sperm. Each developing embryo has its own inner amniotic sac (amnion), outer amniotic sac (chorion), and placenta. Sometimes the two placentas can fuse and appear as one large placenta, but are easily separated after birth. These dizygotic twins are also called *fraternal twins.*

With monozygotic twins, there is one, single, fertilized egg that splits. Monozygotic twins have the same exact genotype, but can have minor differences in phenotype. These twins are also called *identical twins.* There are three different choices of placentation with monozygotic twins. If the embryo splits early within the first 2 days after fertilization, then each fetal twin will develop its own amnion, chorion, and placenta prior to implantation, exactly the same as dizygotic twins (dichorionic/diamniotic, or "di–di"). If the embryo splits between day 3 and day 8 after fertilization, then the twins will develop two amnions (inner sacs) with one chorion (outer sac) with one placenta (monochorionic/diamniotic, or "mono–di"). If the embryo splits between 9 and 12 days after fertilization, the twins will be together in one sac (mono-chorionic/monoamniotic, or "mono–mono") with one placenta. If the embryo splits later than 13 days after fertilization, the twins will be conjoined (Fletcher & Zach, 2015).

With triplets, there can be three separate zygotes, two zygotes in which one splits into two, or one zygote that splits into three identical zygotes. With higher order multiples, most em-bryos occur as a result of ART and are individual zygotes, each with a separate egg and sperm. Occasionally, a zygote can split, producing an identical pair of "twins" within the multiple set.

There are always an increased number of complications when both twins are within the same sac (monochorionic/monoamniotic). This is a relatively uncommon type of twin pregnancy and only occurs in about 1% of monozygotic twin pregnancies (Zach & Fletcher, 2015). With both infants within the same sac, there can be problems with cord entangle-ment, congenital anomalies, and other types of interactions that can compromise the two infants. Monochorionic twins with only one placenta also have an increased risk of TTTS. The two circulations can be intermixed with vascular connections between the two infants. These vascular connections can result in one twin shunting part of its blood flow to the second twin. The twin who receives the blood transfusion is called the "recipient" twin and is usually the larger twin. The recipient also appears plethoric as a result of the hypovole-mia and polycythemia. The infant can exhibit hypertension with signs of congestive heart failure, pulmonary edema, and cardiomegaly (hydrops). This twin also usually presents with polyhydramnios. The "donor" twin is usually small and pale with hypovolemia and hypo-tension. As a result of shunting blood to its twin, the donor is anemic and thrombocytope-nic. Hypoxia from the anemia can also lead to heart failure and hydrops fetalis. This twin usually presents with oligohydramnios, so the donor twin can appear to be "stuck" against the side of the uterine cavity because of lack of fluid.

Chronic TTTS usually occurs early in pregnancy, often with loss of one twin if not treated. Acute TTTS can occur any time during pregnancy with a more sudden occurrence. Arterial-to-venous connections are the most serious because of the difference in BPs be-tween the two systems. These transfusions occur mostly in monochorionic pregnancies (ei-ther diamnionic or monoamnionic); therefore, only in identical twin pregnancies with one outer, chorionic membrane and one placenta. TTTS is rare in fused dichorionic placentas (Revenis, 2016).

Another type of transfusion occurs in these infants as a complication with TTTS. It is called *twin reversed arterial perfusion* (TRAP), in which blood from the recipient twin suddenly reverses back to the donor twin because of hypotension of the donor twin (from acardia, a cardiac defect, or death of the donor twin). Often, both twins do not survive (Revenis, 2016). TRAP results in blood going backward from the umbilical artery to the twins and then back to the placenta through the umbilical vein; this is the opposite of normal circulation (Johnson, Khalek, Martinez-Poyer, & Moldenhauer, 2014).

TTTS is the most common complication of monochorionic twinning. Treatment is considered when ultrasound demonstrates abnormal blood flow and large differences in size or amniotic fluid volume. Options for treatment are as follows:

1. Amniocentesis/amnioreduction to decompress the polyhydramnios in the recipi-ent twin

2. Amniotic septostomy to equalize the pressure between the two amniotic sacs

3. Selective feticide if perinatal survival is expected to be poor

4. Laser photocoagulation to cut off the circulation between the twins (Johnson et al., 2014)

At birth, practitioners need to be concerned if there are significant variations in the weights, amniotic fluid volumes, or umbilical cords of same-sex infants. Observe these infants for any signs of heart failure or hydrops, and evaluate a hematocrit on both infants shortly after birth. Practitioners need to be prepared for an unknown transfusion or severity of TTTS. Usually, these are diagnosed prenatally, but can also occur suddenly at birth. It is important for the practitioner to be aware of any suspected twin-to-twin transfusion and understand the differences between dichorionic and monochorionic twin pregnancies.

Case 1.6

A gravida 1, para 0 (G1P0) Caucasian female at 32 weeks of gestation with limited prenatal care is admitted to the labor and delivery (L&D) unit with a twin pregnancy with polyhydramnios noted on ultrasound. The twins are noted to have diamniotic/monochorionic (di–mono) placentation. Twin A is estimated to be approximately 1,900 g and twin B is estimated to be 1,450 g with intrauterine growth restriction (IUGR). An emergency C-section is performed because of the size disparity of the twins. At birth, Baby A was born with apnea, was bag/mask ventilated with some difficulty, ruddy, and seemed to have a distended abdomen with stiff extremities. Baby was intubated without difficulty and bagged with pressure of 35 mmHg, PEEP = 5, rate = 40. Baby was transferred to the neonatal intensive care unit (NICU) and placed on a ventilator. Chest x-ray showed bilateral pleural effusions and abdominal ascites. Apgar scores were 4 and 6 at 1 and 5 minutes, respectively. Baby B was born with spontaneous cry and respirations, and pinked up in room air. Apgar scores were 8 and 9, and no intervention was required.

1. **Which laboratory study is most important to determine twin-to-twin transfusion risk in these twins?**

   A. White blood count
   B. Hematocrit/hemoglobin
   C. Mean corpuscular hemoglobin (MCH) and mean corpuscular hemoglobin concentration (MCHC)

   ANSWER: B. *Neonatal work-up—a complete blood count with hemoglobin and hematocrit is obtained on multiple-gestation infants to evaluate for anemia and/or polycythemia (Fletcher & Zach, 2015).*

2. **Why do the two infants have very different respiratory requirements?**

   A. They are twins and have different genetic dispositions
   B. One twin has respiratory distress syndrome (RDS) and the other twin does not
   C. One twin has hydrops fetalis and the other twin does not

   ANSWER: C. *Baby A is the larger of the babies and probably has hydrops fetalis with pleural effusions and abdominal ascites. Baby A is the recipient of the blood transfusion and Baby B is the donor. Baby B is the smaller, IUGR donor with oligohydramnios, and is at risk for anemia and hypoxia/acidosis (Revenis, 2016). Baby A is larger with polycythemia, congestive heart failure, hydrops, and poor perfusion from hyperviscosity (Revenis, 2016).*

(continued)

Case 1.6 *(continued)*

3. TTTS usually occurs in which type of twin pregnancies?
  A. Identical twins
  B. Fraternal twins
  C. Both identical and fraternal twins

  ANSWER: A. *There must be a vascular connection for twin-to-twin transfusion syndrome (TTTS) to occur. Fetal blood exchange occurs almost exclusively in monochorionic twins (Revenis, 2016).*

4. Which of the following is a treatment option for TTTS that addresses the actual cause of the disorder?
  A. Umbilical cord ligation of the donor fetus
  B. Serial amnioreduction of the polyhydramnios
  C. Laser photocoagulation of communicating vessels

  ANSWER: C. *"Endoscopic laser coagulation of connecting vessels is used in treating severe TTTS" (Revenis, 2016, p. 381).*

CONCLUSIONS

Maternal status and disorders affect the fetus and neonate because their body systems coexist together for up to 9 months. The woman's body size and health status can cause disorders in the newborn. The woman's previous health status prior to pregnancy can affect the future pregnancy. Disorders, such as hypertension, obesity, diabetes, SLE, or other similar conditions, can have fetal or neonatal effects. Also, maternal problems can develop because of the pregnancy, like an abruption or placenta previa, gestational hypertension or preeclampsia, premature labor, PROM, or infection. Bacterial or viral infections can occur because of problems with the pregnancy (e.g., PROM) or exposure during the pregnancy. Lastly, the specific type of pregnancy (as in multiple gestation) can significantly affect both the mother and the fetus(es). Understanding these maternal complications and their effects on the newborn is imperative for the neonatal caretakers.

ACKNOWLEDGMENTS

To our husbands, John and Tom, for their continuous support of all that we do. To our neonatal nurse practitioner students, who make our lives interesting and fun!!

REFERENCES

Anderson-Berry, A. L., Bellig, L. L., & Ohning, B. L. (2014, February 11). Neonatal sepsis, eMedicine—Medscape. Retrieved from http://emedicine.medscape.com/article/978352-overview
Boh, E. (2004). Neonatal lupus erythematosus. *Clinics in Dermatology, 22*(2), 125–128.
Borchers, A., Naguwa, S., Keen, C., & Gershwin, M. (2010). The implications of autoimmunity and pregnancy. *Journal of Autoimmunity, 34*(3), J287–J299.

Centers for Disease Control and Prevention (CDC). (2016, May 23). *Group B strep (GBS). Neonatal providers guidelines and resources.* Retrieved from www.cdc.gov/groupbstrep/clinicians/neonatal-providers.html

Classen, S., Paulson, P., & Zacharias, S. (1998). Systemic lupus erythematosus: Perinatal and neonatal implications. *Journal of Obstetric, Gynecologic, & Neonatal Nursing, 27*(5), 493–500.

Deering, S. H. (2015, September 15). Abruptio placentae. *Medscape.* Retrieved from http://emedicine .medscape.com/article/252810-overview

Embree, J. E., & Alfattoh, N. I. (2016). Infections in the newborn. In M. G. MacDonald & M. M. K. Seshia (Eds.), *Avery's neonatology: Pathophysiology and management of the newborn* (7th ed., pp. 930–980). Philadelphia, PA: Wolters Kluwer.

Femia, A., Callen, J., & Vleugels, R. (2014, March, 18). Neonatal and pediatric lupus erythematosus. *Medscape.* Retrieved from http://emedicine.medscape.com/article/1006582-overview#a5

Fletcher, G., & Zach, T. (2015, January 13). Multiple births. *eMedicine—Medscape Drugs & Diseases.* Retrieved from http://emedicine.medscape.com/article/977234-overview#a0101

Genetics and Human Traits. (2016, August 30). Help me understand genetics. NIH – U.S. National Library of Medicine, Department of Health & Human Services. Retrieved from http://ghr.nlm .nih.gov

Gifford, R. W., August, P. A., Cunningham, G., Green, L. A., Lindheimer, M. D., McNellis, D., . . . Taler, S. J. (2000). Report of the National High Blood Pressure Education Program Working Group on high blood pressure in pregnancy. *American Journal of Obstetrics & Gynecology, 183*(1), S1–S22.

Gomella, T. (2013). *Neonatology: Management, procedures, on-call problems, diseases, and drugs* (7th ed.). New York, NY: McGraw-Hill.

Hochberg, M. (1997). Updating the American College of Rheumatology revised criteria for the classification of systemic lupus erythematosus. *Arthritis Rheumatology, 40,* 1725.

Johnson, M. P., Khalek, N., Martinez-Poyer, J. L., & Moldenhauer, J. S. (2014, June 13). *Twin reversed arterial perfusion sequence (TRAP sequence).* Philadelphia, PA: Children's Hospital of Philadelphia. Retrieved from http://www.chop.edu/conditions-diseases/twin-reversed-arterial-perfusion-sequence-and-bipolar-cord-coagulation-for-acardiac-acephalic-twins#.VXeld1VViko

Johnston, T., Paterson-Brown, B., & Paterson-Brown, S. (2011). *Placenta praevia, placenta praevia accreta and vesa praevia: Diagnosis and management* (Green-top Guideline No. 27; pp. 1–27), London, UK: Guidelines Committee of the Royal College of Obstetricians and Gynaecologists.

Langenveld, J., Ravelli, A. C., Van Kaam, A. H., Van der Ham, D. P., Van Pampus, M. G., Porath, M., . . . Ganzevoort, W. (2011). Neonatal outcome of pregnancies complicated by hypertensive disorders between 34–37 weeks of gestation: A 7-year retrospective analysis of a national registry. *American Journal of Obstetrics & Gynecology, 205*(6), 540.e1–7. doi:10.1016/j.ajog.2011 .07.003

Lyell, D. (2004). Hypertensive disorders of pregnancy: Relevance for the neonatologist. *NeoReviews, 5*(6), 240–246.

Madazli, R., Yuksel, M., Yilmaz, H., Oncul, M., Imamoglu, M., & Yilmaz, H. (2014). Obstetric outcomes and prognostic factors of lupus pregnancies. *Maternal–Fetal Medicine, 289,* 49–53.

Matsuda, Y., Hayashi, K., Shiozaki, A., Kawamichi, Y., Satoh, S., & Saito, S. (2011). Comparison of risk factors for placental abruption and placenta previa: Case-cohort study. *Journal of Obstetrics and Gynaecology Research, 37*(6), 538–546.

McDonnold, M., & Olson, G. (2013). Preeclampsia: Pathophysiology, management, and maternal and fetal sequelae. *NeoReviews, 14*(1), 4–12.

Moallem, M., & Koenig, J. (2009). Preeclampsia and neonatal neutropenia. *NeoReviews, 10*(9), e454–e459. doi:10.1542/neo.10-9-e454

Neofax. (2015). *Micromedex Clinical Knowledge Suite.* Ann Arbor, MI: Truven Health Analytics.

Potter, C. F. (2013, May 10). Infant of diabetic mother. *Medscape—eMedicine.* Retrieved from http:// emedicine.medscape.com/article/974230-overview

Ramos, G. A., & Moore, T. R. (2012). Endocrine disorders in pregnancy. In C. A. Gleason & S. U. DeVaskar (Eds.), *Avery's diseases of the newborn* (9th ed., pp. 75–87). Philadelphia, PA: Elsevier.

Revenis, M. E. (2016). Multiple gestation. In M. G. MacDonald & M. M. K. Seshia (Eds.), *Avery's neonatology pathophysiology and management of the newborn* (7th ed., pp. 377–384). Philadelphia, PA: Wolters Kluwer.

Rubarth, L. B. (2011). Fraternal or identical: Understanding twin gestation. *Neonatal Network, 30*(3), 196–198. doi:10.1891/0730–0832.30.3.196

Rubarth, L. B. (2013). Infants of diabetic mothers. *Neonatal Network, 32*(6), 416–418. doi:10.1891/0730-0832.32.6.416

Rugolo, L., Bentlin, M., & Trindade, C. (2012). Preeclampsia: Early and late neonatal outcomes. *NeoReviews, 13*(9), 532–541.

Tikkanen, M. (2010). Etiology, clinical manifestations, and prediction of placental abruption. *Acta Obstetricia et Gynecologica Scandinavica, 89*(6), 732–740. doi:10.3109/00016341003686081

Wu, C., Nohr, E., Bech, B., Catov, J., & Olsen, J. (2009). Health of children born to mothers who had preeclampsia: A population-based cohort study. *American Journal of Obstetrics & Gynecology, 201*(3), 269–279.

Yildirim, A., Tunaodlu, F., & Karaabac, A. (2013). Neonatal congenital heart block. *Indian Pediatrics, 50*, 483–488.

Zenk, K. (2003). *Neonatal medications and nutrition: A comprehensive guide* (3rd ed., Appendix A). Santa Rosa, CA: NICU Ink.

2

Identifying Maternal Conditions Affecting Altered Embryologic Development

Cheryl B. Robinson and Donna Campbell Dunn

Chapter Objectives

1. Recognize normal physiology of the placenta and the related role in fetal support and development
2. Determine the embryologic developmental consequences of selected maternal disease processes
3. Apply concepts related to placental physiology to formulate a plan of care for the infant compromised by selected maternal disease processes

The purpose of the chapter is to identify maternal conditions that affect embryologic development. The critical importance of the placenta for fetal support and development is vital to this discussion.

THE PLACENTA

The placenta is derived from both maternal and fetal tissues and performs multiple functions to encourage normal growth and development of a fetus. As the first fetal organ, the placenta (a) facilitates implantation, (b) establishes a mechanism for nutrient and gas exchange, (c) begins the process of maternal physiologic changes associated with pregnancy, (d) affects the immune environment, (e) releases paracrine and endocrine hormones that influence the cardiovascular and metabolic processes in the mother (Cross, 2006).

PHYSIOLOGY

The development of the placenta begins when fertilization occurs between the egg and sperm. Development begins as the morula travels down the fallopian tube toward the uterus. As fluid accumulates around the morula, a blastocyst is formed. The blastocyst is composed of an outer layer of cells called the *trophoblast*, an inner cell mass that will form the embryo, and a fluid-filled cavity. The trophoblast will form the placenta and fetal membranes. Initially, the blastocyst is covered by secretions from the uterus providing oxygen and metabolic substrates. As the requirements for development of the blastocyst increase, attachment to the uterine wall to obtain needed substrates is necessary. The implantation process occurs within 5 to 8 days of fertilization. Once the blastocyst attaches to the uterus, it begins to invade the uterine tissue. The cytotrophoblast cells from the trophoblast invade deeper into the tissue. This space will develop into the intervillous space, which creates the placental blood flow when these spaces are filled with maternal blood. The spiral arteries, which branch from the uterine arteries, deliver the maternal blood to this space. A remodeling of the spiral artery has to occur in order to facilitate the high-volume, low-pressure flow of blood.

FUNCTIONS

The placenta performs multiple functions essential for the development and growth of the fetus. The organ offers endocrine support, a transportation pathway for nutrients and waste materials, sustenance, and an immunologic barrier (Redline, 2015). Uniquely, the placenta functions as an endocrine organ for synthesis of hormones and neurotransmitters and produces peptide and steroid hormones. Peptide hormones, such as human chorionic gonadotropin (hCG), human placental lactogen (hPL), and growth hormones (GH), are produced by the trophoblast of the chorionic villi (Lager & Powell, 2012). Estrogen, progesterone, which helps maintain the pregnancy, and glucocorticoids readily cross the membranes and are produced by the placenta (Lager & Powell, 2012).

The placenta is a vector for exchange of nutrients, oxygen, and waste products between maternal and fetal circulations. Glucose, iron, water, and ascorbic acid utilize placental transport mechanisms (Lager & Powell, 2012). The main site for the exchange of nutrients and gases is the syncytiotrophoblast layer of the placenta.

The placenta provides substances needed to sustain pregnancy as well as protect the fetus from the maternal immune response. Synthesizing glycogen, cholesterol, and fatty acids, the placenta provides energy to the growing fetus (Longo & Reynolds, 2010). As an immunologic barrier between maternal and fetal systems. The placenta prevents the maternal immune system from rejecting the fetus (Longo & Reynolds, 2010). Fetoplacental adaptations are noted to occur depending on the sex of the fetus as well. In preeclampsia, a male fetus demonstrates a normal growth pattern, while a female fetus has a reduction in growth likely due to gene, protein, mRNA, and steroid pathways in the uteroplacenta circulation being sex dependent (Clifton, 2010).

MATERNAL CONDITIONS

Maternal health is crucial to the development of a healthy fetus and, subsequently, a healthy newborn. Varied health conditions are responsible for known complications in embryologic development of the fetus. Conditions that impact maternal oxygenation will impact fetal oxygenation. Conditions that produce maternal inflammation will trigger an inflammatory response in the fetus. Conditions that impact placental blood flow will decrease fetal oxygenation and growth. Every maternal body system can and does have a unique impact on the fetus (Razaee, Lappen, & Gecsi, 2013). Maternal infections, bacterial, viral, or fungal, are not covered in this section. Selected maternal conditions, impacting the placenta and fetus, are discussed.

ASTHMA

An estimated 3% to 12% of all pregnant women have asthma making it the leading pulmonary disease seen in pregnancy (Lin et al., 2012; Rocklin, 2011; Tamási et al., 2011). The severity of symptomatology during pregnancy varies; some women improve, some worsen, and some demonstrate no change in symptoms from their prepregnancy condition. Some estimates suggest, however, that up to 55% of asthmatics will experience an exacerbation during pregnancy (Clifton, 2010). Exacerbations during pregnancy can result in significant increases in the rates of preterm birth, low birth weight (LBW), fetal growth restriction, and preeclampsia with the risk of preeclampsia being increased as much as 50% (Dombrowski & Schatz, 2010; Murphy et al., 2011; Rocklin, 2011; Tamási et al., 2011).

Asthma can lead to hypoxia or hyperventilation, both of which can cause a reduction in the availability of oxygen for the fetus because of alterations in placental function (Blackburn, 2013; Murphy et al., 2011; Rocklin, 2011). The inflammatory processes present with asthma also impact the fetus by decreasing the ability of placental enzymes to metabolize corticosteroids, resulting in an increased level of cortisol reaching the fetus. Increased levels of cortisol, most likely, reduce fetal adrenal activity, which, in turn, decreases fetal growth (Cossette et al., 2013; Murphy et al., 2011). Reducing maternal lung inflammation improves fetal oxygenation.

The common treatment for asthma consists of long-acting B$_2$ agonists (LABAs) and inhaled corticosteroids (ICSs). The first-trimester use of oral corticosteroids has been associated with preeclampsia; preterm birth; LBW; and cleft lip, with or without cleft palate, whereas the use of ICSs appears to be a safer choice (Rocklin, 2011). Lin et al. (2012) concluded there was a moderate risk association between the use of asthma medications and esophageal atresia, anorectal atresia, and omphalocele.

Researchers agree that additional studies need to be conducted to ascertain the significance of the presence of asthma on a pregnancy, the impact of medications, both timing and dosing used to treat asthma, the effect of exacerbations during pregnancy, and the impact on the fetus (Gregersen & Ulrik, 2013). What they do agree on is that maternal hypoxia and maternal inflammation processes lead to adverse outcomes for the fetus and newborn.

Case 2.1

You are called to the newborn nursery to evaluate a patient newly admitted from labor and delivery (L&D) for a baby who will not suck. Review of the history reveals a 22-year-old primigravida mother of baby with documented prenatal care and reports of no significant maternal history other than the as-needed use of a steroid pack for shortness of breath or wheezing. Her admission prenatal labs are negative. The infant was born via spontaneous vaginal delivery without complication with Apgar scores of 8/9.

(continued)

Case 2.1 *(continued)*

Upon examination of the oral pharynx you do not note any cleft, but when you feed the baby you note that milk comes out the baby's nose. You transfer the infant to the neonatal intensive care unit (NICU) and order him to be fed nothing orally (NPO).

1. What could be the cause of this infant's condition?

A. Corticosteroid use
B. Irregular use of an inhaler
C. Maternal hypoxia

ANSWER: A. *The first-trimester use of oral corticosteroids has been associated with pre-eclampsia, preterm birth, low birth weight, and cleft lip, with or without cleft palate, where the use of inhaled corticosteroids (ICSs) appears to be a safer choice (Rocklin, 2011).*

2. The infant is also noted to be small for gestational age (SGA). What placental mechanism could account for this finding?

A. Increased fetal adrenal activity
B. Elevated fetal cortisol levels
C. Use of ICSs

ANSWER: B. *Women not formally diagnosed with asthma may just treat symptoms as needed and not be well controlled. Asthma is an inflammatory process. The placenta responds by decreasing the production of a placental enzyme that helps metabolize corticosteriods. The fetus is impacted by an increased cortisol level which, in turn, reduces fetal adrenal activity, leading to impaired growth (Cossette et al., 2013).*

HYPERTENSION

Cardiovascular disease is the number one cause of death in women older than 25 years of age and its prevalence is increasing among women. One woman in four has some type of cardiovascular disease, such as hypertension, coronary artery disease, heart disease, and stroke. During pregnancy this list includes gestational hypertension, preeclampsia, eclampsia, and HELLP (hemolysis, elevated liver enzymes, and low platelet) syndrome.

Preeclampsia, eclampsia, and HELLP syndrome are associated with defects in vascular development. There is a lack of normal physiological adaptation of the spiral arteries to pregnancy, reduced blood flow into the intervillous space, and relative hypoxia/ischemia.

In a pregnancy without maternal hypertension, the placenta provides sufficient blood flow for the growing fetus's heart and organs. However, when placental flow is decreased, as is the case in maternal hypertension or coronary artery disease, the lack of placental sufficiency leads to slower growth in the embryonic and fetal heart, resulting in heart defects, fetal hypoxemia, hypercapnia, and mild acidemia (Thornburg, O'Tierney, & Louey, 2010). Likewise, additional maternal complications include placental abruption and need for emergent cesarean delivery.

Antihypertensive medications are utilized during pregnancy to promote healthy outcomes for mother and fetus. The use of antihypertensives that improve circulation to mother and fetus may improve fetal outcomes by prolonging pregnancy and reducing the risk for preterm delivery (PTD), SGA, and neonatal death (Orbach et al., 2013; Xu, Charlton, Makris, & Hennessy, 2014). Some women treated with methyldopa or atenolol have experienced higher rates of SGA, PTD, LBW, and intrauterine growth restriction (IUGR) (Orbach et al., 2013).

Understanding the implications of maternal disease and complications on outcomes of the neonate is vital. By collaborating with obstetric providers and effectively treating maternal cardiovascular disease, pregnancies can be prolonged and outcomes improved.

Case 2.2

A 36-year-old female at 30 weeks pregnancy confirmed by a 24-week ultrasound presents to the maternal triage unit complaining of intense abdominal pain—rated as 8 on a scale of 10—with heavy vaginal bleeding, pounding in her ears, and black spots in her field of vision. She reports this started 2 hours ago. While she is being connected to the tocometer in order to assess fetal heart rate and contractions, she proceeds to deliver a 1-kg infant. The infant does not cry and is cyanotic. The neonatal nurse practitioner (NNP) is called emergently to the room for resuscitation and stabilization.

1. **Which of the following is the best explanation of why there was a placenta abruption?**

   A. Maternal medications
   B. Incompetent cervix
   C. Reduced blood flow to the placenta

   ANSWER: C. *When placental flow is decreased, as is the case in maternal hypertension or coronary artery disease, the lack of placental sufficiency leads to fetal hypoxemia, hypercapnia, and mild acidemia. Likewise, additional maternal complications include placental abruption (Orbach et al., 2013; Thornburg, O'Tierney, & Louey, 2010).*

2. **What would explain the neonate's small-for-gestational-age status?**

   A. Oligohydramnois
   B. Increased maternal inflammation
   C. Relative hypoxemia

   ANSWER: C. *When placental blood flow is reduced, the fetus experiences slower growth, fetal hypoxemia, hypercapnia, and mild acidemia all leading to an infant not appropriately grown for gestational age (Thornburg, O'Tierney, & Louey, 2010; Xu et al., 2014).*

MATERNAL WEIGHT

Maternal nutritional status plays a pivotal role in placental–fetal development. Nutrition is an important factor in achieving a positive maternal and fetal outcome. Normal placental function promotes successful transfer of nutrients and substances between the maternal and fetal circulations. However, alterations of nutritional status during pregnancy may negatively impact the maternal and fetal outcomes (Razaee, Lappen, & Gecsi, 2013).

Underweight

Low maternal weight during pregnancy may result in IUGR. This is mostly the result of maternal undernutrition and the reduction in nutrients supplied to the developing fetus. Considering the role of the placenta in the transfer of nutrients from the maternal circulation, if the mother is not obtaining the nutrients needed to encourage proper development, the placenta may not assist the fetus with development.

The weight of the placenta is negatively impacted by poor maternal nutrition. The degree of the impact depends on the timing, degree, and duration of undernutrition. In women with undernutrition, the surface area of the placenta is reduced, providing less opportunity for exchange of nutrients and substances important to the developing fetus (Lakshmy, 2013).

Obesity

Maternal obesity is associated with negative sequelae and the rates of obesity are increasing among mothers. Obesity is associated with additional comorbidities that may put the fetus and neonate at risk for negative outcomes, including type 2 diabetes. Mothers who are obese are more likely to experience macrosomia, PTD, neonatal death, perinatal morbidity, and birth defects (Bloomberg, 2013). Maternal obesity not only impacts the pregnancy but has negative long-term impact on the child, increasing the medical risk of metabolic disease because of a low-grade inflammation (Segovia, Vickers, Gray, & Reynolds, 2014). These findings support the early development of adult disease beginning during fetal development (Freeman, 2010).

Inflammation resulting from maternal obesity impacts not only the pregnancy but the placenta as well. Maternal inflammation, which creates metabolic inflammation, is composed of high levels of adipose tissue and cytokine levels. Maternal obesity exposes the fetus to these elevated levels as well, which contributes to early impact on the risk of the child to experience metabolic disease (Segovia et al., 2014).

THYROID DISEASE

Maternal thyroid disease during pregnancy is as high as 3%. If thyroid disease is not detected and treated, it may lead to fetal loss, PTD, and hypertension (Stagnaro-Green et al., 2011). During development, the fetus depends on maternal thyroid hormone for proper development. Early in pregnancy, the fetus depends completely on the maternal thyroid hormone received through the placenta, because the fetal thyroid does not begin to function until 12 to 14 weeks (Chuang, Gutmark-Little, & Rose, 2015). After the fetal thyroid begins to function, the fetus continues to utilize maternal thyroid hormone.

Hyperthyroidism

Approximately 0.5% of pregnant women are treated for hyperthyroidism. Hyperthyroidism during pregnancy is associated with IUGR and PTD. In addition, hyperthyroidism impacts fetal growth, causing a thyrotoxic and catabolic state in the fetus (Chuang et al., 2015). Once delivered, neonates of mothers with hyperthyroidism are more likely to experience neonatal thyroid diseases (Mannisto et al., 2010).

Hypothyroidism

During pregnancy, an estimated 2.5% of women have hypothyroidism. Low levels of T4 hormones during pregnancy (which is characteristic of hypothyroid) increase neurodevelopmental deficits in the offspring (Henrichs et al., 2010). Hypothyroidism during pregnancy is associated with increased neonatal admission to intensive care units as well as increased risk of respiratory distress syndrome, transient tachypnea, apnea, sepsis, and anemia.

Case 2.3

You are called to the newborn nursery to evaluate a 6-hour-old, full-term infant who is not eating well, is somewhat lethargic, and has a "big" neck. Review of the history reveals a 32-year-old primigravida mother of baby with regular prenatal care, who is taking methimazole. The infant was born via spontaneous vaginal delivery without complication with Apgar scores of 6/8.

Upon examination you note the baby does have a rather large mass in the center of his throat, appears somewhat hypotonic, and the baby's skin appears dry.

1. *Which of the following is the most likely diagnosis for this infant?*

   A. Neonatal Graves' disease
   B. Neonatal thyrotoxicosis
   C. Neonatal transient hypothyroidism

   ANSWER: C. *Most infants with transient hypothyroidism were born to mothers who received goitrogens during pregnancy (Chuang et al., 2015).*

2. *To confirm your diagnosis, which of the following tests should be ordered?*

   A. An x-ray of the neck
   B. Thyroid-stimulating hormone (TSH), T4, and free T4
   C. TSI (thyroid-stimulating immunoglobulin)

   ANSWER: B. *When goiter is present, there should be an elevation of serum TSH and a decrease in serum T4 levels after birth (Chuang et al., 2015).*

REFERENCES

Blackburn, S. (2013). *Maternal, fetal, & neonatal physiology: A clinical perspective* (4th ed.). New York, NY: Elsevier Saunders.

Bloomberg, M. (2013). Maternal obesity, mode of delivery, and neonatal outcome. *Obstetrics & Gynecology, 122*(1), 50–55.

Chuang, J., Gutmark-Little, I., & Rose, S. R. (2015). Thyroid disorders in the neonate. In R. Martin, A. Fanaroff, & M. Walsh (Eds.), *Fanaroff and Martin's neonatal-perinatal medicine: Diseases of the fetus and infant* (10th ed., pp. 1490–1515). Philadelphia, PA: Saunders.

Clifton, V. L. (2010). Review: Sex and the human placenta: Mediating differential strategies of fetal growth and survival. *Placenta, 31*(Suppl. A), S33–S39.

Cossette, B., Forget, A., Beauchesne, M.-F., Rey, E., Lemière, C., Larivé, P., . . . Blais, L. (2013). Impact of maternal use of asthma controller therapy on perinatal outcomes. *Thorax, 68*(8), 724–730.

Cross, J. C. (2006). Placental function in development and disease. *Reproduction, Fertility and Development, 18*, 71–76.

Dombrowski, M. P., & Schatz, M. (2010). Asthma in pregnancy. *Clinical Obstetrics and Gynecology, 53*(2), 301–310.

Freeman, D. J. (2010). Effects of maternal obesity on fetal growth and body composition: Implications for programming and future health. *Seminars in Fetal & Neonatal Medicine, 15*(2), 113–118.

Gregersen, T. L., & Ulrik, C. S. (2013). Safety of bronchodilators and corticosteroids for asthma during pregnancy: What we know and what we need to do better. *Journal of Asthma and Allergy, 16,* 117–125.

Henrichs, J., Jacoba, J., Bongers-Schokking, J. J., Schenk, J. J., Ghassabian, A., Schmidt, H. G., . . . Tiemeir, H. (2010). Maternal thyroid function during early pregnancy and cognitive functioning in early childhood: The Generation R Study. *Journal of Clinical Endocrinology and Metabolism, 95,* 4227–4234.

Lager, S., & Powell, T. L. (2012). Regulation and nutrient transport across the placenta. *Journal of Pregnancy.* doi:10.1155/2012/179827

Lakshmy, R. (2013). Metabolic syndrome: Role of maternal undernutrition and fetal programming. *Review of Endocrine and Metabolic Disorders, 14,* 229–240.

Lin, S., Munsie, J. P. W., Herdt-Losavio, M., Druchel, C. M., Campbell, K., Browne, M. L., . . . National Birth Defects Prevention Study. (2012). Maternal asthma medication use and the risk of selected birth defects. *Pediatrics, 129*(2), e317–e324.

Mannisto, T., Varasma, M., Pouta, A., Hartikainen, A.-L., Ruokonen, A., Helja, A. R., . . . Suvanto, E. (2010). Thyroid dysfunction and autoantibodies during pregnancy as predictive factors of pregnancy complications and maternal morbidity in later life. *Journal of Clinical Endocrinology and Metabolism, 95,* 1084–1094.

Murphy, V. E., Namazy, J. A., Powel, H., Schatz, M., Chambers, C., Attia, J., & Gibson, P. G. (2011). A meta-analysis of adverse perinatal outcomes in women with asthma. *British Journal of Obstetrics and Gynaecology, 118,* 1214–1323.

Orbach, H., Matok, I., Gorodischer, R., Sheiner, E., Daniel, S., Wiznitzer, A., . . . Levy, A. (2013). Hypertension and antihypertensive drugs in pregnancy and perinatal outcomes. *American Journal of Obstetrics & Gynecology, 208*(301), e.1–e.6.

Razaee, R. L., Lappen, J. R., & Gecsi, K. S. (2013). Antenatal and intrapartum care of the high-risk infant. In A. A. Fanaroff (Ed.), *Klaus and Fanaroff: Care of the high-risk neonate* (6th ed., pp. 10–53). New York, NY: Elsevier Saunders.

Redline, R. W. (2015). Placental pathology. In R. Martin, A. Fanaroff, & M. Walsh, (Eds.), *Fanaroff and Martin's neonatal-perinatal medicine: Diseases of the fetus and infant* (10th ed., pp. 365–372). Philadelphia, PA: Saunders.

Rocklin, R. E. (2011). Asthma, asthma medications and their effects on maternal/fetal outcomes during pregnancy. *Reproductive Toxicology, 32,* 189–197.

Segovia, S. A., Vickers, M. H., Gray, C., & Reynolds, C. M. (2014). Maternal obesity, inflammation, and developmental programming. *BioMed Research International.* doi: 1155/2014/418975

Stagnaro-Green, A., Abalovich, M., Alexander, E., Azizi, F., Mestman, J., Negro, R., . . . Wiersinga, W. (2011). Guidelines of the American Thyroid Association for the diagnosis and management of thyroid disease during pregnancy and postpartum. *Thyroid, 21*(10), 1081–1125.

Tamási, L., Horváth, I., Bohács, A., Müller, V., Losonczy, G., & Schatz, M. (2011). Asthma in pregnancy—Immunological changes and clinical management. *Respiratory Medicine, 105,* 159–164.

Thornburg, K. L., O'Tierney, P. F., & Louey, S. (2010). The placenta is a programming agent for cardiovascular disease. *Placenta, 31,* S54–S59.

Xu, B., Charlton, F. C., Makris, A., & Hennessy, A. (2014). Antihypertensive drugs methyldopa, labetalol, hydralazine, and clonidine improve trophoblast interaction with endothelial cellular networks *in vitro. Journal of Hypertension, 32,* 1075–1083.

3

Identifying Factors Influencing Neonatal Transition

Jacqui Hoffman

Chapter Objectives

1. Describe normal fetal and postnatal circulatory patterns
2. Discuss perinatal risk factors that may impact successful postnatal transition
3. Apply identification of potential perinatal risk factors to the postnatal management of the neonate during the transition period

Fetal to neonatal transition is a highly complex process that normally begins prior to delivery of the term infant. The complex processes of adaptation involve almost every system in the body, which enables the dependent fetus to become an independent neonate. Cortisol and catecholamines are the primary mediators that prepare the fetus for this extrauterine transition. This process of transition begins immediately with removal of the placenta; the most important transition time for the neonate is generally thought to be the first 6 to 8 hours after delivery, with mature physiologic postnatal values potentially taking weeks to attain (Verklan, 2002). However, there are many factors that may be present that hinder this successful adaptation and may place the neonate at increased risk of mortality and morbidity.

IN UTERO PLACENTAL SUPPORT

In utero, the fetus obtains oxygenated blood via the umbilical vein from the low-resistance placenta. The fluid-filled lungs are not necessary for gas exchange and receive only 10% or less of the cardiac output, whereas 50% of the cardiac output is sent to the fetal organ of respiration, the placenta (Mercer & Erickson, 2012). Fetal lung fluid is secreted by the airway epithelium by the active transport of chloride, therefore the chloride content is high but the protein content is very low. Production and maintenance of fetal lung fluid is imperative for normal lung growth. The well-oxygenated blood from the intervillous spaces of the placenta goes from the umbilical vein to the liver, with the majority bypassing the hepatic circulation through the ductus venosus. Blood enters the right atrium primarily, going across the foramen ovale into the left atrium after which it is ejected out the left ventricle, which supplies blood to the brain and upper body. Pulmonary vascular resistance (PVR) is high in utero as a result of physiologic fetal hypoxia and resultant vasoconstriction. This high PVR causes the majority of deoxygenated blood flow from the superior vena cava that enters the right atrium and right ventricle to bypass the lungs freely across the dilated ductus arteriosus, with this blood being distributed to the descending aorta and out to the systemic circulation. Because of the presence of fetal hemoglobin (Hgb), which facilitates transfer of oxygen from the mother to the fetus, the fetus has a PaO_2 of approximately 25 to 35 mmHg (Blackburn, 2013). These circulatory shunts in utero are advantageous to the fetus as it provides oxygen to the heart and brain (Figure 3.1). During times of stress, the fetus can shunt blood

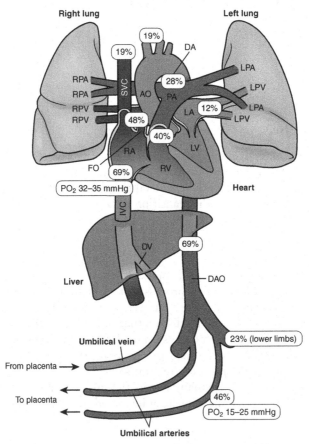

Figure 3.1 Fetal Circulation

Note: The higher fetal PaO_2 values of the blood entering the fetal circulation from the umbilical vein versus the lower PaO_2 as the blood from the systemic circulation returns to the placenta via the umbilical arteries (Blackburn, 2013). Note the percentage of fetal blood flow patterns (Sinha & Donn, 2006).

AO, aorta; DA, ductus arteriosus; DAO, descending aorta; DV, ductus venosus; FO, foramen ovale; IVC, interior vena cava; LA, left atrum; LPA, left pulmonary artery; LPV, left pulmonary vein; LV, left ventricle; PA, pulmonary artery; RA, right atrium; RPA, right pulmonary artery; RPV, right pulmonary vein; RV, right ventricle; SVC, superior vena cava.

away from less critical organs, such as the kidneys, skin, and intestines, to the more critical organs, including the heart, brain, and adrenal glands.

NEONATAL ADAPTATION

CARDIORESPIRATORY FETAL-TO-NEONATAL ADAPTATION

The most dramatic transitional changes from the intrauterine to extrauterine environment involve the cardiorespiratory systems. With removal of the placenta, the first step in neonatal transition is the transfer of gas exchange from the placenta, where the pulmonary circulation is a high-resistance, low-flow circuit, to the lungs. The transitional changes begin with the initiation of respiration. Cardiovascular adaptation requires changes in the circulatory pattern and pressures as well as pulmonary vasodilation. After delivery, the fetal shunts and umbilical vessels are no longer needed in most circumstances. The precise mechanisms for closure of the umbilical vessels are controversial. It is felt that the arterial flow across the umbilical artery rapidly decreases during the first 20 to 25 seconds after delivery and is negligible after 45 seconds, preventing loss of blood from the delivered neonate to the placenta if there is delayed clamping of the cord. With removal of the low-resistance placental circulation, blocking of the umbilical arteries results in a marked increase in left ventricular afterload. The umbilical vein remains open longer allowing transfusion of blood from placenta to neonate and, after 3 minutes, flow becomes insignificant (Kim & Warren, 2015). With removal of the placenta, there is a decrease in blood pressure in the inferior vena cava and right atrium. The sphincter in the ductus venosus begins to constrict soon after cord clamping, allowing all the blood entering the liver to pass through the hepatic sinusoids; the ductus venosus becomes completely obliterated by 2 weeks of age in term infants but may take longer to become obliterated in the presence of pulmonary hypertension (Blackburn, 2013). As the neonate takes its first several breaths, the lungs expand and fetal lung fluid is cleared, the pulmonary arteries dilate with a resultant fall in PVR, leading to increased right ventricular output to the lungs and increasing blood oxygen levels within the first 10 minutes of life (Table 3.1).

As the circulation changes from a "parallel" to a "series" pattern, the right ventricular output equals the left ventricular output. The cardiac output nearly doubles after birth, closely paralleling the rise in oxygen consumption (Hillman, Kallapur, & Jobe, 2012). As a result of the higher oxygen content of the blood, of prostaglandin from the placenta no longer being available, and other chemical changes, in particular bradykinin, the ductus arteriosus begins to constrict, resulting in termination of the right-to-left shunting (Moore, Persaud, & Torchia, 2013). The ductus arteriosus functionally closes within the first 24 hours of life in the term infant; however, persistence is inverse to gestational age, and the younger the gestational age, the more likely the ductus is to remain patent. Anatomical closure of the ductus arteriosus via endothelial and fibrous tissue proliferation usually occurs by 3 months of life (Blackburn, 2013). As pulmonary blood flow increases, there is increased left atrial pressure leading to termination of the right-to-left shunting with functional closure of the foramen ovale. The foramen ovale gradually closes over the first few days to weeks of life as the left atrial pressure becomes higher than the right atrial pressure. Anatomical closure of the foramen ovale may not occur until 30 months of age or older (Blackburn, 2013). It is not unusual for as many as 60% of term infants to have a transient murmur during the first 48 hours, reflecting the cardiovascular changes that are occurring during transition. The closure of the fetal channels is the final result of changing from placental to pulmonary gas exchange, so anything that alters the ability for this to occur can lead to impaired pulmonary gas exchange transition, resulting in either oxygenation or ventilation failure (Table 3.2).

The most essential adaptation at birth is the initiation of breathing. The neonate has to transition from intermittent respiratory effort in the intrauterine environment to a continuous

Table 3.1 Oxygen Saturations in a Healthy Term Infant During the First 10 Minutes of Life

Age of Life (min)	Targeted Preductal S_{PO2} (%)
1	60–65
2	65–70
3	70–75
4	75–80
5	80–85
10	85–95

Adapted from Kattwinkel (2011).

respiratory pattern after delivery. A high negative pressure is initially required for the first spontaneous breaths in order to overcome the viscosity of the fluid-filled airways, the surface tension of the lungs filled with pulmonary fluid, and the elastic recoil and resistance of the chest wall, lungs, and airways (Sinha & Donn, 2006). The required increase in transthoracic pressure generated with the first postnatal breath can lead to a spontaneous pneumothorax in a small percentage of neonates, even in the absence of parenchymal lung disease. This first breath is initiated by several stimuli, including mild physiologic asphyxia, stimulation of aortic and carotid chemoreceptors, stimulation of aortic baroreceptors and the sympathetic nervous system, as well as thermal stimulation (Blackburn, 2013). Gas exchange needs to switch from an air–liquid interface of alveolar epithelium to an air–blood exchange. This postnatal pulmonary gas exchange is determined by the ability to decrease PVR, ability to facilitate pulmonary blood flow by maintaining a more alkaline environ-

Table 3.2 Successful Transition Findings

Mobilization and absorption of lung fluid

Spontaneous respirations with inflation of lungs

Decreased pulmonary vascular resistance

Increased systemic vascular resistance

Constriction of the ductus arteriosus and ductus venosus

Thermal regulation

Glucose stability

ment, the establishment of spontaneous respirations, the ability to maintain an optimal tidal volume, and the secretion of surfactant. As the pregnancy progresses, there is decreased production of fetal lung fluid by the fetal lung epithelium. The process of pulmonary fluid absorption also begins prior to the onset of spontaneous labor and increases during labor as hormonal influences facilitate the secretion of chloride, the absorption of sodium and fluid from the alveoli into the interstitium, and stimulation of alveolar surfactant secretion. After delivery, alveolar fluid absorption is facilitated by the respiratory epithelium, changing from a chloride-secreting membrane to a sodium-secreting membrane (Keene, Bland, & Jain, 2012). In addition, there is a transepithelial protein gradient that facilitates movement of fluid from the alveolar lumen into the interstitial space. Increased transpulmonary pressure, caused by the aeration of the lungs, further drives fluid into the interstitium. Pulmonary fluid absorption through the lymphatic vessels and the pulmonary capillary beds is typically completed within the first few hours of life in the full-term healthy neonate (Sinha & Donn, 2006). Inflation of the lungs leads to a dramatic decrease in PVR and a tenfold increase in pulmonary blood flow. After delivery, there is postnatal remodeling of the pulmonary arterioles as a result of stimulation of the pulmonary stretch receptors that occurs with progressive thinning of the medial musculature of the pulmonary artery walls. The pulmonary arterioles remain very reactive and factors, such as hypoxia, hypercarbia, or acidosis, can result in constriction and increased PVR with resultant right-to-left shunting through the foramen ovale and ductus arteriosus mimicking fetal circulation patterns (Blackburn, 2013).

ENDOCRINE FETAL-TO-NEONATAL ADAPTATION

Fetal cortisol levels increase by half between 35 weeks gestation and term; these levels quadruple during term labor and the first hours after birth. Increase in cortisol levels plays important roles in contributing to a normal fetal-to-newborn transition, including thyroid and glucose metabolism, catecholamine release, digestion properties of the intestines, stimulation of surfactant production, absorption of fetal lung fluid, and increased beta-adrenergic receptors (Hillman et al., 2012). Cortisol, along with increasing thyroid hormones, activates the sodium pump, which facilitates clearing of fetal lung fluid at delivery.

Glucose is the major energy source for placental tissue itself and for the fetus. Fetal energy needs are met not only by maternal transplacental transfer of glucose, but also transplacental transfer of amino acids, fatty acids, and ketones. Fetal blood glucose levels fluctuate with changes in maternal glucose levels and are approximately 60% to 70% of maternal glucose levels (Heck & Erenberg, 1987). Glucose stimulates insulin secretion by the fetal pancreas, which induces lipogenesis and releases insulin-like growth factor. Large amounts of glucose are converted to glycogen. From 36 weeks onward there are increased glycogen stores in the fetal liver, in muscle, and the heart. Infants who are born prior to 36 weeks have lower glycogen stores and less available energy reserves (Sinha & Donn, 2006). In addition, preterm, especially extremely preterm, infants may lack the cerebral defenses against hypoglycemia that exists in term infants, reflecting the importance of early enteral feeding or provision of intravenous (IV) glucose if feeds are not possible. Early protein administration is also important in the extremely preterm infant to help buffer the occurrence of hyperglycemia by stimulating endogenous insulin secretion (Castrodale & Rinehart, 2014). Although fat is not a major source of energy for the fetus, it provides a significant percentage of the energy expenditure in the neonate on the first day of life. Transitional changes also occur related to hormonal and metabolic changes. A catecholamine surge occurs in response to the labor and delivery as well as the cold stress that is experienced immediately after birth. The release of epinephrine and norepinephrine stimulates cardiac function and the release of surfactant, promotes clearance of fetal lung fluid, promotes glycogenolysis and lipolysis, and initiates thermogenesis from brown fat (Hillman et al., 2012; Verklan, 2002). The organ systems in the preterm infant are less responsive, thus more catecholamines are secreted. As the plasma levels of these catecholamines and glucagon increase rapidly during delivery, insulin concentrations fall leading to the mobilization of stored glucagon and fatty acids (Sinha & Donn, 2006). Following umbilical cord clamping, neonatal glucose concentration decreases rapidly. Newborn blood glucose reaches a nadir by about 1 to 2 hours of age and newborn glucose production switches from glycogenolysis to gluconeogenesis. The majority of hepatic glycogen stores are depleted by 10 hours of age (Graves & Haley, 2013).

Calcium is actively transported across the placenta to the fetus and, by term, the serum calcium levels actually exceed maternal serum values. Calcitonin and $24,25(OH)_2$ vitamin D levels are high, facilitating a high rate of deposition of calcium into the bone. Once the neonate is born, the transplacental supply no longer exists, causing the neonate to decrease the rate of bone mineralization and resorb bone to maintain extracellular homeostasis. There is a progressive decline in the serum calcium level in the term neonate over the first 24 hours of life until the parathyroid gland stimulates the synthesis of $1,25(OH)_2$ vitamin D, with levels stabilizing over the next 24 hours and then gradually increasing (Britton, 1998). Infants who are delivered prematurely before these calcium stores are built up will need early parenteral and/or enteral sources of calcium to prevent hypocalcemia.

FETAL-TO-NEONATAL ADAPTATION TO THERMOREGULATION

Fetal thermogenesis is normally inactive as a result of a virtually constant in utero environment; however, fetal basal heat production is twice that of an adult. Because of heat generated by the uterus, placenta, and fetal metabolism, the fetal temperature is approximately 0.5°C higher than the mother's (Bissinger & Annibale, 2010; Hillman et al., 2012). Brown adipose tissue is noted at 29 weeks gestation and increases throughout the third trimester, accumulating in particular around the kidneys and in the intrascapular areas of the back. When infants are born preterm or are growth restricted, they lack the brown-fat stores needed to fully initiate nonshivering thermogenesis and will be at risk for cold stress and hypothermia as they do not have stored brown fat to burn for heat production (Blackburn, 2013). The very thin epidermal layer of skin lacks keratin and these infants are at high risk for transepidermal water loss, which diminishes heat regulation. At the time of delivery, neonates have a high surface area-to-body ratio and will lose heat quickly in the cooler delivery room environments (convection) with the wet amniotic fluid on them (evaporation). Placing the infant skin-to-skin or on a prewarmed surface will result in decreased heat loss by conduction. Drying the infant immediately following delivery will decrease heat loss by evaporation. Keeping the infant away from cold walls or windows will decrease radiation heat losses, while maintaining the room temperature at least at 80°F, minimizing air drafts, and using heated gases for respiratory support will decrease convective heat losses. Utilizing a polyethylene wrap in the delivery room in younger gestational age infants can also minimize evaporative and convective heat losses. In the flexed position, the term neonate can decrease heat loss by reducing his or her surface area. If the infant is not protected from heat loss, the drop in the neonate's temperature will result in increased oxygen consumption, respiratory compromise, utilization of energy sources, in particular brown fat, in which the sympathetic system releases norepinephrine and lipase activity releases fatty acid leading to the production of heat. The presence of hypoxia decreases the process of heat production and results in anaerobic metabolism, which causes metabolic acidosis and pulmonary vasoconstriction that can alter the transition process (Bissinger & Annibale, 2010; Sinha & Donn, 2006). Vernix caseosa covers the skin in utero and offers protection from the amniotic fluid.

As the pregnancy progresses, the vernix layer decreases and is virtually nonexistent in the term infant. If vernix is present at the time of delivery, new evidence supports many benefits of leaving it in place, including protection from the drier extrauterine environment, antimicrobial properties, and decreased fluid and electrolyte loss (Blackburn, 2013).

Gastrointestinal Fetal-to-Neonatal Adaptation

With removal of the placenta, waste products must now be removed by the neonate. At delivery, the intestinal tract is sterile but rapidly becomes colonized with bacteria from breastfeeding or formula feeding. As the neonate cries, air is swallowed and begins to fill the intestines, initiating peristalsis. There is decreased blood flow to the gut in utero, so after delivery there is commonly a delay in gastric emptying and slow motility, which explains why spitting up in the immediate neonatal period is not necessarily the result of protein or lactose intolerance. Sucking stimulates the production of many enteric hormones, including insulin, growth hormone, gastrin, motilin, and lingual lipase, which is helpful in fat digestion. Enteral feeds stimulate postnatal development of the gastrointestinal (GI) tract, including the secretion of specific hormones. The surge in vasopressin levels during labor and after delivery, together with motilin release after feedings, is thought to contribute to increased motility leading to stooling (Van Woudenberg, Wills, & Rubarth, 2012).

Renal Fetal-to-Neonatal Adaptation

Fetal urine production begins between 9 and 10 weeks and tubular reabsorption starts around 12 to 14 weeks gestation. Fetal-fluid homeostasis is maintained by maternal and placental exchange. With the removal of the placenta, the neonate's kidneys must take over the role of fluid and electrolyte balance and removal of body waste products. Although the cardiorespiratory changes are rapid and immediate, the renal system demonstrates slower adaptation to extrauterine life (Botwinski & Falco, 2014). With the increase in systemic vascular resistance, there is an increase in renal blood flow as well as an increase in angiotensin II and renin. The renal vascular resistance begins to fall and there is an increase in glomerular filtration rate (GFR). The GFR increases with advancing gestational age during pregnancy (Blackburn, 2013). Fluid shifts from the intravascular compartment to the interstitium as a result of catecholamine release prior to labor, increased atrial natriuretic factor, and the changes in acid–base levels during labor. The excess fluid in the interstitium is absorbed and excreted, which is reflected in the weight loss normally seen in the first few days of life. This normal diuresis and weight loss may not be seen in the small-for-gestational-age infant. The increase in arginine vasopressin and the increased activity of the renin–angiotensin system of the kidneys affect the ability of neonates to concentrate their urine (Botwinski & Falco, 2014). If the neonate's kidneys cannot concentrate the urine appropriately, electrolyte imbalances will occur. Hypernatremia, hyperglycemia, and hyperkalemia can result as there is a large amount of dilute urine loss. Diuresis and increased insensible water losses place the neonate at risk for hypernatremia and hyperkalemia, whereas fluid overload results in the opposite, hyponatremia and hypokalemia.

Hepatic Fetal-to-Neonatal Adaptation

As the fetus gets closer to term gestation, more blood is diverted to the liver, allowing the liver to begin the role of excretory and detoxification properties at birth (Blackburn, 2013). As gestation increases, glycogen stores increase. Catecholamine release during labor prepares the glycogen to be used in energy production and growth as discussed previously.

HEMATOLOGIC FETAL-TO-NEONATAL ADAPTATION

With increasing gestational age, white blood cell production increases. Stress related to labor and delivery increases white blood cell production even further. Red blood cell volume is determined by the timing of cord clamping; if cord clamping is delayed, a larger amount of placental blood is transferred to the neonate causing increased systolic blood pressure. Increased systolic blood pressure improves renal perfusion as discussed previously. Because of increased PaO_2 levels and the higher concentration of red blood cells, erythropoietin levels will fall. Fetal Hgb, which has an affinity for carrying oxygen, is replaced by adult Hgb over the next few months (Blackburn, 2013). Neonates may appear pale because of blood loss prior to or at the time of delivery. Neonates with high hematocrit levels may appear ruddy and during crying, may appear dusky.

NEUROLOGICAL FETAL-TO-NEONATAL ADAPTATION

In utero, the infant has a warm, dark, wet environment in a confined space within the uterine walls. After delivery, the infant's neurological system must adapt to the cold, bright, dry environment that has no barriers. This is more difficult in the preterm neonate, as the nervous system, including autonomic regulation, sensory perception, motor regulation, and state organization, is not as mature (Van Woudenberg et al., 2012).

SUCCESSFUL FETAL-TO-NEONATAL ADAPTATION

One measure of adequate fetal-to-neonatal transition is an increase in heart rate (HR) after birth as a result of parasympathetic responses. Neonates who are not transitioning well will have a HR of less than 100 beats per minute (bpm). Neonates in secondary apnea, type of maternal anesthesia, mode of delivery, and gestational age are some of the factors that may affect the changes in HR at birth (Baik et al., 2014). Blood pressure is an important indicator of appropriate circulation and can be affected immediately after birth by mode of delivery, gestational age, perinatal asphyxia, maternal antihypertensive therapy, and certain anesthetic agents administered just prior to birth. Recognizing factors that can help or lead to delayed/ unsuccessful transition is imperative for the neonatal nurse practitioner in order to prevent or minimize the potential complications that may occur (Table 3.3). Infants with perinatal, intrapartum, or postpartum factors that hinder transition will require vigilant monitoring for complications and management to establish normal gas exchange as well as circulatory and metabolic functions.

The factors that may facilitate normal newborn transition are as follows:

1. *Avoid induction of labor unless medically necessary.* Waiting for spontaneous labor to occur allows the complex interaction of hormonal processes to begin. Spontaneous labor in term infants typically occurs when lung function has matured, fetal lung fluid absorption has started, and adequate surfactant production is present (Graves & Haley, 2013).

2. *Delay cord clamping or milking the umbilical cord.* The most recent definition of *early versus delayed cord clamping* is early cord clamping (ECC) occurs within 15 seconds after delivery, whereas delayed clamping occurs at 1 minute or later (Raju, 2013). With ECC, the umbilical vein and arteries are blocked simultaneously. If the neonate does not have adequate ventilation present at delivery, ECC increases left ventricular afterload and terminates oxygenated blood from the placenta to the neonatal

Table 3.3 **Factors Affecting Transition**

Factors That May Facilitate Transition	Factors That May Delay/Hinder Transition
Avoiding induction of labor	Elective C-section
Delayed cord clamping or umbilical cord milking	Maternal analgesic/anesthetics, magnesium therapy
Skin-to-skin contact	Acute perinatal events
Antenatal steroids if anticipated preterm delivery	Maternal conditions
	Fetal growth restriction
	Prolonged resuscitation and hypothermia
	Early cord clamping
	Neonatal conditions
	Prematurity
	Congenital heart defects

C-section, cesarean section.

circulation, resulting in decreased left ventricular output. In this circumstance, the infant may present with shock and hypoperfusion, requiring fluid volume administration (Boere et al., 2014; Kim & Warren, 2015). The neonate with a tight nuchal cord that appears compromised at delivery can benefit from delayed cord clamping (DCC). During labor and delivery of the infant with a tight nuchal cord, there is intermittent occlusion of the thin-walled vein leading to decreased oxygenated blood flow from the placenta to the fetus, however, the thicker walled arteries typically are more patent, resulting in continued flow from the neonate to the placenta. In this circumstance if the cord is clamped early, the neonate will present with a reduced amount of circulating blood volume, thereby promoting the development of shock (Raju, 2013). With DCC, the thin-walled umbilical vein remains open after delivery, allowing blood to flow from the placenta to the baby until the cord is clamped or the placental blood flow stops. Recent evidence demonstrates expansion of the blood volume by 20 to 30 mL/kg with DCC. There are several factors that affect the volume of this placental transfusion, including the timing of cord clamping, position of neonate after delivery, uterine contractions, and onset of respirations. It is believed that this expansion of the blood volume may facilitate cardiopulmonary transition in addition to providing additional red cell volume and a large number of hematopoietic stem cells (Kim & Warren, 2015). In the preterm population, hemodynamic stability reflected by a trend toward higher mean arterial blood pressures at birth and at 4 hours of age resulted in less inotropic support after delivery. This hemodynamic stability may reduce fluctuations in cerebral blood flow and decrease intraventricular hemorrhage (Raba, Diaz-Rossella, Dooley, & Deswell, 2012). There are other concerns outside of the extrauterine transition period that do need to be weighed against these potential benefits such as polycythemia and hyperbilirubinemia in both the preterm and term populations. If DCC is not possible, an alternative method is umbilical cord milking, which is defined as milking 20 cm of the umbilical cord two to three times with the infant at or below the level of the placenta at a rate of 20 cm per seconds (Hosono et al., 2008).

3. *Promote skin-to-skin contact.* The most immediate benefit of skin-to-skin contact is thermoregulation. Other evidence has demonstrated less crying, more stable blood sugars, improved behavior organization, and higher rates of breastfeeding (Graves & Haley, 2013).

4. *Administer antenatal corticosteroids when preterm delivery is anticipated.* Based on fetal sheep studies, corticosteroids stimulate production of surfactant as well as increase pulmonary blood flow. Heart function is improved, blood pressure increases, cardiac output and left ventricular contractility increases, thereby demonstrating the benefits of corticosteroids in cardiorespiratory transition (Blackburn, 2013).

Following are the factors that may delay or lead to unsuccessful transition:

1. *Elective cesarean (C)-section.* Incomplete or slow reabsorption of lung fluid can cause delays in transition from a respiratory standpoint. In the hours prior to initiation of labor, there is decreased fetal lung fluid secretion; in those cases in which labor has not occurred, such as routine scheduled C-sections, whether repeat or for maternal or fetal conditions, this process does not occur. When delivery occurs without labor at term, the postnatal rise in cortisol is blunted, and the catecholamine release is depressed. With the onset of labor, adrenaline production is stimulated in the fetus and thyrotropin-releasing hormone production is stimulated in the mother, leading to the beginning of fetal lung fluid reabsorption. Delivery in the absence of labor has a higher association of retained fetal lung fluid, surfactant deficiency, and pulmonary hypertension (Jain & Dudell, 2006).

2. *Maternal pharmacologic factors.* Maternal anesthetics and/or analgesics or maternal magnesium therapy may result in the neonate having decreased, inefficient, or absent respiratory effort, which can delay the initiation of spontaneous respiratory effort.

3. *Acute perinatal conditions.* Acute perinatal events (placental abruption, uterine rupture, prolapsed cord, maternal cardiac arrest) lead to ischemia (impaired perfusion and oxygenation) and asphyxia (hypoxemia and hypercarbia). Severe hypoxemia leads to anaerobic metabolism and lactic acidosis and metabolic acidosis occurs. Oxygen deprivation in utero results initially in rapid breathing by the fetus and, if

this in not successful in reversing the asphyxia, primary apnea occurs. Gasping follows this period of primary apnea and, if the gasping is ineffective and the hypoxia continues, secondary apnea occurs. Infants delivered in secondary apnea do not respond to stimulation and will require resuscitation in the delivery room to initiate respirations (Kattwinkel, 2011). Red flags seen during the perinatal period that may potentially anticipate the infant presenting in secondary apnea include nonreassuring fetal heart tracing (lack of variability, late decelerations), history of an acute event as listed previously, abnormal Doppler flow studies, decreased fetal movements, or meconium-stained fluid. As the PaO_2 drops in utero, chemoreceptors are stimulated causing a release of catecholamines, a fall in the HR, and decreased myocardial conduction (Verklan, 2002). The same response can be seen with umbilical cord compression. Periodic compression of the cord occurs with uterine contractions, leading to stimulation of the chemoreceptors and parasympathetic nervous system stimulation depending on the degree of fetal hypoxia and changes in blood pressure that occur during this time (Verklan, 2002). Both hypoxia and acidosis affect the reactivity of the pulmonary vascular bed and influence the magnitude and direction of blood flow through fetal channels during the transitional period after birth. In the presence of hypoxia and/or acidosis, there is pulmonary arteriolar vasoconstriction, pulmonary hypertension, and decreased pulmonary blood flow. Under these conditions, there is decreased pulmonary venous return to the left atrium leading to decreased left atrial pressure and right-to-left shunting through the foramen ovale and ductus arteriosus persists. There may also be myocardial dysfunction with transient tricuspid insufficiency as a result of perinatal asphyxia, which can also impair the expected transitional changes (Sinha & Donn, 2006). Hypoxic infants may need to rely on anaerobic glycolysis, which is very inefficient and provides energy for only a short period of time. Elevated lactate levels and metabolic acidosis suggest anaerobic glycolysis; therefore, you want to screen these neonates for hypoglycemia.

4. *Maternal conditions.* Maternal conditions, such as pregnancy-induced hypertension, diabetes, oxytocin administration resulting in hyperstimulation of the uterus, and epidural anesthesia, may all lead to uteroplacental insufficiency resulting in impaired blood flow to the fetus (Blackburn, 2013). Infants of diabetic mothers (IDMs) may have cardiomyopathy or other congenital heart defects (CHD) that may alter cardiac transition (Hines, 2013). In addition, IDMs may have surfactant deficiency, which affects the respiratory transition. Finally, IDMs are at risk for hypoglycemia and hypocalcemia that may alter the normal metabolic/endocrine adaptations.

5. *Fetal growth restriction.* Fetal growth restriction that occurs prior to 34 weeks gestational age demonstrates progressive arterial to venous Doppler abnormalities (absence or reversal of umbilical artery end-diastolic flow and abnormal ductus venosus flow velocity waveforms) as the placental function becomes more impaired and myocardial dysfunction occurs. These ultrasound abnormalities should alert the practitioner to the potential of circulatory transition problems and a higher risk for need for pharmacologic support of their blood pressure (Turan et al., 2013).

6. *Prolonged resuscitation and hypothermia.* Prolonged resuscitation places the infant at risk for hypothermia (core temperature < 97.7°F) as a result of hypoxia and inability to metabolize brown fat. In response to hypothermia, the metabolic rate increases

in an attempt to produce and conserve heat leading to increased oxygen consumption, which puts the infant at risk for hypoxemia. There is also increased glucose utilization leading to depletion of glycogen stores putting the infant at risk for hypoglycemia. Norepinephrine is released in response to cold stress and hypothermia, causing peripheral and pulmonary vasoconstriction, which leads to increased PVR and right-to-left shunting through the ductus arteriosus and/or foramen ovale. If the adrenal gland cannot respond to the increased stress, a functional adrenal insufficiency may occur. In the preterm infant, hypothermia can also impair surfactant production worsening respiratory distress syndrome (Blackburn, 2013).

7. *Early clamping of the umbilical cord.* Immediate or ECC may impact the transition to neonatal circulation in preterm and infants with in utero impairment of circulation regardless of the cause. It is theorized that continued flow in the umbilical vessels after delivery by delaying cord clamping may assist these groups of infants as they transition to neonatal circulation (Duley & Batey, 2013).

8. *Neonatal conditions.* Sepsis, congenital diaphragmatic hernia, parenchymal lung disease, or anything that interferes with the normal drop in PVR leads to persistence of the channels (patent foramen ovale [PFO] and patent ductus arteriosus [PDA]), leading to significant mixing and hypoxemia. The right ventricle continues to contribute to a large portion of the cardiac output and the postductal saturations will be significantly lower than the preductal saturations (Hillman et al., 2012).

9. *Prematurity.* The absorptive mechanisms of fetal lung development do not occur until later in gestation, so neonates born prematurely have a limited ability to reabsorb the pulmonary fluid. Preterm infants lack surfactant and have inadequately developed lungs, resulting in difficulties maintaining a normal functional residual capacity to recruit lung volume and alterations in gas exchange. They also have an overly compliant chest wall so they may not be able to consistently or successfully maintain respiratory drive and maintain lung volumes. Finally, because of the immaturity of the respiratory center, an effective respiratory pattern may not be established (Armentrout, 2014; Sinha & Dunn, 2006; Snyder, Walker, & Clark, 2010). In the delivery room, the goal is to support the neonate during adaptation to extrauterine life while minimizing lung injury secondary to ventilation or hyperoxia (Doyle & Bradshaw, 2012). Extremely preterm infants may have a limited ability to increase cardiac output because of a higher resting HR. In addition, shunting through the foramen ovale and the ductus arteriosus may be of higher volume compared to the term infant. Preload, afterload, and contractility are also affected, which may also impact successful circulatory transition (Armentrout, 2014). Preterm infants have minimal glycogen and fat stores placing them at risk for hypoglycemia if carbohydrate sources are not provided either parenterally or enterally. Preterm infants also lack adequate fat and have a higher body surface area placing them at risk for hypothermia (Blackburn, 2013).

10. *CHD.* If the infant has a known diagnosed fetal CHD, alterations in the delivery room and immediate neonatal period need to be considered to promote successful transition. If there is a known large left-to-right shunt, such as truncus arteriosus, it is imperative to not administer 100% oxygen. O_2 causes a significant drop in PVR, stealing essentially all the cardiac output resulting in extremely low diastolic blood pressure, coronary ischemia, and ventricular fibrillation. The neonate with a

known right-to-left shunt (tetralogy of Fallot [TOF], D-transposition of the great arteries [D-TGA], total anomalous pulmonary venous connection [TAPVC]) is able to maintain an adequate cardiac output and adequate oxygen delivery as long as the arterial saturation is not too low and the Hgb remains adequate. In the initial neonatal period, metabolic acidosis and lactic acidosis are signs that O_2 delivery is not adequate and the infant may benefit from volume to increase the cardiac output, packed red blood cell transfusion to increase oxygen-carrying capacity, or a balloon atrial septostomy to increase mixing of the blood (Blackburn, 2013; Hines, 2013).

CLINICAL FINDINGS RELATED TO NORMAL AND ABNORMAL NEONATAL ADAPTATION

The term neonate who starts immediate transitional adaptation will have good tone, good respiratory effort, with a strong cry demonstrating their adaptive response to being born. Transition from intrauterine to extrauterine life occurs mainly in the first few hours after life but in the extremely preterm infant may occur over a longer period of time. Most neonates tolerate this adaptation to extrauterine life but those who do not have altered transition evidenced by respiratory distress, tachypnea, poor perfusion with cyanosis or pallor, need for supplemental oxygen, or, in extreme cases, development of persistent pulmonary hypertension of the newborn (PPHN), hypothermia, and/or hypoglycemia. Prompt recognition of the neonate who has been compromised by previous stress or postdelivery problems that may alter transition to extrauterine life is imperative to allow prompt interventions to decrease mortality and morbidity.

Immediately after delivery, the neonate will have rales or rhonchi upon auscultation until the fetal lung fluid is reabsorbed by the vascular and lymphatic systems. Initially, the neonate will have a shallow, rapid, irregular breathing pattern until the lungs are able to fully expand and fluid is absorbed. Transient grunting, mild retractions, and nasal flaring may be noted right after delivery especially in the presence of no labor or rapid delivery. Tachycardia related to catecholamine release during labor and delivery is common in the immediate delivery period and progressively decreases over the first hour of life. Blood pressure is typically mildly lower in the first few hours of life and, as the fluid shifts into and out of the vascular space, it increases. The appearance of a line of demarcation at the diaphragm is caused by the ductal shunting of blood with mixing of blood as it flows into the descending aorta. A transient murmur is commonly related to ductal closing (Van Woudenberg et al., 2012) (see Table 3.4).

MANAGEMENT TO PREVENT OR TREAT ABNORMAL EXTRAUTERINE TRANSITION

If abnormal transition is noted immediately following delivery, the first step is to follow neonatal resuscitation as outlined in the sixth edition of the *Neonatal Resuscitation Textbook* (Kattwinkel, 2011). In the preterm infant, providing continuous positive airway pressure (CPAP) to maintain lung volumes and early administration of surfactant may help in respiratory transition (Snyder et al., 2010). Following a "golden hour" protocol for preterm infants to decrease long-term sequelae associated with complications of premature delivery is also important. This golden hour starts at the time of birth and ends in the neonatal intensive care unit (NICU). The golden hour focuses on resuscitation, thermoregulation, rapid management of presumed sepsis, prompt protein administration, and IV glucose administration

Table 3.4 Clinical Findings During Transition

Organ System	Findings During Transition
Cardiorespiratory	Shallow, irregular respiratory pattern Rales or rhonchi Tachypnea Transient grunting, mild retracting, nasal flaring may be present Transient murmur Transient tachycardia Perfusion and color changes, acrocyanosis Blood pressure may be at lower end of normal initially
Endocrine	Blood glucose level reaches nadir by 1–2 hours of age but may be sooner in the at risk neonate
Integumentary	Temperature decreases Decreasing vernix with increasing gestational age
Gastrointestinal	Emesis due to delayed gastric emptying and motility Bowel sounds audible May pass meconium
Renal	Increased urine output by 24 hours of age
Hepatic	Jittery if hypoglycemic
Hematologic	Increased white blood cell count Decreased erythropoietin levels Pallor or ruddiness may be abnormalities noted based on hemoglobin/hematocrit
Neurologic	State regulation Increased activity

to prevent hypoglycemia, including insertion of umbilical lines if warranted and admission in the NICU completed by 60 minutes of age (Bissinger & Annibale, 2010; Castrodale & Rinehart, 2014; Doyle & Bradshaw, 2012). A differential diagnosis list should be developed if the infant is displaying potential signs of maladaptation, for example, tachypnea. This should guide your diagnostic workup and management.

Case 3.1

Baby A is a 36-week-gestation White male infant born to a 36-year-old gravida 1, para 0 (G1P0) mother who is B+ with unknown group B *Streptococcus* (GBS) status but otherwise has negative serologies. She was admitted to labor and delivery for further evaluation of chronic hypertension now complicated by preeclampsia. Pregnancy was also remarkable for gestational diabetes that was insulin controlled. Based on maternal labs indicating HELLP (hemolysis, elevated liver enzymes, and low platelet) syndrome, the infant was delivered by emergent primary C-section under epidural anesthesia. At time of delivery, there was artificial rupture of membranes for clear fluid. The infant was delivered in a vertex presentation. There was a spontaneous cry at delivery and the infant developed increasing work of breathing evidenced by grunting, retracting, and nasal flaring within the first few minutes after delivery.

1. *What would you include in your differential diagnoses? Why?*

   ANSWERS: A. Respiratory distress syndrome (RDS)

   B. Transient tachypnea of the newborn (TTN)

   Sepsis resulting from unknown GBS status would not be included on the differential diagnosis list as the C-section was done for maternal indications with intact membranes and no labor.

2. *What are your immediate management plans?*

   ANSWERS: A. Obtain an arterial blood gas (ABG) test and chest x-ray (CXR), support the respiratory status (high-flow nasal cannula [HFNC] or CPAP), provide oxygen as needed to maintain infant within ordered oxygen saturation parameters, consider surfactant based on ordered diagnostic testing findings and clinical course.

   B. Maintain nothing orally (NPO) due to increased work of breathing, provide intravenous fluid (IVF) at 60 to 80 mL/kg/d, and monitor blood sugars because of risk for hypoglycemia.

3. *Is this infant at risk for maladaptation during the transition period? Why (be specific for identified perinatal risk factors and support your response with the associated physiology)?*

   ANSWER: Yes

   1. *Late preterm infant, gestational diabetes, and C-section with no labor can all lead to surfactant deficiency (Jain & Dudell, 2006); inability to decrease pulmonary vascular resistance, to maintain an adequate tidal volume, or to secrete alveolar surfactant all result in alterations in postnatal pulmonary gas exchange (Keene et al., 2012).*

   2. *C-section with no labor results in incomplete or delayed absorption of fetal lung fluid causing delays in pulmonary transition (Jain & Dudell, 2006).*

   3. *Infants of diabetic mothers (IDMs) are at risk of hypoglycemia and hypocalcemia that may alter normal metabolic and endocrine adaptations (Hines, 2013).*

Case 3.2

Baby B is a 39-week-gestation Black female born to a 28-year-old gravida 2, para 1 (G2P1) mother who is A+ with negative serologies, including being group B *Streptococcus* (GBS) negative. Pregnancy was unremarkable. Mother presented to labor and delivery (L&D) unit with spontaneous rupture of membranes (SROM) approximately 2 hours ago for clear fluid and early stages of labor. Labor was augmented with Pitocin. Fetal heart rate (HR) tracing demonstrated deep late decelerations and vaginal delivery was assisted by vacuum extraction. Delivery was remarkable for a tight nuchal cord that required clamping and cutting prior to delivery of the infant and mild shoulder dystocia with delay of 1 minute 20 seconds in delivering the infant. The infant was floppy with no spontaneous respiratory effort and HR of 70 bpm. The infant was dried with wet linen removed and positive pressure ventilation (PPV) was initiated by a T-piece resuscitator with slow improvement in the HR to 120 bpm. Spontaneous respiratory effort was noted approximately 1 minute later at which time PPV was discontinued and continuous positive airway pressure (CPAP) +6 was maintained for increased work of breathing. Assigned Apgar scores were 1, 5, and 7 at 1, 5, and 10 minutes of age. The infant was pale with a capillary refill time of 4 seconds. Tone remained slightly decreased but improved with decreased activity.

1. *What would you include in your differential diagnoses?*

   ANSWERS: A. Transient tachypnea of the newborn (TTN)

   B. Rule out pneumothorax

   C. Hypovolemia

   D. Metabolic acidosis

   E. Rule out subgaleal hemorrhage

2. *What are your immediate management plans?*

   ANSWERS: A. Arterial blood gas (ABG) test, chest x-ray, continue CPAP (intubation/mechanical ventilation if hypercarbia and respiratory acidosis), provide oxygen as needed to maintain infant within ordered oxygen saturation parameters, wean respiratory support as able, if pneumothorax is present evaluate need for needle thoracentesis versus chest tube versus clinical monitoring.

   B. Nothing orally (because of increased work of breathing/CPAP support), intravenous fluid at 60 to 80 mL/kg/d, and monitor blood sugars (at risk for hypoglycemia because of need for resuscitation).

   C. If metabolic acidosis on ABG or prolonged capillary refill time with tachycardia, give 10 mL/kg normal saline bolus, repeat once as needed based on response.

   D. Monitor for signs/symptoms of subgaleal hemorrhage secondary to vacuum application.

(continued)

Case 3.2 (continued)

3. Is this infant at risk for maladaptation during the transition period? Why (be specific for identified perinatal risk factors and support your response with the associated physiology)?

ANSWER: Yes

1. *Tight nuchal cord leads to intermittent occlusion of the umbilical vein and decreased oxygenated blood flow to the fetus; as this occlusion continues, fetal compromise develops as evidenced by deep late decelerations and need for resuscitation at delivery. Fetal lung fluid absorption is impaired and the infant is at risk for postnatal pulmonary maladaptation (Henry, Andres, & Christensen, 2013; Narang et al., 2014).*

2. *Significant hypoxemia and decreased placental blood flow in utero result in hypoxia leading to anaerobic metabolism. Lactic acidosis and metabolic acidosis ensue and secondary apnea develops. Hypoxia and acidosis impair pulmonary vascular bed reactivity and can impair postnatal cardiovascular adaptation. Anaerobic metabolism with elevated lactate levels and metabolic acidosis as well as hypothermia from prolonged resuscitation can lead to hypoglycemia as a result of depleted glycogen stores, affecting metabolic postnatal adaptation (Turan et al., 2013; Verklan, 2002).*

3. *Status at delivery led to early cord clamping (ECC). Tight nuchal cord results in fetal compromise and studies have supported delayed cord clamping to assist in postnatal adaptation. With ECC, this proposed benefit is lost and may alter or delay successful transition (Duley & Batey, 2013).*

Case 3.3

Baby C is a 40.2-week-gestation White female born to a 32-year-old gravida 5, para 4 (G5P4) mother who is O+ with a negative antibody screen. Her serologies were negative with the exception of positive group B *Streptococcus* (GBS). Her pregnancy was remarkable for closely spaced pregnancies and rapid deliveries. She presented to labor and delivery in early labor but rapidly progressed to complete dilation within 2 hours, receiving only one dose of penicillin 30 minutes prior to delivery. There was spontaneous rupture of membranes (SROM) 10 minutes prior to delivery for clear fluid. The infant delivered in a vertex presentation vaginally with no maternal anesthesia. The umbilical cord was short, therefore the infant could not be placed on the mother's chest for delayed cord clamping. Skin-to-skin contact was provided with the infant having copious oral secretions cleared by bulb syringe. The physical exam at 45 minutes of age after attempts at

(continued)

Case 3.3 **(continued)**

breastfeeding were unsuccessful was remarkable for significant facial bruising and a respiratory rate of 84 with no grunting or retracting.

1. *What would you include in your differential diagnoses?*

   ANSWERS: A. TTN

   B. Rule out sepsis/pneumonia

2. *What are your immediate management plans?*

   ANSWERS: A. Monitor respiratory status closely; if increased work of breathing or worsening tachypnea, obtain chest x-ray and arterial blood gas test.

   B. Obtain complete blood count (CBC) and blood culture. If CBC is reassuring and there is no increased work of breathing, monitor clinically (inadequate intrapartum antibiotic prophylaxis, however, short labor and no prolonged rupture of membranes).

   C. Breastfeed ad lib on demand if respiratory status allows, monitor blood sugars as per protocol, consider intravenous fluid of D10 at 60 to 80 mL/kg/d if persistent tachypnea is greater than 80 or poor oral feeding exists.

3. *Is this infant at risk for maladaptation during the transition period? Why (be specific for identified perinatal risk factors and support your response with the associated physiology)?*

   ANSWER: Yes

   1. *With the initiation of labor, the postnatal rise in cortisol and release of catecholamines occurs. With rapid labor, the hormonal influences may not have had a chance to fully occur delaying the secretion of chloride and the absorption of sodium and fluid into the interstitium. If alveolar spaces are not cleared of excess fluid, and pulmonary blood flow does not increase, postnatal pulmonary adaptation may be delayed (Jain & Dudell, 2006; Jain & Eaton, 2006; Keene et al., 2012).*

   2. *If the infant has GBS sepsis or pneumonia, this can interfere with the normal drop in pulmonary vascular resistance and continued patency of the patent ductus arteriosus and patent foramen ovale, resulting in potential delay in circulatory adaptation (Hillman et al., 2012).*

   3. *The provision of skin-to-skin contact has been shown to facilitate neonatal adaptation (Graves & Haley, 2013). This infant did not demonstrate fetal compromise, so early cord clamping secondary to short umbilical cord may not have offered beneficial effects.*

Case 3.4

Baby D is a 38.1-week-gestation Black male born by emergency C-section to an 18-year-old gravida 1, para 0 (G1P0) mother who is AB+. Her serologies were negative, including a group B *Streptococcus* (GBS) status. She has had multiple positive urine drug screens for cocaine and marijuana. On admission to the labor and delivery unit, she reported severe abdominal pain and the fetal heart tones were noted to be in the 60s. An emergent C-section under general anesthesia was done for suspected placental abruption. Artificial rupture of membranes (AROM) at delivery demonstrated grossly bloody fluid with clots. The infant was floppy with no spontaneous respiratory effort and heart rate (HR) of 50 bpm.

1. *What would you include in your differential diagnoses?*

   ANSWERS: A. Rule out hypoxic ischemic encephalopathy

   B. Hypovolemia/acute anemia

2. *What are your immediate management plans?*

   ANSWERS: A. Follow *Neonatal Resuscitation Provider* (NRP) guidelines to include positive pressure ventilation (PPV) and, if after 30 seconds of effective ventilation, HR remains less than 60 bpm, begin chest compressions—call for neonatologist backup and prepare for intubation and emergency umbilical venous catheter (UVC) placement. Response to PPV and/or chest compressions will guide remainder of resuscitation.

   B. Provide respiratory support based on response to ventilation. If infant only required PPV and is now vigorous, he will still need to be monitored for potential complications of resuscitation.

   C. Bag for urine drug screen.

3. *Is this infant at risk for maladaptation during the transition period? Why (be specific for identified perinatal risk factors and support your response with the associated physiology)?*

   ANSWER: Yes

   1. *C-section with no labor results in incomplete or delayed absorption of fetal lung fluid causing delays in pulmonary transition (Jain & Dudell, 2006).*

   2. *Placental abruption leads to ischemia and asphyxia. Severe hypoxemia leads to anaerobic metabolism. Lactic acidosis and metabolic acidosis ensue, with secondary apnea developing as evidenced by extended fetal bradycardia. Hypoxia and acidosis impair pulmonary vascular bed reactivity and can impair postnatal cardiovascular adaptation. Anaerobic metabolism with elevated lactate levels and metabolic acidosis as well as hypothermia from prolonged resuscitation can lead to hypoglycemia as a result of depleted glycogen stores affecting metabolic postnatal adaptation (Turan et al., 2013; Verklan, 2002).*

(continued)

Case 3.4 (continued)

3. *Maternal general anesthesia may result in decreased, shallow, or completely absent respiratory effort delaying the initiation of spontaneous respiratory effort. High negative pressures are required with spontaneous first breaths; when the infant is apneic and PPV is required, this high negative pressure may not be achieved leading to delays in postnatal respiratory adaptation (Sinha & Donn, 2006).*

REFERENCES

Armentrout, D. (2014). Not ready for prime time: Transitional events in the extremely preterm infant. *Journal of Perinatal & Neonatal Nursing, 28*(2), 144–149.

Baik, N., Urlesberger, B., Schwaberger, B., Freidl, T., Schmolzer, G., & Pichler, G. (2014). Cardiocirculatory monitoring during immediate fetal-to-neonatal transition: A systematic qualitative review of the literature. *Neonatology, 107,* 100–107. doi:10.1159/000368042

Bissinger, R., & Annibale, D. (2010). Thermoregulation in very low-birth-weight infants during the golden hour: Results and implications. *Advances in Neonatal Care, 10*(5), 230–238. doi:10.1097/ANC.0b013e3181f0ae63

Blackburn, S. (2013). *Maternal, fetal & neonatal physiology: A clinical perspective* (4th ed.). Maryland Heights, MO: Elsevier Saunders.

Boere, I., Roest, A., Wallace, E., ten Harkel, A., Kaack, M., Morley, C., . . . Te Pas, A. B. (2014). Umbilical blood flow patterns directly after birth before delayed cord clamping. *Archive of Disease in Childhood—Fetal and Neonatal Edition, 0,* F1–F5. doi:10.1136/archdischild-2014-307144

Botwinski, C., & Falco, G. (2104). Transition to postnatal renal function. *Journal of Perinatal & Neonatal Nursing, 28*(2), 150–154.

Britton, J. (1998). The transition to extrauterine life and disorders of transition. *Clinics in Perinatology, 25*(2), 271–285.

Castrodale, V., & Rinehart, S. (2014). The golden hour: Improving the stabilization of the very low birth-weight infant. *Advances in Neonatal Care, 14*(1), 9–14.

Doyle, K., & Bradshaw, W. (2012). Sixty golden minutes. *Neonatal Network, 31*(5), 289–294. doi:10.1891/0730-0832.31.5.289

Duley, L., & Batey, N. (2013). Optimal timing of umbilical cord clamping for term and preterm babies. *Early Human Development, 89,* 905–908. doi:10.1016/j.earlhumdev.2013.09.002

Graves, B., & Haley, M. (2013). Original review: Newborn transition. *Journal of Midwifery & Women's Health, 58,* 662–670. doi:10.1111/jmwh.12097

Heck, L., & Erenberg, A. (1987). Serum glucose levels in term neonates during the first 48 hours of life. *Journal of Pediatrics, 110*(1), 119–122.

Henry, E., Andres, R., & Christensen, R. (2013). Neonatal outcomes following a tight nuchal cord. *Journal of Perinatology, 33,* 231–234.

Hillman, N., Kallapur, S., & Jobe, A. (2012). Physiology of transition from intrauterine to extrauterine life. *Clinics in Perinatology, 39*(4), 769–783. doi:10.1016.j.clp.2012.09.009

Hines, M. (2013). Neonatal cardiovascular physiology. *Seminars in Pediatric Surgery, 22,* 174–178.

Hosono, S., Mugishima, H., Fujita, H., Hosono, A., Minato, M., Okada, T., . . . Harada, K. (2008). Umbilical cord milking reduces the need for red cell transfusions and improves neonatal adaptation in infants born at less than 29 weeks' gestation: A randomized controlled trial. *Archives of Disease in Childhood—Fetal and Neonatal Edition, 93*(1), F14–F19.

Jain, L., & Dudell, G. (2006). Respiratory transition in infants delivered by cesarean section. *Seminars in Perinatology, 30,* 296–304.

Jain, L., & Eaton, D. (2006). Physiology of fetal lung fluid and clearance and the effect of labor. *Seminars in Perinatology, 30,* 34–43.

Kalhan, S., & Devaskar, S. (2011). Metabolic and endocrine disorders: Part 1—Disorders of carbohydrate metabolism. In R. J. Martin, A. Fanaroff, & M. C. Wash (Eds.), *Fanaroff and Martin's neonatal-perinatal medicine: Diseases of the fetus and infant* (9th ed., pp. 1497–1522). St. Louis, MO: Mosby.

Kattwinkel, J. (Ed.). (2011). *Neonatal Resuscitation Provider (NRP) Neonatal resuscitation textbook* (6th ed.). Elk Grove Village, IL: American Academy of Pediatrics and American Heart Association.

Keene, S., Bland, R., & Jain, L. (2012). Lung fluid balance in developing lungs and its role in neonatal transition. In Oh, W., Guinard J.-P, & Baumgart, S. (Eds.), *Nephrology and fluid/electrolyte physiology: Neonatology questions and controversies* (2nd ed., pp. 221–232). Philadelphia, PA: Elsevier Saunders.

Kim, A., & Warren, J. (2015). Optimal timing of umbilical cord clamping: Is the debate settled? Part 1 of 2: History, rationale, influencing factors, and concerns. *NeoReviews, 16*(5), e263–e269.

Mercer, J., & Erickson, D. (2012). Rethinking placental transfusion and cord clamping issues. *Journal of Perinatal & Neonatal Nursing, 26*(3), 202–217.

Moore, K., Persaud, T., & Torchia, M. (2013). Cardiovascular system. In *The developing human: Clinically oriented embryology* (9th ed., pp. 289–342). Philadelphia, PA: Elsevier Saunders.

Narang, Y., Baid, N., Jain, S., Suneja, A., Guleria, K., Faridi, M., & Gupta, B. (2014). Is nuchal cord justified as a cause of obstetrician anxiety? *Archives of Gynecology & Obstetrics, 289,* 795–801.

Raba, H., Diaz-Rosella, J., Dooley, L., & Deswell, T. (2012). Effect of timing of umbilical cord clamping and other strategies to influence placental transfusion at preterm birth on maternal and infant outcomes. *Cochrane Database of Systematic Reviews, 8*(8), CD003248.

Raju, T. (2013). Timing of umbilical cord clamping after birth for optimizing placental transfusion. *Current Opinions in Pediatrics, 25*(2), 180–187.

Sinha, S., & Donn, S. (2006). Fetal-to-neonatal maladaptation. *Seminars in Fetal & Neonatal Medicine, 11,* 166–173. doi:10.1016/j.siny.2006.01.008

Snyder, T., Walker, W., & Clark, R. (2010). Establishing gas exchange and improving oxygenation in the delivery room management of the lung. *Advanced in Neonatal Care, 10*(5), 256–260. doi:10.1097/ANC.0b013e3181f0836d

Turan, S., Turan, O., Salim, M., Berg, C., Gembruch, U., Harman, C., & Baschat, A. (2013). Cardiovascular transition to extrauterine life in growth-restricted neonates: Relationship with prenatal Doppler findings. *Fetal Diagnosis and Therapy, 33,* 103–109. doi:10.1159/000345092

Van Woudenberg, C., Wills, C., & Rubarth, L. (2012). Newborn transition to extrauterine life. *Neonatal Network, 31*(5), 317–322.

Verklan, M. (2002). Physiologic variability during transition to extrauterine life. *Critical Care Research, 24*(4), 41–56.

Assessing Growth Parameters in the Newborn: Identifying Abnormal Findings

Leanne M. Nantais-Smith and Carolyn J. Herrington

Chapter Objectives

1. Describe normal and abnormal intrauterine (IU) growth patterns
2. Identify implications of abnormal IU growth on fetal well-being
3. Assess fetal growth patterns using the information provided in the case studies
4. Determine the effects of maternal and genetic factors on fetal growth
5. Apply knowledge related to IU environment and risk factors for small for gestational age (SGA), average for gestational age (AGA), and large for gestational age (LGA) to corresponding infant outcomes

This chapter focuses on the effects of the prenatal environment on growth and development of the fetus and subsequent neonatal presentation. A broad range of factors has been associated with fetal and neonatal growth and development, including maternal overall health status, pregnancy-specific maternal health issues, genetics, and multiple gestation. It is imperative that the neonatal nurse practitioner (NNP) has an in-depth understanding of these interrelated factors to anticipate the neonatal presentation and formulate appropriate management plans. Knowing what to expect from the SGA infant, or anticipating the problems of the 36-week gestation infant of the diabetic mother, will help the NNP and the health care team anticipate the presenting and potential problems as the neonate begins transition to the extrauterine environment.

Case presentations included in this chapter are designed to assist the student to *integrate* the salient points of the didactic content provided in educational coursework with the maternal history. The student is expected to integrate the information provided in the cases with knowledge gained in didactic courses to develop the differential diagnosis and formulate an appropriate initial plan of care for the infant.

TOPIC CONTENT

NORMAL AND ABNORMAL IU GROWTH PATTERNS AND IMPLICATIONS FOR NEONATAL PRESENTATION

Lubchenco, Hansman, Dressler, and Boyd (1963) published IU fetal weight curve charts based on data extrapolated from the birth weights of 5,635 live-born infants born between 1948 and 1961 in Denver, Colorado. Although the sample included only Caucasian and Spanish American infants whose mothers were predominantly from lower socioeconomic environments, these weight charts have historically provided the foundation for evaluating IU growth patterns. In 1966, length and head-circumference data were added to these weight charts, providing the typical graphs we use in the nursery to determine the growth pattern of neonates (Lubchenco, Hansman, & Boyd, 1966). Although these growth curves have been recalculated from time to time to include other ethnicities, socioeconomic statuses, and geographic areas (Fenton, 2003), these types of charts have remained the gold standard for evaluating IU growth. Currently, individualized growth charts that can be customized based on maternal factors, such as height, weight at first visit, ethnic group, parity, and smoking, are appearing in the literature (Gardosi, Mongelli, Wilcox, & Chang, 1995).

Recognizing alterations in fetal growth as early in pregnancy as possible allows for timely intervention to reduce the severity of the growth alteration if possible, thereby reducing the morbidities that are often seen in the inappropriately grown neonate. Determining whether the neonate is SGA (less than 10th percentile), AGA, or LGA (greater than 90th percentile) alerts the NNP to evaluate the neonate for known comorbidities related to the etiology behind the altered growth pattern.

It is also critical to evaluate weight, length, and head circumference for symmetry when the SGA infant is identified. The symmetrical SGA infant is at greater risk for having congenital viral infections or malformations, including aneuploidies, whereas the infant with asymmetrical SGA is not. Asymmetrical SGA is a consequence of placental insufficiency (Halliday, 2009). The LGA infant of the diabetic mother is at a three- to fourfold greater risk for injury at birth secondary to shoulder dystocia, respiratory distress syndrome (RDS) in the late preterm infant, hypoglycemia, polycythemia, and subsequent hyperbilirubinemia (Schwartz & Teramo, 2000).

In addition to determining whether the infant is SGA, AGA, or LGA, it is critical to determine whether the fetus has experienced intrauterine growth restriction (IUGR). The fetus can experience IUGR and remain within AGA parameters, but still be at risk for significant health problems. IUGR can only be determined from serial fetal measurements that demonstrate a deviation from the fetus's specific previously established growth curve. There are significant comorbidities associated with IUGR, including risk for perinatal acidosis from restricted placental blood flow, hypoglycemia resulting from decreased placental transfer of nutrients, hypothermia caused by decreased subcutaneous fat stores, polycythemia resulting from decreased oxygen delivery at the placental level (Pallotto & Kilbride, 2006).

Case 4.1

Ms. J is a 34-year-old gravida 3, para 2,0,0,2 (G3P2,0,0,2; two term infants, no preterm infants, no pregnancy losses, two living children) woman who presented for a routine prenatal care visit at 24 weeks gestation. Her pregnancy has been complicated by protracted morning sickness. Her pre-pregnancy weight was 125 lb. and she is 5 ft., 5 in. tall. A fetal ultrasound was completed at 20 weeks gestation, which noted that growth parameters were appropriate for the fetus. At 24 weeks, she has gained only 5 lb. Knowing that the expected weight gain by 24 weeks gestation would range from 5 to 8 lb. (IOM, 2009), Ms. J's nurse-midwife advises her that fetal growth is likely adequate.

At her 28-week prenatal visit, Ms. J reports that she is no longer experiencing the morning sickness, but she has only gained an additional pound in the past 4 weeks, for a total 6-lb. weight gain. In addition, her fundal height measurements are now lagging behind the gestational age. A fetal ultrasound is completed that reveals the fetus's estimated weight is 1 kg.

Use the Fenton (2003) growth chart provided here to answer the following questions:

1. *According to the growth chart, at what percentile is this fetus's estimated weight?*

   A. 10th percentile
   B. 30th percentile
   C. 60th percentile

   ANSWER: B.

2. *Which of the following terms characterizes this fetus's weight most appropriately?*

   A. Small for gestational age (SGA)
   B. Average for gestational age (AGA)
   C. Intrauterine growth restriction (IUGR)

   ANSWER: B. *At the 30th percentile, this fetus is AGA for weight. We do not know about the estimated length or head circumference, and thus we can address fetal weight only. To qualify as SGA in weight, the infant would need to weigh less than or equal to approximately 800 g. To apply the term IUGR, we would need to have at least one more estimated fetal weight previous to this weight at 28 weeks, and that weight would need to plot in the greater than 30th percentile to demonstrate a decrease in growth pattern.*

3. *Ms. J's weight gain continued to progressively lag; however, serial nonstress tests and kick counts were reassuring and her nurse-midwife continued to monitor the pregnancy closely. Ms. J went into labor at 38 weeks and delivered Baby J after an uneventful labor. The baby's weight is 2,500 g, head circumference 32.5 cm, and length 46 cm. Plot these measurements on the growth curve that accompanies this case. How would you categorize this infant's growth?*

   A. Asymmetric SGA
   B. Symmetric SGA
   C. Symmetric AGA

(continued)

Case 4.1 (*continued*)

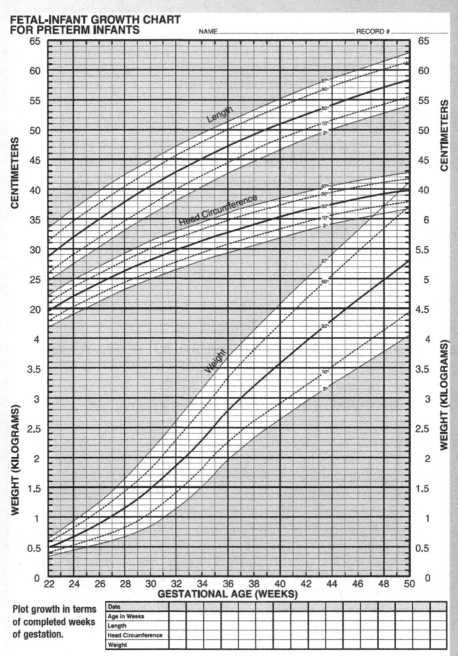

FETAL-INFANT GROWTH CHART FOR PRETERM INFANTS

NAME_____   RECORD #_____

Plot growth in terms of completed weeks of gestation.

Date															
Age in Weeks															
Length															
Head Circumference															
Weight															

(*continued*)

Case 4.1 (continued)

ANSWER: A. *These measurements are consistent with asymmetrical SGA, because two parameters fall below the 10th percentile.*

4. *Based on your classification of Baby J in question 3, which of the following factors is Baby J most at risk for developing in the first few hours of life?*
   A. Hyperglycemia
   B. Hypothermia
   C. Hypoglycemia

ANSWER: C. *Hypoglycemia is the most significant risk factor for this SGA infant because of decreased hepatic glycogen stores, decreased gluconeogenesis, and decreased response of glucose-regulating hormones (Martin, Fanaroff, & Walsh, 2015). If the SGA infant does not have adequate caloric intake in the first hours of life, hypoglycemia will develop quickly. Although the SGA infant is also at risk for hypothermia, and hypothermia can compound the hypoglycemia, avoidance of the development of hypoglycemia is most critical. The SGA infant is not at risk for hyperglycemia at birth, for the same reasons that the SGA is at risk for hypoglycemia.*

5. *Based on your classification of Baby J in question 3, which of the following factors is Baby J most at risk for developing in the first 2 years of life?*
   A. Developmental disabilities related to poor brain growth
   B. Short stature that is likely to normalize in childhood
   C. Baby J would be expected to meet AGA growth curves within the first 2 months of life

ANSWER: B. *Although female infants who are also SGA are at increased risk for remaining short in stature as adults, most SGA infants will catch up in height during childhood. At the 25th percentile, there is adequate brain growth; most infants reach normal AGA growth curves between 6 and 12 months of life (Calkins & Devaskar, 2011; Martin et al., 2015).*

ALTERATIONS IN IU GROWTH PATTERNS AND NEWBORN PRESENTATION SECONDARY TO MATERNAL FACTORS

THE IUGR/SGA INFANT (MATERNAL HYPERTENSION/PREECLAMPSIA)

IU growth is an indicator of fetal well-being and an evaluation of fetal growth as pregnancy progresses and provides insight into the anticipated normal growth and health of the fetus. Maternal well-being has a direct impact on fetal growth by providing nutrient flow via the placenta. Any maternal illness that impacts the quality of nutrient flow can significantly alter fetal growth and lead to immediate and long-term health implications for the neonate (Maulik, 2006b). Careful review of the maternal medical and pregnancy history will provide clues to the timing of the maternal conditions that may have impacted fetal growth during gestation. Any conditions involving altered maternal nutrient supply or adequate placental function will affect nutrient flow. Chronic or pregnancy-induced hypertension and infection, in addition to when these maternal conditions occurred during pregnancy, have different effects on specific growth parameters and thus different risk factors for the neonate.

IUGR alone, whether the infant is AGA or SGA, places the infant at risk for postbirth problems. However, the neonate categorized as SGA has increased risk factors and sequelae as a result of prolonged and significant growth restriction (less than 10th percentile on normal growth curve). Careful physical examination and measurement after birth and plotting of growth parameters (weight, head circumference, and length), with attention to any physical abnormalities that affect reliable measurements, can provide the NNP with valuable information for anticipatory evaluation and management of the neonate.

Case 4.2

Ms. H is a 37-year-old primigravida with no maternal medical risk factors. A 12-week ultrasound showed normal fetal growth. At her 24-week prenatal visit, her blood pressure was 142/92 mmHg and a follow-up 24-hour urine showed 1 + proteinuria and persistent elevated blood pressure. Repeat ultrasound screenings at 28 weeks showed decrease in fetal growth below the normal curve. At 30 weeks gestation, ultrasound screening showed continued decrease in growth and oligohydramnios with a reactive nonstress test. Ms. H presented in the emergency department at 32 weeks gestation in preterm labor with a persistent headache and spots before her eyes. Evaluation by ultrasound showed oligohydramnios and a nonreassuring fetal heart rate pattern. Baby S was delivered by emergent cesarean section, stabilized in the delivery room, and admitted to the neonatal intensive care unit (NICU). Admission statistics included weight 1,250 g, head circumference 31 cm, and length 39 cm.

1. *Based on the maternal medical and pregnancy history, Ms. H had which of the following medical conditions?*

   A. Chronic hypertension
   B. Severe preeclampsia
   C. Eclampsia

   ANSWER: B. *Severe preeclampsia is a type of gestational hypertension that occurs only during pregnancy; onset of elevated blood pressure occurs after 20 weeks gestation. Chronic hypertension is blood pressure elevation that has occurred either prior to pregnancy or before 20 weeks gestation. Eclampsia is a type of gestational hypertension that includes onset of seizures and/or coma (Blackburn, 2013; Verklan & Walden, 2015).*

2. *Maternal preeclampsia affects intrauterine fetal growth by:*

   A. Increasing the diameter of the placental vasculature
   B. Impairing placental blood flow as a result of vasoconstriction
   C. Enhancing normal cytotrophoblast invasion of the uterus

   ANSWER: B. *Elevated blood pressure causes vasoconstriction of the placental vasculature and decreased placental flow, resulting in altered fetal growth. Vascular disorders in general*

(continued)

Case 4.2 (continued)

are associated with abnormal trophoblast invasion; shallow cytotrophoblast invasion has been noted on placental exams of mothers with preeclampsia, which can lead to decreased maternal perfusion of villi and resultant impairment of fetal growth (Blackburn, 2013; Brodsky & Christou, 2004; Maulik, Evans, & Ragolia, 2006).

3. **Two patterns of fetal growth restriction can occur depending on the timing of maternal illness and impairment of growth during gestation. A neonate with asymmetric growth restriction likely had impairment of growth during:**

   A. The third trimester
   B. The first trimester
   C. The second trimester

   ANSWER: A. *Asymmetric growth restriction occurs with impairment during the last trimester. This head-sparing occurs because of fetal adaptation and redistribution of cardiac output to the coronary and carotid arteries (thus enhancing continued growth of the head). Symmetric growth restriction results from problems that occur earlier in pregnancy (first or second trimester) from reduced flow to all organs (i.e., viral infection [cytomegalovirus]; Brodsky & Christou, 2004; Martin et al., 2015).*

4. **Using the Fenton (2003) growth chart in Case 4.1 and the neonatal measurements in this case, the neonatal nurse practitioner determines that Baby S has which of the following diagnosis?**

   A. Symmetric small for gestational age (SGA)
   B. Asymmetric average for gestational age (AGA)
   C. Asymmetric SGA

   ANSWER: C. *Head circumference is AGA but length and weight are SGA; this indicates head sparing. Based on decreasing fetal growth noted at 28 and 30 weeks gestation, this infant is intrauterine growth restriction (IUGR) and is also SGA at birth (Martin et al., 2015; Maulik, 2006a; Verklan & Walden, 2015).*

5. **The SGA infant is at increased risk for:**

   A. Thrombocytosis
   B. Hypercalcemia
   C. Hypoxia and associated sequelae

   ANSWER: C. *The fetus is exposed to a hypoxic IU environment related to placental insufficiency and is at risk for asphyxia and hypoxic insult. The SGA infant is at risk for thrombocytopenia (low platelet production), polycythemia resulting from prolonged IU hypoxia, and hypocalcemia (Blackburn 2013; Martin et al., 2015; Verklan & Walden, 2015).*

6. **The preterm SGA infant has an increased risk for:**

   A. Necrotizing enterocolitis (NEC)
   B. Hyperthermia
   C. Hyperglycemia

(continued)

Case 4.2 (continued)

ANSWER: A. *The preterm SGA infant has an increased risk for NEC because of redistribution of blood flow away from mesenteric circulation with hypoxia. The preterm SGA infant is at increased risk for hypothermia resulting from decreased fat stores and there is an increased risk for hypoglycemia because of decreased glycogen stores and substrate delivery-impaired gluconeogenesis (Martin et al., 2015; Verklan & Walden, 2015).*

ALTERATIONS IN IU GROWTH PATTERNS AND NEONATAL PRESENTATION SECONDARY TO GENETIC/FETAL FACTORS (MULTIPLE GESTATION: DISCORDANT GROWTH)

In addition to maternal and placental risk factors, IU growth can also be affected by genetic and neonatal factors that alter placental flow, nutrient delivery, and IU fetal growth. The multiple-gestation pregnancy is a risk factor for discordant growth and related mortality and morbidities. Although there is some variation in definition, *discordance* has often been defined as a 15% to 25% difference in weight among twins, using the larger of the twins as standard growth (Miller, Chauham, & Abuhamed, 2012). However, current data suggest that a growth difference less than 25% may result from normal variations seen in siblings and that a discordance of greater than 25% is caused by unexpected sibling variation or altered placental blood flow (Martin et al., 2015). Discordance per se places the fetus at risk for IUGR and the comorbidities associated with aberrant growth, in this case, growth restriction.

Several risk factors for discordant growth in the twin pregnancy include monochorionic versus dichorionic twins, placental weight and sharing, vascular anastomoses, and pattern of diastolic blood flow, all with the potential to cause discordant growth and potentially suboptimal growth (Miller et al., 2012). Doppler flow studies are utilized to identify the at-risk IUGR and SGA fetus, distinguishing the "sick" from the "well" IUGR/SGA fetus (Brodsky & Christou, 2004).

Case 4.3

Ms. T is a 35-year-old primigravida with a twin pregnancy diagnosed by ultrasound at 12 weeks. The ultrasound assessment identified monochorionic twins and normal growth of each fetus at the 50th percentile. Routine repeat ultrasound screening at 18 and 22 weeks showed Twin A consistently plotting at the 40th percentile and Twin B plotting consistently at the 45th percentile. At 24 weeks gestation, the ultrasound showed continuing alterations in growth for Twin A, who plotted at the 35th percentile and had a decreased amniotic fluid index. Twin B continued to plot at the 45th percentile. A follow-up biophysical profile (BPP) was 6/10 for Twin A and 8/10 for Twin B.

(continued)

Case 4.3 (continued)

1. *Risk of discordant growth of twins caused by unequal placental sharing or unequally shared placental vessels is:*

   A. Lower in monochorionic twins
   B. Higher in monochorionic twins
   C. Higher in dichorionic twins

   ANSWER: B. *Incidence of uneven placental sharing and unequally shared placental vessels is higher in monochorionic twins and the discordance increases as placental sharing diverges (Blackburn, 2013; Miller et al., 2012).*

2. *Based on the ultrasound and BPP findings at 24 weeks gestation in this case, obstetric management for these twins with identified intrauterine fetal growth restriction would include:*

   A. More intense fetal surveillance, including Doppler flow studies and repeat BPP, to track fetal well-being
   B. Immediate delivery to minimize risk of fetal death
   C. Reevaluation of fetal growth at 32 weeks gestation

   ANSWER: A. *Given the persistent decrease in growth and the borderline BPP, a Doppler flow study can provide important information on placental function and fetal well-being. As long as the BPP is stable and the umbilical artery flow is reassuring, serial evaluation of fetal well-being is appropriate. However, once at the stage of viability and in the presence of decreased placental flow and decreasing amniotic fluid index, fetal evaluation should occur frequently, at least once or twice weekly. Reversed umbilical artery end-diastolic flow warrants immediate delivery (Maulik, 2006c).*

3. *Delivery of the twins in this case occurred at 30 weeks gestation by emergent C-section after Doppler study showed reversed end-diastolic flow. Measurements for Twin A were weight 900 g, head circumference 27 cm, and length 36 cm; measurements for Twin B were weight 1,300 g, head circumference 27.5 cm, and length 39 cm. Based on these findings, the neonatal nurse practitioner determines the following:*

   A. Twins are not discordant; Twin A and Twin B are intrauterine growth restriction (IUGR), but not small for gestational age (SGA)
   B. Twins are discordant; Twin A is SGA, Twin B is SGA
   C. Twins are discordant; Twin A and Twin B were growth restricted, Twin A is SGA, Twin B is average for gestational age (AGA)

   ANSWER: C. *The weight discrepancy between Twin A and Twin B shows a difference greater than 25%; growth curve plotting shows that Twin A is SGA. Although both Twin A and Twin B showed decreasing fetal growth on ultrasound evaluations and are growth retarded, growth restriction in Twin B was not sufficient to result in the diagnosis of SGA (Martin et al., 2015).*

4. *Based on the growth parameters for Twin A and Twin B in this case, what are the risk factors for Twin A and Twin B based on these findings?*

(continued)

Case 4.3 (continued)

A. Only Twin A is at risk for hypoglycemia and hypothermia
B. Twin B is at risk for hypoglycemia, but not hypothermia
C. Both Twin A and Twin B are at risk for hypoglycemia and hypothermia

ANSWER: C. *The IUGR and SGA infants have many of the same risk factors related to growth restriction. Although the SGA infant has had sufficient alteration in growth to plot below the 10th percentile, IUGR alone can result in decreased glycogen stores, decreased delivery of substrate for gluconeogenesis, and decreased fat stores (Martin et al., 2015).*

ALTERATIONS IN IU GROWTH PATTERNS AND NEWBORN PRESENTATION SECONDARY TO MATERNAL FACTORS

THE INFANT OF THE DIABETIC MOTHER

Diabetes is a maternal disease that may also affect fetal growth and development at many levels. The health risks for infants born to mothers with long-standing type 1 and 2 diabetes mellitus (DM) are different from the health risks anticipated for infants born to mothers with gestational diabetes. The duration of maternal disease and the level of glucose control in prepregnancy as well as during the pregnancy itself will all impact fetal outcomes. Understanding the pathology of maternal disease and its effect on the fetus, as well as standards in screening for mother and infant, enables the NNP to anticipate the infant's needs at delivery.

Case 4.4

Ms. K is a 23-year-old primigravida with a history of diabetes mellitus (DM). Initial attempts to manage Ms. K's DM with glyburide during the first trimester were not successful and she was placed on insulin during the 24th week of pregnancy. At that time, ultrasound estimates placed the fetus at the 70th percentile for growth. Ms. K continued to struggle with her glucose management and consistently had elevated fasting blood sugars in the 130 to 140 mg/dL range, despite adjustments in her insulin regimen. At 36 weeks gestation, estimated fetal growth was in the 90th percentile.

1. *Pregestational diabetes carries a high risk for congenital anomalies in the fetus. This risk is related to the level of maternal glucose control. A simple test to estimate average glucose control over a period of 3 months is the hemoglobin A1C test. Hemoglobin A1C levels associated with increased risk for congenital anomalies in infants of diabetic mothers (IDMs) are:*

(continued)

Case 4.4 (*continued*)

A. Hgb A1C 4% to 5.5%
B. Hgb A1C 6% to 7%
C. Hgb A1C 8% to 10%

ANSWER: C. *In nondiabetic individuals, normal Hgb A1C levels are less than 5.7%. Prediabetes is diagnosed with an Hgb A1C of 5.7% to 6.4%. Diabetes is diagnosed with Hgb A1C greater than 6.5%. Hgb A1Cs in women with preexisting diabetes generally run slightly higher than their nondiabetic cohorts. In diabetic women striving for tight preconception glucose control, the recommended Hgb A1C level to achieve prior to conception is less than or equal to 7% (Jensen et al., 2009).*

2. *Fetal macrosomia is a common complication of poor glucose control during diabetes. The mechanism for development of fetal macrosomia is best represented as:*

   A. Fetal hyperglycemia, fetal hyperinsulinemia, enhanced cellular glucose utilization, enhanced protein uptake, increased numbers of fat cells
   B. Maternal hyperglycemia, maternal hyperinsulinemia, secondary fetal hypoglycemia, enhanced cellular glucose uptake, increased fetal subcutaneous fat deposits
   C. Fetal hyperglycemia, increased fetal gluconeogenesis, enhanced glycogen storage

   ANSWER: A. *The driving mechanism for macrosomia is the fetal hyperinsulinemia that results from maternal hyperglycemia. Maternal glucose transfers readily across the placenta, but maternal insulin does not. As fetal insulin levels rise in response to the glucose load, cellular glucose uptake increases, amino acid uptake in the muscles is enhanced, and fat deposits increase in size throughout the body (Martin et al., 2015).*

3. *The longer the duration of maternal diabetes, the greater the likelihood that there are comorbid vascular changes in the mother. These vascular changes affect fetal growth by:*

   A. Limiting the transfer of glucose across the placenta, thus decreasing the incidence of fetal macrosomia
   B. Increasing major-organ perfusion in the mother, thus enhancing fetal growth
   C. Decreasing placental perfusion secondary to hypertension, thus limiting fetal growth

   ANSWER: C. *With advancing type 1 diabetes, the maternal microvasculature become sclerosed and hypertension develops. The effect of hypertension on placental blood flow produces the characteristically small-for-gestational-age infant, thus macrosomia may not be seen in this group of mothers (Martin et al., 2015).*

4. *Hyperinsulinism has a growth-enhancing effect on nearly all tissues in the fetus. Fetal cardiac muscle growth is enhanced by this insulin response, which often results in cardiomyopathy for the infant of the diabetic mother. This diabetic cardiomyopathy may result in compromised perfusion for the newborn. As the newborn insulin levels normalize after birth, when can the neonatal nurse practitioner anticipate the resolution of cardiomyopathy?*

(continued)

Case 4.4 (continued)

A. Within the first few days of life
B. By 6 months of age
C. By 6 weeks of age

ANSWER: B. *Hypertrophic cardiomyopathy secondary to maternal diabetes is a transient condition that generally resolves by 6 months of age (Martin et al., 2015).*

5. *Altered fetal growth resulting in a macrosomic infant, especially the large-for-gestational-age infant, also has comorbidities in many organ systems. Which of the following comorbidities is not associated with the diabetic pregnancy and macrosomic infant?*

A. Shoulder dystocia
B. Respiratory distress syndrome (RDS)
C. Hypercalcemia

ANSWER: C. *Shoulder dystocia is a complication of diabetes in pregnancy and delivery is considered at more than 38 weeks and more than 4,000 g based on this delivery risk. Fetal surveillance of lung maturation is important in the prevention of RDS in any elective delivery; in cases in which delivery is unavoidable, evaluation of respiratory status after birth is imperative. IDMs are at risk for hypocalcemia because of delay in parathyroid hormone synthesis resulting from maternal hypomagnesemia and relative hyperparathyroidism (Blackburn, 2013; Martin et al., 2015).*

6. *Congenital anomalies are a serious comorbidity for the IDM. Which of the following statements correctly describes the congenital malformation risks for the IDM?*

A. Rate of congenital malformations is three to five times higher in IDMs than in infants of nondiabetic mothers
B. Cardiac anomalies are the most common congenital malformations in the diabetic pregnancy
C. Sacral dysgenesis is diagnostic for diabetes
D. Central nervous system anomalies (i.e., neural tube defects) are the least common congenital malformation in infants of a diabetic pregnancy
E. All of the preceding responses are true
F. Only A and B are true

ANSWER: F. *The first two statements are true. Sacral dysgenesis is characteristic, but not diagnostic, for diabetes. Central nervous system malformations are the second most common anomalies in diabetic pregnancies. Note that women with gestational diabetes mellitus (GDM) do not have the same risk for congenital malformations because the malformations occur early in the pregnancy during organogenesis and gestational diabetes does not usually occur prior to 20 weeks gestation (Martin et al., 2015).*

CONCLUSIONS

Prenatal obstetric monitoring of maternal conditions and fetal growth provide important information on IU growth and well-being of the fetus and provide the NNP with data for anticipatory evaluation, potential neonatal medical problems, and short- and long-term comorbidities of altered IU growth. A complete review of maternal medical and pregnancy history, in addition to a thorough physical exam and accurate measurements, is key to expedient assessment, diagnosis, and management of the neonate with abnormal IU growth patterns.

REFERENCES

Blackburn, S. (2013). *Maternal, fetal, & neonatal physiology: A clinical perspective.* Maryland Heights, MO: Elsevier Saunders.

Brodsky, D., & Christou, H. (2004). Current concepts in intrauterine growth restriction. *Journal of Intensive Care Medicine, 19*(6), 307–319.

Calkins, K., & Deveskar, S. U. (2011). Fetal origins of adult disease. *Current Problems in Pediatric and Adolescent Health Care, 41,* 158–176.

Claris, O., Belltrand, J., & Levy-Marchal, C. (2010). Consequences of intrauterine growth and early neonatal catch-up growth. *Seminars in Perinatology, 34,* 207–210.

Fenton, T. (2003). A new growth chart for preterm babies: Babson and Benda's chart updated with recent data and a new format. *BMC Pediatrics, 3*(1), 13.

Gardosi, J., Mongelli, M., Wilcox, M., & Chang, A. (1995). An adjustable fetal weight standard. *Ultrasound in Obstetrics and Gynecology, 6*(3), 168–174.

Halliday, H. L. (2009). Neonatal management and long-term sequelae. *Best Practice & Research: Clinical Obstetrics & Gynaecology, 23*(6), 871–880.

Institute of Medicine and National Research Council. (2009). *Weight gain during pregnancy: Reexamining the guidelines.* Washington, DC: National Academies Press.

Jensen, D. M., Korsholm, L., Ovesens, P., Beck-Nielsen, H., Moelsted-Pedersen, L., Westergaard, J. G., . . . Damm, P. (2009). Peri-conceptual A1C and risk of serious adverse pregnancy outcome in women with Type 1 diabetes. *Diabetes Care, 32*(6), 1046–1048.

Lubchenco, L., Hansman, C., & Boyd, E. (1966). Intrauterine growth in length and head circumference as estimated from live births at gestational ages from 26 to 42 weeks. *Pediatrics, 37,* 403–408.

Lubchenco, L. O., Hansman, C., Dressler, M., & Boyd, E. (1963). Intrauterine growth as estimated from liveborn birth-weight data at 24 to 42 weeks of gestation. *Pediatrics, 32*(5), 793–800.

Martin, R., Fanaroff, A. A., & Walsh, M. C. (Eds.). (2015). *Fanaroff and Martin's neonatal-perinatal medicine: Diseases of the fetus and infant* (10th ed.). Philadelphia, PA: Saunders.

Maulik, D. (2006a). Fetal growth compromise: Definitions, standards, and classification. *Clinical Obstetrics and Gynecology, 49*(2), 214–218.

Maulik, D. (2006b). Fetal growth restriction: The etiology. *Clinical Obstetrics and Gynecology, 49*(2), 228–235.

Maulik, D. (2006c). Management of fetal growth restriction: An evidence-based approach. *Clinical Obstetrics and Gynecology, 49*(2), 320–334.

Maulik, D., Evans, J., & Ragolia, L. (2006). Fetal growth restriction: Pathogenic mechanism. *Clinical Obstetrics and Gynecology, 40*(2), 219–227.

Miller, J., Chauhan, S., & Abuhamad, A. (2012). Discordant twins: Diagnosis, evaluation and management. *American Journal of Obstetrics and Gynecology, 206*(1), 10–20.

Pallotto, E. K. M. D., & Kilbride, H. W. M. D. (2006). Perinatal outcome and later implications of intrauterine growth restriction. *Clinical Obstetrics and Gynecology, 49*(2), 257–269.

Schwartz, R., & Teramo, K. A. (2000). Effects of diabetic pregnancy on the fetus and newborn. *Seminars in Perinatology, 24*(2), 120–135.

Verklan, M. T., & Walden, M. (2015). *Core curriculum for neonatal intensive care nursing.* St. Louis, MO: Elsevier Saunders.

5

Fitting All the Pieces Together: A Summary of Formulating a Differential Diagnosis Based on Assessment Findings

Suzanne Staebler

Chapter Objectives

1. Recognize the significant findings within the infant's history (maternal, intrapartum, neonatal, interim)
2. Integrate findings from the history, physical exam, and supporting documentation (radiology and laboratory findings) to generate a prioritized differential diagnosis list (by systems)
3. Apply clinical issues identified in the problem list to develop a safe and appropriate plan of care for the infant
4. The National Association of Neonatal Nurse Practitioners (NANNP) competencies to be addressed are Domain 9: 1, 2, 3a and b, 4, and 5

This chapter is a bit different from what you have seen thus far in this book. Here, we take the pieces of a mother's history, labor and delivery history, and the infant's history and bring them all together to create a picture or road map for us to follow. Remember, this is not an exact science, but there are some guiding principles that enable us to hypothesize what may be going on. We then take these hypotheses and begin the process of evaluating the plausibility of each, through other diagnostic testing or therapy initiation. For instance, if possible, sepsis is on our list of differential diagnoses, then we would further evaluate by sending a complete blood culture (CBC), maybe a C-reactive protein (to determine presence of inflammatory mediators) and then starting antibiotics (therapy initiation). Or, if we thought a baby was in renal failure, before deciding on the fluid and electrolyte plan for the day, we would want to understand the type of renal failure first, in case further testing would be warranted before devising the plan.

The majority of the "data" we work with in the neonatal intensive care unit (NICU) is objective. Objective data points are observable and measurable; our physical exam findings would fall into this category, as would any laboratory results or diagnostic testing results. Subjective data are information that is reported by the mother or family members. For instance, if you were to ask the mother whether she feels safe at home with her current partner, her answer is subjective data that is incorporated in the holistic care we provide to our NICU patients. These data may prompt social work referral and other resource allocation for the mother to ensure a safe home environment when the baby is discharged. Subjective data may also come from the nurse or respiratory therapist caring for the infant. Usually these data takes the form of "I've had this baby now for the past 3 days and I know something's just not right." Further questioning and probing usually reveal that this team member, based on his or her expertise and experience, is responding intuitively and may not yet be able to quantify his or her concern with specific parameters or data points.

Remember, just because we have all the known pieces in place, the picture may still not be as clear as we would like. Although that may drive you crazy, it's okay . . . the picture will come into focus soon enough, as long as you stay in tune with the evaluation factors. Assessment and evaluation are ongoing and continual—as these processes continue, our diagnosis list and care plan continue to evolve as well. Some problems will be resolved or disproven and fall off; others will be added as care progresses.

PUZZLE PIECE 1: MATERNAL HISTORY

It is important to carefully comb through maternal history as it yields several anticipatory clues to the predispositions of the infant as well as insight into the intrauterine environment of the fetus. If a mother reports that her older child was jaundiced and had to be in the hospital longer, we know that the likelihood of this infant requiring intervention for hyperbilirubinemia is increased. If the mother has chronic hypertension *or* preeclampsia, we know that placental blood flow was compromised/diminished, and this impacts growth of the fetus as well as other organ system functions.

There may be times when an interview with the mother, either before birth (possibly during the prenatal/antepartum consult) or soon after birth, is warranted to gather more specific information. For instance, the obstetric (OB) record reports that the mother is on Synthroid for hypothyroidism. It is imperative to know what kind of hypothyroidism the mother is being treated for and the etiology of her thyroid disease so that we can anticipate issues with the infant's thyroid function. In this example, if the mother had to have a thyroid ablation for hyperthyroidism, and is now in a state of low thyroid, she will still have circulating thyroid-stimulating immunoglobulins (TSIs) that could cross the placenta and impact the fetus's thyroid function after birth (Sperling, 2014).

Mother's social history is also important to review. It gives us clues into the type of home environment she has been living in during her pregnancy and the environment that the infant will be in after discharge home. Social history can be an awkward area for us to venture into especially when we need to have conversations related to legal (alcohol, prescription drug, or marijuana use) or illegal substance use. Even medications such as selective serotonin reuptake inhibitors (SSRIs) can impact the infant after delivery and necessitate more than routine newborn care (Domar, Moragianni, Ryley, & Urato, 2012).

Current pregnancy history rounds out the areas for appraisal in this section. The current pregnancy history helps us anticipate any acute issues that may impact the fetus at delivery. For instance, the mother reports she was treated for a urinary tract infection (UTI) about a month ago. This piece of information elevates our watchfulness over the infant after birth, as we know this could increase the chance of an ascending infection in the fetus. A mother with hypertension who is admitted and given magnesium sulfate to manage her blood pressure is likely to deliver a baby who is somewhat depressed and who may need some intervention right at delivery (for respiratory depression) or a bit later (intravenous [IV] therapy resulting from a functional ileus from a high Mg+ level). So, let us practice identifying "red flags," or important pieces of the maternal history, that we would want to be cognizant of as the neonatal care provider for this mother's infant.

Red Flags 5.1

There are nine in all; see how many you identify. Answers can be found at the end of this chapter.

Mother is a 19-year-old gravida 2, para 0 who is admitted for complaints of chronic headaches and "spots in my eyes." Her pregnancy has been unremarkable up until this point despite a body mass index of 32 prior to pregnancy. She is currently 31 4/7 weeks with prenatal care starting at week 8. Dates are in line with early ultrasound for dating.

Labs: B negative, RPR NR, hep B negative, HIV negative, rubella immune. GTT WNL at 28-week visit.

Past medical history: Unremarkable

Family history: Maternal diabetes and heart disease; maternal grandmother died of cancer; paternal grandmother and aunt with breast cancer

Social history: Mother lives with her boyfriend and is unemployed. She admits to social drinking prior to finding out she was pregnant. Her boyfriend is a marijuana user but she makes him smoke outside. She denies any other substance use and has no active prescriptions.

PUZZLE PIECE 2: INFANT HISTORY

The first aspect we consider under the infant's history is the perinatal history. Much of these data will be obtained from the maternal pregnancy history. Again, it is important to assess the intrauterine environment and factors impacting the fetus/infant during delivery or after birth.

Many times, the neonatal nurse practitioner (NNP) or NNP student is in attendance for the infant's delivery so the delivery history is gathered from firsthand knowledge. Type of delivery (vaginal or C-section), fetal presentation (vertex, breech, face, etc.), and any assistance during delivery (vacuum or forceps) can help the delivery team prepare for issues right after birth. The events that occur after birth in the delivery room can also have some prognostic value. For instance, infants who require chest compression as part of resuscitation measures have higher mortality rates than infants who do not require them (Shah, Shah, & Tai, 2009). Did the infant get intubated in the delivery room and receive surfactant? Again, we would expect these infants to be at risk for complications such as pulmonary hemorrhage or pneumothorax afterward (Lopez et al., 2013).

If the infant is several days or weeks old, these delivery factors are not usually important any longer. So, at this point, we would look to the interval history of the infant. What has been going on with the baby in the past days or weeks. Has the infant had any procedures recently? Does he or she have a central line? What is the baby's respiratory status? What about current problems or diagnosis?

The interval history would look something like this:

You have an ex-24 weeker, who is now 6 months old. He had a tracheostomy tube placed about 2 months ago and is stable on his ventilator settings with a stable O$_2$ requirement at about 40. He has no central lines and is on full gastrostomy tube (G-tube) feedings and is working with speech therapy to improve his oral feeding skills. Over the past 24 hours, the nurses report that he is more irritable but consolable with his pacifier and he has had a low-grade fever (99.0°F–100.4°F [37.2°C–38°C] for the past 6 hours). *Based on this information, what are you thinking is going on with the infant?*

PUZZLE PIECE 3: CURRENT STATUS (OBJECTIVE DATA)

Objective data are those data points we obtain from "technical" sources such as the infant's vital signs. We get heart rate, respiratory rate, blood pressure, and temperature from the monitor or the temperature probe/thermometer. All of these devices are "technological" in nature. The same is true for the laboratory results we analyze or the ventilator settings with measured expired tidal volumes or pressure volume curves.

When we look at classic texts related to assessment and history taking, the subjective data are those things that the patient "says" or reports. But because our patients cannot report to us how they are feeling and what might be hurting, we have to utilize and depend on physiologic and objective data even more. So, we must understand physiologic responses to certain "stress" in order to interpret the data we get. For instance, the physiological responses of a 24-week estimation-of-gestational-age (EGA) infant will be different than those of a 34-week EGA infant. So, that foundational knowledge is absolutely necessary before we can accurately interpret the data we are receiving.

There are also instances when you respond to the data immediately before determining the cause. For instance, you are caring for a 27-week EGA infant who is intubated on the ventilator (patient-controlled ventilation [PCV] mode: 21/6, ×25 and FiO$_2$ of 33%–38%); over the course of the past 6 hours, you have seen progression of her arterial blood gases (ABGs). Her current ABG is: pH 7.21/PaCO$_2$ 39/PaO$_2$ 64/HCO$_3^-$ 16/BE −8. So, what would you do? *What is your interpretation of the ABG?*

Given that this infant is 27 weeks, we do not want to increase the vent rate to "compensate" for the metabolic acidosis because that could alter cerebral blood flow (if the CO$_2$ gets too low) and put her at risk for an intra-ventricular hemorrhage (IVH). But, given that the infant is acidotic, we need to treat the acidosis now, and then do further evaluation to determine why she is so acidotic. What are the possible causes?

Many times in neonatology, we can gain significant data from our physical assessment and by gathering input from the team caring for the baby. If we use the same infant case discussed previously, one of the first things to do would be to assess the infant. This would include both an exam and review of current "technical" data points. In a baby with metabolic acidosis, evaluation of respiratory and cardiovascular status is imperative. What are the baby's vital signs? Are there signs of hypovolemia (such as tachycardia or low blood pressure)? What about assessment of apical pulse? Is there a murmur? What about a dynamic precordium? Are pulses diminished or bounding? Are there palmar pulses? What is the baby's perfusion like?

Physiologic data points would also include urine output and blood pressure trends, especially the mean arterial pressures (MAPs) as well as pulse pressures. Once these questions are answered, we should begin to get an idea of what the cause of the metabolic acidosis is. We can then ask for input from the other team members. For instance, ask the respiratory therapist whether there have been any changes in ventilator parameters, especially those that are measured by the ventilator (minute ventilation, exhaled tidal volume). What about a change in respiratory rate or effort? If the baby has continuous SaO_2 or TCO_2 monitoring, what has the trending over the past several hours been? The bedside nurse can provide invaluable information to help clarify our picture. Changes in assessment, even subtle ones, can be quite helpful. For instance, we have looked in the electronic medical record and the infant's urine output is 2 mL/kg/hr, but the nurse says that the urine output has dropped off over the past 6 hours, so when you look back over the trend, the majority of the urine output was actually in the previous 12 hours with only 0.8 mL/kg/hr in the past 6 hours. This is a completely different picture of renal function than we got from looking at urine output over the past 24 hours.

Lastly, when seeking data and information for team members, do not forget to ask the parents whether they have noticed any changes. This is important for those parents who are actively involved in their child's care and who visit often. As providers, we sometimes forget that parents know their baby, sometimes even better than the nurse who cares for him or her each day. Many times, mothers are intuitively in tune with their babies and although they cannot explain what is going on they know that something is not right.

PUTTING THE PIECES TOGETHER

So, now that we have an understanding of all the pieces of data that are utilized in completing the picture and developing a differential diagnosis list, let us apply what we have learned with the following cases. Once you work through the following cases, you can check your answers with those provided at the end of the chapter.

Case 5.1

Baby girl "Boston" was born to a 31-year-old gravida 2, para 0 (G2P0) Ab1 at 33 weeks, 6 days via C-section as a result of worsening maternal hypertension and superimposed preeclampsia and breech presentation. Maternal labs: O+ blood type/HbSAg neg/HIV neg/ group B *Streptococcus* (GBS) neg/rapid plasma reagin (RPR) nonreactive (NR).

1. *What other questions do you have or would you want to know at this point?*

2. *Based on the history you have thus far, what are your concerns regarding the baby?*

Maternal medications during pregnancy include: Aldomet, hydralazine, Procardia, magnesium sulfate, and Reglan. Betamethasone was received 3 weeks prior to delivery.

(continued)

Case 5.1 (continued)

3. Now, based on mother's medications during pregnancy and perinatal course, what are your concerns for the fetus?

At delivery:
Rupture of membranes (ROM) occurred at delivery with clear fluid. Since the infant was preterm, clamping of the cord was delayed for 1 minute prior to handoff. Initially, the infant cried and was vigorous, but then became apneic and bradycardic—once placed on warmer, the infant was dried, stimulated, and bulb suctioned. She then required bag-mask ventilation and was subsequently transported to the neonatal intensive care unit (NICU) on nasal continuous positive airway pressure (CPAP). Apgar scores were 2 at 1 minute and 8 at 5 minutes.

4. What do you think contributed to the infant's apnea and bradycardia after being initially vigorous?

Upon admission to the NICU:
Vital signs (VS): heart rate (HR), 159; temp, 35.9°C; respiratory rate (RR), 35; SaO$_2$, 95% in room air (RA)
Weight: 1,330 g

5. Based on these data, do you have any new concerns?

Physical exam was unremarkable except for severe intrauterine growth restriction (IUGR).

6. Based on the information presented thus far, what would your initial differential diagnosis list be for this infant?

7. So what orders would you write for this infant?

Admission labs: glucose checks now and every 3 hours until stable; complete blood count w/diff; arterial blood gas? Chest x-ray? Blood culture?

8. Why would you send (or not send) a blood culture and do (not do) a sepsis screen?

9. What else could her respiratory distress be caused by?

Lab results come back:

$$4.2 > \frac{16.6}{52} < 62$$

segs 25/lymphs 52/mono 12/eos 3/baso 6

10. What is the absolute neutrophil count (ANC)?

(continued)

Case 5.1 (*continued*)

11. Does the ANC change your plan of care? Why or why not?

Day of life (DOL) 1:
The infant is weaned to RA and off CPAP by 10 hours of age.
Feeds were started at 20 mL/kg/d.
Intravenous fluids (IVF) changed to total parenteral nutrition (TPN) (D10 with 3 gAA/kg [grams of amino acids per kilogram]) and intralipid (IL; 0.5 g/kg/d).

Labs:

$$10.9 > \frac{21}{65} < 20\text{—repeated at } 66$$

Total bilirubin at 24 hours of age: 10.9

12. Do these labs change your plan of care? Any other pieces of information you would want?

Other labs or points of information on DOL 1:
Baby's blood type is O+ and Coombs negative
Total fluids increased to 100 mL/kg/d
Urine output is 154 mL over past 24 hours; the infant has not been weighed since birth

13. What are your concerns?

DOL 2:
The infant has intermittent increased work of breathing and two episodes of apnea and bradycardia requiring stimulation. Weight at 1,085 g; total fluids at 110 mL/kg/d with feeds (20 mL/kg/d) and TPN/IL. Antibiotics discontinued with report of negative blood culture at 48 hours.

Labs:
Bilirubin: 4.9
Glucose screen: 32

$$6.5 > \frac{19.5}{57} < 68$$

segs 32/bands 1/lymphs 41/mono 9/eos 3/baso 4

(*continued*)

Case 5.1 (continued)

14. What are you concerned about?

Current glucose infusion rate (GIR) was 6 mg/kg/min

15. Is this typically an adequate GIR for preterm infants?

The infant received bolus of D10W (2 mL/kg) with glucose rising to 39; she received an additional bolus and then her GIR increased to 8.7 mg/kg/min (changed dextrose concentration from 10% to 12.5%) with glucose rising to 50.

16. Based on the size of this infant and her current status, what would be a consideration for continued management of hypoglycemia?

Case 5.2

Baby boy "Vegas" is a 4,800-g infant born at 38 weeks gestation by C-section to a 21-year-old G1 mother. Her pregnancy was complicated by a lack of prenatal care (PNC).

Apgar scores were 4 at 1 minute and 8 at 5 minutes. Physical exam was remarkable for large body size, normal head circumference (34 cm), and normal height (21 in.). The infant went skin-to-skin with mother in the recovery room and suckled at the breast.

Baby Vegas did well during the next 48 hours and was discharged home on Monday afternoon with mother breastfeeding exclusively. Follow-up was scheduled for Friday morning with the pediatric provider.

1. Based on the information in this case, as the primary care provider, what would you want to know about this baby's hospital course that is not provided here?

On Thursday morning, Ms. Vegas calls the pediatric office because she is concerned about her baby. He is not waking up for feeds and is not eating well. She cannot remember how many wet or dirty diapers he has had. She can tell her milk has come in but because the baby is not eating well, her breasts are hurting and she wants to just bottle-feed. The nurse tells the mother to bring the baby in for a quick check even though he has an appointment the next day.

2. Knowing this information, before you ever examine baby Vegas, what are your concerns? Create a differential diagnosis list.

Upon examination of baby Vegas you find the following: weight, 4,315 g; heart rate, 164; respiratory rate, 56; temp, 36.7°C.

(continued)

Case 5.2 (continued)

Physical exam: Infant is "sleepy" but arouses. He is notably jaundiced down to his legs with scleral jaundice noted. His tone is slightly diminished but not abnormal, and abdomen is soft and nontender.

3. *What questions would you ask the mother, based on your exam and the infant's history?*

4. *What would you do at this point to further evaluate this infant in the office?*

5. *Based on the data you have currently, what is the most probable diagnosis?*

Case 5.3

A 2,050-g male infant was born at 29 weeks gestation to a healthy 27-year-old mother, with one previous pregnancy and one healthy child. Up until 26 weeks, the pregnancy was uncomplicated and prenatal ultrasounds showed normal growth and development. Per mother's report, there was no alcohol, smoking, or other illicit drugs used during pregnancy. During the last two prenatal visits, the fetal heart tones were noted to be elevated and maternal weight gain had increased exponentially in comparison with previous weight gain.

1. *Based on this history, what are the risk factors for this infant?*

2. *What are you anticipating as far as delivery room support and resuscitation?*

The infant was delivered by cesarean section following rupture of membranes. Fetal heart tones were elevated up to 200 beats per minute up to the moment of delivery. The infant required intubation for respiratory failure. Apgar scores were 2 at 1 minute, 4 at 5 minutes, and 6 at 10 minutes. Physical exam was remarkable for tachycardia (ranging from 184 to 200) and anasarca. He is taken to the neonatal intensive care unit and admitted.

3. *You are asked to write admission orders for the infant. Please make your list.*

Throughout the course of the first day of life, the infant has a urine output of 0.3 mL/kg/hr. The attending neonatologist tells you that the infant needs to be evaluated for causes of renal failure.

4. *Based on the infant's history, and your current management (orders you input earlier), what are the possible causes for the renal failure?*

(continued)

Case 5.3 (continued)

The following additional studies are obtained to evaluate the infant's renal function:

Renal ultrasound is normal—no evidence of hydronephrosis, obstruction, or hypoplasia.

Doppler study of renal blood flow is normal.

Blood culture, urine culture, and cerebrospinal fluid cultures are negative.

Urine is sent for analysis and results are as follows:

- Urine sodium = 36 mEq/L
- Urine creatinine = 17 mg/dL
- 2+ protein
- 1+ blood
- Specific gravity of 1.008

Most recent blood chemistries are:

- Na^+ 122/K^+ 4.9/Cl^- 106/CO_2 19/BUN 31/Cr 3.6

5. *Based on the information you have thus far, what is the most likely etiology for this infant's renal failure?*

6. *Calculate a fractional excretion of sodium for this patient.*

7. *How can this calculation be used to guide fluid and electrolyte therapy until renal function is improved?*

ANSWERS TO RED FLAGS 5.1

1. Age: Mom is young, still a teenager, so she is automatically in a high-risk category.
2. Gravida/Parity: This is mom's second pregnancy but we don't know the outcome of the first. This will require further exploration.
3. Complaint of chronic headache: Could be an indicator of pregnancy-induced hypertension (PIH).
4. Complaint of "spots in my eyes": Could be another symptom of PIH or other vascular issues.
5. BMI: Mom was obese prior to pregnancy; this put her in a high-risk category for maternal complications, especially if she delivers via C-section.
6. Gestational age: Infant is premature at this point; we have good dating and correlation with early ultrasound.
7. Blood type: Mom has a negative Rh factor blood type—if the outcome of her first pregnancy was an abortion (spontaneous or elective) we need to know if she got Rhogam after the first pregnancy was terminated.
8. Risky behavior: Mom is still 19 and so her alcohol use is underage; we need to further explore this area for other at-risk behaviors, even though she denied these to the OB team.
9. Drug exposure: If the boyfriend smokes marijuana, she is exposed as is the fetus and the infant after discharge. Depending on state laws, this may qualify for a referral to child services.

ANSWERS TO PUZZLE PIECE QUESTIONS
PUZZLE PIECE 2

1. *Based on this information, what are you thinking is going on with the infant?*

   ANSWER: While your initial response may be to begin a sepsis workup, remember this is a 6-month-old infant. Maybe he is teething. Check to see if his gums are swollen or inflamed. Or maybe he has otitis media and needs his ears evaluated.

PUZZLE PIECE 3

1. *What is your interpretation of the ABG?*

   ANSWER: Metabolic acidosis

ANSWERS TO CASE QUESTIONS
CASE 5.1

1. *What other questions do you have or would you want to know at this point?*

   ANSWER: Maternal medications during pregnancy and labor and deliver (L&D) course

2. *Based on the history you have thus far, what are your concerns regarding the baby?*

   ANSWER: Prematurity, low birth weight, or small for gestational age (SGA)

3. *Now, based on mother's medications during pregnancy and perinatal course, what are your concerns for the fetus? (allow them to answer)*

   ANSWER: Fetal depression resulting from Mg therapy; low birth weight and poor glycogen stores, risk for alterations in Ca^+ levels; alterations in cardiac contractility (caused by Procardia use in mother)

4. *What do you think contributed to the infant's apnea and bradycardia after being initially vigorous?*

   ANSWER: Maternal Mg use and cold stress affected the neonate

5. *Based on these data, do you have any new concerns?*

   ANSWER: Severe intrauterine growth restriction (IUGR)/SGA, hypothermia, and possible hypoglycemia are possible concerns

6. *Based on the information presented thus far, what would your initial differential diagnosis list be for this infant?*

   ANSWER: IUGR/SGA
   Very low birth weight
   Prematurity
   Respiratory distress
   At risk for hypoglycemia, hyperbilirubinemia, hypothermia

7. *So what orders would you write for this infant?*

   ANSWER: Nasal CPAP (4–6 cm); FiO2 to keep SaO2s between 88% and 95%; admission total parenteral nutrition (TPN) (D10W with 2 gAA/100 mL) at 60 to 80 mL/kg/d; isolette with humidity (60%–80%)—slow rewarming of body temperature

8. *Why would you send (or not send) a blood culture and do (or not do) a sepsis screen?*

   ANSWER: The infant has no risk factors for sepsis except respiratory distress

9. *What else could her respiratory distress be caused by?*

   ANSWER: Hypothermia

10. *What is the absolute neutrophil count (ANC)?*

    ANSWER: 1,050

11. *Does the ANC change your plan of care? Why or why not?*

    ANSWER: If blood culture was not sent earlier, it needs to be sent now and antibiotics started, because of the increased risk for infection with low neutrophil count

12. *Do these labs change your plan of care? Any other pieces of information you would want?*

    ANSWER: Yes. *Need to start phototherapy and increase our total fluid goal to compensate for insensible fluid losses. Also, hematocrit (Hct) is elevated and she is now polycythemic— this may be caused by excessive fluid losses. Other information should include baby's blood type and Coombs/urine output and glucose screens/platelet count*

13. *What are your concerns?*

    ANSWER: The baby's urine output at approximately 5 mL/kg/hr

14. *What are you concerned about?*

    ANSWER: Hypoglycemia—which is new onset at 48 hours

15. *Is this typically an adequate GIR for preterm infants?*

    ANSWER: Yes

16. *Based on the size of this infant and her current status, what would be a consideration for continued management of hypoglycemia?*

    ANSWER: Central-line placement to provide GIR sufficient to maintain euglycemia and normal fluid volumes

Case 5.2

1. *Based on the information in this case, as the primary care provider, what would you want to know about this baby's hospital course that is not provided here?*

   ANSWER: Bilirubin level at time of discharge; any workup or sepsis screen while in the hospital?
   Any issues with hypoglycemia?
   Was a newborn screen sent?

Were mother's labs drawn at hospital and what were they?

Did the mother have breastfeeding support/class while in hospital and did she have support once she was home?

2. *Knowing this information, before you ever examine baby Vegas, what are your concerns? Create a differential diagnosis list.*

ANSWER: Rule out or possible hypoglycemia, hyperbilirubinemia, dehydration, and sepsis

3. *What questions would you ask the mother, based on your exam and the infant's history?*

ANSWER: How did the baby eat while in the hospital?

How often is the baby eating at home?

Do you have a breast pump at home?

When in the hospital, did your baby have any medicines for an infection?

Did your baby have a jaundice check before going home?

Did your baby have any issues with low blood sugar while in the hospital?

Did the baby have any issues in the hospital?

4. *What would you do at this point to further evaluate this infant in the office?*

ANSWER: *Request records from birth hospital; send labs such as a complete blood count, bilirubin level, glucose screen, and electrolytes (if office cannot do these, send to hospital lab)*

5. *Based on the data you have currently, what is the most probable diagnosis?*

ANSWER: The likely diagnosis is hyperbilirubinemia resulting from poor breastfeeding/ dehydration. *Although sepsis is a concern given this case, the significant issues are the significant jaundice on exam, bilirubin level, poor eating, and significant weight loss (over 10%); because the mother is a primigravida, she may not be feeding the infant adequately or is having difficulty getting the infant latched well. The evaluation of electrolytes and bilirubin is imperative here.*

Possible sepsis is also on the list. *Given this infant's history (no prenatal care, group B* Streptococcus *unknown, and unknown prophylaxis course in the hospital) the infant could be lethargic as a result of sepsis, which is causing him to feed poorly and his bilirubin to escalate.*

CASE 5.3

1. *Based on this history, what are the risk factors for this infant?*

ANSWER: Prematurity; fetal tachycardia can be linked to heart defects of supra-ventricular tachycardia (SVT), fetal anemia, and fetal infection. Maternal weight gain could be concerning as well (Why?). Maternal weight gain is a concern as it is an early sign of altered cardiac function. (Is this pregnancy-induced hypertension [PIH], congestive heart failure [CHF], or pulmonary edema?)

2. *What are you anticipating as far as delivery room support and resuscitation?*

ANSWER: Fetal tachycardia is often connected with hydropic presentation of the fetus, so full resuscitation should be with intubation, medications, and possible chest tubes for drainage of pleural effusions.

3. *You are asked to write admission orders for the infant. Please make your list.*

   ANSWER:
   - Admit to humidified isolette (despite his birth weight, he is at risk for insensible water loss through his skin and other mechanisms)
   - Daily weights (given his anasarca, his birth weight is *not* his true weight; we must pay close attention to his weight in order to manage fluid and electrolyte status)
   - Assess VS every hour, with blood pressure (we need to monitor VS and blood pressure so we can anticipate cardiac function and intravascular volume needs)
   - Strict documentation of input and output (I&O) is needed: If no urine in first 8 hours, place a urethral catheter (we need to know what his renal function is and monitor that closely)
   - Intravenous fluids: D10W admission total parenteral nutrition (TPN) with 1g amino acids per 100 mL, total fluids to run at 60 to 80 mL/kg/d (until we know what his renal function is, giving a lot of protein is not wise; yet, he needs some protein to help with the osmotic fluid shifts from the interstitium into the intravascular space); consider central lines for this patient (to help with central blood pressure monitoring and central access for fluid and any blood product administration)
   - Ventilator settings: may need higher positive end-expiratory pressure (PEEP) (distending pressure) and peak inspiratory pressure (PIP) because of chest wall rigidity from anasarca
   - Consider surfactant given gestational age
   - X-ray of chest and abdomen (this can be done before or after umbilical line placement is done—these studies will help us evaluate degree of anasarca [thickness of chest wall], underlying lung disease, heart size, presence of pleural effusions or any other abnormalities)
   - Admission labs:
     a. Complete blood count and blood culture needed because hydrops/anasarca can be related to sepsis [viral or bacterial] we must consider congenital sepsis high on our differential diagnosis list
     b. Arterial blood gas test will help us see acid–base balance and make adjustments to the ventilator and will give an idea of lung function as well
     c. Type and screen; because fetal tachycardia can be associated with anemia, having this done will expedite the process should a transfusion be needed
     d. Assess blood chemistries and renal functions basic metabolic panel (BMP)/comprehensive metabolic panel (CMP) in 12 hours and then every 12 hours × 3 (close monitoring of fluid, electrolytes, and renal function is needed in an infant with this presentation)
     e. Determine immunoglobulin M (IgM) titers; given this infant's presentation, congenital infection is high on the diagnosis list; IgM titers will help rule out viral and other causes of infection that may not grow in a culture
   - Administer ampicillin (50 mg/kg dose every 12 hours)
   - Administer gentamicin (5 mg every 4 to 8 hours); trough level prior to the second dose; because renal function is unknown, we need to make sure that renal function is well established before giving the second dose

4. *Based on the infant's history, and your current management (orders you input earlier), what are the possible causes for the renal failure?*

   ANSWER: Intravascular volume depletion (hypovolemia) resulting from third spacing; urinary tract obstruction; heart failure (caused by arrhythmia or anemia); sepsis

5. Based on the information you have thus far, what is the most likely etiology for this infant's renal failure?

ANSWER: The renal failure is likely the result of prerenal causes such as hypovolemia, hypotension, cardiac failure, hemorrhage, or sepsis

6. Calculate a fractional excretion of sodium for this patient.

ANSWER: 6.144%

$$\frac{\text{Urine Na}^+}{\text{Serum Na}^+} \div \frac{\text{Urine Cr}}{\text{Serum Cr}} \times 100\%$$

$$\frac{36}{122} \div \frac{17}{3.7} \times 100$$

Fractional excretion of Na^+ measures the kidney's ability to reabsorb sodium in the presence of oliguria. Values greater than 3% suggest intrinsic renal damage/failure

7. How can this calculation be used to guide fluid and electrolyte therapy until renal function is improved?

ANSWER: Knowing that this infant's renal dysfunction is "prerenal" in nature allows us to begin interventions to improve function, such as treating hypovolemia, using low-dose dopamine to improve renal perfusion, using low-dose dobutamine to aid in cardiac function and renal perfusion. As renal function starts to improve, the fractional excretion of Na+ should also improve (percentage goes down)

REFERENCES

Domar, A. D., Moragianni, V. A., Ryley, D. A., & Urato, A. C. (2012). The risks of selective serotonin reuptake inhibitor use in infertile women: A review of the impact on fertility, pregnancy, neonatal health and beyond. *Human Reproduction, 28*(1), 160–171. doi:10.1093/humrep/des383

Lopez, E., Gascoin, G., Flamant, C., Merhi, M., Tourneux, P., & Baud, O. (2013). Exogenous surfactant therapy in 2013: What is next? Who, when and how should we treat newborn infants in the future? *BMC Pediatrics, 13,* 165.

Shah, P. S., Shah, P., & Tai, K. F. (2009). Chest compression and/or epinephrine at birth for preterm infants <32 weeks gestational age: Matched cohort study of neonatal outcomes. *Journal of Perinatology, 10,* 693–697. PMID: 19554013

Sperling, M. A. (2014). Disorders of the thyroid in the newborn and infant. *Pediatric endocrinology: Expert consult* (4th ed., pp. 186–208). Philadelphia, PA: Elsevier Saunders.

Diseases/Disorders by Body System

6

Respiratory System Cases: Differential Diagnosis for Respiratory Distress in the Newborn

Mary Beth Bodin

Chapter Objectives

1. Identify abnormalities in newborn normal respiratory function
2. Differentiate respiratory disease states by timing of presentation, clinical signs, and supporting information (blood gas values, chest x-ray [CXR] evaluation)
3. Apply acquired knowledge to solve given case study scenarios to create a safe plan of care for the infant

The respiratory system is a complex and evolving system that can be altered by numerous factors. Some of these influences begin during development of the fetus and some present during labor and delivery or in the immediate newborn period. This chapter focuses on the most common presentations; however, some information is presented on the lower volume, high-risk conditions that require immediate action by the neonatal nurse practitioner (NNP). The author has attempted to provide information to assist the reader in understanding and managing these cases. The first step is developing a differential diagnosis list and taking steps to identify the definitive diagnosis. This approach should always be used in evaluating an infant with respiratory distress.

Respiratory distress in the neonate is a condition exhibited by any difficulty in breathing by the infant. In order to establish a differential diagnosis list, the caretaker must have an understanding of the most common causes for the presentation of respiratory distress in the neonate. This chapter presents these common causes of respiratory distress in the newborn. Case studies are provided to assist the caretaker in determining a definitive diagnosis based on the presentation for a selected number of presentations. General pathophysiology knowledge of the reader is assumed. Please refer to one of the many neonatal pathophysiology texts available for this material if remediation is required.

CONDITIONS THAT RESULT FROM CONGENITAL ALTERATIONS IN ANATOMY

NASAL OR PHARYNGEAL CONDITIONS

Mechanical Blockage

Infants are obligatory nose breathers; therefore, any condition that limits the movement of air through the nasal passages might create a condition of distress for the newborn. The nasal passages may be blocked by blood, mucus, or meconium and simple oral and nasal suctioning may clear the airway and allow for successful breathing to occur. The position of the infant in the birth canal or malposition during the descent into the birth canal may lead to nasal edema, which may create a temporary condition of respiratory distress in the newborn. In these conditions, clearing the nasal passages or creating an alternate route for air exchange, such as opening the infant's mouth, will often eliminate the temporary condition.

Choanal Atresia

A more serious condition may present in which the usual nasal passages are not patent. The most common presentation of this type of blockage is choanal atresia. Choanal atresia is a congenital defect in the development of the bucconasal membrane in which the normal perforation occurs during gestation. It is present more often in females and is bilateral in 50% of cases and may be associated with anomalies such as CHARGE (coloboma, heart defect, atresia choanae [choanal atresia], retarded growth and development, genital abnormality, and ear abnormality) syndrome (Soltau & Carlo, 2014). Assessing for patency of the nares is best done in a quiet state. The NNP looks for the appearance of respiratory distress when the infant has his or her mouth closed. Because infants are obligate nose breathers, they have respiratory distress—particularly retractions and cyanosis and are pink with crying. This can be unilateral, so it is important to assess each nostril separately if choanal atresia is suspected. The usual first diagnostic procedure is to attempt to gently pass a nasogastric (NG) tube. Immediate treatment is placement of an oral airway and, in some situations, intubation. Because the lungs are usually not diseased, the endotracheal tube (ETT) is for establishing an airway. This condition requires surgical correction.

ORAL CAVITY

Macroglossia

Macroglossia, or enlarged tongue, can be congenital or acquired. If localized, it is likely to be secondary to congenital hemangioma. The most common associated condition is Beckwith's syndrome but macroglossia can also be seen with Pompe's disease (Gomella, 2013a). Depending on the severity of the respiratory distress, the infant may need to be intubated. These infants are usually able to breathe through the nose if the nares are patent. Morbidity and mortality depend on the etiology and any associated syndromes.

Pierre Robin Syndrome or Sequence

Micrognathia, or small mandible, may be a familial trait if subtle or it may be associated with a syndrome or sequence. The most common syndrome associated with micrognathia is Pierre Robin syndrome or sequence. Respiratory distress in this case is obstructive in nature and can be severe. Because of the small mandible, the tongue is posteriorly placed into the oropharynx causing obstruction of the airway. There is a very good prognosis for the infant with isolated small mandible because the condition is self-resolving as the mandible grows. As with assessment of any anomaly, it is important for the NNP to assess for associated defects as 60% of patients with Pierre Robin syndrome have a cleft palate. If placing the infant prone does not relieve the distress, a nasal airway device may be needed. There is a good prognosis if the condition is nonsyndromic (Soltau & Carlo, 2014).

In establishing a diagnosis of Pierre Robin syndrome or sequence, the NNP must consider other causes of micrognathia. Many syndromes (e.g., Stickler or Catel-Manzke) have the craniofacial features associated with Pierre Robin syndrome. If noncraniofacial features are the primary defects, a multiple congenital anomaly (MCA) syndrome other than Pierre Robin syndrome should be considered. For example, if an infant presents with small mandible, cleft lip and palate, rocker-bottom feet, and joint abnormalities, this would not lead to a diagnosis of Pierre Robin syndrome.

Oral Teratoma

An oropharyngeal teratoma (epignathus), although rare, may obstruct the airway causing severe respiratory distress that can be difficult to manage at times. Teratomas arise from all three germ layers and may be benign or malignant. If the condition is known prenatally, delivery should occur in a center capable of establishing an emergency airway, such as tracheotomy. Definitive treatment is surgical removal of the teratoma. Prognosis is generally excellent with nonmalignant tumors. Mortality is most commonly the result of airway obstruction (Halterman, Igulada, & Steinicki, 2006).

NECK

Position

Other congenital conditions that may affect the airway leading to respiratory distress include abnormal growths and ineffective positioning of the infant's neck. At times, changing the infant's position will be necessary to open the airway. This is especially important for the infant with a large occipital area or a small mandible. The newborn has little reserve for creating his or her own airway and must rely on the caregiver to establish an effective airway. If no obvious mass is noted, placing the infant in a neutral position with the chin in a "sniffing" position is optimal for air exchange at this level (Katwinkel et al., 2010).

Goiter

Congenital goiter is extremely rare and presents as an asymmetrical mass. The most common cause of neonatal goiter is neonatal Graves' disease, which is a transient condition seen in newborns delivered to mothers with a history of Graves' disease, especially if the mother was treated with antithyroid drugs or has had a thyroidectomy or radioiodine ablation. Any infant delivered to a mother with history of Graves' disease should be examined for presence of a goiter. Neonatal goiter presents as a mass in the anterior neck. Although neonatal goiters may be small, they may be large enough to compress the trachea and lead to respiratory distress. The condition is transient and should resolve by 3 months of age.

If symptomatic hyperthyroidism is present, treatment may be needed. The most common treatments are iodine, antithyroid medications, sedation, and beta-adrenergic blockers (Stokowski, 2011).

Cystic Hygroma

As opposed to the teratoma, which is derived from germ cells, cystic hygroma (CH) is derived from lymphatic tissue. CH is the most common lateral neck mass to occur in the newborn period and should be included in the differential diagnosis when an infant presents with a neck mass. These lesions are usually fairly large and can be quite disfiguring even with surgical repair. The larger lesions can cause disfigurement of the mandible during later gestation as a result of the pressure of the growing lesion against the developing mandible. The immediate concern for the NNP is patency of the airway.

Some experts believe the lesion is present from birth although there have been reports of acquired CH. As with many abnormalities noted at birth, it is important to consider the presence of a congenital chromosomal abnormality. CH has been reported to be more common in infants with trisomy 13, 18, and 21 and in infants with Turner syndrome and Klinefelter syndrome. There have also been reports of increased incidence of CH with certain nonchromosomal disorders such as Noonan syndrome, Fryns syndrome, multiple ptergium syndrome, and achondroplasia (Acevedo et al., 2015).

TRACHEA

Tracheomalacia and Laryngomalacia

Presented with a newborn experiencing wheezing or other noisy airway findings, the NNP must determine the cause in order to treat the condition. Associated findings must be considered in establishing a differential diagnosis. The two most common diagnoses are laryngomalacia and tracheomalacia. Distinguishing between the two is necessary for treatment options. The most reliable initial distinguishing factor is the timing of stridor. In tracheomalacia, expiratory stridor is prominent. In laryngomalacia, course inspiratory stridor, which is worse with agitation, is prominent; although there can be a component of expiratory stridor. Placing the infant in a prone position is often beneficial. Laryngomalacia is the most common cause of congenital stridor and is usually self-limited. This condition is diagnosed by laryngoscopy, in which collapse of the epiglottis with subsequent prolapse into the glottis during inspiration is noted. Conservative treatment is recommended and there is usually spontaneous resolution by 2 years of age. Although tracheomalacia is rare, it can be more difficult to manage. Bronchoscopy demonstrates collapse of the trachea during expiration. Continuous positive airway pressure (CPAP) may be required if air exchange is hindered. In rare cases, tracheostomy is needed. Humidification of inspired air may help thin secretions thereby relieving some distress. The majority of infants experience spontaneous resolution by 6 to 12 months of age (Brodsky & Doherty, 2014a). Secondary tracheomalacia is the result of compression by adjacent structures. Treatment and prognosis are related to the causative diagnosis. Secondary tracheomalacia may be a sequela to esophageal atresia (EA), tracheoesophageal fistula (TEF), vascular rings (double aortic arch), aberrant innominate artery, mediastinal masses, connective tissue disorders, or prolonged mechanical ventilation (Finder, 2016).

Tracheoesophageal Fistula

Although TEF is a defect usually discussed in relation to the gastrointestinal (GI) track because of its common association with EA, this anomaly can and does contribute to respiratory distress in the immediate newborn period as well as later in the neonatal period. Five types of EA are described in the literature based on the Gross classification, with only three associated with TEF. Type A, commonly referred to as pure EA, presents with the esophagus ending in a blind pouch with no connection to the trachea. Type B resembles Type A but has a fistula between the esophageal pouch and the trachea. Type C, the most common form of EA, has a distal connection between the trachea and the esophagus but not the blind pouch. Type D exhibits the connection with the blind pouch and the distal esophagus. Type E, or the H-Type fistula, has a connection between the intact esophagus and the intact trachea (Montrowl, 2014).

All forms of EA, whether or not TEF is present, can lead to respiratory distress in the immediate newborn period or later as there is the possibility of aspiration and subsequent pneumonia in all types. When an infant presents with copious amounts of oral secretions at delivery, the NNP must think about a differential diagnosis immediately. With a history of polyhydramnios and a presentation with large amounts of oral secretions, a differential diagnosis list must include the most common swallowing disorders. The first priority is to establish and protect the airway. Suctioning the oral cavity and passage of an oral or nasal feeding catheter to empty gastric contents is necessary in this case. When a blind pouch is present, the caregiver will be unable to pass the feeding catheter to the estimated depth. A general "rule of thumb" is that inability to pass the catheter more than 9 to 12 cm before encountering resistance suggests EA. Chest radiograph with the catheter in place is always indicated when there is a large amount of oral secretions and/or resistance is met with attempts to pass an oral or nasal catheter. The NNP must note the position of the catheter as well as whether or not gas is present in the bowel. Lack of gas in the GI tract indicates lack of connection between the trachea and the esophagus. Presence of air in the stomach or bowel indicates presence of a fistula (Montrowl, 2014). In the presence of the H-Type fistula, the infant may do well initially with occasional episodes of coughing or choking and recurrent pneumonia. In this case, the NNP should consider the need for bronchoscopy or endoscopy, as contrast studies are associated with aspiration in many cases. Immediate management includes placement of a vented tube, such as a Replogle tube, in the pouch and low intermittent suction. Elevating the head of the bed slightly in an effort to avoid aspiration as well as providing comfort measures to avoid excessive crying are necessary. Surgical repair is the ultimate resolution.

Tracheal Agenesis/Atresia

Tracheal agenesis or atresia is fatal in all but the most rare cases. Presence of a bronchoesophageal fistula may offer some hope for the infant; however, long-term survival is usually not possible. This condition is a rare anomaly with prevalence less than 1:50,000 and a male-to-female ratio of 2:1. Tracheal agenesis or atresia should be considered in the differential diagnosis when there is a maternal history of polyhydramnios, absence of a cry at birth, inability to pass the smallest ETT past the vocal cords, and immediate respiratory distress in the newborn. Although tracheal agenesis or atresia is rare, it is associated with a polymalformative syndrome in 93% of cases (Bertholdt, Perdriolle-Galet, Bach-Segura, & Morel, 2015). Because medical science has little to offer these patients, prenatal diagnosis and parental guidance is the best option for now.

PULMONARY CONDITIONS

Congenital Diaphragmatic Hernia

The typical presentation of congenital diaphragmatic hernia (CDH) is well known. The infant usually presents with a sunken abdomen and respiratory distress. Onset of respiratory distress is related to the extent of the defect and the degree of lung hypoplasia. When a small defect is present, the infant may not have significant respiratory distress and the CDH may be diagnosed when a chest radiograph is obtained for another reason. Whether large or small, surgical repair will be necessary.

Since the defect begins during early gestation (10–12 weeks), lung development is adversely affected. Mainly a result of compression by the herniated bowel, pulmonary hypoplasia is always present to some degree on the affected side, which is usually the left side. There may be some degree of effect on the contralateral side as well as a result of mediastinal shift. In those infants who present with significant respiratory distress, intubation and ventilation via the ETT rather than ventilation via bag and mask is the immediate treatment of choice. Several different support strategies are available depending on the severity of illness. These include conventional mechanical ventilation, high-frequency mechanical ventilation, and nitric oxide. In cases of severe respiratory failure, extracorporeal membrane oxygenation (ECMO) is required prior to surgical repair (Iocono, 2013).

Today, this condition is easily diagnosed by prenatal ultrasound (US); therefore, timing and location of delivery should be coordinated so that delivery occurs in a center equipped to care for this condition. Fetal surgery offers hope when the defect is diagnosed early. The hope is that in utero repair will decrease the risk of pulmonary hypoplasia. Trials continue to determine the best approach (Farrell, 2014).

Congenital Cystic Adenomatoid Malformation

Congenital cystic adenomatoid malformation (CCAM) is the most common thoracic mass noted by fetal US, although the overall incidence is relatively low. A CCAM is usually a benign hamartomatous overgrowth of terminal bronchioles, which leads to a reduction in the number of alveoli (DiPrima et al., 2012). Although CCAM is easily diagnosed prenatally, there are cases in which lack of prenatal care may lead to need for postnatal diagnosis. When the NNP is presented with a neonate exhibiting respiratory distress for which radiograph studies reveal a fluid-filled mass, the differential diagnosis would include pulmonary sequestration, CDH, and bronchogenic cysts. Many pediatric surgeons recommend a "wait and see" plan based on severity of respiratory distress at birth and whether hydrops is present. There is general agreement that the symptomatic infant requires timely surgical removal of the defect. Immediate management of the symptomatic infant by the NNP is supportive and often involves intubation and mechanical ventilation (Farrell, 2014).

Pleural Effusions

Pleural effusions result from accumulations of fluid between the parietal pleura of the chest wall and the visceral pleura surrounding the lung. Increased venous pressure in utero from hydrops fetalis or congestive heart failure (CHF) may lead to pleural effusion. Central venous catheter perforation with fluid leakage into the pleural space is a common cause of iatrogenic pleural effusion. The effusion may also be the result of accumulation of lymphatic fluid (chylothorax) or blood (hemothorax). Pleural effusion or chylothorax should be suspected when the NNP faces difficulty in ventilating a newborn in the delivery room. Emergency thoracentesis or tube thoracostomy for fluid drainage may be life-saving (Soltau & Carlo, 2014).

Pulmonary Hypoplasia or Aplasia

Pulmonary hypoplasia can be used synonymously with pulmonary aplasia and is part of a spectrum of malformations in which incomplete development of the lung is present. Severity is related to the timing of the condition, resulting in alteration of lung development as well as any associated congenital anomalies, such as cardiac, GI, genitourinary, and skeletal anomalies. Pulmonary hypoplasia is most commonly associated with renal defects leading to a lack of fetal urine. The importance of adequate amniotic fluid volume cannot be understated; although this is not the only factor in the pathophysiology of pulmonary hypoplasia. Adequate thoracic space is an important factor and helps to explain the syndrome of pulmonary hypoplasia in the presence of CDH. Other factors that affect lung development include volume of fetal lung fluid and pressure relationships between the lung and trachea. The association of critical composition of fetal lung fluid demonstrates that fetal lung development is a multifactorial event. The role of the kidney in fetal lung growth is one of the factors most commonly related to pulmonary hypoplasia. This accounts for the severe pulmonary hypoplasia seen in the infant with Potter's syndrome (Chin, 2014). Pulmonary hypoplasia is easily diagnosed by radiography. When the hypoplasia is the result of oligohydramnios, the fetus presents with characteristic features, including low-set ears, micrognathia, "flat facies," wrinkled skin, and contractures of the limbs. Potter's syndrome and other syndromes that present with severe hypoplastic lungs are almost universally fatal because of the resultant respiratory failure. Family support is one of the most important roles of the NNP in these cases (Parker, 2014).

Case 6.1

HW, a 32-year-old, G2P1001 female was admitted to the hospital at 26 6/7 weeks gestation for evaluation and treatment of polyhydramnios. Her 12-week ultrasound (US) had indicated a high nuchal lucency with a cystic hygroma (CH) on the fetus's neck. Chorionic villi sampling revealed no chromosomal anomalies. HW was referred to maternal fetal specialists and a fetal cardiac US was negative for cardiac anomalies. After admission to the hospital, the attending physicians remained concerned and serial US evaluations revealed that Baby Cain was edematous but that he was growing. The CH had resolved. Because of the extent of polyhydramnios, a therapeutic amniocentesis was done at 30 weeks. The following day, labor ensued and HW was transferred to the operating room for a cesarean section (C-section) as a result of maternal hypotension and fetal distress.

1. *Which of the following fetal diagnoses are most consistent with polyhydramnios?*
   A. Congenital heart disease (CHD)
   B. Fetal swallowing defects
   C. Renal agenesis

   ANSWER: B. *Polyhydramnios is associated with fetal swallowing defects or gastrointestinal obstruction as the fetus normally swallows amniotic fluid, keeping the amount at an appropriate level (Bertholdt et al., 2015). CHD may be associated with fetal hydrops and renal agenesis leads to oligohydramnios.*

At 1:08 p.m. on that Friday afternoon, a beautiful, well-developed baby boy was born. But he did not cry! The infant required immediate cardiopulmonary resuscitation as respiratory efforts did not result in air exchange and his heart rate was rapidly slowing. Attempts at

(continued)

Case 6.1 (continued)

intubation were unsuccessful because of lack of patency of the trachea. The infant expired after a short time in his mother's arms.

2. **Which of the following conditions would be on the differential diagnosis list for this infant?**

   A. Esophageal agenesis with blind pouch
   B. Pierre Robin syndrome
   C. Tracheal agenesis or stenosis

   ANSWER: A and C. *Both of these differentials are associated with polydramnios (Bertholdt et al., 2015; Montrowl, 2014). Pierre Robin syndrome may interfere with feeding after birth, but does not interfere with swallowing during fetal life.*

3. **What guidance or advice would you offer to these parents in relation to future pregnancies?**

   A. Although this condition is usually the result of a multifactorial etiology, prenatal counseling with a geneticist is warranted
   B. Don't worry. You can get pregnant again after you have had one normal period
   C. With your next pregnancy, you must avoid all caffeine and make sure you take extra prenatal vitamins and folic acid

   ANSWER: A. *This question is related to the appropriateness of advice as much as it is to the accuracy of the reply. It is known that many anomalies are multifactorial and this is one of them (Bertholdt et al., 2015). Prenatal counseling will assist the parents in making decisions related to future pregnancies and may help to relieve them of any feelings of guilt over the outcome. Answers B and C are both inappropriate as they may cause unnecessary feelings of guilt.*

   Note: In memory of Cain Walker, with parental consent. Born and died on September 30, 2011.

CONDITIONS THAT RESULT IN ALTERATIONS IN TRANSITION

NONPULMONARY CAUSES

Congestive Heart Failure

CHF rarely presents in the immediate newborn period. It is important to note that CHF is a sequela of an underlying process rather than a separate entity and presents after compensatory mechanisms fail to maintain adequate cardiac output and function. One of the most common causes of CHF in newborns is anemia. When presented with an infant with severe anemia, the NNP must look at the cardiac status while treating the immediate condition of hypovolemia/anemia. Although not entirely inclusive, other causes include patent ductus arteriosus (PDA), congenital heart defects with obstruction to outflow, myocardial ischemia, volume overload, tachyarrhythmias, and excessive demand as with shock, polycythemia, and myocarditis. Diagnosis of CHF is based on clinical findings as well as radiography. The infant usually presents with respiratory distress, pallor, and irritability. Arterial blood gas (ABG) analysis will reveal a metabolic acidosis with hypoxemia. There may be a respiratory component if pulmonary edema is severe (Lott, 2014). Please refer to Chapter 7 (Cardiovascular System Cases) for treatment options.

Congenital Heart Disease

Discussion of CHD is beyond the scope of this chapter but must be included in a discussion on respiratory distress as a differential diagnosis. Refer to Chapter 7 for a more detailed discussion on specific congenital heart lesions. When faced with a cyanotic newborn, the NNP should be aware that the most common cause of cyanosis in the newborn is respiratory disease followed by sepsis, hypotension and shock, and then cyanotic heart lesions. The challenge for the NNP is to establish a sound differential diagnosis, treat immediate concerns, determine a definitive diagnosis, and, finally, to manage the condition. Maternal history and a thorough physical exam will often lead to a preliminary diagnosis. ABG measurements will determine whether the infant is hypoxic and whether the primary cause of an abnormal ABG has a metabolic or respiratory focus. A complete blood count (CBC) with differential will assist in determining whether anemia or polycythemia might be a precipitating factor and will indicate whether sepsis is likely. A chest radiograph will assist in determining whether a pulmonary process is present and can be informative in diagnosing some congenital heart defects. Observing for increased or decreased pulmonary arterial or vascular markings as well as the size of the heart will help in establishing a preliminary diagnosis. There are certain congenial heart lesions that can also be suggested based on the shape of the cardiac silhouette (Gomella, 2013b). Table 6.1 demonstrates radiologic findings that suggest certain congenital heart lesions.

The hyperoxia test is one of the most helpful early screens for determining whether the cyanosis has a cardiac or pulmonary origin. The typical process of this test is to obtain an ABG in the room, then place the infant in 100% oxygen for 10 to 20 minutes and repeat the ABG. An infant without pulmonary or cardiac disease will usually have a PaO_2 of greater than 300 mmHg. Even with pulmonary disease, the PaO_2 will usually rise to greater than 150 mmHg. In the presence of a cyanotic heart lesion, the PaO_2 will not increase above 100 mmHg and is

Table 6.1 **X-Ray Findings Leading to Suspected Heart Lesion**

Boot-shaped heart	Tetralogy of Fallot, tricuspid atresia
Egg-shaped heart (egg on a string)	Transposition of the great arteries
Large globular heart	Ebstein's anomaly
Dextrocardia/mesocardia	Undetermined association
"Snowman" or "figure 8"	Total anomalous pulmonary venous return

Source: Gomella (2013a).

usually in the range of less than 50 to 70 mmHg. Although this test is an excellent screen and can be useful in sites where a pediatric cardiologist is not available, the definitive test for determining the presence of a cardiac defect is a cardiac echocardiogram (Gomella, 2013b).

Central Nervous System Disorders

The tendency in evaluating the newborn for respiratory distress is to conclude that underlying pulmonary pathophysiology is present. Some of the most common nonpulmonary disorders have been discussed, although the list is not all inclusive. To prevent a delay in treatment by preventing serious diagnostic and therapeutic errors, it is important to have a broad and flexible approach. That is where the differential diagnosis approach is most important. Another group of nonpulmonary disorders that must be considered are the central nervous system (CNS) disorders that present with respiratory distress. This encompasses a wide range of clinical presentations, including apnea, cyanosis, irregular respirations and tachypnea with grunting respirations, nasal flaring, and retractions. These conditions are most commonly associated with cerebral edema or intracranial hemorrhage, usually as a consequence of anoxia or birth trauma. The prognosis depends on the etiology and severity of the initial problem and any ongoing insult. In establishing a differential diagnosis, the NNP must include the most common diseases and disorders while keeping an open mind for the less obvious. Primary CNS disorders affecting respiratory function may include perinatal asphyxia, intracranial hemorrhage or infarct, meningitis, hydrocephalus, increased intracranial pressure, congenital myopathies or neuropathies, congenital malformations of the brain, congenital central hypoventilation syndrome, and other encephalopathies (Gomella, 2013a).

Persistent Pulmonary Hypertension of the Newborn

Persistent pulmonary hypertension of the newborn (PPHN) is a sequela of failed cardiovascular transition from intrauterine to extrauterine patterns, thus it directly affects extrauterine pulmonary physiology. The result is a persistent elevation in pulmonary vascular resistance (PVR) leading to marked pulmonary hypertension with subsequent right-to-left shunting through fetal pathways. PPHN is applied when there is a combination of pulmonary hypertension, right-to-left shunting at the foramen ovale or ductus arteriosus, and a structurally normal heart. The syndrome of PPHN may be idiopathic (of unknown or multifactorial origin) or it may be secondary to perinatal stress from conditions such as meconium aspiration syndrome (MAS), CDH, respiratory distress syndrome (RDS), asphyxia, sepsis, pneumonia, hyperviscosity, or hypoglycemia (Brodsky & Doherty, 2014b; Soltau & Carlo, 2014). More than one disorder may be contributing factors. Certain perinatal factors, such as maternal ingestion of aspirin or indomethacin or other nonsteroidal anti-inflammatory drugs or maternal use of selective serotonin reuptake inhibitors, have been associated with PPHN (Dhillon, 2012). Whether these factors contribute to the idiopathic causes is debatable as there appears to be a direct association.

PPHN is a diagnosis of exclusion; therefore, a sound differential diagnosis is imperative. The differential is usually based on clinical findings, ABG results, supplemental oxygen requirements, and screening tests. The most useful initial screening tool is the simultaneous monitoring of differential preductal and postductal oxygen saturations. This technique involves placement of an oxygen saturation monitor on a preductal and a postductal site and a comparison of the readings, as this is an indicator of right-to-left shunting at the ductal level. A difference greater than 5% is considered evidence of a right-to-left shunt consistent with PPHN. A hyperventilation test may also be of value in ruling out a cyanotic congenital heart lesion as little to no improvement is expected in infants with cyanotic congenital heart lesions. Radiographic images are of little value in diagnosing PPHN but can be useful in determining pulmonary causes of the respiratory distress. Echocardiography is diagnostic and is used to rule out cardiac structural anomalies as well (Alpan, 2013).

Treatment options for PPHN have historically consisted of mechanical ventilation, inhaled nitric oxide (iNO), and ECMO. Prevention is always the best strategy; therefore, optimizing prenatal care and immediate recognition of the conditions leading to development of PPHN are imperative. Optimizing ventilation remains the gold standard, although the best methods may not always be available. In facilities where iNO or ECMO are not available, other treatment options are on the horizon. The safety and efficacy of inhaled and intravenous iloprost, sildenafil, milrinone, and bosentan are being studied as acceptable options (Napolitano & Stoller, 2015).

Respiratory Depression

Neonatal respiratory depression can result from pharmacological agents given to the mother during labor and delivery, CNS defects or disorders, perinatal asphyxia, birth trauma, sepsis, or shock. Regardless of the cause, if an infant does not begin adequate breathing after birth with subsequent establishment of normal functional residual capacity of the lungs, further transition cannot occur. The most effective action by the NNP, when faced with a depressed newborn, is to provide effective ventilation. The most common cause of neonatal respiratory depression at birth is medication given to the mother during labor such as narcotic analgesics for pain control or magnesium sulfate for hypertension or as a means to delay delivery. When there is a known history of narcotic administration to the mother within 4 hours of delivery, a narcotic antagonist may be indicated. Ventilatory support remains the first action for respiratory depression (Bagwell, 2014). In the case of the infant delivered to a narcotic-dependent mother, use of naloxone is contraindicated because of the danger of abrupt reversal of the narcotic effects and immediate withdrawal in the infant. Treatment of choice in this case is assisted ventilation until respiratory drive is adequate to maintain spontaneous respirations by the infant (Katwinkel, 2011).

Magnesium sulfate given to the mother for preeclampsia or as a tocolytics agent is known to have certain adverse effects on the infant and these effects appear to increase as maternal serum magnesium levels increase. The initial effect that is of primary interest to the NNP is respiratory depression and hypotonia. If use of the drug is not known from report of maternal history, the NNP should ask the question when faced in the delivery room with an infant with respiratory depression (Abbassi-Ghanavati, Alexander, McIntire, Savani, & Leveno, 2012). Treatment for respiratory distress related to high serum magnesium levels as a result of magnesium sulfate given to the mother consists of respiratory support in the delivery room. The primary mechanism for decreasing serum magnesium is urinary excretion; therefore, the NNP must follow urine output judiciously. Administration of supplemental calcium in maintenance doses will help to block the neuromuscular manifestations of hypermagnesemia (Inayat, 2013).

Metabolic Influences

Acidosis, whether respiratory or metabolic, can have a significant influence on transition leading to respiratory distress or depression. Metabolic acidosis can be a cause of or a consequence of failure of normal transition. Metabolic acidosis in the immediate newborn period can be a consequence of intrauterine hypoxia with resultant lactic acidosis, maternal acidosis, hypovolemia, and inborn errors of metabolism. Inborn errors in metabolism usually do not present at delivery but can lead to acidosis in the neonatal period. Treatment of neonatal metabolic acidosis consists of supportive care and is directed toward the precipitating cause.

Fluid resuscitation may be successful in treating acidosis precipitated by hypovolemia. Occasionally, cautious administration of sodium bicarbonate may be necessary, although this treatment remains controversial (Gomella, 2013b).

Shock

Shock in the newborn must be distinguished from hypotension when determining the causes and treatment. Hypotension may accompany shock; however, shock is a clinical syndrome associated with inadequate tissue perfusion with the clinical signs shown in Table 6.2.

Treatment for shock in the newborn is directed toward the precipitating cause. The differential diagnosis should include the most common types of shock: hypovolemic, cardiogenic, distributive, obstructive, and dissociative. Hypovolemic shock is the most common type of shock in the newborn. Detailed discussion of the causes and treatment of shock is beyond the scope of this chapter but must be considered when the NNP is faced with a newborn with respiratory distress or depression in the delivery room (Gomella, 2013c).

PULMONARY CAUSES

Looking at the prenatal and antenatal history is important in differentiating pulmonary causes of respiratory distress in the newborn. The NNP would not be as likely to suspect RDS in an infant delivered at 40 weeks gestation by repeat cesarean section (C-section) as he or she would if faced with an infant delivered at 28 weeks gestation by C-section resulting from placental abruption.

Transient Tachypnea of the Newborn

Transient tachypnea of the newborn (TTNB) is a diagnosis of exclusion. When faced with a newborn with unlabored tachypnea, the NNP must establish a differential diagnosis based on the clinical presentation and known history. Risk factors include delivery by C-section

Table 6.2 Clinical Signs of Shock

Tachycardia

Poor/reduced tissue perfusion

Prolonged capillary refill time (> 3–4 seconds)

Respiratory distress

Poor tone

Poor color

Cold extremities (with normal core temperature)

Lethargy

Narrow pulse pressure

Apnea and bradycardia

Tachypnea

Metabolic acidosis

Weak pulses

Source: Gomella (2013e).

without labor, macrosomia, maternal diabetes, multiple gestation, and male gender. TTNB is a common disorder resulting from decreased absorption of fetal lung fluid with resultant pulmonary edema. The etiology is still not fully understood but is thought to be a combination of lack of the mechanical force of the birth canal squeeze and the absence of normal hormonal changes associated with labor and vaginal delivery.

Clinical presentation is consistent, including early onset of respiratory distress with unlabored tachypnea, mildly increased work of breathing, and mild hypoxemia. Chest radiograph reveals increased perihilar interstitial marking with pleural collections of fluid, especially in the horizontal fissures. ABG results often show a mild respiratory acidosis with varying degrees of mild hypoxemia. Respiratory failure requiring mechanical ventilation is rare; however, some infants require supplemental oxygen. As the name suggests, the condition is transient with resolution in all but the most severe cases within 24 to 48 hours.

Meconium Aspiration Syndrome

MAS is the most common aspiration syndrome causing respiratory distress in the newborn. The fetus is capable of expelling intestinal content in the womb in early gestation ending at around 20 weeks gestation when innervation of the anal sphincter occurs. This prohibits the normal passage of meconium between 20 and 34 weeks gestation in most cases. The majority of infants who pass meconium in utero are term or postterm. The etiology of in utero passage of meconium is multifactorial (Crowley, 2015; see Table 6.3 for known risk factors).

MAS occurs when the infant aspirates the meconium-stained amniotic fluid (MSAF) before, during, or after delivery. The respiratory distress exhibited subsequently is diagnosed as MAS if no other factors can explain the symptoms. The NNP should assume MAS, however, and proceed to treat as such until a more definitive diagnosis can be found. Differential diagnoses would include pneumonia, PPHN, CHD, surfactant deficiency, hypoxic encephalopathy, and other pulmonary causes of respiratory distress discussed in this chapter and others.

Diagnosis can be facilitated by clinical history with known MSAF and newborn respiratory distress. Chest radiography demonstrates hyperinflation with course irregular densities. Findings on chest radiography may show a more diffuse picture of decreased aeration with more consistent densities with in utero aspiration. Clinical observation reveals a barrel-shaped chest indicating overinflation with rales audible on auscultation. ABG analysis usually reveals a mixed respiratory and metabolic acidosis with hypoxemia. Respiratory failure requiring mechanical ventilation is common. The NNP should be cognizant of the possibility of development of PPHN (Crowley, 2015; see Table 6.4 for management considerations).

Table 6.3 **Risk Factors for In Utero Passage of Meconium**

Postmaturity (gestational age > 41 weeks)
Small-for-gestational-age status
Fetal distress
Conditions that compromise fetal well-being (placental insufficiency; cord compression)

Source: Crowley (2015).

Other Aspiration Syndromes

The newborn may develop respiratory distress following aspiration of clear (free of meconium) amniotic fluid or maternal blood. The clinical picture can mimic that of MAS but investigation will reveal lack of MSAF. Chest radiography will resemble that of the infant with MAS; the history will help in distinguishing between the two. It is difficult to determine whether the infant has aspirated maternal blood or is experiencing a pulmonary hemorrhage. The NNP can suspect maternal blood aspiration if there is also blood in the stomach with a history of maternal bleeding as with placental abruption (Crowley, 2015). A definitive diagnosis can be assisted by performing the alkali denaturation test (Apt test). This test requires a sample of the blood from the ETT and is more accurate when the specimen is bright red. The specimen remains pink or red in the presence of fetal blood but turns brown in the presence of maternal blood (Gomella, 2013d).

Respiratory Distress Syndrome

RDS is a condition almost always associated with prematurity; however, infants of diabetic mothers or infants who have experienced an asphyxia episode may develop RDS. RDS was formally known as hyaline membrane disease because of the presence of eosinophilic membranes lining the alveolar space on histological exam. Current knowledge of the syndrome implies that RDS is not a separate disease related to the presence of hyaline membranes but is a syndrome of pulmonary surfactant deficiency related to immaturity of the lungs. Fetal pulmonary surfactant is produced by type II alveolar cells, which develop during the latter part of the canalicular phase of lung development. This stage is usually complete at or around 28 weeks gestation. Development of mature lung function continues through gestation and can be altered at any time by premature delivery or other adverse events (Soltau & Carlo, 2014).

Prevention of prematurity is the best method to prevent RDS. Other modalities have been proven to decrease its incidence and severity. Antenatal steroid administration is now

Table 6.4 MAS Management Considerations

Delivery room:

Delivery must occur in a center capable of full resuscitation. Amnioinfusion for MSAF has not been shown to have a benefit in developed countries. Routine oropharyngeal suctioning on the perineum is no longer recommended. Intubation and tracheal suctioning are reserved for the depressed infant.

Neonatal intensive care unit:

Surfactant administration may be beneficial. iNO is indicated for associated PPHN. In facilities in which ECMO is not available, ensure capability to transport with nitric oxide.

Controversial or unresolved issues:

Amnioinfusion for MSAF when routine surveillance is not available as in developing countries. Instillation of pulmonary surfactant as a bolus versus lavage. Administration of anti-inflammatory agents.

ECMO, extracorporeal membrane oxygenation; iNO, inhaled nitric oxide; MAS, meconium aspiration syndrome; MSAF, meconium-stained amniotic fluid; PPHN, persistent pulmonary hypertension of the newborn.
Source: Crowley (2015).

the standard of care for the mother with impending delivery with gestational age between 24 and 34 weeks. After preterm delivery with evidence of RDS, administration of exogenous pulmonary surfactant to the infant requiring endotracheal intubation has been very effective in reducing the incidence of severe disease (Soltau & Carlo, 2014).

The clinical presentation of RDS is difficult to distinguish from many other causes of respiratory distress in the newborn. A history of prematurity leads the NNP to place RDS high on the differential diagnosis list. Ruling out other causes is a priority. Progressive atelectasis with intrapulmonary shunting leads to unventilated areas of the lung and probable hypoxemia. Chest radiograph reveals a characteristic "ground glass" appearance reflective of micro atelectasis with air bronchograms. The NNP should consider group B *Streptococcus* (GBS) pneumonia in the differential diagnosis list, as the two conditions are often indistinguishable by radiograph. ABG analysis is usually consistent with respiratory acidosis with hypoxemia prior to treatment. Treatment is directed toward maintaining functional residual capacity and improving oxygenation. In most cases, CPAP is used to maintain expansion of the alveoli. In the more severe cases, endotracheal intubation with mechanical ventilation is needed (Soltau & Carlo, 2014).

Surfactant B Deficiency

Surfactant protein B (SP-B) deficiency is an autosomal recessive disorder known to cause severe and fatal respiratory disease in term infants. The condition resembles RDS in all ways except gestational age. Recognition and diagnosis of this disorder have significant implications for the parents, as there is a 25% recurrence risk. Management is supportive because these infants do not respond to administration of endogenous pulmonary surfactant, as do infants with RDS (Wilder, 2004).

Pulmonary Air Leaks

Pulmonary air leak syndromes include pneumothorax, pneumomediastinum, pulmonary interstitial emphysema (PIE), pneumopericardium, and less common, pneumoperitoneum and subcutaneous emphysema. Although spontaneous pneumothorax occurs in 1% to 2% of all live births of term infants, pulmonary air leaks are more commonly associated with lung pathology (Crowley, 2015; see Table 6.5).

The underlying pathophysiology of pulmonary air leak syndrome consists of overdistension with subsequent rupture of alveolar sacs leading to dissection of air into extra-alveolar spaces. Air tracks through the perivascular adventitia, causing PIE or the air may dissect along

Table 6.5 Lung Pathology Associated With High Risk for Pulmonary Air Leak

MAS
Pneumonia
RDS
Diaphragmatic hernia
Pulmonary hypoplasia

MAS, meconium aspiration syndrome; RDS, respiratory distress syndrome.
Source: Crowley (2015).

Table 6.6 **Radiographic Findings Related to Pulmonary Air Leaks**

Pneumomediastinum	Classic description = "spinnaker-sail" sign. A lobe or lobes of thymus elevated off the heart.
Pneumothorax	Transillumination may be beneficial in an emergency situation but should not replace the chest x-ray. Air appears in the pleural cavity, which appears hyperlucent and with absence of pulmonary markings. In tension pneumothorax, there will be marked displacement of the mediastinal structures toward the unaffected side.
Pulmonary interstitial emphysema	Linear or cyst-like radiolucencies. May be localized or generalized.
Pneumopericardium	Classic appearance of radiolucent halo completely surrounding the heart. Can be seen in all projections.
Pneumoperitoneum	Presence of free air under the diaphragm. Cross-table lateral decubitus film, in which air collects over the lateral border of the liver, is most helpful.

Source: Solomonia (2013).

vascular sheaths toward the hilum of the lung into the mediastinum. A pneumomediastinum usually precedes development of a pneumothorax. Sudden deterioration in clinical condition, especially when an infant is on mechanical ventilation, should alert the NNP to the possibility of a pulmonary air leak. The NNP may notice a new finding of a barrel-shaped chest with distant heart sounds in cases of pneumomediastinum. When a pneumothorax develops, the infant may suddenly deteriorate with after development of cyanosis and desaturations requiring an increase in supplemental oxygen requirement. The infant may become hypotensive and bradycardic because of the increase in intrathoracic pressure leading to decrease in venous return (Soltau & Carlo, 2014). Definitive diagnosis is made by chest radiograph. Table 6.6 depicts radiograph findings specific to the most common forms of pulmonary air leak.

Management is directed first toward prevention. Attention to distending pressure, positive end-expiratory pressure (PEEP), and inspiratory time (IT) may assist the caregiver in decreasing the incidence of air leak in a given infant. Pneumothorax is the most common air leak and may be asymptomatic. In the term infant with mild symptoms, provision of an oxygen-rich environment may assist in spontaneous resolution. The inspired oxygen facilitates resolution of the pneumothorax by nitrogen washout by establishing a difference in gas tension between the blood in the pulmonary vessels and the free air in the chest. This process usually assists in resolution of the pneumothorax in 1 to 2 hours. In the symptomatic infant, evacuation of the free pleural air by thoracentesis or thoracotomy tube placement may be necessary. Tension pneumothorax is a medical emergency and immediate evacuation of free air is imperative. A pneumomediastinum may be asymptomatic unless accompanied by a significant pneumothorax. The solitary pneumomediastinum usually does not require treatment. Watchful waiting and judicious management of ventilatory settings is necessary for the ventilated infant. PIE is usually a finding in the ventilated premature infant. As with any pulmonary air leak, prevention is the best management. Once PIE is diagnosed, the NNP should attempt to lessen lung trauma by decreasing peak inspiratory pressure (PIP) and PEEP and shortening the IT if possible. In cases of unilateral PIE, positioning the infant with the affected side down has proven beneficial. High-frequency ventilation has been shown to be effective in treating PIE and may help improve survival. More invasive management strategies are reserved for the most severe cases and include surgical resection of the affected lobe. Pneumopericardium can lead to fatal cardiac tamponade. This air leak is a medical emergency and should be treated by placement of a pericardial drain. Even with pericardiocentesis, survival is 75% to 80%. It is rare for a pneumoperitoneum to result from a pulmonary air leak but this can occur. The usual etiology is GI perforation. Management is directed toward the precipitating disorder (Solomonia, 2013).

Pulmonary Hemorrhage

Pulmonary hemorrhage manifests by the presence of blood in tracheal secretions and is rarely an isolated condition. Risk factors include extreme prematurity, surfactant administration, left-to-right shunting through a PDA, multiple birth, male gender, severe systemic illness, coagulopathy, and perinatal asphyxia (Crowley, 2015).

When faced with an infant with blood suctioned from the ETT, the NNP should consider a differential diagnosis, including hemorrhagic pulmonary edema, direct trauma to the airway, aspiration of maternal blood (see aspiration syndromes mentioned earlier), and neonatal coagulopathy. If enough blood is present, checking the hematocrit (Hct) can assist the NNP in narrowing the differential diagnosis. A true pulmonary hemorrhage is suspected if the Hct is close to the infant's venous Hct. The etiology is likely to be trauma, aspiration of maternal blood, or a bleeding diathesis. If the endotracheal blood Hct is 15% to 20% lower than the infant's venous Hct, the NNP can suspect hemorrhagic pulmonary edema. The etiology in this case is more likely to be PDA, surfactant administration, or left-sided heart failure. General management is related to the etiology; however, certain emergency measures will be necessary. Although a controversial measure, endotracheal administration of epinephrine (0.1 mL/kg of 1:10,000) may cause constriction of the pulmonary capillaries and facilitate resolution (Gomella, 2013e; see Table 6.7 for suggested emergency measures).

Table 6.7 **Emergency Measures for Managing Pulmonary Hemorrhage**

Gentle endotracheal tube suctioning	May be necessary every 15 minutes in order to reduce the risk of obstruction of airway.
Supplemental oxygen	Increase in FiO_2 is often necessary to aid in oxygenation.
Mechanical ventilation	Consider mechanical ventilation if not already in use.
Increase mean airway pressure	Increasing PEEP or PIP has the effect of causing tamponade of the pulmonary arteries and may force edema back into the pulmonary bed.

PEEP, positive end-expiratory pressure; PIP, peak inspiratory pressure.
Source: Gomella (2013f).

Case 6.2

Baby boy Blue was delivered at 40 weeks gestation to a 28-year-old G2P1001 female via spontaneous vaginal delivery (SVD) under epidural anesthesia. Maternal prenatal screens and labs were unremarkable with negative group B *Streptococcus* (GBS). (Maternal history obtained after delivery revealed that the mother had taken a baby aspirin each night throughout pregnancy because of a family history of myocardial infarction. She had not revealed this to her obstetrician because she was embarrassed.) Spontaneous rupture of membranes occurred 2 hours prior to delivery with clear amniotic fluid noted. The infant presented with a spontaneous cry with 1-minute Apgar score reported as 8 with 2 points off for color. At 5 minutes, he was still cyanotic with good tone and cry and the Apgar score remained 8. Mild retractions were noted. He was placed on a pulse oximeter and his SpO_2 "oxygen saturation by pulse oximeter" was noted to be 80% in room air. The respiratory therapist (RT) then placed a pulse oximeter probe on his right hand and right foot with a 10% difference noted between the two (the right-hand SpO_2 was 10% higher than the right-foot reading). He was transferred to the neonatal intensive care unit (NICU) with blow-by oxygen at 100% for further evaluation and treatment. Administering supplemental oxygen had no effect on the SpO_2 readings.

1. *Preliminary differential diagnosis list would likely include which of the following?*

   A. Persistent pulmonary hypertension and cyanotic congenital heart disease (CHD)

   B. GBS sepsis and CDH

   C. Respiratory distress syndrome (RDS) and inborn error of metabolism

   ANSWER: A. *Both persistent pulmonary hypertension of the newborn (PPHN) and cyanotic CHD present with cyanosis at birth and should be included in the differential diagnosis (Alpan, 2013; Brodsky & Doherty, 2014b; Soltau & Carlo, 2014). There is no evidence of risk factors for neonatal sepsis with a negative maternal GBS status and rupture of membranes of only 2 hours and there is no evidence of CDH. Although RDS may be seen in term infants, it is too early to have an inborn error of metabolism as a differential at this time.*

2. *An arterial blood gas (ABG) was obtained upon admission to the NICU with the following results: pH 7.22, $PaCO_2$ 48, PaO_2 35, HCO_3 18, and FiO_2 1.0. This ABG demonstrates:*

   A. Metabolic acidosis with hypoxemia

   B. Mixed acidosis with hypoxemia

   C. Respiratory acidosis with hypoxemia

   ANSWER: C. *The first step in ABG interpretation is considering whether acidosis or alkalosis is present. A pH less than 7.25 is considered acidosis. The next step is to consider whether the primary cause is respiratory or metabolic. $PaCO_2$ greater than 45 is considered respiratory in nature. Hypoxemia in the newborn is traditionally identified when the PaO_2 is less than 60, although this varies with gestational age (Soltau & Carlo, 2014).*

3. *What factor(s) can be identified that increased the infant's risk for PPHN?*

   A. Term gestation

   B. Epidural anesthesia given to the mother

   C. Maternal use of aspirin during pregnancy

(continued)

Case 6.2 (continued)

ANSWER: C. *Both term and preterm infants are at risk for PPHN under favorable conditions but gestational age alone is not a risk factor. However, postterm infants may be at increased risk if certain factors are present. There is no evidence that epidural anesthesia given to the mother increases the infant's risk for PPHN. Maternal use of aspirin during gestation is a known risk factor (Dhillon, 2012).*

4. **What is the significance of placing the pulse oximeter probe on the right hand and right foot?**

   A. This ensures that the best area of perfusion is used
   B. This is necessary to obtain a differential between preductal and postductal saturations
   C. This is just the choice of the respiratory therapist

   ANSWER: B. *Determining whether a significant shunt is present requires observing a differential between preductal and postductal oxygen saturations (Alpan, 2013); whereas this may not always be the best area of perfusion. Preference of site has no bearing on the usefulness of this test.*

5. **Which of these steps would best assist the neonatal nurse practitioner in narrowing the differential diagnosis list to a definitive diagnosis?**

   A. Apt test, chest radiogram, and chromosome studies
   B. Chest radiogram, extensive physical exam, and gestational sizing
   C. Thorough maternal history, hyperoxia test, and cardiac echocardiogram

   ANSWER: C. *It is clear that gestational age is not an excluding factor for PPHN and chest radiogram can be misleading so these answers can be excluded (Alpan, 2013).*

CONDITIONS THAT RESULT FROM LATE POSTNATAL EVENTS OR SEQUELAE

PNEUMONIA

Neonatal pneumonia can be classified as early or late pneumonia. The symptoms are the same for early or late pneumonia; the infant presents with respiratory distress, including grunting, nasal flaring, and retractions, often with desaturations requiring supplemental oxygen. Early pneumonia (within the first 3 days) includes congenital pneumonia, which is acquired during late gestation or during labor and delivery. Bacterial, viral, or fungal organisms can cause neonatal pneumonia. The timing of presentation often helps in identification of the organism. Risk factors for early-onset pneumonia include the risk factors for neonatal sepsis; although no risk factors are identified in many cases. Early onset of labor appears to be an important risk factor. The NNP will establish a differential diagnosis for early-onset pneumonia, which will include TTNB, RDS, MAS, and CHD. Radiologic findings are not diagnostic. A high level of suspicion with judicious use of antibiotics after sepsis workup will improve outcome and help to avoid PPHN and possible shock. Tracheal secretion cultures obtained in the first 8 hours are more diagnostic. After that time, colonization begins to

Table 6.8 **Organisms Responsible for Early-Onset Neonatal Pneumonia**

Group B *Streptococcus* (GBS)	Adenovirus
Escherichia coli (E. coli)	Enterovirus
Klebsiella	Mumps
Enterobacter	Rubella
Group A *Streptococcus*	Cytomegalovirus (CMV)
Staphylococcus	Syphilis
Listeria monocytogenes	Toxoplasmosis
Herpes simplex	*Candida*

Source: Crowley (2015).

manifest (Crowley, 2015). Table 6.8 shows the most common organisms causing early-onset pneumonia in the newborn.

Late-onset pneumonia (after 3 days) is usually iatrogenic or hospital acquired and occurs most commonly in the ventilated infant. Late-onset pneumonia is usually a consequence of colonization of the newborn. Table 6.9 lists the most common agents responsible for late-onset neonatal pneumonia. *Chlamydia trachomatis*, as a cause of pneumonia, is acquired during labor but does not manifest as pneumonia until 2 to 4 weeks of life (Crowley, 2015). Whether early or late in onset, neonatal pneumonia may cause significant morbidity and must be treated in a timely manner. The NNP must recognize the symptoms and identify the organism(s) as rapidly as possible. Suspected early-onset pneumonia is usually treated initially with ampicillin and gentamicin. The NNP will pay attention to institutional susceptibility data and may choose to alter this regimen based on these findings. Late-onset neonatal pneumonia is usually treated with empiric therapy consisting of vancomycin and gentamicin. Other drugs are being considered in institutions with known vancomycin-resistant bacteria (Crowley, 2015).

Bronchopulmonary Dysplasia/Chronic Lung Disease

The understanding and definition of bronchopulmonary dysplasia (BPD) has changed over the decades, progressing from a syndrome of severe lung injury in infants receiving long-term mechanical ventilation and high levels of supplemental oxygen to the current theory of the "new BPD" described by Jobe (2006). Clinical diagnosis is currently established at 36

Table 6.9 Organisms Responsible for Late-Onset Neonatal Pneumonia

Staphylococcus species	*Bacillus cereus*
Coagulase-negative staphylococci	*Citrobacter*
Staphylococcus aureus	*Chlamydia trachomatis*
Streptococcus pyogenes	Respiratory syncytial virus (RSV)
Streptococcus pneumoniae	Adenovirus
E. coli	Enterovirus
Klebsiella	Parainfluenza
Serratia	Rhinoviruses
Enterobacter cloacae	Influenza viruses
Pseudomonas	CMV
Candida	

CMV, cytomegalovirus; *E. coli, Escherichia coli.*
Source: Crowley (2015).

weeks postmenstrual age (PMA) and relates to the history of treatment with supplemental oxygen or current treatment with supplemental oxygen and is based less on the pulmonary pathology (see Table 6.10). Treatment modalities have been developed to lessen the effects of mechanical ventilation. These include early use of CPAP, antenatal corticosteroids, exogenous pulmonary surfactant, and improvements in nutrition. These modalities have improved outcome in morbidity and mortality; however, the incidence of BPD in preterm infants has not significantly decreased. The most important factor influencing the continued high incidence of BPD in preterm infants is the increase in survival of extremely low-birth-weight (ELBW) infants. The etiology of the "new BPD" appears to be different, with factors other than mechanical ventilation and oxygen exposure making the most important contribution. These factors include antenatal chorioamnionitis, neonatal sepsis, and PDA (Jobe, 2006).

Long-term outcome remains a major concern for all ELBW infants, even those who have not been diagnosed with BPD. According to Jobe (2006), all ELBW infants have developmental or maturational abnormalities of the lungs. It appears that the ELBW infant with the "new BPD" has the common restrictive airway disease of extreme prematurity as well as remodeling of alveoli and microvascularity. We still have much to learn as these smaller and more immature infants are resuscitated and treated in the NICU (Jobe, 2006).

Table 6.10 **Definitions for Mild, Moderate, and Severe BPD**

New BPD	Treatment With Supplemental Oxygen for 21 days and . . .
Mild BPD	Breathing room air at 36 weeks PMA or discharge
Moderate BPD	< 30% oxygen at 36 weeks PMA or discharge
Severe BPD	> 30% oxygen and/or positive pressure (mechanical ventilation or CPAP) at 36 weeks PMA

BPD, bronchopulmonary dysplasia; CPAP, continuous positive airway pressure; PMA, postmenstrual age.
Source: Jobe (2006).

Case 6.3

Baby boy B is a 3-month-old Caucasian male who was delivered by emergency C-section under general anesthesia to a 21-year-old gravida 1 Caucasian female at 23 weeks gestation because of severe maternal preeclampsia with proteinuria. A fetal monitor at admission revealed the fetal heart rate to be 160 beats per minute with little variability. The mother had received early prenatal care but she had not attended all of her appointments because of a lack of transportation. Maternal prenatal labs were negative with unknown group B *Streptococcus* (GBS) status. The mother stated that she had only taken prenatal vitamins during her pregnancy. She had been healthy and "felt good after the first few weeks" except for a recent "bout" with headache that had been getting progressively worse. Ms. B phoned her obstetrician (OB) because of the intensity of the headache and he directed her to go to the hospital for evaluation. Her blood pressure (BP) was 180/110 mmHg on admission to the labor and delivery unit. Membranes were ruptured at delivery with clear amniotic fluid noted. His birth weight was 480 g.

1. *Which prenatal factors in the preceding case information increased the infant's risk(s) for developing bronchopulmonary dysplasia (BPD)?*

(continued)

Case 6.3 *(continued)*

A. Extreme prematurity
B. Female gender
C. Maternal preeclampsia

ANSWER: A. *Extreme prematurity is a known risk factor for BPD (Jobe, 2006). Although maternal preeclampsia, in itself, may not be a direct risk factor, this often leads to a need for early delivery for maternal health. Female gender is not associated with an increased risk for respiratory distress syndrome or BPD.*

The infant required intubation and mechanical ventilation upon delivery because of poor color and tone with decreased respiratory effort. Transport conventional mechanical ventilation settings were as follows: synchronized intermittent mechanical ventilation (SIMV) 40, peak inspiratory pressure 18, positive end-expiratory pressure +4, and FiO$_2$ 0.60 (adjusted to keep SpO$_2$ 88%–92%).

Hospital Course
Rule out sepsis:
　　Admission labs: Complete blood count: white blood cell 5.9, Hgb 13.5, Hct 39.7, platelets 102K, polys 54, bands 7, metas 1, myelos 1

- #1 Admission blood culture (BC) × 2 as well as endotracheal tube (ETT) secretion cultures were negative at 48 and 72 hours. Baby B was watched expectantly and did not receive antibiotics at admission.
- #2 ETT secretion cultures obtained at 2 weeks of age were positive for Ureaplasma and the infant received 10 days treatment with IV erythromycin.
- #3 Baby B required a sepsis workup twice during hospitalization (once for increased apnea and bradycardia and once for feeding intolerance) with antibiotic therapy each time for 48 hours each. BC, cerebrospinal fluid (CSF) cultures, and urine cultures were negative each time. Vancomycin and Claforan were given for each episode.

　　Respiratory course:
　　Baby B required high-frequency oscillatory ventilation (HFOV) soon after admission to the neonatal intensive care unit as a result of deterioration of respiratory acidosis and inability to oxygenate adequately on maximum conventional ventilator settings. His highest settings were as follows: Amp 40, mean airway pressure (MAP) 14, Hz 12, and FiO$_2$ 1.0. He was weaned to conventional mechanical ventilation at 3 weeks of age but remained intubated and on conventional mechanical ventilation for another month—with two brief attempts to wean to nasal intermittent mandatory ventilation (NIMV). Baby B was successfully weaned to NIMV at 7 weeks of age. On hospital day (HD) #60, he was weaned to high-flow nasal cannula (HFNC) at 2 L/min with FiO$_2$ 0.27 to 0.35. Over the next 30 days, he was weaned to HFNC 1 L/min and, at the time of this case study, he is comfortable in room air except when bottle-feeding. His capillary blood gas this morning is as follows: pH 7.30, PCO$_2$ 59.3, PO$_2$ 32, HCO$_3$ 29.9.

(continued)

Case 6.3 (continued)

2. **Which of the following descriptions best describes the capillary blood gas referred to previously?**

   A. Mild metabolic alkalosis, which is normal for this infant
   B. Mild respiratory acidosis, which is normal for this infant
   C. Severe respiratory acidosis requiring intubation and ventilation

   ANSWER: B. *Although a pH of 7.29 is not generally considered acidosis, it is low for an infant of this age without this diagnosis. The PaCO2 of 59.3, together with the HCO3 of 29.9, indicates a respiratory component (Soltau & Carlo, 2014).*

Cardiovascular:

Baby B was noted to have a continuous, machinery-like murmur with a hyperactive precordium on HD #3. Although he was on HFOV, his BP and oxygenation status were stable. A moderate patent ductus arteriosus (PDA) was diagnosed by a two-dimensional (2D) echocardiogram (cardiac 2D echo). Radiographic findings at 2 weeks of age included increased pulmonary vascularity and cardiomegaly and he was treated with three separate doses of indomethacin. Serial cardiac 2D echo exams continued to demonstrate presence of the PDA (smaller) and the decision was made to treat conservatively with fluid restriction at that time. The ductus arteriosus closed at the time of this case study without further treatment.

3. **Which of the following postnatal factors place the infant at a higher risk for BPD?**

   A. Administration of antibiotics and PDA
   B. Apnea and bradycardia with feeding intolerance
   C. Long-term mechanical ventilation

   ANSWER: C. *Long-term mechanical ventilation has historically been associated with development of BPD. New treatment modalities are available that may lessen the effects (Jobe, 2006). There is evidence that a hemodynamically significant PDA, as well as sepsis, may contribute but the use of antibiotics alone is not associated. Apnea and bradycardia may lead to episodes of hypoxia but feeding intolerance is not known to be a risk factor.*

Medications:

Baby B received three doses of surfactant during the first 2 days of life. See "rule out sepsis" problem mentioned previously for antibiotics; see cardiovascular problem mentioned previously for Indocin. He received Celestone intramuscularly twice at 7 days of age and a short course of Decadron at 6 weeks of age.

Current Medications:

Chlorothiazide
Albuterol
Beclomethasone
Caffeine
NaCl 2 mEq/kg/d and KCl 1 mEq/kg/d supplements orogastric

CONCLUSIONS

Respiratory distress in the neonate almost universally presents as grunting, nasal flaring, and retractions with some degree of supplemental oxygen required. There is no universal treatment that is appropriate for all infants in all situations. In order to manage these infants successfully, the NNP must be able to determine the etiology and most successful treatment options. In order to do this, the NNP should establish a differential diagnosis and apply appropriate methods to narrow the list to a definitive diagnosis. The author has presented the most common conditions seen in the NICU and likely differentials. Use of current and evidence-based literature assists in improving the survival and outcome for these fragile infants.

REFERENCES

Abbassi-Ghanavati, M., Alexander, J. M., McIntire, D. D., Savani, R. C., & Leveno, K. J. (2012). Neonatal effects of magnesium sulfate given to the mother. *Journal of Perinatology, 29*, 795–800. Retrieved from https://www.thieme-connect.com/products/ejournals/pdf/10.1055/s-0032-1316440.pdf

Acevedo, J. L., Shan, R. K., Neville, H. L., Windle, M. L., McClay, J. E., Petry, P. D., . . . Poole, M. D. (2015). Cystic hygroma. Retrieved from http://emedicine.medscape.com/article/994055-overview#a0101

Alpan, G. (2013). Persistent pulmonary hypertension of the newborn. In T. L. Gomella, M. D. Cunningham, F. G. Eyal, & D. J. Tuttle (Eds.), *Neonatology: Management, procedures, on-call problems, diseases, and drugs* (7th ed., pp. 815–822). New York, NY: McGraw-Hill.

Bagwell, G. (2014). Resuscitation and stabilization of the newborn and infant. In C. Kenner, & J. W. Lott (Eds.), *Comprehensive neonatal nursing care* (5th ed., pp. 55–70). New York, NY: Springer Publishing.

Bertholdt, C., Perdriolle-Galet, E., Bach-Segura, P., & Morel, O. (2015, January). Tracheal agenesis: A challenging perinatal diagnosis—Contribution of fetal MRI. *Case Reports in Obstetrics and Gynecology, 2015*, 1–3.

Brodsky, D., & Doherty, E. G. (2014a). *Neonatology: Case-based review* (pp. 28–50). Philadelphia, PA: Wolters Kluwer.

Brodsky, D., & Doherty, E. G. (2014b). *Neonatology: Case-based review* (pp. 65–66). Philadelphia, PA: Wolters Kluwer.

Chin, T. W. (2014). Pediatric pulmonary hypoplasia. Retrieved from http://emedicine.medscape.com/article/1005696-overview

Crowley, M. A. (2015). Neonatal respiratory disorders. In R. J. Martin, A. A. Fanaroff, & M. C. Walsh (Eds.), *Fanaroff and Martin's neonatal-perinatal medicine: Diseases of the fetus and infant* (10th ed., pp. 1113–1136). Philadelphia, PA: Saunders.

Dhillon, R. (2012). The management of neonatal pulmonary hypertension. *Archives of Disease in Childhood—Fetal and Neonatal Edition, 97*, F223–F228. http://dx.doi.org/10.1136/adc.2009.180091

DiPrima, F. A., Bellia, A., Inclimona, G., Grasso, F., Meli, M. T., & Cassaro, N. (2012). Antenatally diagnosed congenital cystic adenomatoid malformations. *Journal of Prenatal Medicine, 6*(2), 22–30. Retrieved from http://www.ncbi.nlm.nih.gov/pmc/articles/PMC3421952/pdf/pag_22-30_prenatl_2_2012.pdf

Farrell, J. A. (2014). Fetal therapy. In C. Kenner & J. W. Lott (Eds.), *Comprehensive neonatal nursing care* (5th ed., pp. 587–607). New York, NY: Springer Publishing.

Finder, N. D. (2016). Bronchomalacia and tracheomalacia. In R. M. Kliegman, B. F. Stanton, J. W. St Geme, & N. F. Schor (Eds.), *Nelson textbook of pediatrics* (20th ed., pp. 2042–2043). Philadelphia, PA: Elsevier.

Gomella, T. L. (2013a). Newborn physical examination. In T. L. Gomella, M. D. Cunningham, F. G. Eyal, & D. J. Tuttle (Eds.), *Neonatology: Management, procedures, on-call problems, diseases and drugs* (7th ed., pp. 43–65). New York, NY: McGraw-Hill.

Gomella, T. L. (2013b). Cyanosis. In T. L. Gomella, M. D. Cunningham, F. G. Eyal, & D. J. Tuttle (Eds.), *Neonatology: Management, procedures, on-call problems, diseases, and drugs* (7th ed., pp. 361–368). New York, NY: McGraw-Hill.

Gomella, T. L. (2013c). Abnormal blood gas. In T. L. Gomella, M. D. Cunningham, F. G. Eyal, & D. J. Tuttle (Eds.), *Neonatology: Management, procedures, on-call problems, and drugs* (7th ed., pp. 325–332). New York, NY: McGraw-Hill.

Gomella, T. L. (2013d). Gastrointestinal bleeding from the upper tract. In T. L. Gomella, M. D. Cunningham, F. G. Eyal, & D. J. Tuttle (Eds.), *Neonatology: Management, procedures, on-call problems, and drugs* (7th ed., pp. 385–390). New York, NY: McGraw-Hill.

Gomella, T. L. (2013e). Hypotension and shock. In T. L. Gomella, M. D. Cunningham, F. G. Eyal, & D. J. Tuttle (Eds.), *Neonatology: Management, procedures, on-call problems, diseases, and drugs* (7th ed., pp. 445–455). New York, NY: McGraw-Hill.

Gomella, T. L. (2013f). Pulmonary hemorrhage. In T. L. Gomella, M. D. Cunningham, F. G. Eyan, & D. J. Tuttle (Eds.), *Neonatology: Management, procedures, on-call problems, diseases, and drugs* (7th ed., pp. 501–506). New York, NY: McGraw-Hill.

Halterman, S. M., Igulada, K. N., & Steinicki, E. J. (2006, March). Epignathus: Large obstructive teratoma arising from the palate. *Cleft Palate-Craniofacial Journal, 43,* 244–246.

Inayat, M. (2013). Magnesium disorders. In T. L. Gomella, M. D. Cunningham, F. G. Eyal, & D. J. Tuttle (Eds.), *Neonatology: Management, procedures, on-call problems, diseases, and drugs* (7th ed., pp. 746–748). New York, NY: McGraw-Hill.

Iocono, J. A. (2013). Surgical diseases of the newborn: Diseases of the airway, tracheobronchial tree, and lungs. In T. L. Gomella, M. D. Cunningham, F. G. Eyal, & D. J. Tuttle (Eds.), *Neonatology: Management, procedures, on-call problems, diseases, and drugs* (7th ed., pp. 885–890). New York, NY: McGraw-Hill.

Jobe, A. H. (2006, October). The new BPD. *NeoReviews, 7,* 531–544. http://dx.doi.org/10.1542/neo.7-10-e531

Katwinkel, J. (Ed.). (2011). *Textbook of neonatal resuscitation* (6th ed.). Elk Grove Village, IL: American Academy of Pediatrics and American Heart Association.

Katwinkel, J., Perlman, J. M., Aziz, K., Colby, C., Fairchild, K., Gallagher, J., . . . Zaichkin, J. (2010). Part 15: Neonatal resuscitation: 2010 American Heart Association guidelines for cardiopulmonary resuscitation and emergency cardiovascular care. *Circulation, 122,* s909–s919. http://dx.doi.org/10.1542/peds.2010-2972E

Lott, J. W. (2014). Cardiovascular system. In C. Kenner & J. W. Lott (Eds.), *Comprehensive neonatal nursing care* (5th ed., pp. 152–188). New York, NY: Springer Publishing.

Montrowl, S. J. (2014). Gastrointestinal system. In C. Kenner & J. W. Lott (Eds.), *Comprehensive neonatal nursing care* (5th ed., pp. 189–228). New York, NY: Springer Publishing.

Napolitano, N., & Stoller, J. (2015, July 30). PPHN: New evidence-based approaches. *eNeonatal Review.* Retrieved from http://eneonatalreview.org/newsletters/2015/volume10_issue10.pdf

Parker, L. (2014). Genitourinary system. In C. Kenner & J. W. Lott (Eds.), *Comprehensive neonatal nursing care* (5th ed., pp. 473–507). New York, NY: Springer Publishing.

Solomonia, N. (2013). Air leak syndromes. In T. L. Gomella, M. D. Cunningham, F. G. Eyal, & D. J. Tuttle (Eds.), *Neonatology: Management, procedures, on-call problems, diseases and drugs* (7th ed., pp. 549–557). New York, NY: McGraw-Hill.

Soltau, T. D., & Carlo, W. A. (2014). Respiratory system. In C. Kenner & J. W. Lott (Eds.), *Comprehensive neonatal nursing care* (5th ed., pp. 133–151). New York, NY: Springer Publishing.

Stokowski, L. A. (2011). Endocrine system. In C. Kenner & J. W. Lott (Eds.), *Comprehensive neonatal nursing care* (5th ed., pp. 253–277). New York, NY: Springer Publishing.

Wilder, M. A. (2004). Surfactant protein B deficiency in infants with respiratory failure. *Journal of Perinatal and Neonatal Nursing, 18*(1), 61–67. Retrieved from http://web.a.ebscohost.com.ezproxy3.lhl.uab.edu/ehost/pdfviewer/pdfviewer?vid=2&sid=3c1b4aa6-f83e-4f57-ad20-499518e16040%40sessionmgr4005&hid=4104

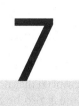

7

Cardiovascular System Cases

Lyn Vargo and Daphne A. Reavey

Chapter Objectives

1. Apply key principles of cardiac physiology to unique neonatal cardiac anatomy and physiology
2. Identify fetal circulation pathways/principles and changes that occur in transitional circulation and understand the effect of these fetal pathways/principles and changes on congenital heart disease (CHD) in the neonate
3. Recognize typical signs/symptoms of CHD in neonates: congestive heart failure (CHF) and cyanosis
4. Identify those cardiac defects that present with cyanosis, including patterns of presentation and management of these defects
5. Identify those cardiac defects that present with acyanosis, including patterns of presentation and management of these defects
6. Identify rhythm disturbances in neonates, including their causes and treatments
7. Formulate a differential diagnosis for an infant presenting with signs and symptoms of CHD
8. Integrate differential diagnostic approaches and appropriate diagnostic studies and management plans for infants presenting with signs/symptoms of different congenital heart defects

The fetal and neonatal cardiac system and regulation of cardiac physiology are unique because of developmental changes found within the system and the fetal shunts that allow the placenta to function as the fetal lung in utero (thus bypassing the fetal lungs). Unique features also include those changes that must occur for successful transition of the circulation at birth from parallel circuitry to a series circulation that provides decreased pulmonary vascular resistance (and increased pulmonary blood flow), increased systemic vascular resistance, and closure of the fetal shunts.

CHD may affect infants before birth, just after birth, or in the weeks and months after birth. It is imperative that practitioners understand neonatal cardiac physiology, normal fetal and neonatal circulation patterns, the cardiac defects and pathologic changes that can alter these patterns and be able to apply this knowledge in developing differential diagnoses and subsequent management plans for infants with CHD. Practitioners must also be able to recognize signs and symptoms of neonatal CHF and rhythm disturbances and integrate that knowledge into care and management.

NEONATAL CARDIAC PHYSIOLOGY

Although fetal and neonatal cardiac output (CO) follow the basic physiologic equation of CO = stroke volume (SV) times heart rate (HR), neonatal cardiac muscle is developmentally immature and because of this does not function the same as the cardiac muscle of children and adults. Unique features of fetal and neonatal CO and neonatal myocardium include:

1. The immature myocardium of both term and preterm infants has fewer contractile units, less well-developed sarcoplasmic reticulum, greater surface/volume ratio, and higher water content (Anderson, 1996).

2. These differences yield increased stiffness and impaired relaxation of the fetal/neonatal heart (Strainic & Snyder, 2015).

3. The three components of SV (preload, afterload, and contractility) are all affected by immature myocardium.

4. Preload and the ability of the heart to pump all blood that enters it within physiologic limits is limited in neonates because of the decreased number of contractile units and the fetal and neonatal heart's inability to stretch sufficiently.

5. Neonatal hearts have a higher baseline contractile state and contractility will rapidly decrease when afterload increases (Noori, Stavroudis, & Seri, 2012).

6. CO is regulated primarily by increases in HR in the neonate and CO will fall dramatically if HR is either too slow or too fast to allow proper filling (Hines, 2013).

7. CO in newborns just after birth is functioning at the high end of the CO curve and there is little reserve to improve CO by increasing SV.

8. The right ventricle predominates in the fetus because it handles more volume than the left ventricle in utero. This causes hypertrophy of the right ventricle in utero and right and left ventricular wall thicknesses are equal as a result (Strainic & Snyder, 2015).

9. Passive filling of the ventricles (especially the right ventricle in the right-ventricle-predominant fetus) is impaired and thus the right ventricle will show signs of dysfunction if preload exceeds physiologic normal volumes as seen in conditions such as atrioventricular (AV) malformations and fetal anemia (Strainic & Snyder, 2015).

All of these differences must be taken into consideration when a neonate presents with issues related to the cardiovascular system as they will significantly affect the newborn's ability to respond hemodynamically.

FETAL CIRCULATION

Fetal circulation is also very unique compared to circulation in children and adults. Most of our knowledge of this circulation comes from fetal lambs. The lungs do not function within the fetus. Instead, the placenta functions as the fetal lung and oxygen and carbon dioxide exchange takes place within the placenta. The fetus's circulation is described as a "parallel circulation" in which both ventricles provide differing volumes of oxygenated blood to different parts of the body as opposed to postnatal and adult circulation, which is considered a "series circulation" because right and left ventricular outputs are generally equal and oxygenated blood is pumped to the organs by the left ventricle only. Because of this, fetal CO is referred to as combined ventricular output (CVO). In the fetus, the left ventricle provides approximately one third of the CVO (with a higher PaO_2) to the upper extremities, brain, and heart, whereas the right ventricle provides approximately two thirds of the CVO to the lungs, lower extremities, and placenta (Brown & Fulton, 2011).

Fetal circulation is possible because of three fetal shunts. These include (a) the ductus venosus (DV), which connects the single umbilical vein to the inferior vena cava (IVC) and allows approximately 50% of the most oxygenated blood from the placenta to bypass the liver and be directed to the right atrium of the fetal heart instead (Moore, Persaud, & Torchia, 2013); (b) the foramen ovale (FO), which is an opening in the atrial wall of the fetus, allows about one third of the blood that has entered the right atrium from the placenta via the IVC (with a higher PaO_2) to be preferentially shunted from the right atrium to the left atrium by the crista dividens, where it is directed through the left ventricle and then to the ascending aorta, the coronary arteries, innominate artery (which branches into the right subclavian artery and right carotid artery), the left carotid artery, and usually the left subclavian artery for oxygenation of the fetus; and (c) the patent ductus arteriosus (PDA), which is a large vessel capable of contraction that connects the pulmonary artery of the fetus to the descending aorta of the fetus (usually just beyond the left subclavian artery). The PDA permits blood coming from the right ventricle (with a lower PaO_2 because it is mixed, desaturated blood from both the IVC and the superior vena cava) to enter the pulmonary artery where it is shunted away from the fetal lungs. Because of the high pulmonary vascular resistance in the lungs only about 10% of CVO from the right ventricle perfuses the lung for growth and development only (Moore et al., 2013). The remainder of the blood coming from the right ventricle (which represents about two thirds of the CVO) shunts across the PDA in a right-to-left direction from the pulmonary artery to the descending aorta (usually just beyond the left subclavian artery), where it perfuses the lower half of the body and then flows back to the low-resistance placenta (via the two umbilical arteries) for oxygen and carbon dioxide exchange (Figure 7.1).

CIRCULATORY CHANGES AT BIRTH

At birth there are several changes that must take place to convert the parallel fetal circulation into the series circulation of the neonate. The events that must occur are the removal of the placenta and expansion of the lungs with the first breath. Removal of the placenta causes decreased blood flow through the umbilical vein, DV, IVC, and thus decreased blood flow into the right atrium. Thus, blood flow and pressure to the right side of the heart decrease. Removal of the low-resistance placenta also concurrently increases systemic vascular resistance. Ventilation and the first breath of the newborn in an oxygen-rich environment and other mechanical factors promote decreased pulmonary vascular resistance and pulmonary vasodilation. Thus, blood flow to the lungs is increased and subsequently blood flow to the left atrium is also increased. When left atrial pressure exceeds right atrial pressure, the flap

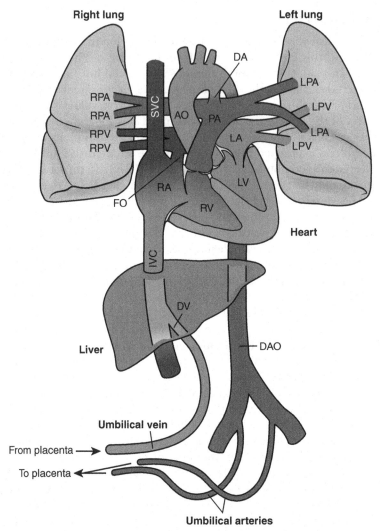

Figure 7.1   Fetal Circulation

AO, aorta; DA, ductus arteriosus; DAO, descending aorta; DV, ductus venosus; FO, foramen ovale; IVC, interior vena cava; LA, left atrium; LPA, left pulmonary artery; LPV, left pulmonary vein; LV, left ventricle; PA, pulmonary artery; RA, right atrium; RPA, right pulmonary artery; RPV, right pulmonary vein; RV, right ventricle; SVC, superior vena cava.

of the FO will functionally close. However, any situation in which right atrial pressure exceeds left atrial pressure can cause the FO to reopen. Although the exact mechanism for closure of the PDA is not known, an increased oxygen environment plays a primary role in promoting active constriction of the PDA after birth. Complete closure of the PDA is a gradual process that generally occurs in the healthy term newborn within the first 48 to 72 hours of life, allowing a small amount of shunting between the aorta and the pulmonary artery during that time.

In infants with persistent hypoxia and in premature infants, the ductus may stay open much longer. In addition, closure of the PDA after birth can be life-threatening for infants with cardiac defects who rely on it remaining open postnatally to provide either blood flow to the lungs (with defects in which blood flow to the lungs is restricted or obstructed) or blood flow to the systemic circulation (when blood flow from the left heart is restricted or obstructed as in critical aortic stenosis or coarctation of the aorta). In those cases, the use of prostaglandin E_1 (PGE_1) via a continuous infusion is necessary to maintain ductal flow.

By the end of the first month of life, the right-sided predominance of the fetal heart (the right ventricle thins) gradually changes to left-sided predominance (the left ventricle thickens) as pulmonary vascular resistance continues to fall and systemic vascular resistance continues to increase (Moore et al., 2013). Pulmonary vascular resistance falls to half of systemic levels within 1 to 2 days but continues to fall over the next several weeks of life, reaching adult levels at about 2 to 6 weeks of age (Brown & Fulton, 2011).

CONGESTIVE HEART FAILURE

The inability of the heart to pump enough blood to meet the metabolic needs of the body is called congestive heart failure. CHF can be the result of many etiologies during the neonatal period, including anemia, birth asphyxia, sepsis, and congenital arteriovenous malformations as well as congenital heart defects. It can present acutely with cardiorespiratory collapse such as in infants with hypoplastic left heart syndrome (HLHS) or other obstructive type defects (Swanson & Erickson, 2016). More commonly, it presents subtly with gradually worsening signs as the CHF worsens.

PRESENTATION

The clinical presentation of CHF represents evidence of decreased CO and decreased tissue perfusion. Because of the neonate's limited ability to increase SV as reviewed earlier, an increase in HR or tachycardia occurs in response to the heart's attempt to increase CO. In addition to CHF, there can be other etiologies for tachycardia in the neonate, including hyperthermia and supraventricular tachycardia (SVT), so careful evaluation is necessary prior to diagnosis of CHF based on HR alone. Cardiomegaly in response to increased pressure or volume overload is another sign of CHF that can be evident on chest radiograph (Park, 2014; Swanson & Erickson, 2016). Other signs of decreased CO and decreased tissue perfusion include decreased or weak peripheral pulses, delayed capillary refill, hypotension, and oliguria. Hepatic venous congestion in the form of hepatomegaly is another classic sign of CHF in the neonate. Tachypnea and increased work of breathing, including retractions, nasal flaring, and head bobbing, are associated signs of respiratory distress noted with CHF. The signs of respiratory distress are related to the increased blood flow to the lungs or an inability of the lungs to drain blood flow adequately. Dyspnea and fatigue, especially with feeding and activity, are also associated with CHF.

MANAGEMENT

It is important to initially evaluate and identify the etiology of the CHF so that proper management can be delineated. In infants who present with CHF and are diagnosed with a ductal dependent lesion, it is critical that a continuous infusion of PGE_1 be initiated. Preload may be augmented with small amounts of fluid boluses and inotropic support may be required to maintain adequate blood pressure and improve contractility.

Other medications that may be helpful in the medical management of CHF include digoxin and diuretic therapy. The digoxin can improve contractility of the heart and diuretic therapy, such as furosemide, decreases pulmonary edema. Other agents that decrease afterload, such as milrinone, captopril, and enalapril, may also be used. The combined use of diuretic therapy, inotropic support, and an afterload reducer may offer more improvement in symptoms than using a single therapy (Park, 2014). The overarching goal in treatment is to maintain a balance between blood flow in the pulmonary system and blood flow in the systemic circulation.

ACYANOTIC DEFECTS

Congenital heart defects that present with signs of no or mild respiratory distress and without evidence of cyanosis are grouped into the category of acyanotic defects. These defects include PDA, ventricular septal defect (VSD), and AV septal defects (AV canals). Coarctation of the aorta, critical aortic stenosis, and HLHS also present without cyanosis so they can be considered an acyanotic defect but they may also have a significant component of hypoperfusion. Acyanotic defects may or may not present with a murmur and either have no effect or cause mild signs of respiratory distress. In some cases, the murmur may present early after birth or later in the first several weeks of life after the pulmonary vascular resistance begins to fall. As the pulmonary vascular resistance falls, increased blood flow occurs across the heart defect from the higher pressured left side of the heart to the lower pressured right side of the heart, which results in more turbulent blood flow and a murmur. The fall in vascular resistance is also responsible for the signs of worsening respiratory distress. The fall in vascular resistance increases the blood flow through the defect resulting in volume overload and increased pulmonary blood flow. The increased blood flow can result in tachypnea and mildly decreased oxygen saturations. Left untreated, symptoms can worsen over time as the pulmonary resistance falls, resulting in worsening pulmonary edema and CHF.

Patent Ductus Arteriosus

The ductus arteriosus (DA), a blood vessel connecting the pulmonary artery to the aorta, is normally open in fetal life. Because the placenta supplies the required oxygen to the fetus, there is minimal need for blood flow through the fetal lungs. Because of the elevated vascular resistance in the fetal lungs, the DA shunts approximately 90% of blood flow from right to left or from the pulmonary artery to the descending aorta thereby bypassing the lungs. Following birth and the removal of the placenta, there is a rapid decrease in the pulmonary resistance with increased pulmonary blood flow. These changes cause blood flow to quickly reverse in the DA resulting in left-to-right blood flow. Once the infant is born, the DA constricts following the increase in arterial oxygen tension. Closure of the DA generally occurs within 48 to 72 hours of life in term, healthy newborns.

If the DA remains patent beyond a few days postnatally, increased left-to-right flow through the PDA occurs as pulmonary vascular resistance further declines. An increase in the left-to-right flow across the PDA results in higher blood flow to the lungs and pulmonary edema. Continuing pulmonary edema results in an increased workload on the left side of the heart. The increased workload can lead to enlargement of both the left atrium and ventricle. Along with the left atrial and ventricular enlargement, increased left-to-right shunting also decreases systemic CO, which potentially can affect blood flow and perfusion to multiple organs, including the kidneys, intestines, and brain.

Clinical Presentation

Signs of a PDA in neonates include a continuous or systolic murmur usually heard at the left upper sternal border (Park, 2014), bounding pulses, palpable palmar pulses, an active precordial impulse or hyperdynamic precordium, and widened pulse pressures. A murmur may not be audible in a large PDA with unrestricted blood flow. Other evidence raising the concern of a symptomatic PDA may include worsening respiratory status and/or increased ventilator requirements. A chest x-ray (CXR) may reveal cardiomegaly, increased pulmonary markings, and pulmonary edema.

Confirmatory diagnosis of a PDA is made by color Doppler echocardiogram. Moderate to large shunts have been characterized by ductal diameter greater than or equal to 1.5 mm, increased ratio of left atrial to aortic root diameter (LA:Ao) of greater than or equal to 1.5 mm, increased diastolic flow velocity in the left pulmonary artery greater than 0.2/ms, and reduced or reversed diastolic flow in the descending aorta (Chen, Tacy, & Clyman, 2010, p. 781; Clyman, 2012). Left ventricular distention has also been described.

Management

Definitive closure of a PDA can be achieved by surgical ligation. Although surgical ligation can permanently reverse the left-to-right shunt via the PDA, it may also initially worsen left ventricular function subsequently requiring escalation of ventilator support and inotropic gtts postoperatively (Teixeira, Shivananda, Stephens, Van Arsdell, & McNamara, 2008). Other complications can include pneumothorax, chylothorax, thoracotomy, and scoliosis (Hutchings et al., 2013; Noori, 2012; Roclawski et al., 2009). Left vocal cord paralysis has also been reported in 40% to 67% of extremely low-birth-weight (ELBW) infants undergoing PDA ligation (Benjamin et al., 2010; Clement, El-Hakim, Phillipos, & Cote, 2008). Potential complications associated with left vocal cord paralysis include bronchopulmonary dysplasia (BPD), reactive airway disease, or need for a gastrostomy tube because of feeding difficulties (Benjamin et al., 2010).

Pharmacologic treatment to close a PDA has also been well described. The two medications primarily used are indomethacin and ibuprofen. Both are cyclooxygenase inhibitors and work by inducing constriction and closure of the PDA. Both indomethacin and ibuprofen have been shown to be effective at closing the PDA. Adverse effects of both medications include renal dysfunction although a meta-analysis suggested that ibuprofen causes less renal dysfunction than indomethacin (Ohlsson, Walia, & Shah, 2013). Urine output and creatinine levels should be monitored closely when using both medications. Indomethacin has also been shown to decrease cerebral blood flow (Austin, Pairaudeau, Hames, & Hall, 1992) but prophylactic indomethacin has also been shown to decrease the rate of severe (grades III and IV) intraventricular hemorrhage (IVH) (Fowlie, Davis & McGuire, 2010), although no differences in neurodevelopmental outcomes were noted at 18 months of age (Fowlie et al., 2010; Schmidt et al., 2001). More recent, paracetamol, or acetaminophen, has also been suggested as a treatment for PDA. Although oral paracetamol has been shown to be as effective as oral ibuprofen in closing the PDA (Oncel et al., 2014), more research is needed before it can be routinely recommended for this indication.

Although multiple studies have shown an association with prolonged patency of the DA and complications, including necrotizing enterocolitis (NEC), BPD, and IVH, there have been no randomized controlled studies to date that showed a clear cause-and-effect relationship between the two. Recent studies have shown spontaneous closure of a PDA to be quite high even in preterm infants, especially those born at 30 weeks gestation or greater (Clyman, Couto, & Murphy, 2012). Because of these recent studies, controversy exists as to whether a PDA should be routinely treated. Experts now suggest supportive management, including modest fluid restriction, diuretic therapy, increased continuous distending pressure (or PEEP [positive end-expiratory pressure]), and possible use of medications to reduce afterload while awaiting spontaneous closure of the PDA (Benitz, 2010, 2015), especially in those infants greater than or equal to 28 weeks gestation. More research is needed, especially in the ELBW infant, to evaluate which neonates would benefit from pharmacologic or surgical ligation for a PDA.

VENTRICULAR SEPTAL DEFECTS

VSDs are openings or defects within the wall or septum separating the right and left ventricles. VSDs can occur anywhere along the septum and are usually classified as inlet, muscular, perimembranous, and outlet VSDs. The size of the defect and the balance or ratio of systemic to pulmonary resistance are the primary factors that determine the degree, if any, of left-to-right shunting and CHF. Small defects will naturally restrict any significant left-to-right flow, whereas larger defects (generally greater than the aortic valve diameter) will not restrict blood flow from the left to the right ventricle. Small defects generally do not have any clinical importance, whereas larger defects can be problematic with development of CHF.

Clinical Presentation

The presenting sign of a VSD is generally a holosystolic, harsh murmur but it is not unusual for the murmur to be absent until several weeks of life. Because of the initial high pulmonary vascular resistance, there is minimal or no shunt across the defect. That changes as the pulmonary vascular resistance falls over the first few days to weeks of life. As the pulmonary vascular resistance falls, there is increased blood flow and turbulence across the defect, resulting in an audible murmur. Increasing pulmonary blood flow also occurs as pulmonary vascular resistance falls, which may result in CHF with large defects. Chest radiographs should be evaluated for heart size as well as pulmonary vascular markings. Worsening pulmonary edema secondary to falling pulmonary vascular resistance can be monitored by serial chest radiographs. Echocardiography is the diagnostic tool used to confirm the presence and size of a VSD but can also be used to determine whether there are other congenital heart defects present. Although an EKG is indicated in all neonates who present with CHD, generally there are no rhythm disturbances indicative of a VSD. Left ventricular hypertrophy can sometimes be seen with moderate to large defects and biventricular hypertrophy may be seen in large VSDs (Park, 2014).

Management

The majority (60%) of muscular VSDs and about 35% of perimembranous VSDs will close spontaneously (Park, 2014). The goal of medical management is to treat the CHF, allowing adequate growth with the hope that the VSD will close without surgical intervention. Pharmacologic management for treatment of the CHF may include furosemide, digoxin, and/or an afterload reducer such as enalapril and/or captopril (Park, 2014; Scholz & Reinking, 2012). Prevention of pulmonary vascular occlusive disease is the overarching goal in both medical and surgical management. Surgical closure should be considered for infants who have poor growth despite maximal medical management of their CHF, evidence of prolonged pulmonary hypertension, and prolapse of the aortic valve cusp into the defect with resulting progressive aortic insufficiency (Park, 2014; Scholz & Reinking, 2012).

ATRIOVENTRICULAR CANAL DEFECTS

AV canal defects have also been described as endocardial cushion defects. The defect is caused by failure of the endocardial cushions, which form the central part of the heart, to fuse or close normally. There is a spectrum of malformations that are grouped under AV canal defects, including the most severe form, which is a complete AV canal. A complete AV canal includes a common AV valve, a large-inlet VSD, and a large ostium primum atrial septal defect (ASD). A transitional AV canal is less severe and includes an ostium primum ASD and small VSD but separate AV valves, although there is a cleft in the mitral valve.

A partial AV canal defect includes an ostium primum ASD with separate AV valves but a cleft of the mitral valve. There is no VSD associated with a partial AV canal defect (Scholz & Reinking, 2012). There is a strong association between complete AV canal defects and trisomy 21 (Park, 2014).

Clinical Presentation

Depending on the degree of pulmonary vascular resistance, desaturation and cyanosis may be present because of right-to-left shunting via the ASD and VSD in the early neonatal period. This is specifically relevant in infants with complete AV canals, including infants with trisomy 21. In the first few months of life, as the pulmonary vascular resistance falls, there is increasing left-to-right flow through the septal defects, leading to signs of CHF. A murmur may or may not be present in the early neonatal period depending on the degree of shunting across the defects. A blowing holosystolic murmur heard best at the lower left sternal border can be heard if AV valve insufficiency is present (Ashwath & Snyder, 2015; Park, 2014). A CXR will reveal normal heart size or cardiomegaly depending on the degree of CHF present; increased pulmonary vascularity is usually present (Swanson & Erickson, 2016). An EKG with "left axis deviation and a counterclockwise loop in the frontal plane, and superior axis" (Swanson & Erickson, 2016, p. 668) is suggestive of AV canal defects. An echocardiogram is diagnostic of the defect.

Management

Management of the defect in the neonatal period consists of treatment of the CHF. Digoxin, furosemide, and medication to reduce afterload are generally used. Oxygen saturations greater than the 75% range are generally acceptable (Swanson & Erickson, 2016). Use of oxygen to improve saturations beyond 75% can actually worsen the CHF as a result of the lowering of the pulmonary vascular resistance. Primary surgical repair generally occurs between 2 and 6 months of age. Earlier surgical repair may be indicated in infants who have persistent pulmonary hypertension and whose pulmonary vascular resistance does not fall.

AORTIC STENOSIS

Stenosis of the aortic value can range from mild to severe. There can also be obstruction below (subvalvular) or above the aortic valve (supravalvular). Aortic valve stenosis is the most common type (Park, 2014) and, if there is inadequate blood supply through the stenotic valve to supply the body's needs, then the diagnosis is critical aortic stenosis. Right-to-left shunting through the PDA can supply adequate blood flow to the body but once the PDA closes, there is inadequate blood flow to the body and cardiac shock occurs in the infant with critical aortic stenosis. Without adequate support and initiation of PGE_1, the infant will die of cardiac failure.

Clinical Presentation

A harsh midsystolic murmur can be heard at the second right or left intercostal space and may radiant to the neck (Park, 2014). A systolic ejection click is generally heard best at the apex of the heart or left lower sternal border (Ashwath & Snyder, 2015; Scholz & Reinking, 2012). In mild to moderate aortic stenosis, especially in the newborn period, a murmur may be the only evidence of a defect. Progression in moderate to severe aortic stenosis can occur over weeks to months. In those infants, as well as infants with critical aortic stenosis, increased workload on the left ventricle can result in ventricular dysfunction with signs of

CHF. In the infant with critical aortic stenosis, signs of hypoperfusion and decreased CO become evident as the ductus arteriosis begins to close. Signs include decreased peripheral pulses; pale, gray color that is cool to the touch; and worsening or prolonged capillary refill.

A CXR may be normal or may reveal cardiomegaly but is not diagnostic of the defect. Pulmonary venous congestion with cardiomegaly may be present in those infants who present with critical aortic stenosis. An EKG may be normal or reveal evidence of left ventricular hypertrophy (Park, 2014). An echocardiogram is diagnostic; the characteristics of the aortic valve can be determined and the gradient across the valve can be evaluated by Doppler flow studies. Evaluation of the left ventricular size and other left-sized lesions are also imperative. Small left ventricular size, small mitral valve, and hypoplastic aortic arch may necessitate a single ventricle repair (Scholz & Reinking, 2012).

Management

Infants with mild aortic stenosis can generally be monitored as outpatients. Infants with moderate to severe aortic stenosis will likely need to undergo a balloon valvuloplasty in the cardiac catheterization laboratory to dilate the aortic valve. Care must be taken to minimize aortic valve insufficiency because that can be a consequence of valve leaflet damage from the procedure (Scholz & Reinking, 2012). It is imperative that infants who present with critical aortic stenosis be managed initially with continuous infusion of PGE_1 to keep the DA open. Medical management should also include inotropic support with dopamine, intubation and mechanical ventilation, and close monitoring for metabolic acidosis as well as signs of CHF. Signs of CHF should be aggressively managed. Once stable, infants will need to undergo a balloon valvuloplasty or surgical intervention (Park, 2014).

Surgical valvotomy is rarely required in the neonatal period. Indications for surgical intervention include failure of the balloon valvuloplasty to improve the pressure gradient across the valve (Park, 2014). Repeated balloon valvuloplasties, which may be needed later in infancy and early childhood, may result in significant aortic regurgitation or insufficiency. The only treatment for significant aortic insufficiency is surgical repair or replacement of the valve (Scholz & Reinking, 2012).

COARCTATION OF THE AORTA

Coarctation or narrowing of the aorta can occur anywhere from the transverse aorta to the abdominal aorta. The most common site of coarctation is in the juxaductal region (Park, 2014), where the DA attaches, distal to the left subclavian artery. Associated defects include bicuspid aortic valves, PDA, and VSDs. Coarctation of the aorta is also associated with Turner syndrome (Scholz & Reinking, 2012).

Clinical Presentation

The location of the coarctation and the presence of associated anomalies determine clinical presentation. With mild coarctation, there may be minimal signs in the newborn period. Generally, the defect is found as part of a diagnostic workup for hypertension. In the most common type of coarctation of the aorta, signs are not immediately seen after delivery but instead develop as the PDA closes. The right-to-left shunt via the PDA supplies blood flow to the descending aorta and, as that closes, signs of decreased perfusion to the lower extremities become evident. Signs include decreased femoral, pedal, and post-tibial pulses as well as a systolic blood pressure gradient greater than 10 mmHg (Swanson & Erickson, 2016) between the upper right arm and lower extremities. In infants who present in circulatory shock, a systolic blood pressure gradient may not be evident until after cardiac function is supported and improved with inotropic agents (Park, 2014). A difference in oxygen saturations can also be seen between the upper and lower extremities. Evidence of CHF may be seen as a result of the increased workload on the left ventricle. A murmur may or may not be present. If present, it is generally a soft murmur audible along the left sternal border with radiation to the left axilla and the back (Scholz & Reinking, 2012). A murmur localized to the back is strongly suggestive of coarctation but is generally not found in neonates (Ashwath & Snyder, 2015). The S2 is single and loud and an S3 gallop may be present (Park, 2014). A CXR may reveal cardiomegaly and increased vascular markings may be seen if CHF is present. Right ventricular hypertrophy can be seen on the EKG, although it is generally only seen in older children. Right ventricular hypertrophy and a normal or rightward QRS axis are seen on the EKG in most infants with coarctation (Park, 2014). An echocardiogram can evaluate the size of the aortic arch. The presence of a PDA makes the precise diagnosis or severity of the narrowing difficult to determine.

Management

Most infants who present in the neonatal period with signs of coarctation have significant narrowing of the aorta and will require PGE_1 to maintain ductal patency to ensure adequate blood flow to the lower body. Medical management also consists of intubation and mechanical ventilation, inotropic support, correction of acid–base abnormalities, and treatment of CHF. Surgical repair of a coarctation, via a lateral thoracotomy incision, is end-to-end anastomosis after resection of the coarctation. In longer segments of coarctation, patch material may be needed to provide an adequate extended end-to-end anastomosis (Scholz & Reinking, 2012).

HYPOPLASTIC LEFT HEART SYNDROME

HLHS is characterized by varying degrees of aortic valve stenosis or atresia, mitral valve stenosis or atresia, coarctation of the aorta, and hypoplasia of the ascending aorta with underdevelopment or severe hypoplasia of the left ventricle. The systemic circulation is dependent on blood flow via the PDA. Retrograde blood flow through the PDA supplies the ascending aorta and anterograde flow through the PDA supplies the descending aorta (Ashwath & Snyder, 2015). Communication through the patent foramen ovale (PFO) or an ASD is required for mixing of oxygenated pulmonary venous blood with blood in the right atrium. Anomalies of the central nervous system (CNS) are common in infants who have HLHS (Ashwath & Snyder, 2015; Park, 2014). The etiology of HLHS is theorized to be related to decreased blood flow to the left side of the heart in utero (Scholz & Reinking, 2012).

Clinical Presentation

Clinical presentation at birth is variable depending on the degree of restriction at the level of the PFO/ASD. Infants with an unrestricted ASD and a PDA may only have mild tachypnea and minimal cyanosis after birth because of the relatively high pulmonary vascular resistance. Infants with a restricted ASD present with marked cyanosis and tachypnea shortly after birth. In both cases, once the DA closes, severe hypoperfusion and multisystem organ failure occur, which results in death if there is no intervention. Most infants are now diagnosed by fetal echocardiogram, allowing for delivery and stabilization at a tertiary unit (Scholz & Reinking, 2012).

A murmur may or may not be present. If a murmur is present, it is usually a nonspecific systolic murmur. A single second heart sound may be heard as well as a third heart sound (Scholz & Reinking, 2012). A chest radiograph may reveal a normal size heart (Scholz & Reinking, 2012) or cardiomegaly, as well as increased pulmonary markings and evidence of pulmonary venous congestion (Ashwath & Snyder, 2015; Park, 2014). An EKG may be normal or it may show right axis deviation and right ventricular hypertrophy (Swanson & Erickson, 2016). An echocardiogram is diagnostic of the disorder with evidence of a small left ventricular cavity, hypoplasia of the ascending aorta, mitral and aortic valve stenosis or atresia, and a dilated right atrium (Park, 2014). It can also provide information on the degree of flow restriction across the PFO/ASD.

Management

If diagnosed prenatally, continuous infusion of PGE_1 should be started immediately after delivery in order to maintain ductal dependency. PGE_1 infusion should also be initiated quickly if an infant presents with signs suggestive of HLHS in the newborn nursery. The goal of medical therapy is to provide balanced systemic and pulmonary blood flow until the infant undergoes a staged surgical palliative repair. Higher oxygen saturations provide evidence of increased pulmonary blood flow but also signal lower systemic blood flow. It will also result in worsening pulmonary edema. Increased systemic blood flow leads to decreased pulmonary blood flow and hypoxia.

Inotropic support, intubation and mechanical ventilation, hyperventilation, and volume expansion have been used in an effort to increase systemic perfusion especially as pulmonary vascular resistance begins to fall. Other therapies that have been used in an effort to increase systemic blood flow include the addition of CO_2 or nitrogen in an attempt to increase pulmonary vascular resistance and increase systemic blood flow at the expense of pulmonary blood flow. The use of milrinone has also been suggested in an effort to decrease afterload and improve systemic blood pressure; its use must be carefully monitored as milrinone can also dilate the pulmonary vascular bed (Scholz & Reinking, 2012). Many centers now minimize aggressive methods to improve systemic vascular resistance, such as intubation, mechanical ventilation, inotropic support, and inhaled nitrogen and CO_2, as long as CO remains adequate. Diuretic therapy has been used to decrease pulmonary edema (Lowry, 2012).

Close monitoring is essential for evaluation of ongoing medical therapy. Goal arterial oxygen saturations of 75% to 85% generally represent a balanced pulmonary-to-systemic blood flow as long as the pH is normal. Other signs of CO in addition to acid–base balance, including urine output and capillary refill, should be routinely monitored. Signs of worsening pulmonary edema, such as tachypnea, hepatosplenomegaly, and worsening pulmonary congestion on chest radiographs, should prompt further evaluation. Oxygen saturations greater than 90% are indicative of increasing pulmonary blood flow and may signify decreased systemic blood flow (Lowry, 2012; Swanson & Erickson, 2016). Near-infrared spectroscopy (NIRS) monitoring may be helpful in identifying decreased CO prior to other changes in clinical status. NIRS measures tissue oxygen saturations of the brain and splanchnic regions and can be useful in monitoring trends, especially in infants with left-sided obstructive lesions like HLHS (Swanson & Erickson, 2016).

Surgical treatment for HLHS includes heart transplantation and a staged, palliative, surgical reconstruction. Because of the relative lack of infant hearts available for transplantation, most infants with HLHS undergo the staged, palliative surgical procedure. The procedure includes a series or stages of three surgeries: stage 1 is the Norwood procedure, which is done in the neonatal period; stage 2 is the bidirectional Glenn procedure generally done some time between 2 and 6 months of age (Park, 2014; Scholz & Reinking, 2012); and stage 3 is the Fontan procedure, which is done in early childhood.

The classical Norwood procedure includes enlargement of the ASD, ligation of the PDA, anastomosis of the pulmonary artery to the ascending aorta, and aortic arch reconstruction. Pulmonary blood flow is supplied by the creation of an aortopulmonary shunt (Blalock-Taussig [BT] shunt; Swanson & Erickson, 2016). The hybrid procedure is an alternative to the classic Norwood procedure in which a stent is placed in the DA and pulmonary artery bands are placed.

The bidirectional Glenn procedure begins the separation of the pulmonary and systemic circulations with anastomosis between the superior vena cava and the pulmonary arteries. The BT shunt is also removed. The Fontan procedure is the last surgery of reconstruction when the IVC is attached to the pulmonary arteries (Swanson & Erickson, 2016). Although the Fontan is the last stage of reconstruction, it is important to remember that the staged procedures do not represent a repair or correction of the defect. Instead, they are palliative procedures and these children will continue to function with a single ventricle.

NEONATAL CYANOSIS

Identifying infants with CHD can be challenging to the practitioner. Many of the signs and symptoms seen with CHD are also present with many other pulmonary, infectious, and metabolic disorders. The two most common signs of CHD are those associated with CHF and the presence of central cyanosis.

Central cyanosis is defined as reduced hemoglobin levels of 5 g/100 mL in the cutaneous veins. It can be associated with arterial desaturation of blood or increased extraction of oxygen by tissues in the periphery (Park, 2014). Central cyanosis (blue coloring of the oral mucosa, tongue, lips, and scrotum in males) must be differentiated from peripheral cyanosis (blue coloring of the hands and feet). Peripheral cyanosis is normal for up to about 2 days in healthy newborns and is not associated with arterial desaturation. One of biggest challenges facing practitioners in caring for infants is ascertaining the cause of central cyanosis when an infant presents with it. The cause of cyanosis must be quickly determined and is best done by establishing a differential diagnosis using an understanding of the findings in the prenatal, birth, and postnatal history; strong assessment skills; and appropriate tests to quickly and safely determine a diagnosis and treatment plan that is appropriate. For infants with CHD, this is especially important as prompt treatment can be life-saving.

There are many common causes of cyanosis in the newborn. Many of the diagnoses can be removed from the differential by examining the maternal and neonatal history, delivery room information, and establishing when the cyanosis presented (at birth, at several hours of age, at 3 days of age, or even later in the newborn period). It is also important to consider infectious risk factors that may be present as sepsis/pneumonia may also present with cyanosis. A careful physical exam should take place. All factors must be carefully examined (although many of these findings are not specific to infants with a cyanotic cardiac defect, they are still critical to a thorough cardiac evaluation).

Respiratory Diagnoses

Note breathing rate, assess for adventitious breath sounds such as rales and rhonchi, and note work of breathing. In infants with grunting, retracting, and flaring, cyanosis is generally related to respiratory diagnoses rather than cardiac diagnoses. An infant with right-sided obstructive lesions or transposition of the great arteries will often present with nonlabored cyanosis that does not respond to oxygen with increasing PaO_2 or saturations. One quick test that can be done at the infant's bedside is the *hyperoxia test*. The hyperoxia test is performed by obtaining an arterial blood gas while the infant is breathing room air; the infant is then placed in a 100% oxygen hood for approximately 15 minutes. The arterial blood gas is then repeated. If the PaO_2 does not increase to at least 150 mmHg in the repeat gas, the etiology of the hypoxemia is more likely caused by cardiac disease as opposed to respiratory disease.

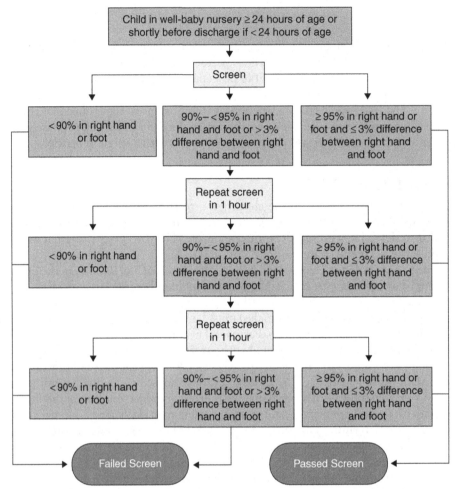

Figure 7.2   Pulse-Oximetry Monitoring Algorithm for Detecting Congenital Heart Disease in Newborns

Note: Percentages refer to oxygen saturation as measured by pulse oximeter.

It is important to obtain preductal and postductal oxygen saturation monitoring for infants with any cyanosis to evaluate differences in preductal and postductal saturations. Most states are now requiring oxygen saturation monitoring for *all* infants at greater than 24 hours of age as a screen for CHD. The American Academy of Pediatrics and the American Heart Association have established an algorithm as an approach for this screening to be done at 24 to 48 hours of age (Figure 7.2). Monitoring should be done in parallel or direct sequence on either foot (postductal), and the right hand (preductal) of the infant. Any infant with positive screening results should have an echocardiogram and a complete examination to determine the cause of the hypoxemia and to rule out CHD.

Cardiac Diagnoses

First, observe precordial activity, noting an especially active precordium if present. With auscultation of heart, note HR, rhythm, and the presence or absence of a murmur. Presence of a murmur (especially murmurs louder than grade II) may indicate cardiac disease, but it is important to remember that many infants who die of CHD never present with a murmur. Blood pressures can be obtained in both upper and lower extremities. Infants with coarctation of the aorta will have systolic blood pressures significantly greater in the upper extremities than in the lower extremities.

PALPATION OF ABDOMEN AND PULSES

Palpating for liver size is an important factor to consider when ruling out CHD. Any liver that is greater than 3 cm below the right costal margin is a good indicator of right-sided cardiac failure. In addition, femoral and brachial pulses should be palpated alone and then palpated simultaneously. It is also better to palpate the right brachial artery because this vessel is always preductal. If the femoral pulses are absent or weak (especially in comparison to the right brachial pulse, which is always preductal), it may indicate a left-sided obstructive lesion.

In evaluating the cause of cyanosis in an infant, there are several other tests that should be undertaken. These include a chest radiograph to examine pronounced or diminished lung field markings and to evaluate for cardiomegaly; an electrocardiogram to determine whether there are typical findings found with CHD; and an echocardiogram, which is the gold standard to determine whether there is CHD. Cardiomegaly on a CXR is generally defined as a cardiac diameter on an anterior–posterior (AP) radiograph of greater than 60% of the thoracic diameter (Weinert & Martinez-Rios, 2015). In addition, blood gases, serum chemistries and blood glucose to rule out electrolyte disturbances and hypoglycemia, and a complete blood count to rule out infection are all imperative.

CYANOTIC DEFECTS

Although infants with the following cardiac defects generally present with cyanosis, the etiology of cyanosis is varied. The etiology can be related to poor mixing or complete mixing of oxygenated and unoxygenated blood as well as restricted blood flow to the pulmonary bed. A discussion of these defects, including anatomy/pathophysiology, clinical presentation, and management of a variety of these cardiac defects, is outlined in the text that follows.

TRANSPOSITION OF THE GREAT ARTERIES

One of the most common cyanotic heart defects in newborns is D-transposition of the great arteries (D-TGA); the majority of infants affected with this defect are boys. In this cardiac defect, there are essentially parallel circulations with the aorta arising from the right ventricle and the pulmonary artery arising from the left ventricle. Without any communication, the oxygenated blood flows from the lungs to the pulmonary arteries and back to the pulmonary bed. Deoxygenated blood flows from the right ventricle to the aorta and back out to the body without any blood flow and thus oxygen from the lungs. For survival, there must be some communication to allow mixing of blood at either the atrial or ductal level.

Clinical Presentation

Infants with D-TGA present with cyanosis at birth or within hours after birth. The degree of cyanosis is related to the number and size of communications that allow mixing of the blood. Infants with a large PDA and a large VSD may only present with mild cyanosis until the ductus begins to close. Infants with restricted PFOs and small PDAs will present with profound cyanosis. The addition of oxygen does not help the cyanosis because the problem is inadequate mixing of oxygenated and deoxygenated blood. A murmur is usually not present but a single, loud S2 is heard. If a murmur is present, it may represent other cardiac defects such as a VSD or pulmonary stenosis. A chest radiograph may be normal or it may have a classic "egg on a string" appearance with a narrow mediastinum (Scholz & Reinking, 2012). Evidence of increased pulmonary vascularity and cardiomegaly can also be seen (Park, 2014). An EKG is usually normal or may show some right ventricular hypertrophy (Park, 2014; Scholz & Reinking, 2012). The diagnosis is made by echocardiogram. Besides the anatomy, it is important to determine the size and degree of shunting at the atrial and ductal levels as well as location of the coronary arteries.

Management

D-TGA is a ductal-dependent defect and it is imperative that a continuous infusion of PGE_1 is started when the diagnosis is suspected. If shunting at the ductal level is inadequate and/ or the infant continues to be hypoxic or acidotic, then an atrial balloon septostomy is recommended. This procedure is done in the cardiac catheterization lab and allows for improved mixing at the atrial level. The surgical repair, an atrial switch procedure, is generally done within the first 1 to 2 weeks of life. In the atrial switch procedure, the aorta and pulmonary arteries are transected and the pulmonary artery is anastomosed to the right ventricle and the aorta is anastomosed to the left ventricle. The coronary arteries are then transplanted to the neoaortic root of the ascending aorta (Ashwath & Snyder, 2015).

TOTAL ANOMALOUS PULMONARY VENOUS CONNECTION

Normally, the pulmonary veins drain into the left atrium. In total anomalous pulmonary venous connection (TAPVC), also called total anomalous pulmonary venous return (TAPVR), the pulmonary veins instead drain into a systemic vein and then into the right atrium. Oxygenated blood flows into the right side of the heart instead of the left side of heart. For survival, an ASD must be present allowing right-to-left shunting of blood to the left side of the heart. Following are the four variants of TAPVC:

1. Supracardiac—all four of the pulmonary veins join together behind the heart, travel superiorly above the heart to the innominate vein, and then drain into the superior vena cava and into the right atrium.

2. Infracardiac—all of the pulmonary veins join together behind the heart and then travel through the diaphragm and the liver, via the portal venous system, then into the IVC and the right atrium.

3. Intracardiac or cardiac—the pulmonary veins drain into the coronary sinus and then into the right atrium or drain directly into the right atrium.

4. Mixed—at least two of the preceding types of TAPVC occur in the same infant.

Any of the these types of TAPVC can obstruct pulmonary venous return but the one that generally presents with significant obstruction is the infracardiac type (Ashwath & Snyder, 2015; Swanson & Erickson, 2016).

Clinical Presentation

Infants with obstructed TAPVC present with marked hypoxia. Both the systemic and pulmonary venous returns occur on the right side of the heart. Systemic cardiac output is supplied via an ASD. Obstruction to the pulmonary venous connection leads to pulmonary venous congestion, which, in turn, causes pulmonary edema as well as decreased pulmonary blood flow. The combination of the pulmonary edema and reduced pulmonary blood flow results in systemic hypoxia. A murmur is not generally heard with this defect (Park, 2014; Swanson & Erickson, 2016). A chest radiograph in obstructed TAPVC will reveal a normal heart size and pulmonary venous congestion (Swanson & Erickson, 2016). An EKG may reveal right ventricular hypertrophy (Park, 2014). An echocardiogram generally reveals the diagnosis, although occasionally cardiac catheterization is needed to determine the exact location of all pulmonary veins.

Unobstructed TAPVC may not be diagnosed in the neonatal period. Signs of CHF develop due to the increased volume on the right side of the heart. A chest radiograph would reveal increased pulmonary vascularity and cardiomegaly. An EKG may reveal right ventricular hypertrophy and right atrial enlargement (Park, 2014). In most cases, an echocardiogram is diagnostic of the defect.

Management

Surgery is the treatment for TAPVC. The exact surgical procedure is dependent on the type of defect. In most cases, reimplantation of the pulmonary venous confluence into the left atrium is done (Scholz & Reinking, 2012). Realignment of the atrial septum and directing the anomalous veins to the left atrial side is the surgical procedure for the cardiac type of TAPVC (Swanson & Erickson, 2016).

TRUNCUS ARTERIOSUS

Truncus arteriosus is defined as one large artery that arises from the left and right ventricles and supplies all of the pulmonary, systemic, and coronary circulation. In the majority of cases, the single arterial trunk overrides a VSD. There are three different types of truncus arteriosus:

1. A short main pulmonary artery arises from the truncus and then bifurcates into the right and left pulmonary arteries.

2. The right and left arteries both arise from the posterior aspect of the truncus.

3. The pulmonary arteries arise from opposite sides or lateral walls of the truncus and are not close together (Ashwath & Snyder, 2015; Swanson & Erickson, 2016).

Mixing of the oxygenated blood from the left ventricle and deoxygenated blood from the right ventricle occurs at the VSD and is supplied to the truncus. Pulmonary and systemic blood flows are determined by the balance of the pulmonary vascular resistance and the systemic vascular resistance.

Clinical Presentation

The amount of pulmonary blood flow at birth determines the degree of cyanosis. In most cases, there is mild tachypnea and mild cyanosis with oxygen saturations around 85% (Ashwath & Snyder, 2015). As pulmonary vascular resistance falls, there is increased pulmonary blood flow and CHF can occur. On physical exam, a single, loud S2 is heard. A loud pansystolic murmur may be audible at the left lower sternal border (Swanson & Erickson, 2016) as well as a low-pitched, diastolic rumble (Scholz & Reinking, 2012; Swanson & Erickson, 2016). Runoff into the pulmonary arteries may occur with decreasing pulmonary vascular resistance; bounding pulses and a widened pulse pressure may be noted. A chest radiograph will exhibit cardiomegaly and increased pulmonary markings. An EKG may reveal right, left, or biventricular hypertrophy (Scholz & Reinking, 2012); left atrial hypertrophy may also be seen (Park, 2014). An echocardiogram is not only diagnostic of the defect but can determine the specific type as well as rule out other associated defects, including dysplastic truncal valve leaflets and right aortic arch. There is an association between truncus arteriosus and DiGeorge syndrome, so genetic evaluation for the syndrome is important (Parks, 2014).

Management

Medical management usually includes anticongestive medications, such as diuretic therapy and digoxin, once evidence of CHF becomes apparent (Ashwath & Snyder, 2015). Oxygen therapy should be avoided because lowering the PVR may worsen the CHF. Calcium levels should be monitored closely until results of genetic testing for DiGeorge syndrome are available.

Surgical repair generally occurs in the first several months of life. The repair consists of closure of the VSD, so the trunk arises from the left ventricle. A right ventricle to pulmonary artery valve homograft conduit is also inserted; this conduit may need to be replaced over the lifetime of the child (Scholz & Reinking, 2012).

TETRALOGY OF FALLOT

Tetralogy of Fallot (TOF) consists of a large VSD, an overriding aorta, a right ventricular outflow tract (RVOT) obstruction, and right ventricular hypertrophy. The degree of cyanosis is directly related to the degree of RVOT obstruction. Infants with a "pink tet" have minimal obstruction to the RVOT, have a left-to-right shunt across the VSD, and therefore will not be cyanotic. Infants with a severe degree of RVOT obstruction will have decreased pulmonary blood flow, right-to-left shunts, and will be cyanotic. Most infants fall somewhere in between and will have adequate blood flow but not develop signs of CHF because of the degree of RVOT obstruction.

Clinical Presentation

Infants with pink TOF may only present with a systolic murmur or mild cyanosis, whereas the infant with severe RVOT obstruction may present with profound cyanosis. A harsh systolic murmur in the mid to upper left sternal border is usually present. The S_2 is single and loud (Parks, 2014). A chest radiograph may reveal a boot-shaped heart resulting from a small or missing main pulmonary artery; the classic finding of the boot-shaped heart is generally not seen in neonates (Park, 2014; Swanson & Erickson, 2016). Pulmonary vascular markings are generally decreased in infants with severe RVOT obstruction; the lungs may appear very dark or black (Park, 2014). An EKG may be normal (Ashwath & Snyder, 2015) or may reveal right ventricular hypertrophy (Parks, 2014; Swanson & Erickson, 2016). An echocardiogram is needed to determine the diagnosis. Doppler flow studies to evaluate the degree of RVOT obstruction, size, and direction of flow across the VSD are important considerations when doing the echocardiogram.

Infants with minimal RVOT obstruction may develop signs of CHF as PVR falls over the first several weeks of life. Signs may include tachypnea, increased work of breathing, hepatomegaly, and fatigue, especially with feedings. Chest radiograph may reveal increased pulmonary markings.

Infants with TOF are also at risk for hypoxic or "tet" spells. Infants and children can become cyanotic, pale, tachypneic, irritable, flaccid, and even lose consciousness during "tet" spells. Spells are thought to be a result of minimal or no pulmonary blood flow secondary to a transient increase in the RVOT obstruction (Swanson & Erickson, 2016).

Management

Medical management depends on the degree of RVOT obstruction. Infants with severe RVOT obstruction who have minimal pulmonary blood flow will require a continuous infusion of PGE_1 to maintain ductal dependency. Those infants will require a systemic-to-pulmonary shunt (BT shunt) in the neonatal period to provide adequate pulmonary blood flow (Swanson & Erickson, 2016).

Infants who have acyanotic defects may develop CHF from a large left-to-right flow through the VSD. They may need medical treatment, including diuretic therapy for treatment of their CHF. For "tet" spells, placing the infant/child into a knee-chest position is recommended as well as administering oxygen, morphine, and fluid boluses (Swanson & Erickson, 2016).

Surgical repair of TOF is generally not done in the neonatal period unless there is inadequate pulmonary blood flow because of severe RVOT obstruction. A modified BT shunt is generally placed in these infants until complete repair is undertaken at a later age (Park, 2014). Surgical repair consists of patch closure of the VSD and relief of the RVOT obstruction; this may be done in a variety of ways. Surgical repair is generally done in the first year of life but may be done sooner if significant "tet" spells are present (Swanson & Erickson, 2016).

TRICUSPID ATRESIA

Tricuspid atresia occurs when there is complete atresia of the tricuspid valve and there is no connection between the right atrium and right ventricle. Blood flow instead goes from the right atrium across the PFO or ASD to the left atrium and then to the left ventricle. Most babies with tricuspid atresia have an associated VSD that allows some blood flow from the left ventricle to the right ventricle and the pulmonary arteries. If there is no VSD present or if the VSD is small, then the right ventricle and pulmonary arteries may be small; a PDA is then required for adequate pulmonary blood flow. There may be pulmonary blood flow if the VSD is large and a PDA may not be required. As PVR falls, increased pulmonary blood flow occurs, especially if there is a large VSD present. There is an association of TGA and coarctation of the aorta with tricuspid atresia (Park, 2014; Scholz & Reinking, 2012; Swanson & Erickson, 2016).

Clinical Presentation

Infants present with cyanosis; the degree of cyanosis is dependent on the amount of pulmonary blood flow. Oxygen saturations are generally greater than 75% (Swanson & Erickson, 2016). Murmurs associated with other defects like a VSD, PDA, or pulmonary stenosis may be present. A chest radiograph may be normal or have cardiomegaly. Pulmonary vascularity is determined by the amount of pulmonary blood flow; increased pulmonary vascularity can be seen with excessive pulmonary blood flow and decreased pulmonary vascularity with inadequate or decreased pulmonary blood flow (Swanson & Erickson, 2016). EKG reveals left ventricular hypertrophy and left axis deviation (Scholz & Reinking, 2012). An echocardiogram is done for diagnostic purposes and also to evaluate right-to-left flow at the atrial level, across the VSD and the PDA, as well as to identify other associated anomalies.

Management

A continuous infusion of PGE_1 is recommended until echocardiogram evaluation can determine the size of the VSD and adequacy of pulmonary blood flow. If there is restriction at the atrial level, a balloon septostomy may be performed in the cardiac catheterization lab to improve blood flow from the right atrium to the left atrium (Park, 2014). If the defect is ductal dependent, then a systemic-to-pulmonary shunt (BT shunt) is placed in the neonatal period. At a later point, the child will undergo a bidirectional Glenn procedure at or before 6 months of age and then a Fontan procedure at 2 to 3 years of age (Park, 2014; Scholz & Reinking, 2012). These procedures do not surgically correct the defect; instead, they offer a single ventricle palliative repair.

EBSTEIN'S ANOMALY

Dysplastic leaflets of the tricuspid valve result in Ebstein's anomaly. The tricuspid valve is displaced down into the right ventricle, which results in a functionally large right atrium but small right ventricle. Because of the small right ventricle, there is decreased blood flow to the pulmonary arteries. Right ventricular outflow is also affected by the degree of tricuspid regurgitation. Infants with significant or severe tricuspid regurgitation only have a small volume of blood that can be ejected to the pulmonary arteries, thus resulting in inadequate blood flow. These infants will require a PDA for adequate pulmonary blood flow. Infants with minimal tricuspid regurgitation generally have good pulmonary blood flow (Swanson & Erickson, 2016). As PVR falls over the first several weeks of life, pulmonary blood flow will be increased and symptoms may improve. Wolff–Parkinson–White (WPW) syndrome and SVT have been associated with Ebstein's anomaly (Park, 2014; Swanson & Erickson, 2016).

Clinical Presentation

Clinical presentation depends on the amount of tricuspid valve (TV) displacement and the amount of tricuspid regurgitation. Some infants with minimal TV displacement and mild tricuspid regurgitation may only have minimal symptoms. Infants with severe tricuspid regurgitation will present with significant cyanosis. A holosystolic murmur is generally present as is hepatomegaly (Park, 2014). A chest radiograph will reveal cardiomegaly and decreased pulmonary vascularity in severe cases. Massive cardiomegaly can be seen in cases of severe tricuspid regurgitation (Park, 2014; Swanson & Erickson, 2016). Normal heart size and normal pulmonary vascularity are common in mild cases (Park, 2014). The EKG is suggestive of right ventricular dilation (Ashwath & Snyder, 2015).

Management

Medical management of the infant with mild tricuspid insufficiency consists of close observation and follow-up. Diuretic therapy and digoxin may be used in infants who develop CHF (Park, 2014). Infants with severe tricuspid regurgitation may require continuous infusion of PGE_1 to maintain ductal dependency and adequate blood flow. High FiO_2, nitric oxide, and mild respiratory alkalosis have been used to decrease PVR and improve antegrade pulmonary blood flow. As PVR gradually falls, attempts are made to wean medical support, including PGE_1 (Scholz & Reinking, 2012; Swanson & Erickson, 2016).

Surgical treatment is generally considered only in the infant with significant tricuspid regurgitation. Procedures may include a BT shunt in order to improve pulmonary blood flow and discontinue PGE_1. Repositioning of the tricuspid valve and annuloplasty or complete replacement of the valve may be considered. Plication of the atrialized ventricle has also been done. Surgical procedures in the neonatal period may be controversial (Swanson & Erickson, 2016).

RHYTHM DISTURBANCES IN NEONATES

Arrhythmias may occur in the fetus and newborn period and involve abnormalities in rate or rhythm of the heart. Many occur with specific cardiac lesions and some occur following corrective surgery for congenital heart defects. Many arrhythmias are benign during the neonatal period but there are a few that can be life-threatening. If the rhythm originates from the sinus node (as demonstrated by a positive P wave in leads I and AVF on an electrocardiogram), it is rare that a cardiac problem is causing it (Cannon, Kovalenko, & Snyder, 2015).

Term neonates generally have an HR between 120 and 140 beats per minute (bpm). However, normal physiological rates may vary from 70 bpm in deep sleep to approximately 170 bpm with crying or agitation. Premature HRs are generally slightly higher (Vargo, 2015). HRs that are too slow or too fast may be a significant problem for newborns whose CO is primarily dependent on HR.

SINUS BRADYCARDIA (RATES < 80 BPM)

Sinus bradycardia can occur transiently in newborns without significant consequences because of the predominance of the parasympathetic nervous system. Most benign episodes are related to abrupt increases in vagal tone. However, infants with persistent bradycardia must be assessed for congenital AV block that is caused by primary sinus node dysfunction (Cannon et al., 2015).

SINUS TACHYCARDIA (RATES APPROXIMATELY 180–200 BPM)

Sinus tachycardia is commonly seen in newborns and can occur with any stimulus such as fever, crying, and anemia. It is also seen as a sign/symptom of CHF in the newborn with CHD. It is rarely pathologic and there is generally no treatment required for it as long as it is transient. However, when associated with CHF, it may require treatment of the CHF.

There are many other arrhythmias in newborns that are benign. These include premature atrial contractions (PACs), which are early beats that originate in the atria in a focus that is not the SA node. Travel beyond this focus is normal and there is a normal ventricular contraction and QRS complex. Treatment for these arrhythmias is generally not needed. However, they may not be benign when related to electrolyte abnormalities or structural cardiac disease. Occasional premature ventricular contractions (PVCs) can also occur in newborns and they are also usually benign. These contractions originate spontaneously from an ectopic focus, do not follow the normal conduction pathway, and thus have unusually wide QRS complexes. PVCs are rarely pathologic in the newborn.

SUPRAVENTRICULAR TACHYCARDIA

Supraventricular tachycardia (SVT; generally defined as sustained rates greater than approximately 220 bpm) is a very fast rhythm that originates in an ectopic focus above the ventricle (not the SA node). The most common form of this rhythm in the neonate is caused by a reentrant pathway. With a reentrant pathway, there are two individual conducting pathways that are connected around an area of tissue that does not conduct. If one of these pathways does not conduct the electrical impulse, the impulse will reverse in the opposite pathway, creating a loop and a subsequent tachycardia (Cannon et al., 2015). There are several different types of SVT. One form of SVT is caused by WPW preexcitation syndrome, which results from an anomalous accessory pathway (bundle of Kent) that conducts an impulse from the atria to the ventricles bypassing the AV node. WPW has a unique area of early ventricular activation on an electrocardiogram called a *delta wave*, which is an initial slurring of the QRS complex. There is also a very short PR interval and a widened QRS complex (Park, 2014; Webb, 2012).

SVT that is sustained in an infant or in a hemodynamically unstable newborn is a medical emergency. That is because the ventricles do not have enough time to fill and CO is greatly diminished. Treatment for a stable infant with SVT includes ice placed within a washcloth and carefully applied to the entire infant's face for a few seconds to create vagal stimulation and slow conduction through the AV node, and/or adenosine given by rapid intravenous (IV) push in a dose of 0.1 to 0.3 mg/kg/dose. Both methods will often convert the SVT, but adenosine is much more effective (Cannon et al., 2015).

Propranolol is generally first started as a maintenance therapy for SVT, especially if caused by WPW excitation. Digoxin has fallen out of favor as first-line treatment for SVT that is not caused by WPW preexcitation because many cardiologists feel that it is ineffective (Cannon et al., 2015). If the rhythm is diagnosed as WPW, digoxin should not be used and propranolol is the drug of choice because some cardiologists feel that digoxin may increase the antegrade conduction of the impulse through the accessory pathway with WPW. Verapamil for long-term treatment of SVT should also be avoided in infants for this reason (Park, 2014). Other maintenance drugs that might be used if propranolol is not effective include flecainide, sotalol, or amiodarone (Webb, 2012). But these are best used under the guidance of a pediatric cardiologist. Finally, some unstable infants might require the use of synchronized cardioversion. However, synchronized cardioversion may not be immediately available and generally should be done with the guidance of a pediatric cardiologist.

Ventricular Tachycardia

Ventricular tachycardia (VT) is tachycardia that originates in the ventricles (not the SA node). Infants with VT will have a widened and bizarre-looking QRS complex. The pattern may have a flutter or saw-tooth appearance. VT can greatly reduce CO because the ventricles cannot properly fill. Fortunately, true VT is extremely rare in newborns.

Complete AV Block

In complete AV block, there is no association between electrical conduction of the atria and the ventricles as a result of a block at the AV node, bundle of His, or bundle branches. This causes the atria to contract at their own rate and the ventricles to activate independently at a site below the block.

This disorder is sometimes seen in fetuses and newborns of mothers with a history of Sjögren's syndrome antibodies (anti-Ro and anti-La antibodies). Mothers with these antibodies often have systemic lupus erythematosus, rheumatoid arthritis, or other connective tissue disorders, although they may also be asymptomatic (Hull, Binns, & Joyce, 1966; Wren, 2011).

Fetuses with congenital AV block may develop hydrops or poor ventricular function in utero because of the low resting HR and the CHF that ensues. These infants may need to be delivered when this becomes evident (although some neonates can tolerate rates in the 50s–60s without compromise; Cannon et al., 2015). They then may need temporary pacemakers placed and eventually permanent pacemakers placed when they are bigger to maintain their CO.

Electrolyte Abnormalities

Electrolyte abnormalities can also cause electrocardiogram changes and arrhythmias. For example, hypokalemia of levels less than 2.5 mEq/L will produce a prominent U wave, prolongation of the QTc, diphasic T waves and ST segment depression, and finally prolonged PR intervals and sinoatrial block can occur. On the other hand, hyperkalemia will initially create a tall, tented T wave, prolonged PR interval, P wave disappearance and, with severe levels of hyperkalemia, may result in ventricular fibrillation and eventually asystole (Park, 2014). Infants with hypocalcemia may have prolonged QTc intervals and longer ST segments. Hypercalcemia will cause shortening of the ST segment and shorter QTc intervals (Park, 2014).

Case 7.1

You are called to attend a repeat cesarean delivery of a 38-year-old female who was admitted this morning in preterm labor at 32 weeks gestation. Mother is a gravida 2, para 1 female whose prenatal labs included a blood type of A positive, antibody screen negative, Venereal Disease Research Laboratory (VDRL) test nonreactive, HBsAg negative, rubella immune, HIV negative, and group B *Streptococcus* (GBS) unknown. Mother refused other labs. She has received one dose of betamethasone and is on ampicillin because of the preterm labor. Labor progressed despite tocolysis and a decision was made to proceed with a repeat cesarean section. The infant is delivered, has a good cry, and is transferred to the radiant warmer after the cord is clamped at 1 minute of age. The infant is dried and stimulated with a good response. As you examine the infant, you notice the following features: upward slanting palpebral fissures, epicanthic folds bilaterally, bilateral single palmar creases, and hypotonia. You discuss your concerns of trisomy 21 with the parents. In addition to your recommendations for high-resolution chromosomes, you also recommend an echocardiogram.

1. *Your recommendation of an echocardiogram is appropriate because all infants with Down syndrome have some type of cardiac defect. True or False?*

    ANSWER: False. *There is an increased risk of congenital heart disease (CHD) in infants with Down syndrome but that risk is approximately 40% (Park, 2014, p. 174).*

2. *You recommend an echocardiogram because there is a known association of trisomy 21 and which of the following?*

    A. Atrioventricular canal
    B. Ebstein's anomaly
    C. Hypoplastic left heart syndrome

    ANSWER: A. *Approximately 70% of patients with complete AV canals also have Down syndrome. There is a 40% risk of CHD in children with Down syndrome. Of those, 50% of the defects are atrioventricular canals (Park, 2014, p. 174).*

The infant is admitted to the neonatal intensive care unit (NICU) for prematurity. The infant breathes room air without evidence of respiratory distress. Enteral feedings via nasogastric route are initiated and advanced to full-volume feedings over several days without difficulty. At 35 weeks gestation, oral feedings are begun with the assistance of occupational therapy. At 4 weeks of age, you are asked by the RN to examine the infant because the infant is "breathing hard" and not wanting to orally feed. On your exam, the infant is breathing 70 to 80 times per minute, has retractions, diaphoresis, hepatomegaly, and a heart rate of 175 bpm. The oxygen saturation level is 80% to 85%.

3. *Based on your exam, the infant is exhibiting signs of which of the following?*

    A. Congestive heart failure (CHF)
    B. Necrotizing enterocolitis (NEC)
    C. Supraventricular tachycardia (SVT)

(continued)

Case 7.1 (continued)

ANSWER: A. *Symptoms of CHF include tachycardia, tachypnea, decreased peripheral pulses and skin mottling, decreased urine output, edema, diaphoresis, hepatomegaly, hypotension, decreased activity, failure to thrive and feeding problems, and diminished cardiac output (Swanson & Erickson, 2016, p. 652). Although NEC may be a concern given that the infant is preterm, several of the symptoms that the infant is exhibiting are not symptoms of NEC, including diaphoresis and hepatomegaly. The infant also has tachycardia but the heart rate is not high enough to warrant concern for SVT.*

4. **You order a chest x-ray as part of your evaluation. What findings would you expect to see in this particular infant?**

   A. Cardiomegaly and decreased pulmonary markings
   B. Cardiomegaly and increased pulmonary markings
   C. Small heart size and increased pulmonary markings

   ANSWER: B. *Cardiomegaly is generally seen, although the heart size can sometimes be normal. Pulmonary vascularity is generally increased (Swanson & Erickson, 2016, p. 668).*

5. **The RN questions you about why the infant is only now having symptoms of heart disease if the defect has been there since birth. You explain that the reason the infant is now having symptoms is because:**

   A. The pulmonary vascular resistance is now decreasing, thus allowing a right-to-left shunt via the defect
   B. The pulmonary vascular resistance is now decreasing, thus allowing a left-to-right shunt via the defect
   C. The pulmonary vascular resistance is now increasing, thus allowing a right-to-left shunt via the defect

   ANSWER: B. *As the pulmonary vascular return (PVR) falls, there is increased flow from left to right at the atrial and ventricular levels. As the degree of shunting increases, the infant's symptoms will increase (Swanson & Erickson, 2016, p. 668).*

6. **It would be appropriate to give supplemental oxygen to this infant to keep the oxygen saturation greater than 90%. True or False?**

   ANSWER: False. *Giving oxygen would potentially decrease the PVR even further, thus increasing pulmonary overcirculation thereby making the infant's symptoms worse. Keeping oxygen saturations greater than 75% should be accepted (Swanson & Erickson, 2016, p. 668).*

7. **As part of your treatment plan, which medical therapy should you order?**

   A. Diuretic medication
   B. Inotropic support
   C. Prostaglandin gtt

   ANSWER: A. *Diuretic therapy is indicated as treatment of the pulmonary overcirculation and edema (Park, 2014, p. 178; Swanson & Erickson, 2016, p. 668). A prostaglandin gtt is not indicated because this is not a ductal dependent lesion. Although hypotension can be a symptom of CHF, management of the CHF should resolve this problem.*

Case 7.2

You are asked to examine an infant in the newborn nursery because the RN is concerned about the infant's "gray color." The RN reports that the infant is a 37-week-gestation female who was born earlier today and is now about 18 hours old. The mother, a 25-year-old, gravida 1 female was admitted in spontaneous labor with spontaneous rupture of membranes (SROM) that occurred approximately 3 hours prior to delivery. Maternal labs included a blood type of A+, HBsAg negative, rapid plasma reagin (RPR) nonreactive, rubella immune, HIV negative, and group B *Streptococcus* (GBS) culture that was positive. Her pregnancy was complicated by diet-controlled gestational diabetes. The infant was delivered by spontaneous vaginal route and did not require resuscitation in the delivery room. Apgar scores were 8 and 9 at 1 and 5 minutes of age, respectively. The infant has been rooming in with mother, although the nurse reports that she has not been feeding well. On your exam, the infant has a grayish-blue color, has a heart rate in the 170s, retractions with a respiratory rate in the 60s to 70s range, and decreased capillary refill at 4 to 5 seconds. Her brachial and posttibial pulses are 1+/4 bilaterally. The right arm blood pressure (BP) is 55/28 mmHg with a mean of 33 and the right leg BP is 50/25 mmHg with a mean of 30. There is no murmur but her S2 is loud and single. Included in your differential diagnosis is congenital heart disease (CHD).

1. *Based on the history and your exam, which cardiac lesion should be highest on your differential diagnosis list?*

   A. Coarctation of the aorta
   B. Hypoplastic left heart syndrome (HLHS)
   C. Ventricular septal defect (VSD)

   ANSWER: B. *Infants with HLHS present with signs of poor perfusion, including weak peripheral pulses and vasoconstriction of their extremities as the patent ductus arteriosus (PDA) closes. They also may have tachycardia and dyspnea (Park, 2014). Although infants with coarctation of the aorta can present with respiratory distress and circulatory shock as the PDA closes, they generally have decreased femoral, posttibial, and pedal pulses as compared to brachial and radial pulses. In coarctation of the aorta, there is usually a systolic BP gradient of greater than 10 mmHg between the right arm and lower extremities (Swanson & Erickson, 2016). Infants with a VSD present with congestive heart failure (CHF) (Swanson & Erickson, 2016) and not with signs of shock.*

2. *As part of your workup, you order an arterial blood gas (ABG) test. What type of blood gas would support the diagnosis of HLHS on your differential?*

   A. Metabolic acidosis
   B. Metabolic alkalosis
   C. Respiratory acidosis

   ANSWER: A. *Severe metabolic acidosis is seen as a result of the significantly decreased cardiac output (CO) as the PDA closes (Park, 2014, p. 259).*

3. *The chest x-ray (CXR) that you ordered is now available. What findings on the CXR would support the diagnosis of HLHS?*

(continued)

Case 7.2 (continued)

A. Cardiomegaly and decreased pulmonary vascularity
B. Cardiomegaly and increased pulmonary vascularity
C. Normal heart size and decreased pulmonary vascularity

ANSWER: B. *The heart size can be normal or cardiomegaly can be present but there is evidence of increased pulmonary vascularity and/or pulmonary edema on the CXR (Park, 2014, p. 259; Swanson & Erickson, 2016, p. 680).*

4. *What medication should be your first priority in starting treatment?*

A. Digoxin
B. Furosemide
C. Prostaglandin gtt

ANSWER: C. *A prostaglandin gtt is required to maintain ductal dependency because CO to the systemic circulation is dependent on the PDA (Park, 2014, p. 259; Swanson & Erickson, 2016, p. 680).*

5. *An oxygen saturation level of 95% is acceptable in an infant with HLHS and signifies that the infant is doing well. True or False?*

ANSWER: False. *Saturations greater than 90% can signify increased pulmonary blood flow and decreased systemic blood flow (Swanson & Erickson, 2016, p. 680).*

6. *Neuroimaging is recommended in infants with HLHS because there is an increased risk of central nervous system anomalies. True or False?*

ANSWER: True. *Neurologic evaluations, including imaging of the brain, should be done because of the high prevalence of brain abnormalities that have been reported in infants with HLHS (Park, 2014, pp. 258–259).*

7. *In discussion with parents regarding the long-term outcomes of patients with HLHS, it is important to remember that once children undergo the three-stage repair, they will have normal cardiac function. True or False?*

ANSWER: False. *Even children who survive the three-step repair will function with a single ventricle (O'Connor, Goldberg, & Rychik, 2012).*

Case 7.3

You are called to the delivery room following a vaginal birth that has just occurred for a 41 1/7-week-gestation male infant for persistent central cyanosis. The RN states that the mother is a gravida 1, now para 1, 27-year-old female who came in for induction of labor postdates. The mother is group B *Streptococcus* (GBS) positive, Venereal Disease Research Laboratory (VDRL) nonreactive, HBsAg negative, rubella immune, HIV negative. The RN states that the infant "has not pinked up since birth but has not been grunting or retracting."

(continued)

Case 7.3 (*continued*)

On your arrival at about 12 minutes of age, you note a centrally cyanotic infant with O_2 saturations of 78% via the right wrist receiving free-flow O_2 that the labor and delivery nurse has just increased to 70% for persistent low saturations.

The infant appears to be a well-nourished term male without obvious abnormalities. The infant is centrally cyanotic but has nonlabored respiratory effort and appears to be in no acute distress. Perfusion is normal and capillary refill is approximately 2 seconds. The breath sounds are equal bilaterally with a few scattered rales noted bilaterally. Aeration is good. Respiratory rate is 80. O_2 saturations remain 78% despite increasing free-flow oxygen to 100%. No murmur is auscultated. HR is 120 bpm. The nurse states that the mother's membranes ruptured 19 hours ago (clear fluid), the mother received three doses of penicillin while in labor and developed a temperature of 100.4°F 1 hour prior to delivery. Fetal monitor tracings were normal during labor. The birth was a spontaneous vaginal delivery. The mother is a type 1 diabetic on insulin. Prenatal medications include prenatal vitamins and insulin. The obstetrician (OB) states that the infant has a two-vessel umbilical cord noted on the ultrasound but otherwise the ultrasound was normal. Congenital heart disease (CHD) is included in your differential for this infant.

1. *Which of the following congenital heart defects is the most likely to be the confirmed diagnosis for this infant?*

   A. Complete atrioventricular (AV) canal
   B. D-transposition of the great arteries (D-TGA)
   C. Ventricular septal defect

   ANSWER: B. *The infant is presenting with cyanosis that does not respond to oxygen and with signs or symptoms of a cyanotic heart defect. TGA is the only cyanotic defect noted on the list presented (Kenney, Hoover, Williams, & Iskersky, 2011). Complete AV canal and ventricular septal defect (VSD) both present with signs/symptoms of congestive heart failure (CHF) and neither generally have symptoms of cyanosis that occur at birth.*

The infant has a chest x-ray (CXR) and echocardiogram immediately after admission to the neonatal intensive care unit (NICU). The echocardiogram demonstrates TGA.

2. *The CXR for this infant would most likely demonstrate:*

   A. An egg-on-a-string heart
   B. A boot-shaped heart
   C. A small heart with pulmonary venous congestion

   ANSWER: A. *D-TGA generally presents with an egg-shaped heart (although this may not be seen in the newborn period; Aswath & Snyder, 2015).*

3. *When auscultating heart sounds on an infant with TGA, you will generally hear:*

   A. An S3 gallop
   B. A single S2
   C. Splitting of S2

   ANSWER: B. *S2 is generally single in infants with TGA (Kenney et al., 2011).*

(*continued*)

Case 7.3 (continued)

4. **An infant with TGA who has a higher oxygen saturation level (or less cyanosis) generally has:**
   A. An intact ventricular septum
   B. No collateral circulation
   C. A VSD

   ANSWER: C. *Infants with an associated VSD, atrial septal defect (ASD), patent ductus arteriosus (PDA), or collateral circulation will have more mixing of oxygenated and unoxygenated blood and thus less cyanosis (Williams & Iskersky, 2011).*

5. **The arterial switch operation done for TGA is generally:**
   A. Done at 6 to 9 months of age
   B. Done at 1 to 2 weeks of age
   C. Done in two stages at birth and then 6 to 9 months of life

   ANSWER: B. *The arterial switch operation is done within the first 2 weeks of life so that the left ventricle is capable of taking on the role of the systemic pumping chamber (Ashwath & Snyder, 2015).*

Case 7.4

You are the neonatal nurse practitioner called to the delivery room at approximately 10 minutes of age for an infant who is grunting and retracting following a repeat cesarean section at 39 2/7 weeks gestation. Mother is a gravida 2, now para 2, 27-year-old afebrile female. Maternal prenatal labs include maternal group B *Streptococcus* (GBS) negative, rubella immune, VDRL negative, HIV negative, and HBsAg negative. Pregnancy was unremarkable. Rupture of membranes (ROM) occurred at delivery with clear fluid. Infant's Apgar scores were 8 and 9, respectively. RN states that the infant began grunting at approximately 5 minutes of age. An O_2 saturation monitor was placed, indicating oxygen saturation levels of 85%, therefore oxygen was not initiated. Saturations drifting to the low 80s prompted initiation of free-flow oxygen at approximately 30% to maintain adequate saturations. On your arrival, the infant is receiving oxygen at 30% with oxygen saturation levels of 88%. The infant has moderate substernal and intercostal retractions. Breath sounds are equal with fair to good aeration. You note scattered rhonchi bilaterally. In auscultating the heart, you note that the heart rate (HR) is approximately 230 bpm. No murmur is appreciable. Capillary refill is slightly delayed at 4 seconds.

The infant is transported to the neonatal intensive care unit (NICU) and placed on a 30% high-humidity nasal cannula. O_2 saturations on this support are 92% to 93%. The infant is placed on a cardiac monitor and the HR is noted to be 138 bpm. Grunting and retracting are now subsiding. Perfusion and capillary refill are now within normal limits. A bedside screening glucose level is 62 mg/dL.

(continued)

Case 7.4 (continued)

A chest x-ray (CXR) is done and indicates increased perihilar infiltrates and fluid in the right fissure. There are no focal infiltrates and the heart size is within normal limits (wnl).

The infant is about 30 minutes of age and has weaned to room air with O_2 saturations of 95% to 96%. Grunting and retracting have subsided. HR and respiratory rate are wnl.

At approximately 40 minutes of age, the cardiac monitor alarm goes off with an HR of 248 bpm. The infant begins grunting and retracting and oxygen saturations drop to the mid-80s on room air. The infant's perfusion is diminished and capillary refill is approximately 5 seconds. The nurse is unable to obtain a blood pressure.

1. **What are the upper limits for normal heart size on a neonatal CXR?**

   A. 50% of the total diameter of the chest
   B. 55% of the total diameter of the chest
   C. 60% of the total diameter of the chest

   ANSWER: C. *The upper limit for normal heart size on a chest radiograph of an infant is up to 60% of the diameter of the heart compared to the total diameter of the chest (Weinert & Martinez-Rios, 2015, p. 536).*

2. **The most likely etiology of the clinical deterioration of this infant is:**

   A. Acute signs of heart failure
   B. Pulmonary insufficiency
   C. Hypoplastic left heart syndrome (HLHS)

   ANSWER: A. *This infant has supraventricular tachycardia (SVT) with an HR of 248 bpm and is hemodynamically unstable most likely as a result of diminished cardiac output and the heart's inability to empty or fill appropriately (Hines, 2013).*

3. **The specific findings on the electrocardiogram of an infant with Wolff–Parkinson–White (WPW) preexcitation are:**

   A. An area of late ventricular activation
   B. A prolonged PR interval and a narrow QRS
   C. A short PR interval and widened QRS

   ANSWER: C. *The electrocardiogram of an infant with WPW preexcitation has a unique area of early ventricular activation on an electrocardiogram called a delta wave, which is an initial slurring of the QRS complex. There is also a very short PR interval and a widened QRS complex (Park, 2014; Webb, 2012).*

4. **The initial treatment of SVT may include vagal stimulation done by:**

   A. Ocular pressure
   B. Applying ice to entire face
   C. Carotid pressure

   ANSWER: B. *Ice in a glove placed on the entire face of the infant for 10 to 15 seconds may induce the diving reflex and cardiovert the infant (Cannon et al., 2015). Occular pressure, gagging, anal stimulation, and carotid pressure should be avoided.*

(continued)

Case 7.4 (continued)

5. Appropriate long-term treatment of infants with WPW preexcitation may include:

A. Digoxin
B. Propranolol
C. Verapamil

ANSWER: B. *For infants with WPW preexcitation, digoxin should not be used and propranolol may be used (Park, 2014).*

REFERENCES

Anderson, P. A. (1996). The heart and development. *Seminars in Perinatology, 20*(6), 482–509.

Ashwath, R., & Snyder, C. S. (2015). Congenital defects of the cardiovascular system. In R. J. Martin, A. A. Fanaroff, & M. C. Walsh (Eds.), *Fanaroff and Martin's neonatal-perinatal medicine: Diseases of the fetus and infant* (10th ed., pp. 1230–1249). Philadelphia, PA: Saunders.

Austin, N. C., Pairaudeau, P. W., Hames, T. K., & Hall, M. A. (1992). Regional cerebral blood flow velocity changes after indomethacin infusion in preterm infants. *Archives of Disease in Childhood, 67,* 851–854.

Benitz, W. E. (2010). Treatment of persistent patent ductus arteriosus in preterm infants: Time to accept the null hypothesis? *Journal of Perinatology, 30,* 241–252.

Benitz, W. E. (2015). Patent ductus arteriosus. In R. J. Martin, A. A. Fanaroff, & M. C. Walsh (Eds.), *Fanaroff and Martin's neonatal-perinatal medicine: Diseases of the fetus and infant* (10th ed., pp. 1223–1229). Philadelphia, PA: Saunders.

Benjamin, J. R., Smith, P. B., Cotton, C. M., Jaggers, J., Goldstein, R. F., & Malcolm, W. F. (2010). Long-term morbidities associated with vocal cord paralysis after surgical closure of a patent ductus arteriosus in extremely low birth weight infants. *Journal of Perinatology, 30,* 408–413.

Brown, D. W., & Fulton, D. R. (2011). Congenital heart disease in children and adolescents. In V. Fuster, R. Walsh, & R. Harrington (Eds.), *Hurst's the heart* (13th ed., pp. 1827–1883). New York, NY: McGraw-Hill.

Cannon, B., Kovalenko, O., & Snyder, C. S. (2015). Disorders of cardiac rhythm and conduction in newborns. In R. J. Martin, A. Fanaroff, & M. C. Walsh (Eds.), *Fanaroff and Martin's neonatal-perinatal medicine: Diseases of the fetus and infant* (10th ed., pp. 1259–1274). Philadelphia, PA: Elsevier Saunders.

Chen, S., Tacy, T., & Clyman, R. (2010). How useful are B-type natriuretic peptide measurements for monitoring changes in patent ductus arteriosus shunt magnitude? *Journal of Perinatology, 30,* 780–785.

Clement, W. A., El-Hakim, H., Phillipos, E. Z, & Cote, J. J. (2008). Unilateral vocal cord paralysis following patent ductus arteriosus ligation in extremely low-birth-weight infants. *Archives of Otolaryngology—Head and Neck Surgery, 134*(1), 28–33.

Clyman, R. I. (2012). Patent ductus arteriosus in the preterm infant. In C. A. Gleason & S. U. DeVaskar (Eds.), *Avery's diseases of the newborn* (9th ed., pp. 751–761). Philadelphia, PA: Elsevier.

Clyman, R. I., Couto, J., & Murphy, G. M. (2012). Patent ductus arteriosus: Are current neonatal treatment options better or worse than no treatment at all? *Seminars in Perinatology, 36,* 123–129.

Fowlie, P. W., Davis, P. G., & McGuire, W. (2010). Prophylactic intravenous indomethacin for preventing mortality and morbidity in preterm infants. *Cochrane Database of Systematic Reviews, 2010*(7), CD000174. doi:10.1002/14651858.CD000174.pub2

Hines, M. H. (2013). Neonatal cardiovascular physiology. *Seminars in Pediatric Surgery, 22,* 174–178.

Hull, D., Binns, B. A., & Joyce, D. (1966). Congenital heart block and widespread fibrosis due to maternal lupus erythematosus. *Archives of Disease in Childhood, 41*(220), 688–690.

Hutchings, K., Vasquez, A., Price, D., Cameron, B. H., Awan, S., & Miller, G. G. (2013). Outcomes following neonatal patent ductus arteriosus ligation done by pediatric surgeons: A retrospective cohort analysis. *Journal of Pediatric Surgery, 48,* 915–918.

Kenney, P. M., Hoover, D., Williams, L. C., & Iskersky, V. (2011). Cardiovascular diseases and surgical interventions. In S. L. Gardner, B. S. Carter, M. Enzman-Hines, & J. A. Hernandez (Eds.), *Merenstein & Gardners handbook of neonatal intensive care* (7th ed., pp. 678–716). St. Louis, MO: Elsevier Mosby.

Lowry, A. W. (2012). Resuscitation and perioperative management of the high-risk single ventricle patient: First-stage palliation. *Congenital Heart Disease, 7,* 466–478.

Moore, K. L., Persaud, T. V. N., & Torchia, M. G. (2013). *The developing human: Clinically oriented embryology* (9th ed., pp. 289–342). Philadelphia, PA: Elsevier Saunders.

Noori, S. (2012). Pros and cons of patent ductus arteriosus ligation: Hemodynamic changes and other morbidities after patent ductus arteriosus ligation. *Seminars in Perinatology, 36,* 139–145.

Noori, S., Stavroudis, T. A., & Seri, I. (2012). Principles of developmental cardiovascular physiology and pathophysiology. In C. Kleinman, I. Seri, & R. Polin (Eds.), *Hemodynamics and cardiology* (2nd ed., pp. 3–27). Philadelphia, PA: Elsevier Saunders.

O'Connor, M. J., Goldberg, D. J., & Rychik, J. (2012). Single-ventricle congenital heart disease. In M. Gleason, J. Rychik, & R. Shaddy (Eds.), *Pediatric practice: Cardiology* (pp. 195–214). New York, NY: McGraw-Hill.

Ohlsson, A., Walia, R., & Shah, S. S. (2013). Ibuprofen for the treatment of patent ductus arteriosus in preterm and/or low birth weight infants. *Cochrane Database of Systematic Reviews, 2013*(4), CD003481. doi:10.1002/14651858.CD003481.pub5

Oncel, M. U., Uirttutan, S., Erdeve, O., Uras, N., Altug, N., Suna, S., . . . Dilmen, U. (2014). Oral paracetamol versus oral ibuprofen in the management of patient ductus arteriosus in preterm infants: A randomized controlled trial. *Journal of Pediatrics, 164,* 510–514.

Park, M. K. (2014). *Pediatric cardiology for practitioners* (6th ed.). Philadelphia, PA: Elsevier Saunders.

Schmidt, B., Davis, P., Moddemann, D., Ohlsson, A., Roberts. R., Saigals, S., . . . Wright, L. L. (2001). Long-term effects of indomethacin prophylaxis in extremely-low-birth-weight infants. *New England Journal of Medicine, 344,* 1966–1972.

Scholz, T. D., & Reinking, B. E. (2012). *Congenital heart disease.* In C. A. Gleason & S. U. DeVaskar (Eds.), *Avery's diseases of the newborn* (9th ed., pp. 762–788). Philadelphia, PA: Elsevier.

Strainic, J., & Snyder, C. S. (2015). Prenatal diagnosis of congenital heart disease. In R. J. Martin, A. Fanaroff, & M. C. Walsh (Eds.), *Fanaroff and Martin's neonatal-perinatal medicine: Diseases of the fetus and infant* (10th ed., pp. 1215–1229). Philadelphia, PA: Saunders.

Swanson, T., & Erickson, L. (2016). Cardiovascular diseases and surgical interventions. In S. L. Gardner, B. S. Carter, M. E. Hines, & J. A. Hernandez (Eds.), *Merenstein & Gardner's handbook of neonatal intensive care* (pp. 644–688). St. Louis, MO: Elsevier.

Teixeira, L. S., Shivananda, S. P., Stephens, D., Van Arsdell, G., & McNamara, P. J. (2008). Postoperative cardiorespiratory instability following ligation of the preterm ductus arteriosus is related to early need for intervention. *Journal of Perinatology, 28,* 803–810.

Vargo, L. (2015). Cardiovascular assessment. In E. P. Tappero & M. E. Honeyfield (Eds.), *Physical assessment of the newborn* (5th ed., pp. 93–110). Petaluma, CA: NICU Ink.

Weinert, D. M., & Martinez-Rios, C. (2015). Diagnostic imaging of the neonate. In R. J. Martin, A. Fanaroff, & M. C. Walsh (Eds.), *Fanaroff and Martin's neonatal-perinatal medicine: Diseases of the fetus and infant* (10th ed., pp. 536–558). Philadelphia, PA: Saunders.

Wren, C. (2011). *Concise guide to pediatric arrhythmias.* Hoboken, NJ: Wiley-Blackwell.

8

Neonatal Head, Ears, Eyes, Nose, and Throat System Cases

Roxanne R. Stahl

Chapter Objectives

1. Explore dysmorphology and pathophysiology related to the head, ear, eyes, nose, and throat (HEENT) in the neonate
2. List malformations of the ears that can be seen at birth and recognize their associated genetic syndromes
3. Discuss nasolacrimal duct obstruction and apply pathophysiology to clinical presentation in the newborn period
4. Apply pathophysiology of cleft lip and palate to challenges of ventilation and feedings in the newborn
5. Relate pathophysiology of the neonatal throat to appropriate differential diagnosis

This chapter provides opportunities for students to understand and review physiology/pathophysiology of the neonatal HEENT system(s) and to apply this knowledge to case studies and several simulated "real-life" clinical problems in the nursery/neonatal intensive care unit (NICU). In these cases, clinicians will be able to move through a clinical neonatal problem, delve into its corresponding anatomy, pathology and physiology, and arrive at a diagnosis.

NORMAL HEENT DEVELOPMENT AND PHYSIOLOGY

Clinicians perform a thorough physical examination of infants shortly after birth to look at physical characteristics, which determine overall health. Many problems can be identified, corrected, and prevent further disability. Clusters of abnormal findings may indicate syndromes. This chapter focuses on HEENT pathophysiology.

Normal Development and Physiology

Head

The newborn's head is inspected for shape and symmetry. It may be asymmetric as a result of in utero positioning or molding during labor and delivery as the head moves through the cervix and vagina (see Figure 8.1).

Normally, the anterior fontanel is open and flat, not tense, and measures up to 4 cm in diameter. If the anterior fontanel is tense (when the newborn is not crying), it can be a sign of increased intracranial pressure. The sagittal sutures can be open (separated) or overriding. The posterior fontanel is usually small and similar in size to an adult fingertip.

Eyes

The eye of the newborn differs from the adult eye primarily in function (Martin, Fanaroff, & Walsh, 2015). The growth of the eye parallels the growth of the brain and continues at a rapid rate for the first 3 years of life. Clinicians must be skilled in assessing and recognizing eye abnormalities so that intervention can be made to promote optimal visual outcome. Inspection should include eye shape, size, positioning on the face, visual fixation, red-light reflex, and ocular movements.

Ears

Normal ear development begins 24 days after conception. During the last 2 weeks of the embryonic period (at about 6 weeks gestation), the ears become distinct but are low set on the head. Rapid growth of the fetus occurs between 13 and 16 weeks, with the eyes and ears moving to more normal positions. Infant's ears are inspected for location of the pinna on the head, size and shape of the ear, abnormal folds of the pinna, skin tags, pits, and ear canal openings. The external ear consists of the pinna and ear canal; it conducts sound to the

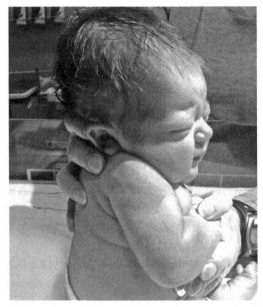

***Figure* 8.1** Infant With Molded Head From Vaginal Delivery

Photographs used with permission from R. Stahl.

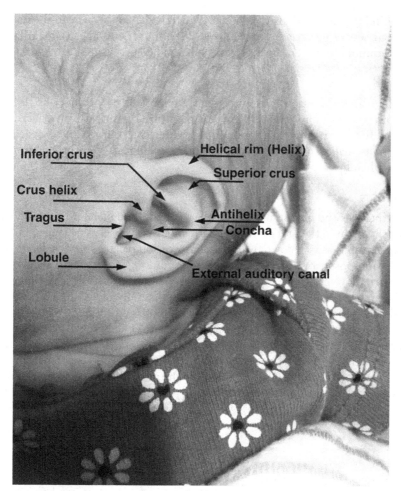

Figure 8.2 Infant Ear

Photographs used with permission from R. Stahl. Graphics by D. Stahl.

inner ear (see Figure 8.2). Ear tissue in the pinna and ear canal is soft and flexible, including the tympanic membrane. Neonates have proportionately smaller ears than adults, which will grow from 14 mm long to 23 mm long over time.

Nose

In normal anatomy, the nasal root is where the nose starts at the level of the eyes. Proceeding down the face, the nasal bridge is the bony structure between the eyes. The nostrils, or nares, are separated by epidermal, mucosal, and cartilaginous tissue called *columella* (small column). The columella supports the tip of the nose and must be long enough to keep the nose at a normal slope. The nasal septum sits behind the columella and divides the nasal cavity in half. The nasal septum should be straight but it is often deviated in normal patients. The nasal turbinates are bony structures in the nasal cavity. They are long and narrow, curving to increase air flow, or turbulence, over the nasal muscosal lining over the bones. The nasal turbinates have three functions: the muscosal lining traps particulates and acts as a filter, they warm and humidify inspired air, and they deflect air in order to enhance the sense of smell. Behind the turbinates is the choana, which is the passageway to the nasopharynx. There are four sets of paranasal sinuses: frontal (behind the forehead), maxillary (behind the cheeks), ethmoid (between the eyes), and sphenoid (deep in the skull; Kummer, 2014).

Upper Lip

The philtrum is an indentation that goes from the columella to the upper lip. It has philtral ridges on both sides, which were the embryologic suture lines that formed as the upper lip developed and fused. The top of the upper lip should be well curved and is called the *cupid's bow* because of its shape. In normal anatomy, the upper lip rests slightly over and in front of the lower lip when lips are closed.

Mouth/Palates

The mouth includes the oral structures of the tongue, the faucial pillars, and the palate. The tongue should fit in the oral cavity when the mouth is closed. The faucial pillars are the muscular structures that arch down from the velum, or soft palate. They are bilaterally paired into anterior and posterior faucial pillars that contain muscles that manage velopharyngeal and lingual movements (see Figure 8.3). The tonsils are lymphoepithelial tissue located between the anterior and posterior faucial pillars bilaterally. The lingual tonsils are also lymphoid tissue at the base on the tongue to the epiglottis (Kummer, 2014).

The palate consists of the hard palate and soft palate. The hard palate is bony and separates the oral from the nasal cavity. It makes an arch we call *the roof of the mouth* but it also is the floor of the nasal cavity. The alveolar ridge, or gum line, on the hard palate is where the teeth will erupt. The soft palate, or velum, is the musculature palate in the back of the mouth posterior to the hard palate. Furthest back, posteriorly to the velum, hangs the uvula. The normal uvula should be long and tear-dropped shaped. It is interesting to note that the

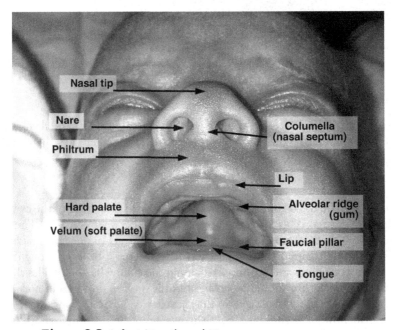

Figure 8.3 Infant Mouth and Nose
Photographs used with permission from R. Stahl. Graphics by D. Stahl.

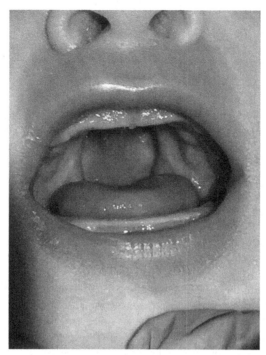

Figure 8.4 Infant Cleft Palate
Photographs used with permission from R. Stahl.

uvula has no known action and does not contribute to velopharyngeal function. If the infant has no uvula upon inspection, this infant likely is missing part of the soft palate. This may be your first clue to a soft palate cleft (Kummer, 2014; Polin, Fox, & Abman, 2010; Tewfik, 2013) (see Figure 8.4).

Throat

The throat consists of the pharynx, Eustachian tube, and adenoids. The pharynx is divided into three sections. Proceeding down from the nasal cavity to the oral cavity is the nasopharynx. The oropharynx is directly behind the mouth, or oral cavity. The hypopharynx extends from below the oral cavity and epiglottis to the esophagus. The back of the throat is termed the *posterior pharyngeal wall* and is where the adenoids (or pharyngeal tonsils) lie just behind the velum. Adenoids are present in children and atrophy with age by adulthood. The Eustachian tube is a membrane-lined tube connecting the middle ear with the pharynx bilaterally. Its function is to allow middle ear ventilation and pressure equalization with external air pressure and drainage of fluid and debris from the middle ear. In infants, the Eustachian tubes are horizontal with small pharyngeal openings. As the child ages and grows, these tubes slant increasingly downward from ear to pharynx and have larger openings that allow improved function and drainage (Kummer, 2014).

The lungs and trachea develop early in embryonic life from the primordial lung bud at the fourth week of gestation. The diverticulum of the ventral foregut contains a pair of folds that fuse to form the tracheoesophageal septum. The main stem bronchus is formed by the division of grooves between the lung bud and the esophagus with the lung bud elongating. Further branching of the bronchial tree from bronchi to bronchioles to terminal bronchioles happens by 8 to 18 weeks. Alveolar sacs are formed by 23 weeks (Blackburn, 2013).

Case 8.1

Baby boy Ethan Jones was born on April 10, at 07:14 at Community Hospital X. The mother is Stephanie Jones, a 16-year-old, gravida 1 woman weighing 215 lb. Pregnancy was complicated by a lack of prenatal care; this is a case of teen pregnancy with denial of pregnancy. Maternal labs are unknown (no prenatal care) and drawn on admission to the labor and deliver (L&D) unit and revealed: blood type O+, antibodies negative, rapid plasma reagin (RPR) nonreactive (NR), hepatitis B pending, HIV pending, gonorrhea and chlamydia (G/C) unknown, GBS (group B *Streptococcus*) unknown. She smokes one pack of cigarettes per day but denies any alcohol or drug use. Maternal medications included Zyrtec for seasonal allergies. She reports a poor diet when questioned, typical of a teenager with a lot of fast-food and limited fresh fruits and vegetables. Her mother and stepfather were in shock to find out about the pregnancy; her father and brother live in another state. The father of the baby is identified as 18 years old and on active duty in the Army. Stephanie is in high school and works a part-time job.

Stephanie presented on the evening of April 9, to the emergency department with her mother for abdominal pain. She was given a brief ultrasound to confirm that she was pregnant and taken to the L&D unit. Stephanie was 6-cm dilated and an ultrasound revealed her pregnancy to be approximately 37 to 40 weeks by fetal measurements. Decreased amniotic fluid was observed. She denied knowing when her water had broken but said she "peed herself" earlier that day at suppertime. She progressed rapidly and delivered vaginally with an epidural. Stephanie pushed for 1.5 hours. A few variables and late decelerations were noted on the fetal heart tracing (FHT).

The neonatal nurse practitioner (NNP) was called to delivery for unknown dates and teen pregnancy. The baby cried on the perineum and was placed on the mother's chest and dried. The L&D unit RN brought the baby to the NNP within 20 seconds of life and both the RN and obstetrician (OB) asked the NNP to take a close look at the baby. Facial expressions by the OB suggested to the NNP that something was wrong with this baby. At 1 minute of life, the baby was noted to have the following: easy respirations, heart rate (HR) 130 beats per minute (bpm), color pink with acrocyanosis, increased nuchal skin fold, short neck, decreased and floppy tone, narrow and high-arched palate with grimace noted upon palpation, large tongue protruding slightly from mouth, normal- sized chin, small ears, flattened nose, flat head, up-slanting palpebral fissures of the eyes with inner epicanthal folds.

1. *What is your Apgar score?*

   ANSWER: Easy respirations = 2, HR 130 bpm = 2, color pink with acrocyanosis = 1, floppy tone = 1, grimace noted = 1. Use of the Virginia Apgar scoring system provides a trustworthy method for reporting the status of the newborn infant immediately after birth and the response to resuscitation if needed (AAP & ACOG, 2015).

2. *List two abnormal findings from this brief physical exam.*

   ANSWER: The following list indicates the abnormal findings: increased nuchal skin fold, short neck, decreased and floppy tone, narrow and high-arched palate, large tongue protruding slightly from mouth, small ears, flattened nose, flat head, up-slanting palpebral fissures of the eyes with inner epicanthal folds.

(continued)

Case 8.1 (continued)

3. *What is your differential diagnosis based on these abnormal findings?*

   ANSWER: This infant has a syndrome, likely Down syndrome. *The differential diagnosis of Down syndrome is based on clinical findings. The clinician must consider: hypothyroid, XXXXY syndrome, penta-X syndrome, and Zellweger syndrome (Hennekam, Allanson, & Krantz, 2010).*

4. *Do you have a preliminary diagnosis for this baby?*

   ANSWER: Down syndrome (trisomy 21). *Based on the clinical finding of Ethan, increased nuchal skin fold, short neck, decreased and floppy tone, narrow and high-arched palate, large tongue protruding slightly from mouth, small ears, flattened nose, flat head, and upslanting palpebral fissures of the eyes with inner epicanthal folds.*

The baby is stable in room air (RA) with SpO$_2$ 90% at 5 minutes of life, probe on right hand. Identification bands were placed on the baby and footprints were taken; the NNP notes sandal-grooved toes bilaterally. Grandma is taking pictures; you weigh the baby and he is 3,585 g and 51 cm long. You wrap the baby and take him to his mother. You congratulate Stephanie on her beautiful baby and ask his name. Stephanie states, "I think Ethan." You then indicate that there are some abnormal features of Ethan and proceed to show Stephanie and her mom. "These abnormal things with Ethan lead me to think that he might have Down syndrome but we won't know for sure until we draw his blood and look at his chromosomes." Give a brief summary of how long it will take to get chromosomal analysis results. Tell Stephanie how alert and strong Ethan is. Always tell the parent and family that nothing could have caused or prevented Down syndrome. Mothers tend to blame themselves for any problems in their children and can carry guilt for the rest of their lives. Stephanie is a teenager and needs to know that she did not cause Ethan to have problems or a syndrome.

Genetic diseases occur from a problem with gene structure or a chromosome disorder. Chromosomes are structures in the cells that contain genes. Genetic problems can be inherited, caused by new mutations, or by chromosomal alterations. If an entire chromosome is changed, it manifests in much more symptomology than does a single-gene defect. In this case, we will focus on trisomy 21, or Down syndrome, a chromosomal disorder with aneuploidy. Following the path of normal conception, an individual inherits 23 chromosomes from the mother's egg and 23 from the father's sperm, which form a fertilized egg containing 46 chromosomes. Most trisomy 21 cases occur before fertilization in the developing egg or sperm from aneuploidy nondisjunction during the first meiotic division when both members of a homologous pair of chromosomes move to one gamete. This error in cell division results in one gamete having 22 chromosomes and the other having 24. Once the gamete with 24 chromosomes pairs with a normal gamete with 23 chromosomes, the total is 47 chromosomes. There is now an extra set or copy of chromosomes on number 21. Down syndrome is the most common chromosomal disorder generally resulting from trisomy of chromosome 21 with the first meiotic division. This type of trisomy 21 more typically occurs from the effect of advanced maternal age. It can also happen after fertilization during the second meiotic division when sister chromatids fail to separate, causing some cell lines to have the normal number of 46 cells and others the abnormal number of 47. This is mosaicism and accounts for 1% to 2% of Down syndrome cases (Blackburn, 2013). Trisomy 21 can also be caused by duplication or translocation of a specific region of chromosome 21 (Hennekam et al., 2010).

Trisomy 21 is the most common congenital anomaly syndrome, occurring in about one in 650 to 1,000 live births with physical findings of hypotonia, poor or absent Moro reflex, flat facial profile and occiput, up-slanting palpebral fissures, Brushfield spots, small anomalous ears, excess nuchal skin, sandal-groove/gap toes, single palmar creases/simian creases (Hall, 1964). Congenital heart defects occur in about 50% of cases and are most commonly atrioventricular canal defects (Gomella, 2013).

Case 8.1 *(continued)*

Ethan is stable and pink, so you leave him with the family and send the nursery RN to check on him. She brings him to the nursery at 30 minutes of life and says that Stephanie wants him to get "that blood drawn so we'll know for sure."

A more thorough examination of Ethan is performed in the nursery. The clinician examines Ethan's head and notes a flat head, a third fontanel in the sagittal suture line, increased nuchal skin fold, and a short neck.

ABNORMAL FINDINGS OF THE HEENT SYSTEM SEEN IN DOWN SYNDROME INFANTS

Head

Flat occiput, brachycephaly, and/or microcephaly in Down syndrome children result from delayed fetal brain growth. Decreased total brain weight arises specifically from a smaller cerebellum and inadequate development of nuclei in the brain stem. The fontanels are large and closure can be late. A third fontanel is often present in the sagittal suture. The eye, ear, and forebrain begin embryologic development approximately 4 weeks postconception. The forebrain (diencephalon, referring to two outpouchings) expands laterally to form the optic vessels (Polin, Fox, & Abman, 2010; Volpe, 2008).

Eyes

Ocular findings associated with Down syndrome can include amblyopia, nystagmus, strabismus, nasolacrimal duct obstruction, epicanthus, telecanthus, upward slant of palpebral fissures, blepharitis, keratoconus, glaucoma, iris nodules (Brushfield spots), cataract, and optic nerve swelling (Martin, Fanaroff, & Walsh, 2015). Because genes control development of the eye, chromosomal anomalies show up with significant alteration of genetic materials. Ocular abnormalities are extensive in trisomy 21.

Case 8.1 (continued)

The more thorough physical examination of Ethan includes inspection and an oph-thalmologic exam. The size, shape, position, and slant of the eyes should be noted. Ethan has a negative red reflex bilaterally and Brushfield spots bilaterally in the iris. The clinician had already noted up-slanting palpebral fissures of the eyes with inner epicanthal folds. She now notes strabismus when Ethan gazes out from his crib.

Eyelid abnormalities seen in trisomy 21 are blepharophimosis and epicanthus. *Blepharophimosis* refers to narrow eyelids, both vertically and horizontally. There is usually an associated ptosis (drooping). Epicanthus is the most common eyelid abnormality seen in infants and involves a skin fold starting in the upper lid and extending over the medial end of the upper lid, the medial canthus and the caruncle, and ends in the skin of the lower lid. Telecanthus describes a disproportionate increase in distance between the medial canthal angles.

Teardrops can occur at birth and are as a result of irritants. Emotional tearing (crying) begins at about 2 to 3 months. Newborns have a strong blink reflex that can be elicited with light and stimulation to the lids, lashes, and cornea. At birth, the eyes should appear straight, but because of developing newborn musculature, many eye movements can be seen. Strabismus or misalignment of the eyes is common in newborns but constant strabismus after 4 months of age warrants investigation. Down syndrome children frequently have central nervous system (CNS)-associated esotrophia. Abnormal CNS esotrophic children are characterized by continual or intermittent inward deviation of the eye or eyes. Strabismus detection, classification, and treatment are especially important in pediatrics to prevent a loss in visual functioning, which develops from inadequate or abnormal visual system stimulation. In children, strabismus needs to be corrected to maximize potential for straightening of the eyes. Uncorrected strabismus accounts for approximately 30% of amblyopia in children (Lorenz & Brodsky, 2010). Nystagmus is evident by jerking or oscillating contractions of the eye, either unilateral or bilateral.

Abnormal (negative) red reflex in the child in the case study was seen as cloudy. A cataract is any opacity of the lens or white pupil (leukocoria). Congenital cataracts are present at birth and can be responsible for 10% of all blindness. Etiology of cataracts can be hereditary, metabolic, traumatic, and those seen with chromosomal abnormalities. The size and shape of the cataract varies with fetal eye development and when the damage occurred. Early embryonic damage results in opacifications in the center of the lens, later damage produces ring-like opacifications surrounded by clear areas (zonal; Martin et al., 2015).

Ears

Visual inspection of the ears notes size, shape, and position on the head. Ears should be positioned on each side of the head in a normal location. The clinician can draw an imaginary line from the infant's eye's inner to outer canthus; extend the line, and the helix should be at this location, where it attaches to the head. The helix is below this line with low-set ears. An examination of the ears of Ethan, the baby in the case study, noted they were small with a deformed helix bilaterally. An auditory canal was visible upon visual inspection bilaterally. Newborns with syndromeic craniofacial anomalies often have microtia (small ears), absent ear lobes, and malformation of the pinna (overlapping rim of the helix), making ears seem square shaped. The more severely malformed the external ear, the increased likelihood of middle and inner ear problems. According to Mitchell and Pereira (2009), Eustachian tube dysfunction can manifest with recurrent effusions and often require tympanostomy tubes. Hearing loss prevalence is 70% in Down syndrome children and stenotic canals are present in 50% of these infants.

Children with Down syndrome are described by their families as good and happy babies who are not easily disturbed. This is likely a result of a diminished response to external stimuli from hearing loss and decreased tone/reflexes (Hennekam, Allanson, & Krantz, 2010).

Maternal smoking directly dysregulates cytotrophoblast expression and differentiation, which helps to explain the mechanisms by which smoking negatively impacts pregnancy outcome (Polin, Fox, & Abman, 2010). Maternal smoking has been linked to sensori-neural hearing loss.

Nose/Throat

Bony midface hypoplasia manifests in hypotelorism, small nose, flattened nasal bridge, high-arched palate, and mandibular protrusion (prognathism). These children have auditory, short-term memory, speech (articulation, language development), and visual (color retention, shape identification) problems. Mental retardation and hypotonia affect motor ability and language, which leads to delayed developmental milestones (Bull, 2011).

Neck

The neck is inspected for abnormalities. Redundant skin over the posterior neck is seen in Down syndrome. A webbed neck is a feature of Turner syndrome.

Case 8.1 (*continued*)

The NNP was called to the nursery to see Ethan at 2 hours of life for poor feeding and glucose of 35 mg/dl. The nurse was attempting to bottle-feed formula to Ethan but he had an ineffective suck with frequent tongue thrusting. The mother did not want to breastfeed.

1. *What do you know about trisomy 21 that would cause the feedings to be difficult for Ethan?*

   ANSWER: Trisomy 21 infants likely have hypotonia, macroglossia, and poor muscle control. *Hypotonia is one hallmark of trisomy 21. In the neonate at birth, CNS organization and integration are dependent on in utero environment and genetic structural makeup. Organization is how we are "wired" and shows our capacity to operate integrated as a whole. Infants with Down syndrome have alterations in organization in fetal neurodevelopment. Ethan will have poor head control as a result of hypotonia in addition to his large tongue, which makes positioning him during feedings difficult. Poor muscle control also manifests in the perioral muscles, lips, tongue, and masticatory muscles, which makes sucking, swallowing, and breathing more difficult. Care must be taken not to overextend his*

(continued)

Case 8.1 (continued)

neck and increase risk of aspiration. Regurgitation can occur from a weak musculature of the soft palate, resulting in poor closure at the nasopharynx. The infant may also have a small mouth and flat tongue, which makes cupping the nipple difficult.

2. ***How can you support him with his bottle feedings?***

   ANSWER: Ethan could benefit from feeding in the side-lying or straddle positions and with pacing. *Feeding via breast or bottle can often be easier in side-lying or seated straddle positions to optimize support for the infant's neck. Pacing is often needed because of poor muscle control in Down syndrome children.*

Mothers who are breastfeeding are taught to support the breast with their hand using the Dancer hand position (head supported with one hand, cheek pressure exerted by using her other hand to cup the baby's chin with her thumb on one cheek and her fingers on the other cheek, thereby providing counter pressure). Sucking will improve with age as these children progress beyond the neurodevelopmental delay present at birth (Wilson-Clay & Hoover, 2013).

Case 8.1 (continued)

Ethan responds to feeding strategies and can take 30 mL of formula every 3 hours orally when in the seated position in front of the mother. She learns how to support Ethan's hypotonic neck and body. When Ethan thrusts the nipple out of his mouth, Grandmother is coached to encourage the mother to hold the bottle/nipple firmly in Ethan's mouth and not let him spit it out repetitively. Repeat blood sugar test on Ethan at 3 hours of life is 45 mg/dl and at 6 hours of life is 52. Ethan is discharged home on day of life (DOL) 3 with his mother, who lives with Ethan's grandmother. Home visits are arranged for follow up on this first-time teen mom and social services are offered. Preliminary chromosomal analysis reveals (47XY + 21) trisomy 21. Follow-up is arranged with a pediatrician well versed in children with Down syndrome, and if available, referral to a children's hospital with a Down syndrome clinic. According to the American Academy of Pediatrics, Health Supervision for Children With Down Syndrome (Bull, 2011), children with Down syndrome have lifelong special needs and health care issues that need support.

NEONATAL EAR MALFORMATIONS

Ears may also be referred to as *auricles* and *pinna*. Skin tags and/or pits located anterior to the ear are called *preauricular* and must be inspected and noted. They are the most commonly occurring ear malformations and occur in 0.5% live births. Small skin tags may be benign and isolated, especially if unilateral. Complex skin tags may be a clue to a more complex syndrome or hearing disorder. Any variety of ear abnormalities can be seen by the clinician. In Figures 8.5 and 8.6, the infant presented with bilateral ear deformities of the helix, antihelix, and lobule. No family history of ear deformities or hearing loss was established. Renal ultrasound of this baby was normal. Hearing testing of acoustic brain response (ABR) was referred in both ears and subsequent follow-up was arranged at the nearby children's hospital for neurology, genetics, and auditory consults.

Ear malformations can be associated with other familial disorders, history of deafness, maternal history of diabetes, and an increased risk of renal abnormalities. Plastic surgeons will need to be consulted for cosmetic and functional correction of ear deformities. Splinting can often improve minor eye deformities to avoid surgery.

Low-set ears, melotia, can be seen in syndromes such as Treacher–Collins; triploidy; and trisomy 9, 13, 19, and 21. Hairy ears can be seen in infants of diabetic mothers and mothers of Hispanic, Latin, or Mediterranean backgrounds. *Anotia* refers to complete absence of the pinna or external ear and is associated with thalidomide and retinoic acid teratogens.

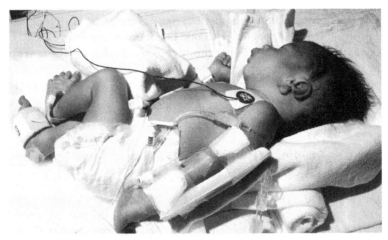

Figure 8.5 Infant With Bilateral Ear Deformities
Photographs used with permission from R. Stahl.

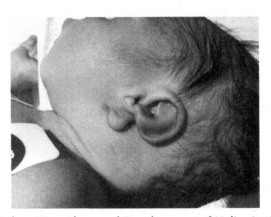

Figure 8.6 Ear Deformities: Abnormal Development of Helix, Antihelix, and Lobule
Photographs used with permission from R. Stahl.

Bilateral anotia can be seen in offspring of consanguineous parents. Microtia, small ears, can be seen in trisomy 13, 18, and 21; triploidy; thalidomide; and retinoic acid teratogens. Macrotia, large ears, are commonly bilateral and symmetric and can be seen in Marfan, Fragile X, and DeLange syndromes. Lop ears have a folded-down helix and cup ears stand away from the head. If the ear is hypoplastic, it may indicate a disorder of the inner ear.

A renal ultrasound should be considered in infants with ear malformations, especially if multiple congenital anomalies exist. Previous thinking was that ear and kidney development coincided in utero. We have evidence that fetal kidney and ears primordial arise at different times and develop at different rates. Strong evidence links ear malformations with renal anomalies. Wang, Earl, Ruder, and Graham (2001) observed 42 patients with ear anomalies. Of the 12 patients with renal anomalies, 92% had a diagnosis of multiple congenital anomaly (MCA) syndrome. Infants with isolated ear anomalies have an 11% incidence of a renal anomaly, and infants with MCA syndrome had 33% incidence of a renal anomaly.

EYE ABNORMALITY IN NEWBORN INFANT

Case 8.2

You are called by the nursery RN to the bedside of a 2-day-old infant because of a "bump by the eye and the eye has drainage." Upon your inspection, you note a clear bluish mass overlying the lacrimal sac. The mass can be decompressed with digital pressure and results in purulent discharge.

1. **What is this condition called?**

   ANSWER: Nasolacrimal duct obstruction. *Nasolacrimal duct obstruction manifests in the first few days of life as a sticky mucoid eye discharge, either unilateral or bilateral. It may resolve spontaneously or, if prolonged, can derive from blocked or incomplete canalization of the nasolacrimal duct.*

2. **What is the differential diagnosis for eye drainage?**

   ANSWER: Conjunctivitis. *Conjunctivitis presents with erythematous, swollen eyelids, and purulent discharge. Gonococcal infection can present on day of life (DOL) 1 but routine administration of erythromycin eye ointment prevents infection in the United States. Chlamydia presents around DOL 3 to 14 and is also treated with erythromycin eye ointment.*

Nasolacrimal duct obstruction may manifest with a mucocele. If the mucocele becomes infected and dacryocystitis occurs, there is swelling and erythema over the lacrimal sac with a palpable mass. Purulent drainage can be seen through the lacrimal puncta. If the dacryocystitis is severe, rupture of the abscessed sac through the skin can occur.

Congenital nasolacrimal duct obstruction occurs in approximately 5% of normal newborn infants (Figure 8.7). The blockage most commonly occurs at the valve of Hasner at the distal end of the duct. There is no sex predilection and no genetic predisposition. The blockage can be unilateral or bilateral. The rate of spontaneous resolution is estimated to be 90% within the first year of life. Treatment is aimed at comfort, therefore eyes may be cleansed with sterile water (Gomella, 2013).

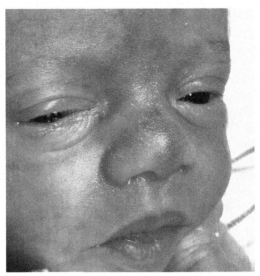

Figure 8.7 Nasolacrimal Duct Obstruction
Photographs used with permission from R. Stahl.

Case 8.3

Baby boy Jacob Steel was born on October 4, at 00:31 at County Medical Center Y. The mother is Andrea Steel, a 35-year-old, gravida 4, term 2, preterm 0, abortion 1, living children 2, now 3. She weighs 155 lb. Pregnancy was complicated by prenatal diagnosis of cleft lip. Good prenatal care was obtained. Obstetric history is significant for abnormal Pap smear and loop electrosurgical excision procedure (LEEP) in 2013, and spontaneous vaginal deliveries (SVDs) in 2000 and 2008. Maternal labs were drawn at 12 weeks gestation and revealed: blood type O+, antibodies negative, syphilis (RPR) nonreactive, hepatitis B negative, HIV negative, G/C negative, GBS unknown. Andrea smokes five to 10 cigarettes per day and denies any alcohol or drug use. Maternal medications included prenatal vitamins. Andrea is married but tells you that the father of the baby is not her husband. Andrea works and cares for her two small children. She is unsure whether she will tell her husband that this is not his baby. She is still having a relationship with the father of her baby but he is not planning to come to the hospital.

Andrea was admitted October 3, at 23:41 for observation in questionable preterm labor at 32 1/7 weeks gestation. The obstetrician (OB) consulted with a neonatologist about this patient and discussed her prenatal diagnosis of cleft lip. Ultrasound scans at 18 weeks had shown unilateral cleft lip on the right and no cleft palate identified by scan. Parents stated they were very optimistic that the cleft lip is "very small" and had not gone to the regional medical center where they were instructed to go for maternal–fetal medicine (MFM) consult and delivery. In preparing the patient for transfer to the regional

(continued)

Case 8.3 *(continued)*

medical center, she dilated from 3 to 7 cm and spontaneously ruptured her membranes with clear fluid. Transfer was canceled and labor progressed. The neonatal nurse practitioner (NNP) asked the OB to repeat maternal labs as Andrea has had multiple sex partners and preterm delivery is eminent. Maternal labs of hepatitis B, HIV, RPR, and G/C were drawn. Andrea denied any history of herpes or any vesicular lesions on her perineum. Penicillin was given prior to delivery. SVD occurred on October 4, at 00:31 with an NNP and RN present. Jacob had a rapid delivery with two pushes only. He had a weak cry at delivery and was placed on the warmer. Neonatal Resuscitation Program (NRP) protocol was followed and Jacob received 1 minute of positive pressure ventilation (PPV), then 3 minutes of mask continuous positive airway pressure (CPAP). He was shown to his "parents" briefly, then transported to the Level II neonatal intensive care unit (NICU) on blow-by 40% oxygen. SpO$_2$ was 92% on 40% oxygen at 5 minutes of age. Jacob weighed 1,500 g. He received erythromycin ophthalmic ointment and vitamin K per protocol on admission. On brief physical examination, he had a severe right cleft lip and palate, wide forehead, hypertelorism, slightly cupped ears, deformed nose with extension of cleft into right nare. Jacob also had nasal flaring, grunting, and intercostal retractions (G/F/R). Parents were visibly upset and crying.

1. *What options are available to treat Jacob's respiratory distress?*

   ANSWER: Options to treat respiratory distress in the delivery room may be: free-flow blended oxygen per face mask, CPAP via face mask with or without oxygen, PPV with a bag and mask or T-piece resuscitator, and/or intubation with PPV. *Resuscitation of the newborn always follows NRP guidelines (Weiner & Zaichkin, 2016). It is important to ensure Jacob has a patent airway, free from secretions. The NNP may need to open or close Jacob's mouth if ventilating him with a mask to establish a good airway or intubate.*

2. *What is the critical thinking of the NNP caring for him on the optimal mode of respiratory support?*

   ANSWER: Critical thinking of the NNP notes that Jacob is a preterm, White male at 32 1/7 weeks gestation with no previous preterm labor, had rapid labor and delivery, who did not receive antenatal steroids, and was in respiratory distress at delivery. He is expressing G/F/R and severe facial, mouth, and airway anomalies—evidence-based reasons for moderate to severe respiratory distress syndrome. For the purpose of this HEENT chapter, we focus on the facial deformities and how they dictate certain treatment modalities. In this Level II NICU, respiratory distress is treated with (a) high-flow nasal cannula flow and oxygen, (b) Vapotherm (high-flow humidification system), (c) nasal CPAP, and (d) mechanical ventilation. Since Jacob has a nasal and palate deformity with absent upper lip, a nasal cannula would potentially be difficult to place and flow would have no normal anatomy to get into the lungs for distending pressure. An oxygen hood could be very useful to deliver oxygen without disturbing the face but Jacob is having G/F/R indicating a need for pressure support of some kind. Vapotherm and nasal CPAP also depend on normal facial and palate anatomy. *Critical*

(continued)

Case 8.3 *(continued)*

thinking must include quick assessment of the patient and his condition in order to intervene optimally.

The NNP continues mask CPAP and gets an immediate chest x-ray that reveals a seven-rib expansion (RE) reticulogranular pattern bilaterally. She decides to carefully intubate Jacob and give him surfactant and keep him on the ventilator for now.

Once he is stable, the clinician completes a physical examination of Jacob. She notes abnormal findings of severe right cleft lip extending into the right nare, hard and soft palate missing (possibly up into the sinus), deformed nose with extension of cleft into right nare, left nare obstructed from defect, wide forehead, hypertelorism, slightly cupped ears measuring 3.5 cm in length. Jacob has improved on the ventilator with resolved nasal flaring and grunting but he continues with mild intercostal retractions.

The anatomy of the face is reviewed to enhance understanding of anomalies and clefts. We review the nose, lips, palates, and mouth to understand neonatal pathophysiology in the infant born with cleft lip and palate.

1. ***When does the lip begin to develop in embryologic life?***

   A. 4 to 5 weeks gestation
   B. 6 to 7 weeks gestation
   C. 10 to 12 weeks gestation

   ANSWER: B. *Cleft lip and palate are frequently a result of improper fetal development; these structures fuse early in gestation. The lip begins embryologic development at about 6 to 7 weeks gestation and the palate at 8 to 9 weeks gestation (Blackburn, 2013).*

2. ***Do infants with cleft lip and palate have ear problems?***

   A. Yes
   B. No

   ANSWER: A. *Infants with cleft lip and palate can have associated ear problems such as otitis media and hearing loss. The Eustachian tubes do not align properly and cannot drain from the middle ear to the pharynx. This leads to improper ventilation and buildup of bacteria in the middle ear that can impair the conduction of sound through the ossicles. Breast milk has been proven to reduce the occurrence of otitis media (Wilson-Clay & Hoover, 2013).*

Andrea asks, "Why does my baby have this awful face … what happened?" You know that clefts vary in size and can be hypoplastic as a result of poor embryologic development.

Clefts do contain all normal underlying structures but appear abnormal because of improper fusion. Etiology of cleft lip and/or palate can be genetic as seen in syndromes or caused by something that occurred during the pregnancy such as amniotic banding or teratogens. Because clefts are caused by disruptions in development, they follow fusion lines in the formation of the face, oral cavity, nose, and eyes. If the newborn has a congenital cleft lip and/or palate and other anomalies, there is often a genetic origin and likely a syndrome to diagnose. Maternal smoking has been linked to cleft lip and/or palate and Andrea smokes. It would not be beneficial to point this out to Andrea as it would only increase her guilt and could interfere with bonding and enhance postpartum depression. According to Hennekam, Allanson, and Krantz (2010), obesity and maternal diet lacking in B6 have been associated with clefts. Folic acid deficiency was thought to be linked to clefts, but folic acid supplementation in childbearing women has not been proven to be beneficial in preventing clefts. Most clefts are caused by multifactorial inheritance.

Classification of clefts falls into two categories as described by Kernahan and Stark: clefts of the primary palate and clefts of the secondary palate. The primary palate is the front of the hard palate, called the alveolar process, and the lip. These structures are anterior to the incisive foramen and fuse at approximately 7 weeks gestation (Kummer, 2014).

Posterior to the incisive foramen is the secondary palate, which fuses at 9 weeks gestation. This includes the hard and soft palate (velum). More complicated classification systems have been identified by specialists, such as those of the ear, nose, and throat (ENT).

Case 8.3 (continued)

1. What is Jacob's cleft classification and how severe is his defect?

ANSWER: Jacob has a complete unilateral cleft on the right. *The severity of his clefting is dictated by the extent of his palate, gum, nostril, and dentition involvement. Jacob has a cleft into the right nare and his left nare is obstructed from his defect on exam.*

A complete cleft lip includes deformation of the lip, nostril sill, and alveolus to the incisive foramen. These are all parts of the primary palate. The primary cleft palate can be unilateral or bilateral. Unilateral clefts more often occur on the left side. Bilateral cleft lip can extend through the lips, incisive suture lines in the alveolus (gumline) to the incisive foramen, which can cause damage to the premaxilla bone. This gives the infant the appearance that the defect extends from the tip of the nose.

The nose can appear very wide and flat because the orbicularis muscle is divided and distorted. In unilateral defects, the nose columella is usually short on the cleft side and deviated toward the noncleft side. The nasal cavity itself is also affected in primary and secondary palate deformities. The nasal cavity is usually smaller in size, even more so in unilateral versus bilateral cases. The underlying dysplagia of the tissues in the nasal and oral cavities can result in dental, tongue, and chin movement problems because of crowding in the small cavities. Speech may be greatly affected.

The hard and soft palates appeared to be missing in Jacob on earlier careful inspection with a tongue blade and light in his mouth. Various degrees of severity can be seen when looking at his hard and soft palates. Clefting of the hard palate is further categorized as complete or incomplete.

Case 8.3 *(continued)*

2. *How would the NNP know whether the soft palate was also affected by the cleft?*

ANSWER: The NNP must inspect the uvula. *A slight line in the uvula or a bifurcated uvula demonstrates an incomplete cleft secondary palate. Extension of the cleft into the velum or part of the hard palate is a more severe form of incomplete cleft of the secondary palate. If a complete secondary palate cleft is diagnosed, the cleft passes through the uvula, velum, and hard palate to the incisive foramen. The uvula could be missing entirely in soft palate clefting. Numerous muscles attach to the structures of the mouth, so when there is a major deformity, there is extensive musculature deformity and hypoplasticity as well.*

3. *Can cleft secondary palate occur without cleft primary palate?*

ANSWER: Yes, a cleft palate can occur with or without a cleft lip. *An isolated cleft palate without lip involvement is suspect for genetic syndromes and warrants further investigation for other defects in the infant.*

Three days after delivery, a different NNP takes over Jacob's care. She receives a report that the maternal labs were repeated at delivery per request of her colleague, who noted that the mother admitted to two sexual partners. Maternal labs drawn at delivery are reported as hepatitis B negative, HIV negative, RPR negative, gonorrhea negative, chlamydia positive.

4. *What does this mean for the baby now?*

ANSWER: Jacob's mother could have been infected with chlamydia later in pregnancy. *Andrea had lab work early in her pregnancy that reported chlamydia as negative. Lab reporting from the day of Jacob's delivery reported Andrea as chlamydia positive.*

The nurse calls the NNP and asks her to come to the bedside and see Jacob. She states, "Jacob seems to have more frothy secretions and his breathing is still distressed on the ventilator. Couldn't he have pneumonia from his mom's chlamydia? He also has some watery discharge from his right eye but he got his eye medicine at birth so that would treat the chlamydia, right?" On your exam, you note copious clear secretions from Jacob's eyes, nose, and mouth and mucous secretions around his right eye. Increased secretions have been noted around his cleft lip and palate defect since birth.

5. *How do you respond to the nurse?*

ANSWER: Jacob had a chest x-ray this morning that revealed seven-RE bilateral hazy pattern without streaks. This suggests underinflated lungs typically seen in preterm lung disease. If Jacob had pneumonia, we would see hyperinflation of the lungs to nine-RE with diffuse bilateral interstitial or alveolar infiltrates; let me show you the x-rays. It may be that he has an eye infection so I will order some cultures for you to obtain.

6. *What lab tests would you order?*

ANSWER: Jacob would need tissue cultures of the eyes, specifically the tarsal conjunctiva and, if pneumonia is suspected, cultures from nasopharyngeal aspiration or deep

(continued)

Case 8.3 (continued)

endotracheal suctioning. *The NNP would consult the neonatologist and the American Academy of Pediatrics* Red Book *(Kimberlin, Brady, Jackson, & Long, 2015) of infectious diseases for further instructions.*

7. **Would you order any treatment for Jacob's eye drainage at this point? Jacob's cultures are pending.**

   ANSWER: The NNP should go ahead and treat for possible conjunctivitis based on symptoms of his clear eye drainage and positive maternal chlamydia late in pregnancy. *Neonatal ophthalmia is defined as conjunctivitis that occurs within the first 4 weeks of life. It is relatively common, occurring in 1% to 12% of neonates. The NNP knows that* Neisseria gonorrheae *accounts for 1% and chlamydia 1% to 12% of conjunctivitis, which is acquired from the vagina and cervix during delivery. Eye prophylaxis at birth with erythromycin ophthalmic ointment treats conjunctival infection and is required by all states (Gomella, 2013). Timing and symptoms can assist in diagnosis with ophthalmia neonatorum.* Neisseria gonorrheae *typically manifests in the first 5 days postbirth and is associated with marked bilateral purulent discharge and local inflammation. Conjunctivitis secondary to infection with chlamydia produces conjunctivitis on DOL 3 to 14. The discharge is usually more watery in nature (mucopurulent) and less inflamed. Babies infected with chlamydia can develop pneumonitis at a later stage (2 weeks to 19 weeks postdelivery). Conjunctivitis is easily treated with oral erythromycin for 14 days. Topical treatment is ineffective. When the mother is infected at the time of delivery, the risk of neonatal conjunctivitis due to chlamydia can be high (between 18% and 40%). Treatment can be stopped if the eye cultures come back negative but delaying treatment could be harmful and, if untreated, could cause blindness (Kimberlin et al., 2015).*

One week later in the NICU, Jacob is on an oxygen hood at 30% blended oxygen and orogastric tube feedings. The mother is concerned about "fixing him as soon as possible" and asks you what can be done for him surgically. The goal of cleft palate surgery is to repair the defects in the muscles, palates, and face. The muscles are corrected to achieve normal orientation but, because of the extent of the defects, the muscles may never be completely fixed. An estimated 25% of patients with cleft palate will have velopharyngeal insufficiency and therefore abnormal speech and resonance. Jacob will need to be followed by a multidisciplinary craniofacial team at a large hospital. Andrea also wants to breastfeed and asks why Jacob cannot start breast- and bottle-feeding.

8. **What other problems will Jacob face in the next few weeks as he learns to nipple feed?**

   ANSWER: Infants with cleft lip and/or palate are at extremely high risk for early feeding problems and nasal regurgitation. *The oral and nasal cavities are small with possible tongue misalignment causing difficulty in latching and sucking. Breathing can be difficult at rest and exacerbated during feedings because of the reduced nasal cavity size and nasopharyngeal depth contributing to upper airway obstruction and mouth breathing in infants with clefts (Kummer, 2014).*

Breast milk is the best nutrition for all infants. Infants with cleft lip and palate are at high risk for failure to thrive from inadequate intake. The anatomical problems inherent with cleft lip and palate make sucking difficult, sucking is often so tiring that the infant does not get near the intake needed while expending great effort. Breastfeeding is encouraged to facilitate maternal–infant bonding and milk production. When breastfeeding, most of the defect is obstructed by the breast and may give the baby a somewhat more normal appearance. Supplemental feedings with a special bottle or an SNS (supplemental nursing system) will usually provide adequate intake. Infants with cleft lip/palate often need increased caloric intake because of this inadequate intake of volume. Mothers must be taught to pump the breasts even after breastfeeding to adequately empty the breasts to ensure a full milk supply. If expressing breast milk is not done after breastfeeding, the mother will dry up. Mothers are encouraged to work with lactation consultants for the continued challenges that they face while feeding the infant over the next few years as the baby undergoes numerous cleft surgeries.

Case 8.4

The neonatal nurse practitioner (NNP) is called to the nursery for evaluation of an infant. The nurse states, "Baby boy Beckett was born yesterday and is making noise with his feedings and chokes a lot when he swallows." The NNP performs a physical examination on Brady Beckett and notes the following: Well developed, slightly small for gestational age (SGA). Head appears of normal size and shape with mild molding from delivery, head circumference is 34 cm, anterior fontanel open and flat, sagittal suture open, eyes appear normal, red reflex positive bilaterally, ears appear normal in placement and size, auditory canal visible bilaterally, palate intact, neck appears normal with good range of motion, no neck mass, lungs clear to auscultation bilaterally, resting quietly in room air (RA), no respiratory distress but mild tachypnea and striderous noises when feeding. Heart rate is regular with grade 1-2/6 murmur, strong brachial and femoral pulses, color pink with slight jaundice, normal tone and reflexes, testes descended bilaterally, good tone. Nasal patency is assessed by placing a glass slide or metal instrument under each nare (while occluding the other with your finger) and looking for fogging. Infants are obligate nose breathers and nasal patency must be established before further workup is considered.

1. *What information would you research for further evaluation purposes?*

ANSWER: Maternal history, labor, delivery, and nursery course. *A thorough history and physical provides information that is key in caring for any patient. Maternal history is especially important in neonatology as the neonate's development or "history" has been in utero.*

The mother is Alyssa Beckett, 36-year-old gravida 5, full term 2, preterm 0, spontaneous abortion 2, living children 2, now 3. She is African American and is married. Maternal labs: B+, syphilis negative, group B *Streptococcus* (GBS) negative, hepatitis B negative, HIV refused testing, rubella immune, G/C negative. Maternal history is positive for herpes with no outbreaks for 5 years. Alyssa denies drug use or smoking. She takes prenatal vitamins. She had spontaneous rupture of membranes on April 2 at 07:00 with clear fluid, came to hospital and labored for 7 more hours with Pitocin augmentation. Obstetrician noted

(continued)

Case 8.4 (continued)

poor fetal heart tracing (FHT) so C-section was performed on the same day at 14:48, gestational age 36 6/7weeks. Apgar scores were 8 and 9 and birth weight was 2,470 g. Vital signs were stable at delivery but respiratory rate is increasing over the past 4 hours to 70 to 80 breaths per minute (bpm). She is formula feeding every 3 hours and Brady has eaten eight times in the past 24 hours, five voids and one stool are noted. Pediatrician's note is unremarkable but you call her with your findings and suggest a chest x-ray for increasingly evident tachypnea, stridor, and choking with feedings.

Chest x-ray reveals: eight of 12 RE with streaks in bases showing possible microaspirations. You call the pediatrician and discuss the chest x-ray and decide to move the infant to the neonatal intensive care unit (NICU) so you can monitor the patient and treat the respiratory distress. Brady is placed on room air and SpO_2 reads 97% to 100%, heart rate 140 bpm, blood pressure 78/29 mmHg with a mean of 46. It is now time to feed Brady.

2. ***Would you feed Brady or start intravenous fluids and keep him as nothing per os (NPO)?***

   ANSWER: I would order Brady to be fed orally as tolerated. *Since Brady's vital signs and physical examination at rest are essentially normal, it would be helpful to see for yourself how he feeds and what his vital signs are on the monitors.*

You ask your experienced NICU RN to bottle-feed Brady while you watch to assess his sucking and swallowing abilities. Brady was eager to nipple feed and had a good suck, he did have three desaturation episodes to SpO_2 in the 70% range that resolved with pacing of the feedings in the first few minutes. He choked once but had a good cough. He was able to take 30 mL of formula. On the next two feedings, Brady continued to cough, choke, and have stridor with his feeds. He remained intermittently tachypneic between feedings; SpO_2 remains 97% to 100%. Parents report that Brady has been making these noises since birth but they thought it was because of his dry nares. They are concerned because they feel that Brady's feedings and breathing are getting more striderous.

3. ***As the clinician what would you order next?***

   ANSWER: It would be prudent to obtain a blood culture, complete blood count (CBC), and possibly C-reactive protein (CRP) and follow trends of these over the next few days. It would certainly be thorough to start antibiotics in case Brady is aspirating. Follow-up chest x-rays would be warranted at least daily. *Baseline and serial testing provide information to assess and treat patients. Brady is possibly aspirating and could develop aspiration pneumonia. Lab work could reveal possible infection. Chest x-ray can demonstrate lung opacities suggestive of aspiration and serial x-rays show progressive states.*

4. ***What is your differential diagnosis for microaspiration, choking, and coughing with feedings?***

   ANSWER: The clinician should be thinking about basic newborn issues such as airway congestion, airway obstruction, or infection. Other considerations must be tracheoesophageal fistula (TEF) and tracheomalacia. *TEF occurs from incomplete division of the*

(continued)

Case 8.4 (continued)

foregut at 4 to 5 weeks gestation. It results in TEF with or without esophageal atresia. Brady does not have oxygen desaturations when feeding and he does not vomit so esophageal atresia can be ruled out. Brady does have symptoms that could be explained by TEF (coughing, choking when feeding). Since stridor has been noted with feedings, the clinician should be thinking about other airway problems that can frequently occur in newborns. Tracheomalacia is seen in infants, especially newborns, from weak musculature and tracheal cartilage. This abnormality may allow the tracheal walls to collapse. Airway resistance in the term newborn is very high (20–40 cm H20/L/sec; Blackburn, 2013) due to smaller nares, shorter airways with multiple bifurcations, and peripheral airway diameter. Cartilage gives structure and support to the airways. Newborns have an increase in the number of cartilage rings during the first 2 months of life. Any airway congestion, obstruction, or infection can lead to respiratory distress, muscle fatigue, and respiratory failure. Tachypnea is the most efficient mechanism for the infant to improve ventilation and compensate for hypoxia and hypercarbia. Neonates with tracheomalacia present with expiratory stridor, wheezing, and coughing (Mitchell & Pereira, 2009).

The NNP discusses her suspicions of tracheomalacia with the neonatologist and pediatrician. The team decides to continue Brady's feedings via nasogastric (NG) tube to assess his respiratory status through the night and, if NG feedings improve his respiratory status, they will obtain an ear, nose, and throat (ENT) consult tomorrow for a possible flexible bronchoscopy to look for tracheomalacia and/or laryngomalacia.

Tracheomalacia will often resolve as cartilage in the trachea grows and becomes less floppy. This may take from several days up to 2 years as the child and trachea grow. Infants with respiratory distress from tracheomalacia can benefit from continuous positive airway pressure to essentially splint the airway open. Laryngomalacia is the most common cause of stridor in the newborn at 75%. Stridor in laryngomalacia is inspiratory as opposed to tracheomalacia with expiratory stridor. Stridor is caused by collapse of the epiglottis and artenoid mucosa and can be high pitched or musical in sound. Laryngomalacia is thought to occur as a result of a floppy larynx with neurologic immaturity. Gastroesophageal reflux disease (GERD) is also caused by immature neurologic development of the larynx and is highly correlated with laryngomalacia.

Case 8.4 (continued)

The ENT consults on Brady Beckett and reports: trachea/laryngeal malacia and, because of the heart murmur, suggests an echocardiogram to rule out a vascular sling, which could cause the tracheomalacia. Vascular rings and slings can be complete or incomplete

(continued)

Case 8.4 (continued)

and arise from abnormal development of the aorta arch. Stridor and respiratory distress result from tracheal compression by these abnormal vascular formations. They can cause compression on the trachea, esophagus, or both. Brady's echocardiogram results are normal for his age. The ENT suggests keeping Brady in the NICU for a few days to teach his parents how to pace him with his feedings. Brady should outgrow this in a few weeks to 2 months as the trachea develops more cartilage rings and becomes stronger. The instructors must emphasize to the parents that any respiratory infection could potentially make Brady's breathing very difficult and distressed. They must keep him away from any sick children and take care to implement good hand washing in their family.

ACKNOWLEDGMENTS

I would like to acknowledge numerous NNP colleagues who have mentored me over 30 years; specifically, Karen Gannon, APRN, NNP-BC, and Suzanne Staebler, APRN, NNP-BC. Special appreciation is offered to the National Association of Neonatal Nurses (NANN) and National Association of Neonatal Nurse Practitioners (NANNP) for professionalizing the field of graduate-level neonatal nursing. I am proud to serve on numerous committees and the NANNP Council. Additional thanks go to my medical colleagues, especially two dedicated neonatologists, Dr. Barbara Engelhardt and Dr. Bradley Stancombe.

REFERENCES

American Academy of Pediatrics Committee on Fetus and Newborn, American College of Obstetricians and Gynecologists Committee on Obstetrics Practice. (2015, October). The Apgar Score. *Pediatrics, 136*(4).

Blackburn, S. T. (2013). *Maternal, fetal, & neonatal physiology: A clinical perspective.* Maryland Heights, MO: Elsevier Saunders.

Bull, M. J. (2011). Health supervision for children with Down syndrome. Retrieved from pediatrics .aappublications.org/content/128/2/393.full

Gomella, T. L. (2013). *Neonatology: Management, procedures, on-call problems, diseases and drugs* (7th ed.). New York, NY: McGraw-Hill.

Hall, B. (1964). Mongolism in newborns: A clinical and cytogenetic study. *Acta Paediatrica Scandinavica, 154*(Suppl.), 1–95.

Hennekam, R., Allanson, J., & Krantz, I. (2010). *Gorlin's syndromes of the head and neck* (5th ed.). New York, NY: Oxford University Press.

Kimberlin, D. W., Brady, M. T., Jackson, M. A. & Long, S. S. (2015). *Red book: 2015 report of the Committee on Infectious Diseases* (30th ed.). Elk Grove Village, IL: American Academy of Pediatrics.

Kummer, A. W. (2014). *Cleft palate and craniofacial anomalies: Effect on speech and resonance* (3rd ed.). Clifton Park, NY: Delmar.

Lorenz, B., & Brodsky, M. (2010). *Pediatric ophthalmology, neuro-ophthalmaology, genetics: Strabismus—New concepts in pathophysiology, diagnosis, and treatment.* Berlin, Germany: Springer.

Martin, R. J., Fanaroff, A. A., & Walsh, M. C. (2015). *Fanaroff and Martin's neonatal-perinatal medicine: Diseases of the fetus and infant* (10th ed.). Philadelphia, PA: Saunders.

Mitchell, M. B., & Pereira, K. D. (2009). *Pediatric otolaryngology for the clinician.* Dordrecht, the Netherlands: Springer.

Polin, R. A., Fox, W. W., & Abman, S. H. (2010). *Fetal and neonatal physiology* (4th ed.). Philadelphia, PA: Elsevier Saunders.

Tewfik, T. L. (2013). Cleft lip and palate and mouth and pharynx deformities. Retrieved from Emed icine.medscape.com

Volpe, J. J. (2008). *Neurology of the newborn* (5th ed.). Philadelphia, PA: Saunders.

Wang, R. Y., Earl, D. L., Ruder, R. O., & Graham, J. M. (2001, August). Syndromic ear anomalies and renal ultrasounds. *Pediatrics, 108*(2). Retrieved from http://www.pediatrics.org/cgi/content/full/108/2/e32

Weiner, G. M., & Zaichkin, J. (2016). *Textbook of neonatal resuscitation* (7th ed.). Elk Grove Village, IL: American Academy of Pediatrics and American Heart Association.

Wilson-Clay, B., & Hoover, K. (2013). *The breastfeeding atlas* (5th ed., pp. 200–204). Manchaca, TX: LactNews Press.

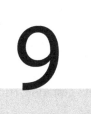

9

Hematologic System Cases

Catherine Witt

Chapter Objectives

1. Describe the physiology of anemia of prematurity
2. Identify three causes of anemia
3. Interpret the components of a complete blood count (CBC) and differential
4. Describe three causes of thrombocytopenia
5. Formulate a treatment plan for the jaundiced infant with a blood group incompatibility
6. Explain the signs of vitamin K deficiency bleeding in the newborn
7. Generate a treatment plan for the infant with disseminated intravascular coagulation (DIC)
8. Identify indications for a blood transfusion in the neonate
9. Apply concepts related to hematologic disorders to select cases presented

Hematologic disorders are a common occurrence in the newborn population. Caregivers must be knowledgeable about the development and function of blood cells and the coagulation system. This chapter discusses common hematology problems in the newborn. Following the presentation of this content, the student is provided with several case studies through which the student will engage in active learning to build critical-thinking skills.

DISORDERS OF ERYTHROCYTES

ANEMIA

Anemia is defined by a low concentration of hemoglobin or a decreased number of erythrocytes (red blood cells [RBCs]). This decrease limits the oxygen-carrying capacity of blood and the level of oxygen that is delivered to the tissues.

The hemoglobin level increases with increased gestational age (Juul, 2012). The hemoglobin level rises during the first 24 to 48 hours after birth, likely as a result of fluid shifts as extra cellular water is shed, then decreases slightly over the first week. In term infants, the hemoglobin levels average 17 to 21 g/dL, with hematocrit averaging 51% to 61% (Christenson, Henry, Jopling, & Wiedmeier, 2009; Diehl-Jones & Fraser, 2015). Preterm infants exhibit hemoglobin levels that are up to 10 points lower at less than 28 weeks gestation, rising with gestational age (Christenson et al., 2009).

There are three major causes of anemia in the newborn. These include hemorrhage, hemolysis (destruction of RBCs), and decreased production of erythrocytes.

Anemia Caused by Blood Loss

Approximately 5% to 10% of neonatal anemia is caused by blood loss (Aher, Malwatkar, & Kadam, 2008). Blood loss resulting from obstetrical complications includes fetal–maternal hemorrhage, twin–twin transfusion, placental abruption, placental previa, and umbilical cord accidents. Neonatal hemorrhage can include intracranial hemorrhage, subgaleal hemorrhage, or organ rupture (from liver, adrenal glands, or kidney). Iatrogenic causes of blood loss, such as arterial line malfunctions or excessive blood draws, may also lead to anemia (Diehl-Jones & Fraser, 2015).

Chronic blood loss may be asymptomatic or present with mild pallor. Over a longer period of time it may lead to congestive heart failure and hepatomegaly.

Acute blood loss presents with signs of hypovolemic shock, including pallor, cyanosis, tachycardia, hypotension, weak pulses, and respiratory distress. The hemoglobin concentration may be normal initially, then decrease rapidly over the next few hours (Diehl-Jones & Fraser, 2015).

Hemolytic Anemia

Hemolysis refers to the destruction or breakdown of RBCs. In the neonate, RBCs have a normal life span of 60 to 90 days at term and 30 to 50 days in the preterm infant. This is in contrast to the 120-day life span of the RBC in adults (Diab & Luchtman-Jones, 2015). Accelerated destruction of blood cells can lead to anemia accompanied by an increased reticulocyte count and elevated indirect bilirubin.

Alloimmune Hemolytic Anemia

Blood group incompatibilities are a common cause of hemolysis in the neonate. Rh disease can result in significant hemolysis and anemia in the fetus and neonate.

Hemolysis resulting from ABO incompatibility is seen in mothers with O type blood and an A or B fetus. Typically, it is less severe than the anemia caused by Rh incompatibility. Maternal exposure to A or B antigens leads to maternal production of anti-A or anti-B antibodies. These antibodies may be produced as a result of exposure to A or B substances found in food, bacteria, or pollen as well as to previous pregnancies; therefore, the disease may be seen in an initial pregnancy (Diab & Luchtman-Jones, 2015).

Hemolysis can also be caused by minor blood group incompatibilities. Antigens E, c, Kell, Kidd, or Duffy can all cause erythrocyte hemolysis with Kell being the most severe.

Nonimmune Hemolytic Anemia

Several disorders can cause red cell hemolysis. Hereditary spherocytosis and elliptocytosis are examples of abnormally shaped RBCs that are more susceptible to lysis. Enzymatic defects, such as glucose-6-phosphate dehydrogenase (G6PD) deficiency or pyruvate kinase deficiency, can cause increased hemolysis.

ANEMIA RESULTING FROM DECREASED PRODUCTION

Physiologic Anemia in Neonates

As the neonate transitions from an in utero environment, the hemoglobin saturation increases from approximately 50% to more than 90% (Aher et al., 2008). Fetal hemoglobin, which has a high affinity for oxygen, is gradually replaced by adult hemoglobin, which has a lower oxygen affinity. This adult hemoglobin more readily releases oxygen to the tissues, and this increase in oxygen levels suppresses erythropoiesis. The hemoglobin concentration decreases over the first few weeks after birth until eventually tissue needs for oxygen are greater than the amount of oxygen delivered. In term newborns, this point is typically reached by 6 to 12 weeks of age, with hemoglobin concentrations of 9.5 to 11 g/dL (Aher et al., 2008; Juul, 2012).

Anemia of Prematurity

The neonatal RBC has a shorter half-life (60–90 days for term infants; 30–50 days in the preterm infant) compared to 120 days in the adult. In addition, the infant has a blunted response to hypoxia in terms of synthesis of erythropoietin. In the preterm infant, the hemoglobin levels fall more quickly, reaching a nadir at 4 to 6 weeks with hemoglobin levels of 7 to 9 g/dL (Juul, 2012). Other factors that may contribute to anemia of prematurity include frequent laboratory tests, decreased iron intake, and deficiencies in folate and vitamins B_{12}, A, C, and E (Aher et al., 2008; Strauss, 2010). Adequate protein intake is also important for erythropoiesis (Carroll & Widness, 2012).

Other Causes of Decreased Erythropoiesis

Some congenital disorders of erythrocyte production exist. Fanconi's anemia is an autosomal recessive disorder that results in bone marrow failure (Aher et al., 2008). Diamond–Blackfan anemia causes bone marrow suppression and failure of erythropoiesis, likely caused by a defect in stem cell differentiation (Aher et al., 2008).

Clinical Presentation

Anemia may present with pallor, poor perfusion, and cyanosis. The infant may have signs of shock such as lethargy, tachycardia, hypotension, and extended capillary refill time. Respiratory distress, including tachypnea, may accompany anemia, particularly if severe.

Diagnostic Studies

A hemoglobin and hematocrit, reticulocyte count, and a peripheral blood smear are important in the diagnosis. Hemoglobin concentration may be normal at first, then decrease over 4 to 6 hours if blood loss is acute. The reticulocyte count will be elevated in the face of ongoing RBC destruction or with chronic anemia. Examination of the red cell will detect abnormalities in size, shape, or structure of the RBC and may indicate cells that are more readily destroyed. A blood type and Coombs test may be indicated to look for antibodies. A positive direct Coombs test indicates maternal immunoglobulin G (IgG) antibodies on the surface of the infant's RBC. A positive Coombs indicates antibodies are present in the serum.

A Kleihauer–Betke test may be indicated if fetal maternal hemorrhage is suspected. A positive Kleihauer–Betke indicates the presence of fetal hemoglobin in the maternal blood.

Prevention of Anemia

Acute blood loss resulting from obstetrical events or hemorrhages cannot always be prevented. Delayed cord clamping for preterm infants at delivery has been shown to be beneficial in limiting the need for transfusions for anemia or hypotension (Christensen, Carroll, & Josephson, 2014). Limiting phlebotomy losses in the first few days after birth has also been shown to significantly decrease the need for blood transfusion in preterm infants (Caroll & Widness, 2012; Henry et al., 2015).

Treatment

For acute, significant blood loss, transfusion with type O, Rh negative blood, 10 to 20 mL/kg will help to restore blood volume. If emergency blood is not available, normal saline, 10 to 20 mL/kg, may be used while waiting for blood to become available.

For nonemergent anemia, the decision to administer a blood transfusion depends upon the gestational and postnatal age of the patient, the hemoglobin level, the reticulocyte count, and the presence of signs of anemia or significant illness (Christensen et al., 2014; Jawdeh, Martin, Dick, Walsh, & DiFlore, 2014).

Erythropoiesis-stimulating agents, such as darbepoetin alfa (Darbe) or erythropoietin (Epogen), have been used in the neonatal intensive care unit (NICU) in an effort to decrease the number of RBC transfusions in preterm infants. Use of these products has been limited because of a concern for an increase in retinopathy of prematurity as an adverse effect (Aher & Ohlsson, 2012). However, some evidence suggests that these products can decrease the number of transfusions required and they may be of benefit when used judiciously (Aher & Ohlsson, 2012; Christensen et al., 2014; Ohls et al., 2013).

Optimal nutrition, including adequate protein and iron intake, is important for the production of RBCs in the neonate (Carroll & Widness, 2012). Iron supplementation is necessary, particularly in the preterm infant, as most iron stores are accumulated in the third trimester of pregnancy.

POLYCYTHEMIA

Polycythemia is defined as a hemoglobin level of 2 standard deviations above the mean for gestational age. This translates to a venous hematocrit greater than 65% in a term newborn (Diab & Luchtman-Jones, 2015). An increase in hematocrit can cause an increase in blood viscosity, which can interfere with blood flow to the organs. Capillary blood samples typically display a higher hemoglobin level than venous or arterial samples.

Etiology

Polycythemia occurs in approximately 2% to 5% of term infants (Diab & Luchtman-Jones, 2015). It can occur secondary to transfusion of blood to the fetus in a twin–twin or maternal–fetal transfusion or with delayed clamping of the umbilical cord at delivery. It may also occur as a result of intrauterine hypoxia secondary to placental insufficiency, maternal hypertension, maternal diabetes, maternal smoking, or postmaturity.

Clinical Presentation

Many infants are asymptomatic. Neonates may present with plethora, cyanosis, respiratory distress, hypoglycemia, hyperbilirubinemia, and poor feeding (Diehl-Jones & Fraser, 2015). Central nervous system abnormalities, such as lethargy, jitteriness, or seizures, may occur.

Treatment

Treatment is mainly supportive. Treatment of hypoglycemia and providing oxygen as needed may be all that is required. If symptoms are severe, a normal saline bolus of 10 mg/kg may be of benefit (Diehl-Jones & Fraser, 2015). Partial exchange transfusions are controversial and likely to be of limited benefit, particularly in the asymptomatic infant (Diab & Luchtman-Jones, 2015).

DISORDERS OF NEUTROPHILS

Leukocytes, or white blood cells (WBC), are the primary cells for defense against invading organisms. They include granulocytes (basophils, eosinophils, and neutrophils), lymphocytes, and monocytes. The total WBC count is the number of circulating WBCs per cubic millimeter of blood and varies by gestational age. Premature infants have a WBC count approximately 30% to 50% lower than term infants (Christensen, Del Vechio, & Henry, 2012; Diehl-Jones & Fraser, 2015). The normal white count in term infants varies from 10,000 to 26,000 mm^3 and from 6,000 to 19,000 mm^3 in preterm infants (Blackburn, 2013). The total WBC count increases for the first 24 hours after birth, then decreases over the next 2 to 3 days.

NEUTROPENIA

Neutrophils are the primary WBCs responsible for protecting the body from infection. Neutrophils typically make up approximately 50% to 60% of the total WBC count (Diab & Luchtman-Jones, 2015). Term and preterm infants have neutrophil levels approaching that of adults; however, preterm infants have smaller bone marrow reserves (Del Vecchio & Christensen, 2012). Neutrophils in preterm infants exhibit decreased phagocytosis and chemotaxis, leading to a decreased response to infectious organisms.

Neutrophils may appear in the blood in mature or immature forms. Mature forms are referred to as *neutrophils*, but are sometimes called *segmented neutrophils* (segs) because of their segmented nucleus, or *polymorphonuclear neutrophils* (PMNs). Immature neutrophils are referred to as *bands* because of their unsegmented nucleus, which appears in a band form. Very immature neutrophils are metamylocytes and mylocytes.

To determine the concentration of neutrophils in the CBC, an absolute neutrophil count (ANC) may be calculated by multiplying the number of WBCs by the percentage of immature and mature neutrophils. This can then be compared to reference ranges for newborns of similar age. Manroe (1979) published reference ranges for ANCs in newborns (Figure 9.1). Manroe included very few low-birth-weight infants in that study and subsequent authors have found that immature neonates may have a wider range of ANCs during the first week after delivery (Christensen, Henry, Jopling, & Wiedmeier, 2009; Maheshwari, 2013).

Neutropenia is defined as an ANC less than 2 standard deviations below the mean value or below the fifth percentile for postnatal age (Nittala, Subbarao, & Maheshwari, 2012). Depending on the author, an ANC of less than 1,000 to 1,500 mcL can be considered neutropenia (Del Vecchio & Christensen, 2012; Nittala et al., 2012).

Etiology of Neutropenia

Neutropenia can be caused by decreased production of neutrophils, increased destruction of neutrophils, or the result of drug-induced granulocytosis.

Decreased production can be seen in infants born to mothers with hypertension or preeclampsia for reasons that are not entirely clear. It may also be seen in neonates with Rh hemolytic disease (likely the result of increased production of RBCs), infants with intrauterine growth restriction, or in the donor twin of twin–twin transfusion syndrome (Maheshwair, 2013). Viral infections, such as cytomegalovirus, rubella, or enterovirus, may cause bone marrow suppression leading to neutropenia.

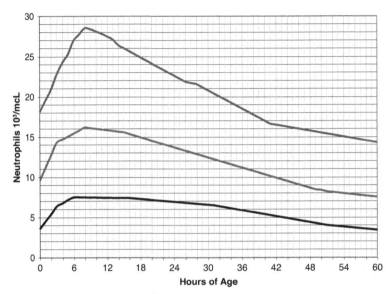

Figure 9.1 Manroe Chart Indicating Range of Neutrophil Counts in Neonates up to 60 Hours After Delivery

Reprinted with permission from Macmillan Publishers Ltd, *Journal of Perinatology*, 28(4), 2008.

Increased neutrophil destruction is most often the result of bacterial sepsis, fungal infection, and inflammatory disorders such as necrotizing enterocolitis. Neutropenia on the neonatal CBC should alert the caregiver to the possibility of sepsis. Further evaluation can be made by a comparison of immature neutrophils to the total number (I:T ratio). As neutrophils respond to a foreign antigen, an increased number of immature neutrophils may be released from the bone marrow. This left shift suggests that the number of mature neutrophils is being depleted and may heighten the concern for infection. The I:T ratio can be calculated by dividing the sum of the immature neutrophils (bands, metamylocytes, and mylocytes) by the total number of neutrophils (segs, bands, metamylocytes, and mylocytes).

Management of Neutropenia

Methods for increasing production of neutrophils in the neonate are limited. Recombinant granulocyte colony-stimulating factor (rG-CSF) stimulates release of neutrophils from the bone marrow and will raise the neutrophil count but the benefits of this have not been well established in clinical trials (Del Vecchio & Christensen, 2012). Infants with neutropenia secondary to pregnancy-induced hypertension (PIH) or intrauterine growth restriction will usually increase their neutrophil count without intervention.

HEMOSTATIC DISORDERS IN THE NEONATE

Thrombocytopenia

Thrombocytopenia, or low platelet count, has traditionally been defined as a platelet count of less than 150,000/mm³. Thrombocytopenia occurs in 1% to 2% of healthy term neonates and in up to 35% of ill neonates (Holzhauer & Zieger, 2011). In well newborns, mild to moderate thrombocytopenia resolves spontaneously without intervention. In infants who are ill or have severe thrombocytopenia (< 50,000 mm³), additional surveillance and diagnostic studies may be required.

Etiology

Thrombocytopenia in the newborn can occur for a number of reasons, originating in either the mother or the newborn, and can put the newborn at risk for bleeding complications. Thrombocytopenia can be caused by decreased production of platelets or increased consumption or destruction of platelets. Platelets that function inadequately (thrombocytopathy) may also be seen in the newborn.

Mild cases of thrombocytopenia may be seen in infants born to mothers with HELLP (hemolysis, elevated liver enzymes, and low platelet count) syndrome, infants of diabetic mothers, and infants with intrauterine growth restriction. Typically, these cases of thrombocytopenia resolve spontaneously and do not present a problem for the neonate.

Severe thrombocytopenia can occur as a result of chronic fetal hypoxia, congenital viral infections, immune-mediated thrombocytopenia, DIC, or a variety of congenital or hereditary disorders.

PLATELET DESTRUCTION

Immune-Mediated Thrombocytopenia

Neonatal Alloimmune Thrombocytopenia

Neonatal alloimmune thrombocytopenia occurs in approximately 1:700 to 1:1,100 neonates (Holzhauer & Zieger, 2011; Kamphuis, Paridaans, Porcelijn, Lopriorie, & Oepkes, 2014; Risson, Davies, & Williams, 2012). Thrombocytopenia results from fetal platelets entering the maternal circulation and stimulating the formation of maternal antibodies to antigens on the platelet's surface. These antibodies cross the placenta and coat the fetal platelets causing destruction of the platelets. Thrombocytopenia can occur in the fetus as early as 20 weeks gestation and can lead to intracranial hemorrhage in the fetus or the newborn. Platelet counts may be as low as 20,000 mm^3. Diagnosis is made by the presence of human platelet antigens (HPA) in the mother and neonate. Treatment consists of platelet transfusions, preferably with maternal platelets. Intravenous immunoglobulin (IVIG) may be used, but should not delay platelet transfusions (Holzhauer & Zieger, 2011). A cranial ultrasound should be done to evaluate for bleeding.

Autoimmune Thrombocytopenia

Mothers with idiopathic thrombocytopenic purpura (ITP) secondary to systemic lupus erythematosus can pass antiplatelet IgG antibodies to the fetus through the placenta. This can result in neonatal thrombocytopenia, although it is typically less severe than alloimmune thrombocytopenia and intracranial hemorrhage is rare. Maternal platelet count does not necessarily correlate with the fetal/neonatal platelet count. Treatment is with IVIG if platelet counts are less than 20,000 mm^3. Those with higher platelet counts may be observed. Infants with active bleeding should receive platelet transfusions (Diab & Luchtman-Jones, 2015; Holzhauer & Zieger, 2011).

Other Causes of Platelet Destruction

Platelet destruction in the neonate can result from a number of other disorders. Infection from gram-negative bacteria or viruses, such as cytomegalovirus, herpes, and enterovirus, can cause platelet consumption and destruction. Infants with congenital viral illnesses may present with petechia, hepatosplenomegaly, and jaundice. Thrombocytopenia secondary to viral illness is typically not severe and usually resolves within the first week or 2 after birth (Holzhauer & Zieger, 2011). Infection from gram-negative bacteria may result in DIC and severe thrombocytopenia requiring platelet transfusion.

Decreased Platelet Production

Disorders that cause decreased platelet production are rare and are usually hereditary or associated with congenital malformations or chromosomal abnormalities. Neonates with trisomies, such as trisomy 13 or 18, may have bone marrow hypoplasia resulting in decreased platelet production (Diehl-Jones & Fraser, 2015). Fanconi's anemia, absent radii syndrome, and other disorders can occur.

Diagnosis of Thrombocytopenia

Diagnosis of thrombocytopenia is made based on the platelet count on the CBC. A blood smear should be performed, looking particularly at platelet size and red cell morphology. A complete history, including family and obstetrical history, should be obtained. Symptoms may include bleeding, petechia or bruising, and hepatosplenomegaly.

Treatment

Transfusion guidelines vary, but most authors agree that platelet transfusions should be performed for platelet counts less than 20,000 mm^3 or with active bleeding. This can vary depending on the diagnosis and clinical presentation.

DISSEMINATED INTRAVASCULAR COAGULATION

ETIOLOGY

DIC is a secondary process triggered by a disease or disorder such as sepsis, hypoxia, acidosis, or tissue damage. It is characterized by activation of the coagulation mechanism, resulting in consumption of platelets and formation of microthrombi in small vessels, along with systemic hemorrhage (Schwartz & Rote, 2014). This formation of thrombi leads to decreased blood flow to vital organs, and consumes platelets and other clotting factors. This leads to uncontrolled bleeding and organ failure. Neonates are at increased risk of DIC because of their decreased levels of antithrombin and protein C and hepatic immaturity, which delays synthesis of clotting factors (Blackburn, 2013).

PRESENTATION

Symptoms of hemorrhage, such as petechiae, bruising, and bleeding from puncture sites or umbilicus, may be seen. Pulmonary or gastric hemorrhage may occur (Diehl-Jones & Fraser, 2015). Laboratory tests will reveal a low fibrinogen level and the presence of fibrinogen degradation products and D-dimers. The prothrombin time (PT) and the partial thromboplastin time (PTT) may be normal initially and then become prolonged. The platelet count will decrease as platelets are consumed.

TREATMENT

Treatment should focus on treating the underlying disease, preventing organ damage, and controlling ongoing thrombosis. Replacement of clotting factors is important. Fresh frozen plasma (FFP) will replace the clotting factors and a small amount of fibrinogen (Diehl-Jones & Fraser, 2015). Platelet transfusions should be given if the platelet count is low. Cryoprecipitate may be given to replace fibrinogen and factor VIII. Heparin infusions are generally not recommended in cases of DIC caused by sepsis or hypoxia (Schwartz & Rote, 2014).

VITAMIN K DEFICIENCY BLEEDING

ETIOLOGY

Vitamin K is a fat-soluble vitamin that is necessary for synthesis and activation of clotting factors II, VII, IX, and X (Schulte et al., 2014; Schwartz & Rote, 2014). Neonates are relatively deficient in vitamin K because of limited placental transfer of vitamin K, limited hepatic stores, and decreased enteral intake after birth. There are limited amounts of vitamin K in human milk and altered gastrointestinal flora leads to decreased production of vitamin K for the first 3 months after birth (Schulte et al., 2014). Prophylactic vitamin K given after birth prevents the development of early, classic, or late vitamin K deficiency bleeding in the neonate (American Academy of Pediatrics [AAP], 2015).

Vitamin K deficiency bleeding occurs in three forms: early, occurring within 23 hours after delivery; classic, which is seen within the first week after birth; and late, which occurs at 2 to 12 weeks after birth. Early vitamin K deficiency bleeding is usually caused by the mother taking certain anticonvulsants, or warfarin, which is a vitamin K antagonist (Diehl-Jones & Fraser, 2015).

PRESENTATION

Infants with vitamin K deficiency bleeding present with localized or diffuse bleeding, primarily from umbilicus, puncture sites, circumcision, or gastrointestinal sources. Intracranial bleeding may also occur; this is more common in late onset (Diab and Luchtman-Jones, 2015). The PT and PTT are prolonged. The platelet count and fibrinogen are normal. Vitamin K-dependent clotting factors may be measured and are low. Diagnosis is also affirmed with improvement upon administration of vitamin K.

TREATMENT

Treatment is administration of vitamin K either intravenously or subcutaneously and should be done immediately, even before the diagnosis is confirmed. FFP may be given if active bleeding is present. Transfusion of packed RBCs may be necessary if there is significant blood loss.

HYPERBILIRUBINEMIA

DEFINITION

Hyperbilirubinemia is an elevated level of bilirubin in the serum. Bilirubin is a byproduct of the breakdown of RBCs. Total serum bilirubin is the total of conjugated (direct) and unconjugated (indirect) bilirubin. For the purposes of this chapter, only indirect hyperbilirubinemia is described.

ETIOLOGY AND RISK FACTORS

The increased number and shorter life span of RBCs in the neonate, along with decreased albumin-binding capacity, makes hyperbilirubinemia common in the newborn period.

Approximately 90% of term infants will have hyperbilirubinemia (levels more than 2 mg/dL in the first week after birth; Blackburn, 2013). *Physiological jaundice* refers to the normal increase in bilirubin seen in the neonate during the first few days after birth (Kaplan, Wong, Sibley, & Stevenson, 2015). Typically, physiologic jaundice peaks at around 5 to 6 mg/dL at 3 to 4 days of age in the term infant. Preterm infants typically display a higher level (10–12 mg/dL), which peaks around day 5 (Kaplan et al., 2015).

Preterm infants, including late preterm infants, are at increased risk for hyperbilirubinemia because of decreased conjugation in the immature liver, decreased enteral feeding intake, and lower uridine 5'-diphospho-glucuronosyl transferase (UGT) enzyme activity. The UGT gene is responsible for coding enzymes necessary for conjugation of bilirubin and the UGT activity does not reach full adult levels until approximately 6 to 12 weeks of age (Kaplan et al., 2015).

Isoimmunization increases the risk of hyperbilirubinemia because of increased hemolysis of RBCs. A positive direct antibody test (DAT) indicates the presence of maternal antibodies on the red cell, resulting from Rh disease or ABO incompatibility. An indirect antibody test indicates that the antibodies are present in the serum. Additional causes of hemolysis were discussed earlier in the chapter.

Other risk factors include being of East Asian or Mediterranean descent, increased hemoglobin levels, hepatic dysfunction, infection, or delayed feeding. Sequestration of blood from bruising, cephalohematomas, structural abnormalities of erythrocytes such as spherocytosis, or biochemical defects such as pyruvate kinase deficiency or G6PD deficiency can also lead to increased levels.

DIAGNOSIS

Physical examination will reveal jaundice with a serum bilirubin of approximately 5 mg/dL. Jaundice progresses in a cephalocaudal pattern as the serum level rises (AAP, 2004). Laboratory evaluation of bilirubin should be done on every baby who appears jaundiced in the first 24 hours of life, or if jaundice appears excessive for the age of the infant (AAP, 2004). Physical assessment should include examination for hepatosplenomegaly, which may indicate the presence of liver disease or viral illness.

The serum bilirubin can be plotted on a nomogram and evaluated in the presence of risk factors (Figure 9.2). Additional information collected by the clinician should include maternal blood type, infant blood type and DAT if mother is O+ or Rh negative, weight loss, feeding method, voiding and stooling pattern, and if baby is of East Asian or Mediterranean decent. Male infants and those with previous siblings with jaundice are also at higher risk. Babies who are exclusively breastfeeding should be assessed for excessive weight loss, and breastfeeding should be evaluated for adequate milk transfer. A hematocrit, red cell smear, and reticulocyte count may be indicated to evaluate for hemolysis.

Serial measurements are helpful in determining the rate of rise—or how fast the bilirubin level is increasing over time. An increase of more than 5 mg/dL or more over 24 hours indicates more than physiologic jaundice.

COMPLICATIONS

Unconjugated bilirubin that is not bound to albumin (free bilirubin) is able to cross the blood–brain barrier and penetrate neuronal cell membranes. The resulting bilirubin encephalopathy is characterized by lethargy, poor feeding, hypotonia, and changes in the brainstem auditory evoked response (BAER). A high-pitched cry may be present in some infants (Kaplan, Bromiker, & Hammerman, 2014). Early in the course, bilirubin encephalopathy may be reversible, but if untreated, may progress to permanent neurological damage, or kernicterus.

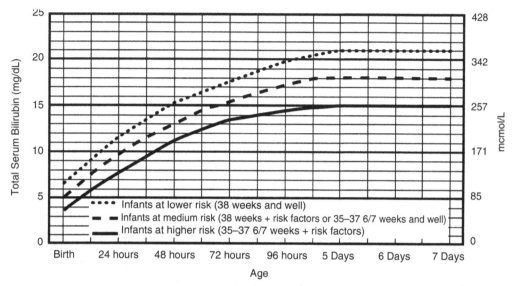

- Use total bilirubin. Do not subtract direct reacting or conjugated bilirubin.
- Risk factors = isoimmune hemolytic disease, G6PD deficiency, asphyxia, significant lethargy, temperature instability, sepsis, acidosis, or albumin less than 3.0 g/dL (if measured).
- For well infants 35–37 6/7 weeks can adjust TSB levels for intervention around the medium risk line. It is an option to intervene at lower TSB levels for infants closer to 35 weeks and at higher TSB levels.
- It is an option to provide conventional phototherapy in hospital or at home at TSB levels 2–3 mg/dL (35–50 mmol/L) below those shown but home phototherapy should not be used in any infant with risk factors.

Figure 9.2 Bilirubin Nomogram

TSB, total serum bilirubin.

Reprinted with permission from the American Academy of Pediatrics from *Pediatrics,* 114, 297–316, 2008.

TREATMENT

The goal of treatment is to prevent the toxic effects of bilirubin, including bilirubin encephalopathy and kernicterus. The level of indirect hyperbilirubinemia at which bilirubin encephalopathy occurs is not known.

Monitoring neonates for risk factors and identifying jaundice is the first step in preventing significant hyperbilirubinemia. Frequent feedings, including breastfeeding, will aid in removal of meconium and therefore bilirubin. Comprehensive discharge education should be documented and should include signs of jaundice and information about hyperbilirubinemia. Plans for follow-up after discharge must be in place.

Phototherapy is the main treatment for hyperbilirubinemia. Guidelines for treatment with phototherapy for neonates greater than 35 weeks gestation have been published by the AAP (2004) and can be found on the AAP website. Treatment is based on age (in hours) and risk factors. Phototherapy works on bilirubin that is in the subcutaneous tissues and converts it to a water-soluble form that can be excreted through the liver into the bile without being conjugated (Stokowski, 2011). It can be used to reduce bilirubin levels or prophylactically to slow the rate of rise of serum bilirubin.

If phototherapy is unsuccessful in controlling the serum bilirubin level, or if the infant presents with signs of bilirubin encephalopathy, an exchange transfusion is indicated. This is most common in infants with isoimmunity or other hemolytic disorders. The neonate's blood is removed in small amounts (5–10 mL) and replaced in equal aliquots until a volume twice that of the neonate's estimated blood volume is reached. The procedure usually takes approximately 2 to 3 hours. This will reduce the serum bilirubin level by approximately 50% (Kaplan et al., 2015). Complications include hypocalcemia, hyper-kalemia, and hypoglycemia; careful monitoring during and after the exchange transfusion is required.

Case 9.1

You are called to a delivery of a term neonate for fetal distress. Upon delivery you note the neonate has a heart rate of 180 beats per minute (bpm) and a respiratory rate of 70. The neonate is pale with a capillary refill of 5 to 6 seconds. You note weak pulses in all extremities. A pulse oximetry probe is placed on the right wrist and indicates saturations of 100% in room air. Apgar scores are 7 at 1 minute (1 off for tone and 2 off for color) and 8 (1 off for tone and one off for color). You admit the baby to the neonatal intensive care unit (NICU).

1. *What is the most likely explanation for the neonate's appearance?*

   A. Acute blood loss
   B. Asphyxia
   C. Sepsis

   ANSWER: A. *Pallor, tachycardia, and weak pulses are signs of anemia in the newborn (Aher et al., 2008).*

2. *What other information would be helpful in making your diagnosis?*

   A. Blood pressure
   B. Cerebral function monitoring
   C. Pre- and postductal saturations

   ANSWER: A. *Blood pressure, although a late sign of severe blood loss, can be helpful in making the diagnosis (Diehl-Jones & Fraser, 2015).*

3. *What laboratory test(s) would be most helpful initially?*

   A. Calcium and electrolytes
   B. Complete blood count (CBC)
   C. Lactate level

   ANSWER: B. *A CBC will provide a hemoglobin measurement helping to determine if the neonate is anemic. Keep in mind that the initial hemoglobin may not reflect acute blood loss, therefore serial hemoglobins may be beneficial (Diehl-Jones & Fraser, 2015).*

4. *What is your most likely first intervention?*

   A. Apply a cool cap
   B. Obtain a blood culture and start antibiotics
   C. Transfuse with O negative uncross-matched blood

   ANSWER: C. *The most effective treatment for acute blood loss is a blood transfusion. O negative blood can be used in emergency situations while waiting for a blood type and cross match to be done (Diehl-Jones & Fraser, 2015).*

Case 9.2

You are called to see a baby with respiratory distress in the well-baby nursery. You find the baby to be plethoric, with a respiratory rate of 70 and mild grunting. The nurse tells you that the parents requested delay of cord clamping until the cord stopped pulsating, approximately 5 minutes after delivery. His glucose is 45 mg/dL.

1. **What other laboratory test do you need?**

   A. Blood culture
   B. Hematocrit
   C. Platelet count

   ANSWER: B. *Polycythemia may result in respiratory distress, hypoglycemia, and plethora. An elevated hematocrit will confirm the diagnosis (Diehl-Jones & Fraser, 2015).*

2. **You obtain the following laboratory results: White blood cells 12.4, Hgb 23%, Hct 70%, plts 245,000, 65 segs, 0 bands, 32 lymphs, 2 monos, 1 eosinophil. Repeat glucose at 1 hour of age is 40 mg/dL. Oxygen saturations are 90% in room air and mild grunting continues with respiratory rate of 70. Your next intervention is to:**

   A. Begin nasal continuous positive airway pressure (CPAP)
   B. Feed 30 mL of formula
   C. Give a bolus of 10 mL/kg of normal saline

   ANSWER: C. *A hemoglobin level of 23% indicates polycythemia. While it is important to address the hypoglycemia, treating the underlying cause will be necessary to resolve the problem (Diehl-Jones & Fraser, 2015).*

3. **Your most likely diagnosis is:**

   A. Anemia
   B. Polycythemia
   C. Transient tachypnea of the newborn

   ANSWER: B. *The hemoglobin of 23%, along with the symptoms displayed by the neonate, indicate polycythemia (Diehl-Jones & Fraser, 2015).*

Case 9.3

The nurse in the well-baby nursery calls to report a bilirubin level of 10.2 at 36 hours of age. Upon review of the history you see that the baby is 40 weeks gestation, born to a G2P1, O+ mother.

(continued)

Case 9.3 (continued)

1. **What additional laboratory data do you want from the baby?**

   A. Blood culture
   B. Blood type
   C. Electrolytes

   ANSWER: B. *Blood incompatibilities are a common cause of hyperbilirubinemia and should be tested for, particularly in infants born to a mother who is O positive (AAP, 2004).*

2. **The mother is of Mediterranean descent. What additional laboratory test might be helpful?**

   A. G6PD
   B. Galactosemia
   C. Sickle cell disease

   ANSWER: A. *G6PD is more common in mothers of Mediterranean descent and can be a cause of hyperbilirubinemia (Kaplan et al., 2014).*

3. **At 48 hours of age, the bilirubin level is 14.8. Your next intervention would be to institute:**

   A. A bilirubin blanket in the mother's room
   B. Home phototherapy
   C. Intensive phototherapy

   ANSWER: C. *The rapid rate of rise is best treated by intensive phototherapy. Home phototherapy or a bilirubin blanket in the mother's room may not result in a level of intensity required to treat the accumulation of bilirubin (AAP, 2004).*

4. **What other laboratory test(s) should be done?**

   A. Calcium level
   B. Complete blood count (CBC) and smear
   C. Glucose

   ANSWER: B. *A CBC and smear will provide a hematocrit, which if low may indicate hemolysis. An examination of the red cell will determine any abnormally shaped red cells that may contribute to hemolysis (AAP, 2004).*

Case 9.4

A 31-week, 1,500-g male infant is born to a 28-year-old, G1P0, O+ mother after spontaneous onset of labor and premature rupture of membranes 15 hours prior to delivery. The neonate was intubated in the delivery room and received one dose of surfactant and is on a ventilator. A complete blood count (CBC) was obtained with the following results:

(continued)

Case 9.4 (continued)

White blood cells 4.2, Hgb 14, Hct 42, plts 152,000, segs 22%, bands 8%, lymphocytes 55%, monos 5%, basos 2%, eos 3%, metamylocytes 5%.

1. **What is your absolute neutrophil count?**

    A. 1,260
    B. 1,470
    C. 1,680

    ANSWER: B. *The percentage of neutrophyllis is 35%, which equals an absolute neutrophil count of 1,470 (Diehl-Jones & Fraser, 2015).*

2. **What is the immature to total (I:T) ratio?**

    A. 0.26
    B. 0.37
    C. 0.77

    ANSWER: B. *There are a total of 35% neutrophils of which 13% are immature. The ratio of immature to total neutrophils is 0.37 (Diehl-Jones & Fraser, 2015).*

3. **This result is most likely caused by:**

    A. Bone marrow suppression resulting from prematurity
    B. Maternal disease process
    C. Neonatal sepsis

    ANSWER: C. *The history of preterm labor and premature rupture of membranes, respiratory distress, a low absolute neutrophil count and an elevated I:T ratio indicates possible sepsis in the newborn (Nittala et al., 2012).*

Case 9.5

As the neonatal nurse practitioner (NNP), you are called to the emergency room to see a 4-day-old male infant with a history of irritability, poor feeding, and pallor for the past 12 hours. The parents report that the pregnancy was uncomplicated and the baby was born at home with no problems with delivery. The mother is a gravida 2, para 1, A+ mother. She reports no signs or symptoms of illness in herself or other family members. The baby has been breastfeeding well prior to onset of symptoms that day.

Upon exam you note that the heart rate is 170 bpm, respiratory rate is 66 breaths per minute, and the oxygen saturations are 98% in room air. The baby is pale and lethargic with decreased tone but is irritable when aroused. Oozing of blood from the umbilical cord is present. A complete blood count (CBC) and differential is significant for a hematocrit

(continued)

Case 9.5 (continued)

of 31%. A disseminated intravascular coagulation (DIC) screen is sent and is significant for a prolonged prothrombin time (PT) and partial thromboplastin time (PTT).

1. Treatment for this infant should include:

A. Blood transfusion with packed red blood cells

B. Parenteral vitamin K administration

C. Transfusion with fresh frozen plasma

ANSWER: B. *Classic vitamin K deficiency most often presents in the first week of life. A prolonged PT and PTT are consistent with vitamin K deficiency (Diab & Luchtman-Jones, 2015).*

Case 9.6

You are called to see a 2-hour-old term neonate with petechiae and oozing of blood from a heel stick and the injection site from administration of vitamin K. A complete blood count (CBC) and differential is significant for a platelet count of 19,000. The baby otherwise appears well. The mother is a 29-year-old gravida 1, para 0, B+ mother. Pregnancy was uncomplicated and baby was born by spontaneous vaginal delivery with Apgar scores of 9 and 9 at 1 and 5 minutes, respectively.

1. The most likely diagnosis is:

A. Disseminated intravascular coagulation

B. Neonatal alloimmune thrombocytopenia

C. Neonatal autoimmune thrombocytopenia

ANSWER: B. *This is the most common cause of low platelets and bleeding in an otherwise uncomplicated pregnancy (Holzhauer & Zieger, 2011).*

2. Treatment for this infant should be:

A. Administration of fresh frozen plasma

B. Administration of maternal platelets

C. Administration of random donor platelets

ANSWER: B. *The neonate should be treated with maternal platelets if possible, due to platelet antibodies from the mother adhering to fetal platelets expressing paternal antigens (Holzhauer & Zieger, 2011).*

REFERENCES

Aher, S. M., Malwatkar, K., & Kadam, S. (2008). Neonatal anemia. *Seminars in Fetal & Neonatal Medicine, 13*, 239–247.

Aher, S. M., & Ohlsson, A. (2012). Early versus late erythropoietin for preventing red blood cell transfusion in preterm and/or low birth weight infants. *Cochrane Database of Systematic Reviews, 10*, CD004865. doi:10.1002/14651858.CD004865.pub3

Aher, S. M., & Ohlsson, A. (2014). Late erythropoietin for preventing red blood cell transfusion in preterm and/or low birth weight infants. *Cochrane Database of Systematic Reviews, 23*(4), CD004868. doi:10.1002/14651858.CD004868.pub4

American Academy of Pediatrics (AAP). (2004). Management of hyperbilirubinemia in the newborn infant 35 or more weeks of gestation. *Pediatrics, 114*, 297–316. doi:10.1542/peds.114.1.297. Retrieved from http://pediatrics.aappublications.org/content/114/1/297.full.pdf

American Academy of Pediatrics (AAP). (2015). AAP publications reaffirmed or retired. *Pediatrics, 135*(2), 135e. Retrieved from http://pediatrics.aappublications.org/content/135/2/e558.full.pdf+html

Blackburn, S. T. (2013). Hematology and hemostatic systems. In *Maternal, fetal, and neonatal physiology: A clinical perspective* (4th ed., pp. 216–251). Philadelphia, PA: Elsevier.

Carroll, P. D., & Widness, J. A. (2012). Nonpharmacological blood conservation techniques for preventing neonatal anemia—Effective and promising strategies for reducing transfusion. *Seminars in Perinatology, 36*, 232–243.

Christensen, R. D., Carroll, P. D., & Josephson, C. D. (2014). Evidence-based advances in transfusion practice in neonatal intensive care units. *Neonatology, 106*, 245–253.

Christensen, R. D., Del Vecchio, A., & Henry, E. (2012). Expected erythrocyte, platelet, and neutrophil values for term and preterm neonates. *Journal of Maternal-Fetal & Neonatal Medicine, 25*, 77–79.

Christensen, R. D., Henry, E., Jopling, J., & Wiedmeier, S. E. (2009). The CBC: References ranges for neonates. *Seminars in Perinatology, 33*, 3–11.

Del Vecchio, A., & Christensen, R. D. (2012). Neonatal neutropenia: What diagnostic evaluation is needed and when is treatment recommended? *Early Human Development, 88*(Suppl. 2), S19–S24. doi:10.1016/S0378-3782(12)70007-5

Diab, Y., & Luchtman-Jones, L. (2015). Hematologic and oncologic problems in the fetus and neonate. In R. J. Martin, A. A. Fanaroff, & M. C. Walsh (Eds.). *Fanaroff and Martin's neonatal-perinatal medicine: Diseases of the fetus and infant* (10th ed., pp. 1303–1374). Philadelphia, PA: Saunders.

Diehl-Jones, W., & Fraser, D. (2015). Hematologic disorders. In M. T. Verklan & M. Walden, (Eds.), *Core curriculum for neonatal intensive care nursing* (5th ed., pp. 662–688). Philadelphia, PA: Elsevier.

Henry, E., Christensen, R. D., Sheffield, M. J., Eggert, L. D., Carroll, P. D., Minton S. D., . . . Ilstrup S. J. (2015). Why do four NICUs using identical RBC transfusion guidelines have different gestational age-adjusted RBC transfusion rates? *Journal of Perinatology, 35*, 132–136.

Holzhauer, S., & Zieger, B. (2011). Diagnosis and management of neonatal thrombocytopenia. *Seminars in Fetal & Neonatal Medicine, 16*, 305–310.

Jawdeh, E. G. A., Martin, R. J., Dick, T. E., Walsh, M. C., & DiFlore, J. M. (2014). The effect of red blood cell transfusion on intermittent hypoxemia in ELBW infants. *Journal of Perinatology, 34*, 921–925.

Juul, S. (2012). Erythropoiesis and the approach to anemia in premature infants. *Journal of Maternal-Fetal & Neonatal Medicine, 25*, 97–99.

Kamphuis, M. M., Paridaans, N. P., Porcelijn, L., Lopriorie, E., & Oepkes, D. (2014). Incidence and consequences of neonatal alloimmune thrombocytopenia: A systemic review. *Pediatrics, 133*, 715–721. doi:10.1542/peds.2013-3320

Kaplan, M., Bromiker, R., & Hammerman, C. (2014). Hyperbilirubinemia, hemolysis, and increased bilirubin toxicity. *Seminars in Perinatology, 38*, 429–437.

Kaplan, M., Wong, R. J., Sibley E., & Stevenson, D. K. (2015). Neonatal jaundice and liver disease. In R. J. Martin, A. A. Fanaroff, & M. C. Walsh (Eds.). *Fanaroff and Martin's neonatal-perinatal medicine: Diseases of the fetus and infant* (10th ed., pp. 1618–1673). Philadelphia, PA: Saunders.

Maheshwari, A. (2013). Neutropenia in the newborn. *Current Opinions in Hematology, 21*, 43–39.

Monroe, B. L., Weinberg, A. G., Rosenfeld, C. R., & Browne, R. (1979). The neonatal blood count in health and disease. *Journal of Pediatrics, 95*(1), 89–98.

Nittala, S., Subbarao, G. C., & Maheshwari, A. (2012). Evaluation of neutropenia and neutrophilia in preterm infants. *Journal of Maternal-Fetal and Neonatal Medicine, 25*(55), 100–103. doi:10.3109/14767058.2012.715468

Ohls, R. K., Christensen, R. D., Kamathy-Rayne, B. D., Rosenberg, A., Wiedmeier S. E., Roohi, M., . . . Lowe, J. R. (2013). A randomized, masked, placebo-controlled study of darbepoetin alfa in preterm infants. *Pediatrics, 132*, e118–e127.

Risson, D. C., Davies, M. W., & Williams, B. A. (2012). Review of neonatal alloimmune thrombocytopenia. *Journal of Paediatrics and Child Health, 48*, 816–822.

Schulte, R., Jordan, L. C., Morad, A., Naftel, R. P., Wellons, J. C., & Sidonio, R. (2014). Rise in late onset vitamin K deficiency bleeding in young infants because of omission or refusal of prophylaxis at birth. *Pediatric Neurology, 50*, 564–568.

Schwartz, A., & Rote, N. S. (2014). Alterations of leukocyte, lymphoid and hemostatic function. In S. E. Huether & K. L. McCance (Eds.), *Pathophysiology, the biologic basis for disease in adults and children* (7th ed., pp. 1008–1054). Philadelphia, PA: Elsevier.

Stokowski, L. (2011). Fundamentals of phototherapy for neonatal jaundice. *Advances in Neonatal Care, 11*, S10–S21.

Strauss, R. G. (2010). Anemia of prematurity: Pathophysiology and treatment. *Blood Reviews, 24*, 221–225.

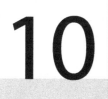

10

Neurologic System Cases

Bresney Crowell

Chapter Objectives

1. List the elements of a basic neurologic examination
2. Discuss the pathophysiology, neuroimaging findings, and potential causes of intraventricular hemorrhage (IVH) in a preterm infant
3. Recognize potential complications and outcomes of neonates with IVH
4. Interpret upcoming studies and treatments and apply to current practice for infants with IVH and posthemorrhagic hydrocephalus (PHH)
5. Explain the etiology of hypoxic ischemic encephalopathy (HIE)
6. Describe the criteria used to diagnose, evaluate, and treat HIE
7. Discuss differential diagnoses of an infant with seizures
8. Examine the primary etiology of neonatal seizures and classifications
9. Apply basic strategies for evaluating and treating seizures
10. Describe the assessment and care of infants with brachial plexus injury
11. Summarize optimal patient outcomes that may be achieved through evidence-based management of infants with neurologic system disorders

Recognizable neural tissue begins developing in the fetus approximately 18 days after fertilization. Development of the central nervous system continues to mature and change over 6 years. The immature, developing brain is vulnerable and is at risk for a large range of injury that may have devastating effects on structure and function. It is important to note that brain injury can affect preterm and term infants differently because of the different developmental stages that occur at various gestational ages. Practitioners are faced with numerous challenges when caring for an infant with neurological damage and must work as a multidisciplinary team in order to provide differential diagnoses, determine cause, and decide on appropriate treatment for the infants affected. Advances in technology and knowledge surrounding neonatal neurology have enhanced the clinician's ability to evaluate and manage neurologic disorders. As more information is learned, controversies and uncertainties emerge surrounding ethical dilemmas and treatment options for infants with neurological damage. In this chapter, the most prominent and challenging neurologic conditions are discussed in case format and the pathophysiology of each is reviewed.

INTRAVENTRICULAR HEMORRHAGE

In the United States every year, approximately 12,000 new cases of IVH are diagnosed in preterm infants (Ballabh, 2010). IVH is a major concern in the preterm population and can cause major neurologic sequelae. IVH is predominantly diagnosed in preterm infants and is an intracranial hemorrhage that starts in the subependymal region of the germinal matrix, resulting in entrance of blood into the ventricular system. IVH is associated with risks that increase with the severity of the lesion and cause adverse neurodevelopmental outcomes.

The pathogenesis of IVH is multifactorial and is both anatomical and pathophysiologic and largely related to the immature and weak structure of the germinal matrix and disturbances in cerebral blood flow (CBF). The most common origination of IVH is in the germinal matrix and is caused by the fragility of the vasculature and lack of structural support as a result of immaturity. This is compounded by the paucity of CBF. The venous system that drains the delicate capillary network of the germinal matrix is thought to be prone to venous congestion and stasis, which contributes to the risk of IVH. The greatest risk period for IVH is the first 3 days of life, after which the germinal matrix becomes less friable (Adcock, 2012).

The susceptibility of the germinal matrix in the first 3 days of life is compounded by the physiological instability of the preterm infant after birth (Annibale, 2014). Autoregulation and cerebral vasoreactivity mechanisms are poorly developed in the preterm infant's brain. This poor autoregulatory mechanism causes instability of systemic blood pressure and results in a pressure-passive cerebral circulation and CBF disturbances. Positive pressure ventilation, spontaneous movements, sleep cycles, noxious stimuli, and rapid volume infusion are some of the factors that may cause alterations in blood pressure, causing variations in CBF. Changes in carbon dioxide levels can also disrupt the cerebral autoregulation. CBF fluctuations can be caused by hypotension, hypoxemia, acidosis, patent ductus arteriosus, and irritability. Increase in cerebral venous pressure caused by mechanical ventilation, pneumothorax, and positive pressure ventilation can decrease cerebral perfusion and put the brain at risk for reperfusion injury.

The risk of IVH can be magnified by multiple prenatal factors. Complications, such as chorioamnionitis, Von Willebrand disease, anticoagulation therapy, cocaine abuse, seizures, abdominal trauma, amniocentesis, and febrile illness, increase the risk for prenatal IVH. Fetal risk factors include congenital tumors, immune thrombocytopenia, clotting factor deficiencies, fetomaternal hemorrhage, twin-to-twin transfusion, and co-twin death. Another factor that increases the risk for IVH in the preterm infant is disturbances in coagulation. Studies have shown that thrombocytopenia as well as coagulopathies can increase the risk for IVH, although the mechanism is not completely understood.

The pathogenesis of grades I, II, and III IVH are thought to be related to the disruption of autoregulation that leads to pressure passive CBF, which is controlled by blood pressure. Fluctuations in blood flow result in local hemorrhage at the site of the germinal matrix. The hemorrhage can cause edema and vascular congestion locally, leading to increased venous pressure. The hemorrhage can then continue and spread into the ventricles.

Pathogenesis of grade IV hemorrhage is believed to result from the lower grade hemorrhages because of the increased cerebral pressure. The increased cerebral pressure in the area of the germinal matrix hemorrhage leads to increased venous pressure. Blood flow is then impaired in the medullary veins that drain the cerebral white matter into the terminal vein. This increased venous pressure results in periventricular hemorrhage infarction (PVI), also referred to as grade IV IVH, with the destruction of periventricular white matter.

Since the early 1980s, the incidence of IVH in very low-birth-weight (VLBW) infants (< 6,500 g) has decreased to 20% to 35%, and remains a major complication of prematurity (Ballabh, 2010). In the extremely low-birth-weight (ELBW) infants (< 1,000 g), the incidence of IVH increases to around 45% (Ballabh, 2012). A total of 10% to 15% of VLBW infants suffer from severe grades of IVH, and about three fourths of these infants will be affected by mental retardation and/or cerebral palsy at various severity levels (Annibale, 2014).

Most IVH occurs within the initial 5 postnatal days, with 50% occurring within the first day, 25% in the second, and 15% in the third (Polin, 2015). Clinical presentation of IVH can vary. A total of 25% to 50% of infants with IVH are diagnosed by routine brain sonography and have no symptoms (Martin, 2011). This presentation is called *silent syndrome*. Saltatory syndrome can evolve over hours or days and is characterized by an altered level of consciousness, hypotonicity, and subtle changes in positioning and eye movements. Catastrophic presentation is the least common and can develop rapidly. Symptoms include stupor, coma, irregular respiration, seizures, or posturing. The infant may also demonstrate a bulging fontanel, hypotension, bradycardia, anemia, and metabolic acidosis.

Cranial sonography is the procedure of choice for diagnosis of IVH because of its high resolution, portability, and nonradiating abilities. Guidelines from the American Academy of Neurology and the Practice Committee of Child Neurology Society suggest that screening should be performed routinely on infants less than 30 weeks gestational age or infants less than 1,500 g. The initial screen should be done at 7 to 14 days postnatal age and repeated at 36 to 40 weeks postmenstrual age (Annibale, 2012). The grading system for IVH was initially described by Papile and later modified by Volpe (Table 10.1).

Table 10.1 **Table Comparing IVH Grading Scale Between Authors Papile and Volpe**

Grade	Papile	Volpe
I (Figure 10.1)	IVH is subependymal and is limited to the germinal matrix	There is minimal or no intraventricular blood
II (Figures 10.2 and 10.3)	IVH is in the lumen of the lateral ventricle(s), without ventricular distention	The hemorrhage occupies 10%–50% of the ventricle
III (Figures 10.4 and 10.5)	IVH is within the lumen of the lateral ventricle(s) with dilation of the ventricle(s)	The hemorrhage occupies greater than 50% of the ventricular volume
IV (Figures 10.6 and 10.7)	IVH is a combination of blood within the ventricle(s) and an echogenic area in the periventricular tissue	Referred to as a periventricular infarction (PHI)

IVH, intraventricular hemorrhage.

Source: Papile et al. (1978) and Volpe (2008).

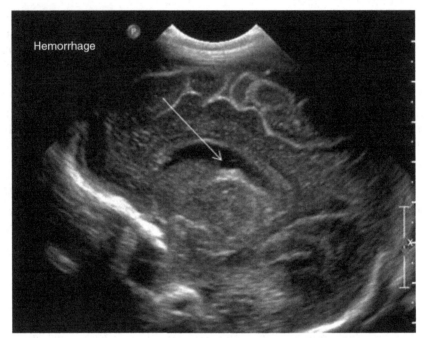

Figure 10.1 Germinal Matrix Hemorrhage

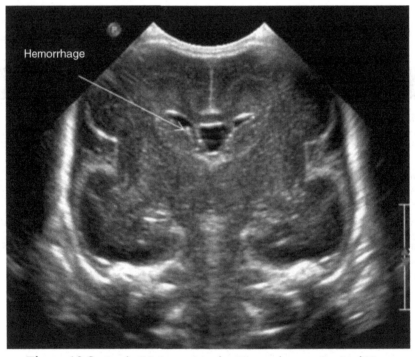

Figure 10.2 Grade II Intraventricular Hemorrhage—Sagittal View

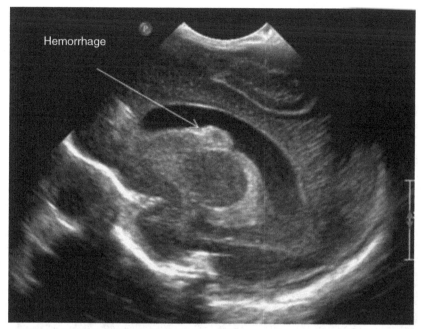

Figure 10.3 Grade II Intraventricular Hemorrhage—Coronal View

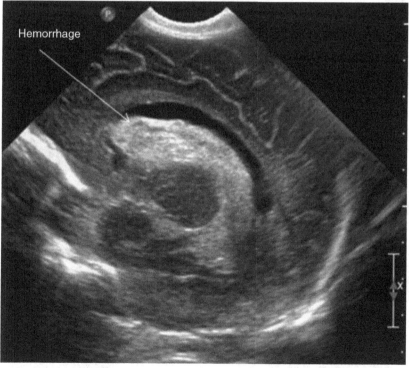

Figure 10.4 Grade III Intraventricular Hemorrhage—Sagittal View

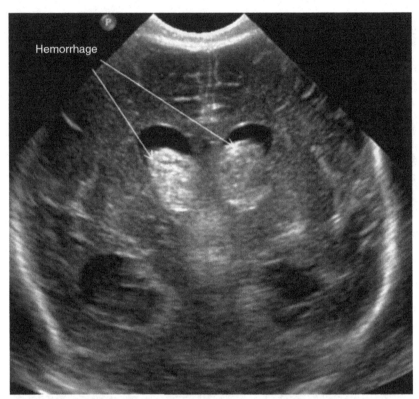

Figure 10.5 Grade III Intraventricular Hemorrhage—Coronal View

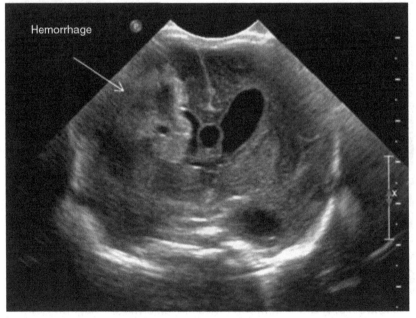

Figure 10.6 Grade IV Periventricular Hemorrhage Infarction—Coronal View

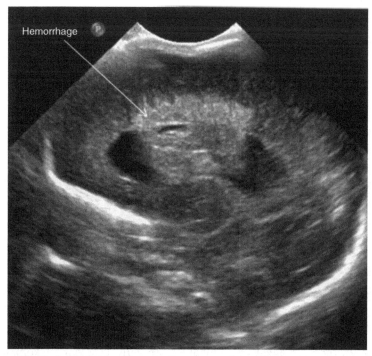

Hemorrhage

***Figure* 10.7** Grade IV Periventricular Hemorrhage Infarction—Sagittal View

Treatment of IVH is supportive and should be aimed at preventing further injury, preserving cerebral perfusion, and identifying associated complications. Maintaining blood pressure, oxygenation, and ventilation is important, as are adequate nutrition and fluid support. It is also important to be aware of associated complications and lesions. Periventricular hemorrhagic infarction (PHI) is a direct complication of IVH and affects 10% to 15% of infants with IVH (Robinson, 2012). PHI is an area of hemorrhagic necrosis in the white matter around the ventricles and is usually asymmetrical. Ischemia and further hemorrhage are caused when pressure is exerted on the periventricular terminal drain from IVH, leading to venous congestion. Periventricular leukomalacia (PVL) is also associated with IVH and refers to the necrosis of the white matter in the brain (Figure 10.8). It is nonhemorrhagic and is usually bilateral. It is described as an ischemic injury caused by vascular insults and 87% of infants with severe PVL have major deficits and impaired cognitive function. Although PVL is often found in association with IVH, it can occur independently and has a high association with maternal chorioamnionitis.

PHH is a major complication of IVH and is found in approximately 50% of infants with IVH and 75% of infants with more severe grades of IVH (Figures 10.9 and 10.10) (Annibale, 2014). A rapidly increasing head circumference with ventricular dilation and signs of increased intracranial pressure are signs of PHH. Symptoms may take weeks to present after the initial hemorrhage. The two types of PHH are called *communicating* and *noncommunicating*. Communicating PHH is the most common and is caused by the inability to resorb cerebral spinal fluid (CSF) as a result of inflammation. Noncommunicating PHH is caused by obstruction caused by a clot or scarring in the ventricular system. Some PHH can resolve spontaneously without intervention. Progressive PHH requires intervention,

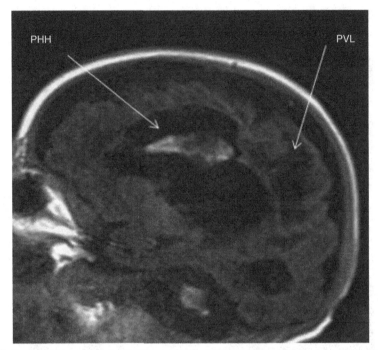

***Figure* 10.8** Posthemorrhagic Hydrocephalus With Periventricular Leukomalacia—MRI

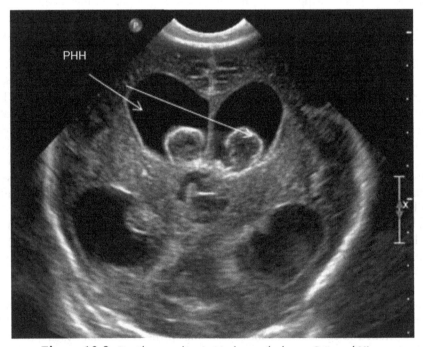

***Figure* 10.9** Posthemorrhagic Hydrocephalus—Coronal View

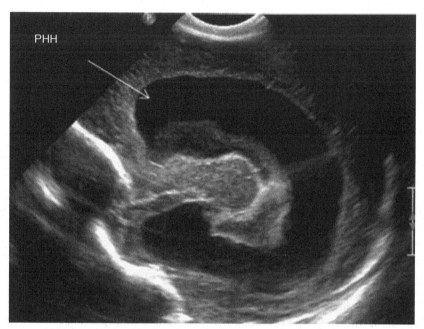

Figure **10.10** Posthemorrhagic Hydrocephalus—Sagittal View

although treatment options have significant risks. Close surveillance for symptoms of PHH is important. Head growth should be monitored closely and signs of increasing intracranial pressure should be evaluated. Infants with rapidly increasing head growth or significant changes on head ultrasound (HUS) should have a neurosurgery consultation for further recommendations and treatment options. Management of PHH is controversial and is treated differently in different medical centers, including optimal time to intervene and temporizing mechanisms for symptomatic infants with PHH who are too small or too unstable for shunt placement. Historically, lumbar and ventricular taps are the most common short-term therapies for early stages of slowly progressing, communicating hydrocephalus. In recent literature reviews, serial lumbar punctures to avoid shunt placement or to slow the progression of hydrocephalus in preterm infants are not recommended. Ventricular access devices to remove CSF have been shown to reduce morbidity and mortality rates and allow effective decrease in intracranial pressure. External ventricular drains (EVD) are also treatment options in the management of PHH and have low infection rates, but do have complications associated with them such as blockage, over drainage, and surgical revisions. The incidence of needing a permanent shunt after EVD is approximately 64% to 68% (Annibale, 2014; Shooman, 2009). Ventriculoperitoneal (VP) shunting remains the most common long-term treatment of PHH. Infants greater than 2 kg are candidates for this procedure. There are multiple problems and risks associated with this method of treatment, including high revision rates with complicated surgeries, infection rates as high as 5% to 15%, and risk for shunt failure caused by obstructions (Annibale, 2014). The mortality rate of infants requiring a VP shunt for PHH is 25% (Robinson, 2012). Only approximately 30% of infants with VP shunts will have a normal outcome.

Although shunt technology and surgical techniques have improved, an increasing number of neurosurgeons are recommending endoscopic third ventriculostomy (ETV) in hopes of deferring shunting. With the development of endoscopy, this approach became a viable treatment option in select cases. The goal of ETV is to make a small perforation in the floor of the third ventricle to allow CSF to flow into the interpeduncular cistern. This is an attempt to bypass an obstruction and relieve pressure. This should normalize pressure in the brain and avoid shunt placement. The most common complications of ETV are fever, bleeding, and transient endocrine dysfunction (Hydrocephalus Association, 2010). Isolated ETV is appropriate for patients greater than 6 months of age. For infants, ETV should be combined with choroid plexus cauterization (CPC). Tissue is cauterized from the choroid plexus to decrease CSF production. ETV combined with CPC has shown to be more effective in avoiding permanent shunt placement. More studies are needed to continue to evaluate these procedures and outcomes to develop reliable statistics.

IVH and PHH are a major concern for preterm infants. Mental retardation caused by IVH accounts for approximately 3,600 new cases a year according to data from the U.S. Census Bureau, the National Institute of Child Health and Human Development (NICHD) Neonatal Network, and the Centers for Disease Control and Prevention (Annibale, 2014). Long-term outcomes are inversely related to birth weight and gestational age as well as extent and location of the lesion. IVH is associated with a mortality rate of 20% with PHH increasing the rate to 55% (Robinson, 2012). Major cognitive defects affect 45% to 85% of infants with moderate to severe IVH, including cerebral palsy and mental retardation (Ballabh, 2012). Predictors of outcome include PVI, cystic PVL, and need for VP shunt placement. Shunt infections and revisions also can predict poor outcomes.

Advances in prenatal and postnatal care have helped to decrease the incidence of IVH and its associated lesions and complications. Prevention of preterm delivery is the most effective prenatal intervention. According to Cochrane Reviews, antenatal corticosteroids can reduce the risk of respiratory distress syndrome, which, in turn, decreases the risk for IVH and magnesium sulfate administration prenatally has been shown to have a neuroprotective effect (Roberts & Dalziel, 2006). The International Liaison Consensus on Cardiopulmonary Resuscitation's (ILCOR) 2015 systematic review confirmed that delayed cord clamping is associated with decreased risk of IVH. The American Academy of Pediatrics and ILCOR now recommend the practice of delayed cord clamping for 30 to 60 seconds in preterm and term infants not requiring resuscitation after birth. Because of insufficient evidence, this is not recommended for infants who require resuscitation as well as preterm infants less than 29 weeks gestational age. Postnatal interventions should include prompt and appropriate resuscitation measures that avoid hemodynamic instability and impaired cerebrovascular autoregulation. Synchronized ventilation should be used and suction should be limited. A neutral head position should be maintained. Avoidance of metabolic abnormalities as well as hypo- or hypertension should also be a priority.

Despite major advances and efforts to elucidate and prevent IVH, it still remains a major complication of prematurity. Infants with severe IVH and associated lesions and complications are at risk for neurodevelopmental deficits and increased morbidity and mortality.

HYPOXIC ISCHEMIC ENCEPHALOPATHY

HIE is a serious birth complication with an incidence as high as one to eight per 1,000 live births (Douglas-Escobar, 2015). HIE can have devastating effects on the late preterm and term infant and, despite recent advances in therapy, HIE remains a major cause of long-term neurologic disabilities. HIE is characterized by a brain injury that is caused by a hypoxic–ischemic event during the prenatal, intrapartum, or postpartum period that prevents adequate blood flow and oxygen to the brain. Risk factors include maternal cardiac arrest, severe anaphylaxis, placental abruption, umbilical cord prolapse, tight nuchal cord, acute blood loss, uterine rupture, placental abruption, uterine infection, twin-to-twin transfusion, maternofetal hemorrhage, severe isoimmune hemolytic disease, and cardiac arrhythmia.

Injury associated with HIE is a result of impaired CBF and oxygen delivery to the brain. The effect of the initial insult is pathophysiologically complex and evolves over time. Conditions resulting in decreased placental perfusion or disruption of oxygen delivery eventually lead to hypoxia, which leads to decrease in fetal cardiac output and causes decreased CBF. With moderate decrease in cerebral perfusion, the cerebral arteries redistribute blood to the posterior circulation, maintaining adequate perfusion to the brainstem, basal ganglia, and cerebellum. There is then focal damage to the cerebral cortex and the watershed areas in the cerebral hemispheres. With decreased perfusion, a cascade of injury occurs, which is divided into phases.

The acute phase, or primary energy failure, is described as the reduction of blood flow leading to decreased oxygen and glucose delivery to the brain, causing anaerobic metabolism. The production of adenosine triphosphate decreases and lactic acid production increases (Figure 10.11). Low levels of ATP lead to failure of the NA^+/K^+ pumps and reduce transcellular transport and causes intracellular accumulation of sodium, water, and calcium. With the influx of sodium ions, depolarization occurs in the neurons. Accumulation of NA^+, combined with the failure of energy-dependent enzymes, leads to cytotoxic edema and necrotic cell death. Excitatory amino acid receptor overactivation plays a large role the in the pathogenesis of HIE. The release of glutamate, the primary excitatory amino acid neurotransmitter in the brain, follows depolarization of the neuron and binds to glutamate receptors. The efflux of glutamate concentration and activation of receptors triggers excitotoxic cascade.

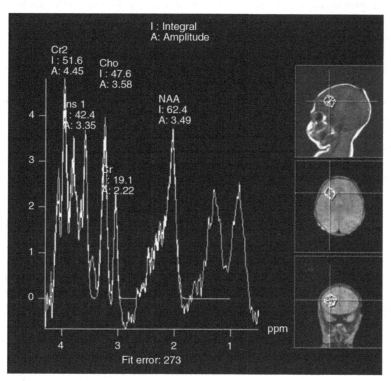

***Figure* 10.11** Magnetic Resonance Spectroscopy—Lactate Peak

This leads to further increase in water and increased calcium and sodium flow into the cell. Intracellular accretion of CA^+ results in cytoskeletal and DNA damage, free radical production, and nitric oxide production. Cellular rupture causes inflammation because of the cell contents released and the activation of inflammation mediators, which increases damage to white matter.

Approximately 30 to 60 minutes after the initial injury, there is a recovery phase. The latent period or recovery phase begins when blood flow is restored to the brain. The length of reperfusion determines the severity of the hypoxic ischemic insult and can last 1 to 6 hours. During this time, there is recovered cerebral metabolism and this is the optimal time for intervention. Although reperfusion is required for the reversal of injury, it can simultaneously cause additional injury and mitochondrial dysfunction.

With moderate to severe injury, a second deterioration phase occurs and is referred to as "the secondary energy failure phase." This phase occurs 6 to 48 hours after the initial insult (Allen & Brandon, 2011). The exact mechanism of this phase remains unclear, but is thought to be related to continued oxidative stress and excitotoxicity, cytotoxic edema, and inflammation. There is secondary energy failure with complete failure of mitochondrial activity leading to cell death and clinical deterioration. With mitochondrial damage, signals are released that lead to programmed cell death. Oxidative stress is caused by the overproduction of free radicals and is particularly harmful to the neonatal brain. Damage to neuronal tissue is exacerbated by the decreased ability of the neonatal brain to eliminate free radicals and the neonate's increased susceptibility to the free radicals. Excitotoxic injury continues, causing further cell death and damage.

Diagnosis of HIE is imperative for timely treatment and decreasing brain injury, but can be challenging. A comprehensive evaluation should be performed and should include all factors that potentially can contribute to the neonate's clinical status, including maternal history, medications, intrapartum history, and placental pathology. HIE is diagnosed on the presence of neurologic dysfunction. Neonatal encephalopathy presents as alterations in the level of consciousness, including respiratory effort, muscle tone, cranial nerve function, and seizures. According to the American Academy of Pediatrics (1992), in addition to neurological dysfunction, low Apgar scores (0–3 for greater than 5 minutes) and metabolic or mixed acidosis (pH < 7.0 from umbilical arterial sample), and multiple organ involvement should be demonstrated. The Sarnat staging system is used to classify infants with suspected HIE and should be used in combination with other clinical factors to determine severity and prognosis.

To form a diagnosis and prediction of outcome neuroimaging is imperative. MRI is the modality of choice for diagnoses as well as follow-up for infants with HIE and is useful in predicting outcomes. MRI sequences can provide information on the development of the brain and can demonstrate the pattern of injury in the brain at days 7 to 10. Injury may be seen as hyperintense areas on the images (Figure 10.12). A central pattern of injury is seen in the brain after a severe hypoxic–ischemic event with deep gray matter injury involving the bilateral basal ganglia and thalami as well as parasagittal injury of the cerebral cortex. In less severe injuries, subcortical white matter injury in the arterial watershed distribution is commonly present and is associated with limb weakness or spasticity. Diffusion weighted imaging (DWI) should be done in the first week after injury to look for abnormal signal intensity as well as abnormal lesions. A magnetic resonance spectroscopy should also be done and can serve as a biomarker for brain injury with the measurements of metabolite levels in the brain (Figure 10.11). The ratio of elevated lactate to N-acetyl aspartate in the basal ganglia can be a negative predictor for long-term neurological impairments. Both MRI and DWI have a positive predictive value in estimating death or major disability at

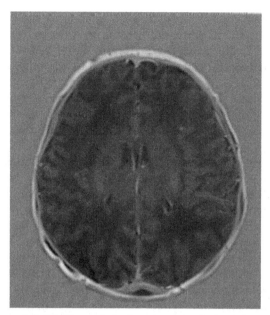

***Figure* 10.12** Hypoxic Ischemic Encephalopathy—MRI

age 2. Neuroimaging can also be useful to identify other underlying causes of neonatal encephalopathy such as infarction, hemorrhage, and brain malformations.

Electroencephalography (EEG) can be useful in evaluating the extent of brain injury. The abnormalities seen in infants with moderate to severe HIE may include discontinuous tracing, burst suppression, continuous low-voltage pattern, inactive pattern without cortical activity, and seizures. Results should be interpreted cautiously and should be assessed for improvements over time.

Treatment of HIE and reduction of the severity of brain injury is aimed at decreasing the effects of the secondary energy failure phase and supportive management. Systemic support remains the foundation for care for neonates with HIE. Restoration of cerebral perfusion and avoidance of secondary injuries that occur due to other organ impairment is the goal of supportive treatment. Metabolic changes that occur during HIE lead to less carbon dioxide production and can put the infant at risk for hypocapnia, which can be associated with death and poor long-term neurodevelopmental outcomes. Hyperoxia can also have detrimental effects with the increase in oxidative stress and free radical production. Infants with HIE are at increased risk for pulmonary hypertension. Initial respiratory resuscitation should be adequate but managed cautiously. Up to 50% of infant with HIE can have myocardial dysfunction (Zanelli, 2015). Hypotension should be avoided if possible and treated if present to avoid decrease in cerebral perfusion and further injury. Up to 20% of asphyxiated infants will have acute renal failure (Zanelli, 2015). Fluid and electrolyte management can be complex and should be managed carefully. Fluid overload should be eluded to avoid cerebral edema. HIE is one of the most frequent causes of neonatal seizures and usually occur between 12 and 24 hours after insult and can be difficult to control. Other complications include elevated liver function tests and coagulopathy.

Moderate hypothermia is considered the standard of care for infants with HIE. The exact neuroprotective mechanism of hypothermia is not fully understood, but is thought to be effective due to the reduction in free radicals and glutamate levels, decreased oxygen and metabolic demand in the brain, decrease in edema, vascular permeability, and decreased programmed cell death. In 2013, a Cochrane Review found that therapeutic hypothermia resulted in a decrease in mortality and major neurological disability at 18 months. According to the International Liaison Committee on Resuscitation in infants equal and greater than 36 weeks gestational age, with evolving moderate to severe encephalopathy, hypothermia should be offered according to a strict protocol in the postresuscitation period. Therapeutic hypothermia has been shown to reduce the risk of death and improve long-term neurologic outcomes.

Cooling should begin as early as possible and within 6 hours after insult. Hypothermia involves decreasing the neonate's temperature to between 33.0°C and 35.0°C. Most protocols aim at cooling infants for 48 to 72 hours and slowly rewarming the infant over 6 to 8 hours to prevent complications. Optimal duration of cooling has not been established and ongoing investigations are in the planning phases. Two methods have been used in clinical trials for hypothermia in neonates. Selective head cooling is done via a cooling cap with circulating cool water with temperature monitored via nasopharyngeal or rectal temperature probes (Gluckman, 2005). For total body cooling, the infant is placed on a commercially available cooling blanket with circulating cool water. Meta-analysis has not shown any difference in long-term developmental outcome when comparing the two methods. A 2013 Cochrane Review showed significant adverse reactions of therapeutic hypothermia were limited to sinus bradycardia and thrombocytopenia. Hypothermia should be performed under strict protocols in a regional referral center with comprehensive multidisciplinary care teams. Therapeutic hypothermia is the only therapy currently available that improves the outcomes of infants with moderate to severe HIE. Due to the complexity of the pathophysiological features of HIE, there are many opportunities for therapeutic intervention and new therapies to be developed.

Due to the association with death and poor neurological outcomes, HIE is a major clinical concern. In severe HIE, the mortality rate is as high as 25% to 50%, with many dying in the first week of life due to multisystem organ failure (Zanelli, 2015). Eighty percent of infants who survive HIE experience serious complications with only 10% being healthy (Zanelli, 2015). Infants with mild HIE have better long-term outcomes and are usually without serious complications. In the most recent hypothermia trials, approximately 25% of infants with severe HIE died prior to hospital discharge, and approximately 38% died by the age of 18 months after discharge home. Of the surviving infants at 18 months with severe HIE, 30% experience cerebral palsy, 16% had epilepsy, approximately 15% experienced blindness, and 6% had severe hearing impairments (Shankaran, 2012; Zanelli, 2015). Precise prediction of outcome can be difficult, although certain criteria have been shown to be useful in expecting likely outcomes. Apnea at 20 to 30 minutes of life is associated with death, seizures have been associated with worse neurological outcomes, and abnormal neurological exams past the first 7 to 10 days and difficult feedings can be suggestive of neurologic impairment. MRI is one of the most useful tools in determining prognosis. Studies have shown that infants with injury to the basal ganglia and thalamus have a worse prognosis when compared to infants who have prominently white matter damage and were associated with motor impairment at 2 years of age. Decreased or abnormal signals in the posterior limb of the internal capsule (PLIC) have been shown to be correlated with the inability to walk independently by 2 years of age (Martinez-Biarge, 2011). Follow-up is required for infants with HIE. The goal is to detect deficits and provide early intervention for infants who need it.

NEONATAL SEIZURES

Neonatal seizures represent an age-specific disorder and are defined as a paroxysmal alteration in the neurologic function, including motor, behavior, and/or autonomic functions occurring in term infants less than 28 days of life and preterm infants less than 44 weeks adjusted age (Vinayan, 2014). The presence of a seizure in the neonate is usually the first sign of neurological dysfunction and can reflect underlying brain injury. The risk of symptomatic seizures is the highest in the first year of life and is thought to be caused both the relative excitability in the neonatal brain and the high risk for brain injury in the perinatal period. Most seizures occur within the first 2 days to first week of life. The incidence of neonatal seizures has not been clearly defined, but is estimated to occur in one to two of every 1,000 term infants, with rates even higher in preterm births.

Determining the etiology is critical and helps to guide treatment strategies. Etiology is also a determining factor of prognosis and outcomes. HIE remains the most common cause of neonatal seizures and accounts for approximately 80% of all seizures in the first 2 days of life (Panayiotopoulos, 2005); these seizures are often persistent and difficult to control. Seizures caused by HIE are usually transient and pharmacological therapy is usually short term. Meningitis is commonly responsible for neonatal seizures in the first few days of life, with the most common organisms being group B *Streptococcus* (GSB) and *Escherichia coli*. Seizures associated with meningitis are indicators for risks of an abnormal neurological outcome. Other infections that can present with seizures include herpes simplex virus (HSV) type 2, which results in encephalitis and congenital cytomegalovirus. Structural malformations of cortical development and metabolic disorders constitute a large portion of neonatal seizures. Persistent metabolic disorders should also be considered when seizures are present. Overall these disorders are rare, but among these disorders, urea cycle defects, organic acidurias, and aminoacidopathies are the most common causes of seizure. Epilepsy disorders are very rare, such as epileptic encephalopathy and benign familial neonatal convulsions. Other etiology categories include intracranial hemorrhage; transient metabolic disturbances such as hypoglycemia, hypocalcemia, hypomagnesemia, hyponatremia, and hypokalemia; drug withdrawal; and intrauterine infections (such as cytomegalovirus [CMV], toxoplasma, HIV, and rubella).

Neonatal seizures have many characteristics that are different from seizures in other age groups and usually present with subtle or focal features. This is thought to be the result of the immature nervous system and the incomplete myelination patterns in the brain. The most widely used classification scheme divides neonatal seizures by clinical presentation (Vinayan, 2014). Clonic seizures are most commonly seen with electrographic seizures and occur predominately in term infants. They often involve one extremity or one side of the body or face and are characterized by slow, rhythmic, and repetitive shaking or movement of the body part. Focal clonic seizures usually involve one part of the body and multiclonic seizures involve several parts simultaneously. Tonic seizures may involve one extremity or the whole body and can be focal or generalized and occur primarily in preterm infants. Focal tonic seizures involving one extremity are often associated with electrographic seizures and are usually transient. Generalized tonic seizures often present with extension of the upper and lower limbs bilaterally and are often triggered by stimulus or changes in state. The majority of generalized tonic seizures are not associated with electrographic seizures. Myoclonic seizures may occur focally in one extremity or in several body parts, including the face. They may be focal or generalized. These seizures are typically not associated with electrographic seizures and usually appear as brief jerks. Subtle seizures consist of other paroxysmal activities, such as eye deviation, oral–buccal movements, or patterned movements of the extremities, and are the most common in the neonatal period, but can frequently be overlooked. Autonomic changes, such as apnea, tachycardia, and changes in blood pressure, may be signs of subtle seizures. Seizures should be differentiated from nonconvulsive movements such as jitteriness and benign neonatal sleep myoclonus.

An epileptic seizure is transient and is caused by excessive or synchronous neuronal activity. Other paroxysmal behavior may be generated from subcortical brain structures. These types of seizures do not have ictal EEG changes and are considered a type of primitive reflex. Electroencephalographic seizures, or subclinical seizures, are common in the neonatal period because of the immaturity of myelination in the newborn's brain, which leads to minimal seizure expression (Panayiotopoulos, 2005).

Detecting seizures has become easier in this population because of advances in technology. EEG is essential in diagnosis and management of seizure in the neonate. In the 1980s, it was discovered that not all clinical seizures were true electrographic seizures. Only 10% of neonates with suspected seizures have ictal EEG activity. Most clonic, myoclonic, and focal tonic seizures have electrographic correlates. Generalized tonic seizures and many forms of subtle seizures do not have electrographical correlates. Infants may also demonstrate an electrographic seizure without any clinical evidence. EEG can be analyzed not only for ictal activity, but also background activity, which is important in predicting prognosis and risk for seizures (Vinayan, 2014). MRI scanning can determine the presence and the extent of ischemic injury and of parenchymal brain injury, but is not a diagnostic study for determining the presence of seizures. The dissociation between clinical and electrographical seizures also causes controversies on how to monitor and treat neonatal seizures.

Neonatal seizures require urgent treatment to prevent or reduce brain injury. Adequate ventilation and perfusion should be established immediately and any metabolic disturbances should be corrected quickly because of the risk of injury to the brain. The World Health Organization (WHO) published treatment guidelines and recommendations in 2011. Neonates demonstrating any seizure activity should be evaluated for electrolyte abnormalities and infection. Hypoglycemia and other electrolyte abnormalities should be ruled out and treated prior to administration of an antiepileptic drug. Infants having clinical seizures lasting longer than 3 minutes, serial seizures, or electrographical seizures without treatable metabolic disturbances should be treated immediately with an antiepileptic drug. Phenobarbital is the first-line antiepileptic drug of choice for treating neonatal seizures. If seizure cessation is not achieved after the maximum tolerated dose of phenobarbital has been administered, a benzodiazepine, phenytoin, or lidocaine can be used as a second-line treatment. Cessation of pharmacological treatment remains controversial and unclear. The current treatment practices vary widely in different settings. The WHO published the recommendation that if a neonate has achieved seizure control on a single antiepileptic therapy, the drug can be discontinued without tapering the dose. In neonates requiring multiple antiepileptic therapies for seizure control, the drugs should be stopped one at a time with phenobarbital being the final drug to be removed. More studies are needed to evaluate these current recommendations.

Early recognition and appropriate management of seizures and underlying disease or injury may protect the brain and improve outcomes. Infants with neonatal seizures are at an increased risk for cerebral palsy, epilepsy, behavior problems, and abnormal cognitive outcome. The best prognostic factor in determining outcomes in patients with neonatal seizures is the underlying etiology and the timing of the insult. Patients with the worst prognosis are infants with HIE, intracranial hemorrhage, meningitis, and structural cerebral anomalies (Wong, 2012). Seizures in ELBW infants are associated with higher risks for cerebral palsy, cognitive impairment, and epilepsy when compared to more mature neonates.

The mortality rate of neonatal seizures is approximately 15%, with a morbidity rate of 30% (Panayiotopoulos, 2005). Fifty percent of neonates with seizures will have long-term neurologic complications, including epilepsy, mental retardation, and cerebral palsy (Wong, 2012). Neonatal neurological exams have been shown to be a good predictor of outcomes. The severity of EEG abnormalities is also a good predictor of outcome. Infants with burst suppression, severe low-voltage and multifocal abnormal discharges on EEG, are associated with abnormal outcomes in 80% of the cases (Wong, 2012).

Seizures are a relatively common but serious risk in the neonatal period. Etiology is the main determinate of outcome and should be identified promptly. The clinical and EEG features of neonatal seizures can differ from seizures in other patient population groups and are often a sign of severe underlying neurological or systemic diseases. An extensive workup is necessary to identify the underlying cause of the seizures and to direct appropriate treatment.

BIRTH TRAUMA

BRACHIAL PLEXUS INJURY

Birth traumas comprise two categories: fractures and neurological injury. *Neonatal brachial plexus palsy* (NBPP) refers to damage to the group of nerves that supply the arm and hand. This group of nerves stimulates muscles and controls sensitivity to the upper extremity. The brachial plexus is a group of nerve fusions and divisions that come from cervical (C5) nerve roots through thoracic (T1) nerve roots and end as combined peripheral nerves. Mechanisms of injury are thought to include compression, stretching, traction, oxygen deprivation, and infiltration. The most common mechanism of injury is stretching caused by excessive lateral traction on the head of the infant during delivery or during labor. The stretching of these nerves manifests as weakness or complete paralysis of the upper extremity in the newborn.

NBPP is rare and occurs in less than 1% of births and can be transitory or have long-term complications (Chauhan, 2014). Risk factors include shoulder dystocia, macrosomia, malpresentation, large for gestational age (LGA), uterine abnormalities, and mechanical assistance during delivery (Ouzounian, 2014). NBPP is most commonly seen with shoulder dystocia in LGA infants during vertex deliveries. Measures for prevention and prediction of NBPP have not been proven effective. Careful physical assessment is important when an injury is suspected, as is maternal and delivery history. Most cases of NBPP are unilateral and five patterns of nerve injury have been described. In practice, NBPP is usually divided into the three more common brachial plexus injuries. Erb's palsy, or upper brachial plexus injury, involves injury to C5, C6, and sometimes C7. This is the most common injury and accounts for 90% of all NBPP. The arm is typically adducted and internally rotated at the shoulder and there is extension and pronation at the elbow and flexion at the wrist and fingers. This position is commonly referred to as the "waiter's tip" and hand function is preserved. The Moro reflex will be absent and a weak grasp reflex will be seen on the effected side and sensation may or may not be affected. Total brachial plexus injury (global plexus palsy) accounts for 10% of brachial plexus injuries and affects the entire arm, including the hand, and involves all the nerve roots from C5 to T1. The arm will be flaccid and all reflexes and sensation are absent. Klumpke palsy (lower brachial plexus injury) is the rarest and involves C7, C8 to T1. It accounts for less than 1% of all brachial plexus injuries. The lower arm is affected with paralysis of the muscles in the hand, wrist, and fingers and sensory impairment on the ulnar side of the forearm and the hand. The bicep and radial reflexes, however, are still present, however, the grasp is absent. As a result of the first thoracic root injury, there may be ipsilateral Horner's syndrome, which interrupts the sympathetic nerve supply to the eye. In addition, sensation over the hand may be lost because of damage to the cervical sympathetic nerves.

Newborns with brachial plexus palsy are also at risk for other injuries and should be carefully examined. These injuries include clavicle and humerus fractures, spinal cord injury, shoulder injuries, facial palsy, and diaphragmatic paralysis caused by involvement of the phrenic nerve. Diagnosis includes obtaining a complete history and a good physical examination. The exam should include assessment of hand grasp, Moro and fencing reflexes, along with the presence or absence of Horner's syndrome. A detailed neurological exam should be done to observe and assess spontaneous movements, positioning, passive and active range of motion, reflexes, and other neurological defects. Radiographic studies may be required to rule out fractures and further imaging studies may be considered to evaluate root avulsion. Assessments should be ongoing during the first 6 months of life to assess the return of bicep function, which is one of the most important signs of NBPP recovery. NBPP has a 95% chance for normal function if there is return of bicep function in the first 3 months (Gleason, 2012). Any neonate with NBPP should have a referral to a pediatric orthopedist.

Management of these injures remains controversial, but should focus on avoiding contractures of the shoulder, arm, and hand, along with muscle atrophy. It is important to keep the arm in a neutral position and begin therapy within the first week of life. Physical and occupational therapy and observation are common initially. The goal of treatment is to maintain range of motion, improve muscle strength, and regain functionality (Yang, 2014). Some infants may require hand or elbow splints because of muscle tightness. Botulinum toxin injections are used in the treatment of contractures. Surgical intervention may be considered in infants who have had no recovery within 3 to 9 months after injury. A total of 50% to 90% of brachial plexus injuries resolve in 2 to 3 months (Hale, 2010). Full recovery rates in NBPP are estimated to be around 65%. Functional impairment lasting greater than 1 year is considered permanent and occurs in 10% of NBPP. Early assessment and management give the infant the best opportunity to improve function, movement, and sensation. Research is ongoing to clarify treatment options and outcomes of infants with all ranges of NBPP.

SUBGALEAL HEMORRHAGE

A subgaleal hemorrhage (SGH) is a rare but potentially life-threatening birth injury in newborns. SGH most frequently occurs during delivery when forceps or a vacuum are used to assist in the extraction and can also occur in nontraumatic births of infants with coagulation disorders. Risk factors also include LGA, prolonged second stage of labor, and cephalopelvic disproportion (Swanson et al., 2012). It is important to note that SGHs can occur spontaneously with no risk factors. It is caused by sheer force during delivery, leading to rupture of the emissary veins, which connect the dural sinuses and scalp veins. Blood accumulates between the epicranial aponeurosis of the scalp and the periosteum (Figure 10.13). The subgaleal space has no anatomical boundaries and can result in hemorrhage of the infant's total circulating blood volume. This can result in anemia, hypovolemic shock, and death. The hemorrhage can be sudden or gradual and may not be apparent in the first few hours following delivery (Fakih, 2014). Diagnosis is made by physical exam and presents as a fluctuant mass over the scalp that crosses suture lines and may extend into the nape of the neck and behind the ears. It is important to differentiate between an SGH and other extracerebral hemorrhages such as caput succedaneum and a cephalohematoma. Clinical symptoms include pallor, tachycardia, hyperbilirubinemia, tachypnea, hypotension, coagulopathy, and changes in neurological status. Management includes early diagnosis, careful observation,

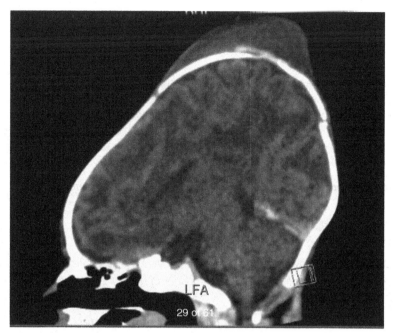

Figure 10.13 CT of Subgaleal Hemorrhage
LFA, left frontoanterior.

and aggressive treatment of symptoms. The progression of the hematoma should be followed as well as the head circumference of the infant. Vital signs should be monitored frequently. Therapy should include the treatment of shock, replacing blood volume, and correcting coagulopathies. Other injuries should be assessed and ruled out, such as skull fractures and other intracranial hemorrhages. A head and brain CT or MRI is the preferred imaging to clinically diagnose SGH. SGH is estimated to occur in one of 2,000 vaginal births without instrumental assistance and increases to one of 200 births with vacuum assistance (Fakih, 2014). Newborns who survive the acute hemorrhage and symptoms have good outcomes without neurologic sequela.

Case 10.1

A 25 6/7-week-gestation male infant was born to a 27-year-old gravida 2, para 1 as a result of severe preeclampsia. The mother received two doses of betamethasone and received magnesium sulfate. Maternal labs were significant for unknown group B *Streptococcus* (GBS) and type 1 diabetes. The infant was patted dry, leads were applied, and thermoregulation was initiated. The infant required resuscitation at birth, including positive pressure ventilation and intubation. Surfactant was delivered at 13 minutes of life and the infant subsequently needed a total of four doses of surfactant. On day of life (DOL) 2, the infant had

(continued)

Case 10.1 (continued)

significant respiratory acidosis requiring high-frequency ventilation with severe hypoxemia. On day 3, he continued to have worsening hypercapnia and developed significant hypotension requiring maximal support with pressors as well as significant volume expansion with normal saline boluses, fresh frozen plasma, and blood transfusions. After acute decompensation, an initial head ultrasound (HUS) showed grade IV IVH on the right side and grade III intraventricular hemorrhage (IVH) on the left.

1. **What is the most common site of origin of IVH in the preterm neonate?**
   A. Cerebellum
   B. Cerebral cortex
   C. Germinal matrix

   ANSWER: C. *The most common origination of IVH is in the germinal matrix and is caused by the fragility of the vasculature and lack of structural support as a result of immaturity.*

2. **When is the greatest risk period for IVH in a preterm neonate?**
   A. First 3 days of life
   B. First 4 to 5 days of life
   C. After the first week of life

   ANSWER: A. *The greatest risk for IVH in the preterm neonate is in the first 3 days of life after which the germinal matrix becomes less friable. The susceptibility of the germinal matrix in the first 3 days of life is compounded by the physiological instability of the preterm infant after birth. Autoregulation and cerebral vasoreactivity mechanisms are poorly developed in the preterm infant's brain.*

3. **According to the American Academy of Neurology, when should routine screening for IVH be performed?**
   A. Less than 30 weeks gestational age
   B. Infants less than 2,000 g
   C. Infants less than 32 weeks gestational age

   ANSWER: A. *Less that 5% of IVH occurs in infants delivered after 30 weeks gestational age.*

Head circumferences and bi-weekly HUS were followed carefully. The hemorrhages continued to evolve. At 3 weeks of life, a repeat HUS showed developing hydrocephalus and neurosurgery was consulted. The head circumference continued to enlarge and the infant started having increasing apneic events. At 4 weeks of life, a right frontal intraventricular reservoir was placed and taps to remove approximately 10 mL/kg/d of cerebral spinal fluid (CSF) were performed twice a day and cultured for bacteria. The infant had improved respiratory patterns with this intervention.

Serial HUSs were continued and the ventricles remained stable with reservoir tapping. At 3 months of age, it was decided to decrease the amount of reservoir tapping and evaluate the ventricles closely in hopes of avoiding shunt placement. HUS after 1 week

(continued)

Case 10.1 (continued)

showed an increase in ventricular size. As a result of the returning hydrocephalus, the decision was made to perform an endoscopic third ventriculostomy (ETV) with choroid plexus cauterization (CPC) in hope of avoiding shunt placement. A large amount of scarring was noted during the procedure.

The patient did well after surgery and was discharged home after 2 weeks with stable ventricular size and head circumferences. One month after discharge, the patient had a slow increase in head circumference with increase in fontanel tenseness. The mother noticed decreased movement with difficulty in eye movements and decreased feeding. An MRI was obtained and showed progressing posthemorrhagic hydrocephalus (PHH). The decision was made to perform a ventriculoperitoneal (VP) shunt placement.

4. What is a major complication of a VP shunt?

   A. Infection
   B. Ventriculitis
   C. Both A and B

   ANSWER: C. *Infection is a common complication after VP shunt placement, occurring in approximately 5% to 15% of procedures. This may lead to ventriculitis, may promote the development of loculated compartments of CSF, and may contribute to impaired cognitive outcome and death.*

Case 10.2

A term infant was delivered via emergent cesarean section after persistent fetal bradycardia of less than 60 beats per minute. The pregnancy was complicated by gestational diabetes. The infant was floppy, apneic, and bradycardic after delivery. Resuscitation was started per Neonatal Resuscitation Program guidelines and the infant was intubated. Subsequent Apgar scores were 1, 3, and 7 at 1, 5, and 10 minutes, respectively.

1. What should the clinician ask the labor and delivery staff to do?

   A. Obtain a cord gas
   B. Place infant on cooling blanket
   C. Turn off the radiant warmer

   ANSWER: A. *Diagnosis of hypoxic ischemic encephalopathy (HIE) is imperative for timely treatment and decreasing brain injury, but can be challenging. In addition to neurological dysfunction, low Apgar scores (0–3 for greater than 5 minutes) and metabolic or mixed acidosis (pH < 7.0 from umbilical arterial sample), and multiple organ involvement should be demonstrated.*

(continued)

Case 10.2 (*continued*)

The cord blood gas obtained showed pH 6.80, PCO$_2$ 90, bicarb 16 with a base deficit of 20. A detailed neurological exam was done and showed poor response to stimulation, hypotonia without spontaneous movement, pupils restricted and nonreactive, no suck or gag appreciated, no deep tendon reflexes, and minimal Moro reflex.

2. *How soon should hypothermia be initiated?*

    A. By 6 hours of life
    B. By 8 hours of life
    C. By 12 hours of life

    ANSWER: A. *Approximately 30 to 60 minutes after the initial injury, there is a recovery phase. The latent period or recovery phase begins when blood flow is restored to the brain. The length of reperfusion determines the severity of the hypoxic ischemic insult and can last 1 to 6 hours. During this time, there is recovered cerebral metabolism. By 6 hours after the insult is the optimal time for intervention. Although reperfusion is required for the reversal of injury, it can simultaneously cause additional injury and mitochondrial dysfunction.*

The infant was transferred to the neonatal intensive care unit (NICU) for continued care. He was placed on a cooling blanket and labs and vital signs were monitored closely per protocol. The parents were updated and had a lot of questions regarding the extent of brain injury and long-term outcomes.

Case 10.3

A term infant was delivered via spontaneous vaginal delivery to a 33-year-old gravida 3, para 2 mother with unremarkable prenatal labs. Pregnancy was complicated by gestational diabetes that was diet controlled and gestational hypertension requiring treatment with Aldomet. There was a maternal history of distant herpes simplex virus (HSV) with maternal HSV 2 antibodies without lesions and treatment with Valtrex. The infant required only warmth, drying, and stimulation after delivery and Apgar scores were 8 and 9 at 1 and 5 minutes, respectively. The infant was noted to have a temperature of 101.5°F after delivery that improved shortly after transfer to the nursery. The mother was afebrile without signs of chorioamnionitis. At approximately 15 hours of life, the infant had a cyanotic and apneic spell requiring positive pressure ventilation via mask for 1 minute. At this time, the infant began having repetitive movement of the right lower extremity for 3 minutes.

1. *What type of seizure is this infant presenting with?*

    A. Clonic
    B. Subtle
    C. Tonic

(continued)

Case 10.3 (continued)

ANSWER: A. *Clonic seizures predominately occur in term infants. They often involve one extremity or one side of the body or face and are characterized by slow, rhythmic, and repetitive shaking or movement of the body part.*

2. **What is the first-line antiepileptic drug of choice for neonatal seizures?**
   A. Lorazepam
   B. Phenobarbital
   C. Phenytoin

   ANSWER: B. *Guidelines established in 2011 by the World Health Organization recommend phenobarbital as the first-line antiepileptic drug to treat neonatal seizures.*

Glucose at that time was 91 mg/dL. Fifteen minutes after the initial episode, the infant had generalized tonic–clonic movements of all four extremities that lasted 4 minutes; a 10 mg/kg dose of phenobarbital was administered and the infant was transferred to the neonatal intensive care unit. The infant had a third episode of seizure activity and a second 10 mg/kg dose of phenobarbital was given. Labs were obtained and were reassuring. A sepsis evaluation was done and antibiotics were started. Serum and cerebral spinal fluid were sent for bacterial culture and remained negative. HSV polymerase chain reaction was sent and was negative. A pediatric neurologist was consulted and a continuous-video EEG was started. The EEG revealed continued seizure activity; the phenobarbital level was checked and was 23. The infant was placed on phenytoin, which immediately stopped the seizure activity. A head CT on day of life 1 showed a large, nonhemorrhagic acute infarct in the left mid-cerebral artery (MCA) territory and loss of gray–white matter differentiation and sulcal effacement involving the left parietal, posterior temporal, and occipital lobes. MRI/MRV (magnetic resonance venography) and MRS (magnetic resonance spectroscopy) demonstrated similar findings. An anticoagulation workup was completed and was negative. Phenytoin was discontinued after about 5 days of therapy and the infant was transitioned to Keppra for home therapy. The patient was discharged on Keppra with no seizures noted 3 to 4 days prior to discharge.

Case 10.4

A 35 5/7-week-gestation female infant delivered vaginally after induction of labor for polyhydramnios, fetal macrosomia, chronic hypertension, obesity, and uncontrolled type 1 diabetes. The mother is a 31-year-old gravida 2, para 1 and was on an insulin drip to control diabetes. During delivery, there was a right shoulder dystocia with difficult extraction. The McRoberts maneuver, suprapubic pressure, and Rubin maneuvers were used. The infant was finally extracted after delivery of the posterior arm. The infant was noted

(continued)

Case 10.4 (*continued*)

to be large for gestational age (LGA) (> 95th percentile). On assessment, the right arm was well perfused but the infant had very limited spontaneous movement. Moro reflex was absent on the right side and the palmar grasp was noted to be weak but present. On day of life 3, the infant continued to have no spontaneous movement of the right arm. The arm was held adducted and internally rotated.

1. *What is one risk factor that puts this infant at risk for birth injury?*

   A. Gestational age
   B. Infant of a diabetic mother
   C. Maternal age

   ANSWER: B. *Infants of diabetic mothers are at increased risk for birth injury due to increased incidence of macrosomia and LGA.*

2. *Brachial plexus injury usually affects which nerve segments?*

   A. C8–T11
   B. C5–C6
   C. C3–C4

   ANSWER: B. *Erb's palsy, or upper brachial plexus injury, involves injury to C5, C6, and sometimes C7. The arm is typically adducted and internally rotated at the shoulder, and there is extension and pronation at the elbow and extension at the wrist and fingers. This position is commonly referred to as the "waiter's tip" and hand function is preserved.*

Case 10.5

A 3,752-g, term infant is delivered via spontaneous vaginal delivery to a 23-year-old gravida 2, para 1 mother with limited prenatal care. The mother has a history of chlamydia and human papillomavirus (HPV), whereas other prenatal labs were normal. The infant was delivered in a vertex presentation after vacuum assistance after vacuum pop off × 2. After delivery, the infant was warmed, dried, and stimulated and received Apgar scores of 7 and 9 at 1 and 5 minutes, respectively. The infant was taken to the newborn nursery where he received routine newborn care. He was noted to have some scalp edema with excoriation from the vacuum. At 8 hours of life, the infant had an increase in head circumference from 35 to 37.5 cm.

The infant showed no abnormal neurologic symptoms. On assessment, the infant had a prominent occipital and parietal soft tissue induration, with boggy fluid quality with light palpation. A fluid wave was present with shifting fluid.

(continued)

Case 10.5 (continued)

1. What is not a preferred imaging method to diagnose subgaleal hemorrhage (SGH)?
   A. CT scan
   B. Head ultrasound
   C. MRI

ANSWER: B. *CT scan or MRI is the preferred method of diagnosing a subgaleal hemorrhage. Using these methods, the provider can assess the extent of the hemorrhage as well as any other hemorrhages or fractures.*

The pediatric neurology team was consulted and a head CT was ordered. Coagulation labs were normal and hematocrit was 34%. The head CT showed a large subgaleal hematoma, small subdural hematoma, as well a left parietal hairline skull fracture. Head circumference increased slightly over the next 24 hours with edema. The hematocrit remained stable. The total bilirubin at 24 hours was elevated and the infant required multiple days of phototherapy. The subgaleal hemorrhage did not progress, and no further intervention was required.

CONCLUSIONS

As research and technologies continue to develop, more knowledge regarding neonatal neurology will continue to be gained. Neonatal neurology is a complex field of medicine and injury or abnormalities can be convoluted. Infants with suspected neurological compromise or abnormalities require a multidisciplinary team to diagnose and provide appropriate treatment modalities.

REFERENCES

Adcock, L. (2012). Clinical manifestations and diagnosis if intraventricular hemorrhage in the newborn. Retrieved from http://www.uptodate.com/contents/clinical-manifestations-and-diagnosis -of-intraventricular-hemorrhage-in-the-newborn?source=search_result&search=head+ultraso unds+screening+for+ivh&selecteditle=2%7E150

Allen, K., & Brandon, D. (2011). Hypoxic ischemic encephalopathy: Pathophysiology and experimental treatments. *Newborn and Infant Nursing Reviews, 11*(3), 125–133.

American Academy of Pediatrics. (1992). Relation between perinatal factors and neurological outcome. In *Guidelines for perinatal care* (3rd ed., pp. 221–234). Elk Grove Village, IL: American Academy of Pediatrics.

Annibale, D. (2012). Periventricular hemorrhage–intraventricular hemorrhage. Retrieved from http:// emedicine.medscape.com/article/976654-overview

Annibale, D., Bissinger, R., Burke, C., Byrd, F., Carlson, C., Cavaliere, T., . . . Vargo, L. (2014). *Golden hours: Care of the very low birth weight infant.* Chicago, IL: National Certification Corporation.

Ballabh, P. (2010). Intraventricular hemorrhage in preterm infants: Mechanism of disease. *Pediatric Research, 67*(1), 1–8.

Chauhan, S., Blackwell, S., & Ananth, C. (2014). Neonatal brachial plexus palsy: Incidence, prevalence, and temporal trends. *Seminars in Perinatology, 38,* 210–218.

Douglas-Escobar, D., & Weiss, M. (2015). Hypoxic-ischemic encephalopathy: A review for the clinician. *JAMA Pediatrics, 169*(4), 397–403.

Fakih, H. M. (2014). Spontaneous neonatal subgaleal hematomas after caesarian section. *Journal of Case Reports, 4*, 359–362.

Gleason, C. (2012). Common neonatal orthopedic ailments. In *Avery's disease of the newborn* (9th ed., pp. 1359–1360). Philadelphia, PA: Saunders.

Gluckman, P. D. (2005). Selective head cooling with mild systemic hypothermia after neonatal encephalopathy: Multicenter randomised trial. *Lancet, 365*, 663–670.

Hale, H., Bae, D., & Waters, P. (2010). Current concepts in the management of brachial plexus birth palsy. *Journal of Hand Surgery, 35A*, 322–331.

Hydrocephalus Association. (2010). Fact sheet: Endoscopic third ventriculostomy (ETV). Retrieved from http://www.hydroassoc.org/docs/FactSheets/FactsheetETV.pdf

Martin, R., Fanaroff, A., & Walsh, M. (2011). *Neonatal perinatal medicine diseases of the fetus and infant*. St. Louis, MO: Elsevier.

Martinez-Biarge, M., Diez-Sebastian, J., Kapellou, O., Ginder, D., Allsop, J. M., Rutherfod, M., & Cowan, F. (2011). Predicting motor outcome and death in term hypoxic ischemic encephalopathy. *Neurology, 76*(24), 2055–2061.

Ouzounian, J. (2014). Risk factors for neonatal brachial plexus palsy. *Seminars in Perinatology, 38*, 219–221.

Panayiotopoulos, C. P. (2005). Neonatal seizures and neonatal syndromes. In *The epilepsies: Seizures, syndromes and management* (Chapter 5). Oxfordshire, UK: Bladon Medical Publishing. Retrieved from http://www.ncbi.nlm.nih.gov/books/NBK2599

Papile, L. A., Burstein, J., Burstein, R., & Koffler, H. (1978). Incidence and evolution of subependymal and intraventricular hemorrhage: A study of infants with birth weights less than 1,500 gm. *Journal of Pediatrics, 92*(4), 529–534.

Polin, R., & Ditmar, M. (2015). *Pediatric secrets* (6th ed.). Philadelphia, PA: Elsevier.

Roberts, D., & Dalziel, S. R. (2006). Antenatal corticosteroids for accelerating fetal lung maturation for women at risk of preterm birth. *Cochrane Database of Systematic Reviews, 2006*, CD004454.

Robinson, S. (2012). Neonatal posthemorrhagic hydrocephalus from prematurity: Pathophysiology and current treatment concepts. *Journal of Neurosurgery: Pediatrics, 9*(3), 239–241.

Shankaran, S., Laptook, A. R., Ehrenkranz, R. A., Tyson, J., McDonald, S., Donovan, E., . . . Jobe, A. (2005). Whole-body hypothermia for neonates with hypoxic-ischemic encephalopathy. *New England Journal of Medicine, 353*(15), 1574–1584.

Shooman, D., Portess, H., & Sparrow, O. (2009). A review of the current treatment methods for posthemorrhagic hydrocephalus of infants. *Cerebrospinal Fluid Research, 6*(1).

Swanson, A. E., Veldman, A., Wallace, E. M., & Malhotra, A. (2012). Subgaleal hemorrhage: Risk factors and outcomes. *Acta Obstetricia et Gynecologica Scandinavica, 91*, 260–263.

Vinayan, K. P., & Moshé, S. L. (2014). Neonatal seizures and epilepsies. *International Journal of Epilepsy, 1*(2), 75–83.

Volpe, J. J. (2008). Intracranial hemorrhage: Germinal matrix intraventricular hemorrhage. *Neurology of the newborn* (5th ed.). Philadelphia, PA: Saunders.

Whitelaw, A. (2011). Core concepts: Intraventricular hemorrhage. *NeoReview, 12*(2), e94.

Wong, M. (2012). Neonatal seizures. Retrieved from https://neuro.wustl.edu/patient-care/pediatric-neurology/pediatric-epilepsy-center/patient-family-and-physician-information/neonatal-seizures

World Health Organization (WHO). (2011). *Guidelines on neonatal seizures*. Geneva, Switzerland: Author. Retrieved from http://www.ilae.org/visitors/centre/documents/Guide-Neonate-WHO.pdf

Yang, L. (2014). Neonatal brachial plexus palsy—Management and prognostic factors. *Seminars in Perinatology, 38*, 222–234.

Zanelli, S. (2015). Hypoxic ischemic encephalopathy. Retrieved from http://emedicine.medscape.com/article/973501-overview

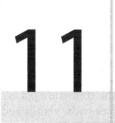

11

Dermatology Cases

Amy Jnah, Desi Newberry, and Tracey Bell Robertson

Chapter Objectives

1. Review the physiology and structural composition of neonatal skin
2. Explain the protective functions of neonatal skin
3. Define medical terminology used to characterize neonatal dermatologic findings
4. Differentiate benign, infectious, vascular, and other neonatal skin lesions
5. Identify evidence-based diagnostic and treatment regimens for common neonatal skin lesions
6. Evaluate clinical scenarios using the diagnostic reasoning process
7. Apply evidence-based diagnostic, management, and treatment plans to neonates with skin lesions

Examination, both visual and tactile, of the skin is primary to identifying congenital, postnatal, or emerging skin lesions. A primary understanding of basic dermatologic concepts, along with the definitions of key descriptive terminology specific to skin lesions, encourages accurate communication and diagnostic reasoning. Careful consideration of the prenatal history, ethnicity, and any genetic predispositions is a necessary complement to all examination findings. These essential steps, in addition to a collaborative and interprofessional approach to diagnosis and treatment, will ensure the provision of best practices and vigilant care to the vulnerable neonatal population.

PHYSIOLOGY OF SKIN DEVELOPMENT IN UTERO

Neonatal skin comprises three main layers: the epidermis, dermis, and a subcutaneous layer. The epidermis contains an outer layer called the *stratum corneum* and an inner layer composed of keratin-forming cells and melanocytes (Verklan & Walden, 2015). The dermis layer contains blood and nerve endings, sweat glands, sebaceous glands, and hair shafts and the subcutaneous layer contains fatty tissue (Verklan & Walden, 2015).

Early in the embryonic period, during weeks 5 to 8, the primitive epidermis has two layers: the basal and periderm (Martin, Fanaroff, & Walsh, 2015). The basal cells give rise to the future epidermis and the periderm interacts with the amniotic fluid to provide nutrition (Martin et al., 2015). An intermediate cell layer is formed during the transition period between the embryonic and fetal zones (Martin et al., 2015). Formation of sweat glands and synthesis of melanin begin at the end of the first trimester (Martin et al., 2015). Future hair, sebaceous glands, apocrine glands, eccrine glands, and nails form from appendages formed in the embryonic period (Martin et al., 2015).

Two to three intermediate layers of skin cells are added during the second trimester. Keratinization, or filling of epithelial skin cells with keratin, begins at 22 to 23 weeks gestation (Martin et al., 2015). Shortly thereafter at approximately 23 to 24 weeks gestation, the stratum corneum begins to evolve, eventually forming the outermost keratinized layer of the epidermis (Hoath & Narendran, 2001).

Further development of the stratum corneum and vernix caseosa occurs in the third trimester as does accumulation of subcutaneous fat (Martin et al., 2015; Verklan & Walden, 2015). Differentiation of brown fat begins around 28 weeks gestation (Verklan & Walden, 2015). The epidermal layer is not well established until the third trimester and is close to adult maturation by 34 weeks gestation (Martin et al., 2015; Verklan & Walden, 2015). After birth, the neonate's skin continues to mature over the first few weeks of life.

PRIMARY PROTECTIVE FUNCTIONS OF NEONATAL SKIN

Neonatal skin has four main protective functions, including provision of a physical barrier, prevention of transepidermal water losses (TEWL), immune protection, and thermoregulation. The skin provides physical protection by serving as a barrier to chemicals and insensible water loss resulting from the effective water-impermeable membrane of the stratum corneum (Hoath & Narendran, 2001). The skin also provides tactile discrimination via blood vessel and nerve endings, which carry sensations of heat, touch, pain, and pressure to the brain to protect from injury (Verklan & Walden, 2015). The subcutaneous layer provides insulation to protect the internal organs (Verklan & Walden, 2015). The melanocytes found in skin produce melanin to protect the skin against ultraviolet light radiation (Verklan & Walden, 2015).

The skin is covered and protected in utero and immediately after birth by vernix caseosa, a waxy, white biofilm. Vernix caseosa protects fetal skin from the amniotic fluid and neonatal skin from environmental elements. In addition, it facilitates skin maturation after birth and has endogenous anti-infective and cleansing functions (Association of Women's Health, Obstetric and Neonatal Nurses [AWHONN], 2013; Hoath & Narendran, 2001; Verklan & Walden, 2015). Maintenance of the vernix caseosa also assists in infection control through the acidification of the surface (acid mantle formation); the pH of the skin is acidic to prevent bacterial invasion (Larson & Dinulos, 2005; Tollin et al., 2005; Visscher et al., 2005).

Constant sloughing of dead epidermal skin cells helps prevent bacterial colonization on the skin (Hoath & Narendran, 2001; Martin et al., 2015; Verklan & Walden, 2015). Langerhans cells, produced in the dermis, provide immunosurveillance (Hoath & Narendran, 2001).

The skin assists in thermoregulation through sweat production and evaporation, constriction and dilation of blood vessels, and via subcutaneous and brown fat (Hoath & Narendran, 2001; Martin et al., 2015; Verklan & Walden, 2015).

UNIQUE CHARACTERISTICS OF THE SKIN OF PREMATURE INFANTS

The protective function of the skin in premature infants is decreased because of overall decreased thickness of the skin and a higher surface area–body weight ratio (AWHONN, 2013; Verklan & Walden, 2015). Premature skin lacks a well-developed stratum corneum and is more gelatinous, which predisposes it to skin breakdown and tears associated with lead pads and adhesives required in the neonatal intensive care unit (NICU; AWHONN, 2013; Hoath & Narendran, 2001; Lund & Keller, 2007; Verklan & Walden, 2015).

The immaturity of the stratum corneum and higher surface area–body weight ratio leads to increased TEWL, which, in turn, can lead to hypernatremia, dehydration, hypotension, and other electrolyte imbalances (Bhatia, 2006; Verklan & Walden, 2015). TEWL is inversely proportional to gestational age, making neonates less than 1,000 g particularly vulnerable (Hoath & Narendran, 2001; Verklan & Walden, 2015).

Structural and functional immaturity of premature skin puts the infant at risk for multiple comorbidities, including infection and increased absorption of topical drugs and chemicals. This is mainly caused by the absence of vernix caseosa, a thinner stratum corneum and dermis, and higher surface area–body weight ratio (Verklan & Walden, 2015). The lack of a vernix caseosa coating over the epidermis increases the risk for bacterial invasion through the skin and resultant infection (Verklan & Walden, 2015). The immature epidermis and dermis and decreased amount of subcutaneous fat and brown fat decrease the premature neonate's ability to regulate temperature and can negatively impact glucose homeostasis (Bhatia, 2006; Verklan & Walden, 2015). In addition, the sweat glands, though present, do not function properly before 34 weeks gestation (Verklan & Walden, 2015).

BEST PRACTICES FOR CARE OF THE SKIN OF PREMATURE INFANTS

Premature skin is vulnerable to chemical burns, tears, blistering, lacerations, extravasations, and bruising and edema. Care of the premature infant's skin must be focused on maintaining thermoregulation, forming the acid mantle, avoiding breakdown, cleansing during sterile procedures, and decreasing TEWL.

Premature infants should be placed in polyethylene wraps or bags immediately after birth to avoid heat and fluid loss (Bissinger & Annibale, 2010; Hoath & Narendran, 2001; Knobel, Wimmer, & Holbert, 2005; Vohra, Roberts, Zhang, Janes, & Schmidt, 2004). Premature infants should be bathed infrequently with warm water (AWHONN, 2013). Warmed sterile water can be used if skin breakdown exists (AWHONN, 2013). The vernix caseosa should be left intact to decrease TEWL, moisturize the skin, help form the acid mantle, and to encourage wound healing (AWHONN, 2013). Premature infants should be handled gently to avoid trauma (AWHONN, 2013). The use of tape, adhesives, and adhesive solvents (i.e., benzoin) should be minimized to avoid skin tears and burns; instead, the use of gelled adhesives, pectin-based barriers, or hydrocolloid layers is encouraged (AWHONN, 2013).

Cleaning agents, such as betadine and chlorhexidine gluconate, used in sterile procedures should be completely removed with sterile water after invasive procedures to decrease topical absorption or burns (AWHONN, 2013). Isopropyl alcohol use should be discouraged because of its drying effect (AWHONN, 2013).

To decrease TEWL and skin breakdown, the use of heated, humidified isolettes is recommended (Gaylord, Wright, Lorch, Lorch, & Walker, 2001; Kim, Lee, Chen, & Ringer, 2010). Preservative, perfume-free emollient creams/skin protectants can also be utilized to decrease TEWL; however, concerns regarding the risk for infection have been raised (AWHONN, 2013; Beeram, Olvera, Krauss, Loughran, & Petty, 2006). Lastly, transparent

Box 11.1 *Descriptive Categories for Skin Lesions*

- *Type* (primary/secondary)
- *Number of lesions*
- *Color*
- *Shape* (borders/symmetry)
- *Surface area distribution*
- *Texture* (rough/smooth)
- *Size*

adhesive dressings can be used to protect abrasions and to secure intravenous catheters and central lines (Bhandari, Brodsky, & Porat, 2005; Mancini, Sookdeo-Drost, Madison, Smoller, & Lane, 1994).

DERMATOLOGY-SPECIFIC TERMINOLOGY AND ASSOCIATED DEFINITIONS

Identification of a skin lesion is the first step toward diagnosis, management, and treatment (if applicable). Once recognized, a clinician is expected to comprehensively and accurately describe the lesion as well as communicate those findings to other members of the interprofessional team. Box 11.1 describes the essential features that should accompany any written or verbal description of a skin lesion.

Characterizing the lesion by *type*, as primary or secondary, aids in narrowing the differential diagnosis and quickly identifying the need for further evaluation, management, and treatment, as in the case with infectious skin lesions. Primary lesions are most suggestive or characteristic of a disease process. Secondary lesions evolve after rupture of a primary lesion and are often described as scales, crusts, erosions, ulcerations, or fissures. The assessment of *color* (red, white, yellow, black/gray/brown/blue) and *shape* (borders, symmetry or asymmetrical presentation) offers additional details that aid diagnostic reasoning. An assessment of *number* of lesions and the *surface area distribution* helps quantify the amount of skin affected by the lesion(s), the likelihood that the lesion may be associated with a genetic aberration, as well as the extent of treatment required with lesions at-risk for eruption and scarring. Articulation of the *texture* and precise measurement of the *size* of the lesion(s) (documented as length and width) are required to assess for morphologic changes or spontaneous regression. These data should be provided with as much precision and specificity as possible. Table 11.1 provides clinicians with a brief overview of key dermatology-specific terms, their definition, diagnostic association(s), and characterization as primary or secondary types of lesion.

BENIGN SKIN ANOMALIES

One or more benign skin lesions are observed in most newborns. In order to avoid unnecessary, costly, and painful testing, a scrupulous clinical examination is necessary to properly identify and differentiate benign from infectious or other skin lesions. This section of the chapter provides an overview of common benign skin lesions. Table 11.2 provides a ready reference for clinicians seeking to describe and diagnose these findings.

Table 11.1 **Key Dermatology-Specific Terminology**

	Brief Description	Examples of Association(s)	Primary or Secondary
Bulla	Small, fluid-filled vesicles often <1 cm in diameter; associated with both benign or severe disease processes	Sucking blisters, bullous impetigo	Primary
Cicatricial	Fibrous and contracted scar tissue	Congenital varicella zoster virus (VZV)	Primary
Crusted ulcerations	Crusted skin lesions comprising dried exudate (blood, pus, or other serous or serosanguinous fluid) found on the epidermal layer of the skin	Trauma, viral/infectious etiologies, genetic or congenital syndromes, or vascular or other malformations	Secondary
Erythema	Redness of the skin that can occur in any one or more location(s) and covers a small to large volume of surface area of the skin	Erythema toxicum, periumbilical erythema (omphalitis or funusitis), erythema multiforme, and staphylococcal scalded skin syndrome	Secondary
Exanthem	Widespread rash	Toxoplasmosis, herpes simplex virus (HSV)	Primary
Fissures	Linear breaches at the skin surface, resulting in an often painful separation of the epidermal layer	Keratodermas, eczema	Secondary
Macules	Small, flat areas of discoloration	Neurofibromatosis, treponema pallidum, transient neonatal pustular melanosis	Primary

(continued)

Table 11.1 **Key Dermatology-Specific Terminology (*continued*)**

	Brief Description	**Examples of Association(s)**	**Primary or Secondary**
Nodules	Tender, palpable, sometimes moveable raised lesions located within the subcutaneous tissue; range in size from 1 to 5 mm in diameter; commonly found on the legs, buttocks, forearms, face, or trunk region	Subcutaneous fat necrosis, systemic lupus erythematosus, and nephrocalcinosis	Primary
Papules	Small (<1 cm in diameter) raised, circular lesions that are solid in composition	Granuloma	Primary
Patches	Circumscribed, flat skin lesions often referred to as *macules*; variable size (can exceed 1 cm in diameter); can be found scattered throughout the body	Nevi, Mongolian spots	Primary
Scaling	Heaping of the stratum corneum with resultant shedding upon exfoliation	Ichthyoses, seborrheic dermatitis	Secondary
Scarring	Permanent, fibrotic alteration in skin integrity incurred as a result of trauma or tissue injury	Congenitally acquired infections, epidermolysis bullosa, infantile acne	Secondary
Vesicles	Small, round, elevated, and fluid-filled lesions, typically <1 mm in diameter	HSV	Primary
Wheals	Reddened, raised areas caused by serous fluid collection	Infantile acropustulosis, herpes simplex, staphylococcal impetigo, congenital candidiasis, and transient neonatal pustular melanosis	Secondary

Table 11.2 **Summary of Key Descriptive and Diagnostic Factors Associated With Benign Skin Lesions**

Name of Benign Skin Lesion	Key Characteristics	Diagnostic Associations (Examples)
Acrocyanosis	Bluish discoloration of hands and feet, often observed within first 24–48 hours after birth	Congenital cyanotic heart defect(s)
Congenital melanocytic nevus	Pigmented skin lesion caused by accumulation of nevomelanocyte cells; may be "hairy"	Nonhairy nevus: malignant melanoma "hairy nevus": spina bifida, meningocele
Diaper dermatitis	Most common cutaneous eruption in the diaper region, often associated with candida	Contact dermatitis, miliaria, atopic dermatitis, seborrheic dermatitis, psoriasis, nutritional and metabolic abnormalities (acrodermatitis enteropathica, zinc deficiency, biotin deficiency, multiple carboxylase deficiency), epidermolysis bullosa, histiocytosis X (Letterer–Siwe disease), granuloma gluteale infantum, phyoderma, candidiasis, dermatophytosis, syphilis, and scabies
Epstein pearls	Small, firm epidermal oral milia; also known as Bohn nodules or gingival cysts	Epidermolysis bullosa, HSV, contact dermatitis, congenital syphilis, and staphylococcal scalded skin syndrome
Erythema toxicum	White papules encompassed by a wheal of erythema	HSV, impetigo varicella, candidiasis, transient pustular melanosis, miliaria rubra, or incontinentia pigmenti
Milia	Small < 3 mm superficial keratinous papules, typically white or yellow in color	Sebaceaous hyperplasia

(continued)

Table 11.2 Summary of Key Descriptive and Diagnostic Factors Associated With Benign Skin Lesions (*continued*)

Name of Benign Skin Lesion	Key Characteristics	Diagnostic Associations (Examples)
Miliaria	Small, clear vesicular lesions located directly under the stratum corneum, of variable severity	Chorioamnionitis, infantile acne, infectious skin lesions
Mongolian spot	Blue-black or blue-gray lesion often found on shoulders, lower back, or sacrum	Inborn errors of metabolism (mucopolysaccharidosis, GM1 gangliosidosis)
Neonatal acne	Erythematous papules or pustules scattered over the face and cheeks	Miliaria rubra, seborrheic dermatitis
Seborrhoeic dermatitis	Greasy, scaly, yellow plaques found on the scalp	Erythroderma, erythema desquamativum, psoriasis, atopic dermatitis, neonatal immunodeficiencies, diaper dermatitis
Sucking blisters	Self-inflicted bullous lesions found on the mouth, lips, arms, or hands	HSV, varicella, congenital syphilis, congenital candidiasis, and group B streptococcal infection
Transient neonatal pustular melanosis	Erythematous pustules that rupture and convert to small, pinpoint scales	None

HSV, herpes simplex virus.

ACROCYANOSIS

Acrocyanosis (Figure 11.1) is a common, benign, transient condition caused by slow capillary bed perfusion, or vasomotor instability (Steinhorn, 2008; Tappero & Honeyfield, 2014). This phenomenon can also occur as a result of vasoconstriction of peripheral areas from exposure to cold temperatures (Eichenfield, Frieden, Zaenglein, & Mathes, 2015). Acrocyanosis is most commonly observed in newborn infants over the first 24 to 48 hours after birth.

Clinical manifestations include a bluish discoloration of the skin limited to the hands and feet. Management and treatment are often limited to clinical observation. However,

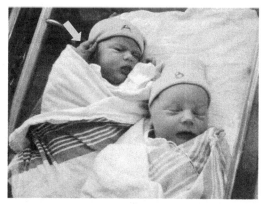

***Figure* 11.1** Newborn Twins Hours After Birth; Note Right Hand (*Arrow*) Displaying Acrocyanosis

acrocyanosis that persists beyond the first 24 to 48 hours warrants further investigation. In this case, a differential diagnosis is indicated and includes etiologies for peripheral cyanosis, including polycythemia, low cardiac output, or sepsis.

CONGENITAL MELANOCYTIC NEVUS

Congenital melanocytic nevus (CMN; Figure 11.2) is considered a pigmented skin lesion that primarily appears at birth or within the neonatal period. The incidence of CNM is 1:20,000 to 500,000 with a female-to-male ratio of 3:2 (Alikhan, Ibrahimi, & Eisen, 2012). Small, incidental CMN comprise the majority of cases, with large and hairy nevi less common.

Clinical manifestations of the CMN include a light- to dark-brown and flat to slightly raised, tan-appearing skin lesion with irregular borders. The lesion is mottled and heterogeneous, most commonly appearing on the trunk (Alikhan et al., 2012; Verklan & Walden, 2015). Over time, the lesion raises and forms a plaque, some are so large they impose psychosocial strain on the afflicted individual later in life. Some may present with hairs contained within the plaque and are termed a "hairy nevus."

The differential diagnosis for small CMN includes café au lait (CAL) spots, benign acquired nevi, and neurofibromatosis (when associated with CAL spots). Giant CMN are associated with lipoma, lymphangioma, capillary hemangioma, Mongolian spots, rhabdomyosarcoma, neuroblastoma, and other rare diseases and syndromes that may or may not be obvious at birth (Alikhan et al., 2013). Giant CMN (> 20 cm) carry risks for melanoma and neurocutaneous melanosis (Alikhan et al., 2012; Verklan & Walden, 2015).

Size, symptomology and associated and psychosocial risks must be considered when developing a follow-up, management, and treatment plan for the CMN. Small CMN may require only routine follow-up. Giant CMN require closer observation through childhood and adolescence with routine measurements to assess for changes in size, shape, or appearance. Imaging studies may be indicated in some cases. Close neurodevelopmental follow-up is essential, including routine head circumference measurements, to promptly identify any deviations in normal development. Laser therapy or surgical excision may be considered.

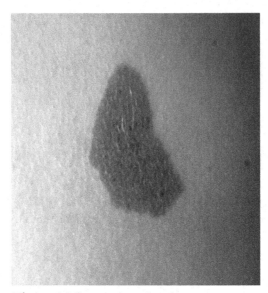

Figure 11.2 Congenital Melanocytic Nevus

DIAPER DERMATITIS

Diaper dermatitis is defined as the most common cutaneous eruption occurring in the diaper region (Eichenfield et al., 2015). It is estimated that up to 50% of all newborns and infants develop some degree of diaper dermatitis within the first year of life, and more than 30 diagnoses, or etiologies, for diaper dermatitis are identified in the literature (Eichenfield et al., 2015; Klunk, Domingues, & Wiss, 2014). Most cases of diaper dermatitis are attributed to irritant contact dermatitis, with candida noted as the second most common type of diaper dermatitis (Eichenfield et al., 2015). Allergic contact dermatitis is estimated to be as high as 55% to 77%, the result of allergic sensitization to dye(s) contained in infant diapers (Klunk et al., 2014).

Irritant diaper dermatitis has a multifactorial etiology. The infant's urine mixes with fecal matter causing an increase in pH, which activates the fecal enzymes lipase and protease. These enzymes strip the epidermis and increase the relative risk for skin irritation and breakdown exacerbated by frictional forces, including rubbing of skin folds in the groin area as well as from the diaper itself (Eichenfield et al., 2015; Klunk et al., 2014).

The differential diagnosis may include contact dermatitis, miliaria, atopic dermatitis, seborrheic dermatitis (SD), psoriasis, nutritional and metabolic abnormalities (acrodermatitis enteropathica, zinc deficiency, biotin deficiency, multiple carboxylase deficiency), epidermolysis bullosa (EB), histiocytosis X (Letterer–Siwe disease), granuloma gluteale infantum, phyoderma, candidiasis, dermatophytosis, syphilis, and scabies (Wolf, Wolf, Tuzun, & Tuzun, 2000). Therefore, accurate clinical assessment is essential to avoid unnecessary testing and treatment.

Management and treatment for irritant diaper dermatitis is best described using Klunk and associates' (2014) ABCDE pneumonic. "A" refers to the provision of air, or periods of time when the infant wears no diaper at all. "B" refers to the application of barrier creams, ointments, or pastes. "C" refers to gentle cleansing of the diaper area with products containing a neutral pH. "D" refers to the use of diapers capable of wicking fluid away from the stratum corneum. Finally, "E" calls for parental education meant to encourage long-term best practices and the maintenance of optimal skin integrity.

ERYTHEMA TOXICUM

Erythema toxicum (ET) is a benign, common form of erythema observed on approximately 50% to 70% of all full-term neonates (Eichenfield et al., 2015; Monteagudo, Labandeira, Cabanillas, Acevedo, & Toribio, 2012; Tappero & Honeyfield, 2014). The typical presentation is observed within the first 48 to 72 hours after birth and can last through the first 7 postnatal days (Eichenfield et al., 2015). Possible etiologies include systemic absorption of endotoxins, allergic responses to environmental or transplacental allergens (medications, vaginal fluid, milk), negative responses to thermal, mechanical, or chemical stimuli, or graft-versus-host disease (Monteagudo et al., 2012). More likely than not, ET is a cutaneous response to microbial colonization of neonatal hair follicles shortly after birth (Monteagudo et al., 2012).

The classic presentation of ET includes small, yellow to white papules surrounded by a wheal of erythema (Eichenfield et al., 2015; Tappero & Honeyfield, 2014). ET is found on all parts of the body with the exception of the hands and feet. Diagnosis is primarily by clinical observation, but can be confirmed by Wright stain analysis and a resultant elevated eosinophil count (Monteagudo et al., 2012). The differential diagnosis may include infectious and noninfectious skin diseases such as herpes simplex virus (HSV), impetigo, varicella, candidiasis, transient pustular melanosis, miliaria rubra, or incontinentia pigmenti (Monteagudo et al., 2012). No specific treatment is indicated and the lesions usually resolve spontaneously in a matter of days.

MILIA

Milia are defined as small, less than 3 mm superficial keratinous skin lesions (Eichenfield et al., 2015; Tappero & Honeyfield, 2014). Primary (congenital) milia occur in 40% to 50% of newborns (Berk & Bayliss, 2008). They originate from vellus hairs and contain layers of stratified squamous epithelial cells (Berk & Bayliss, 2008). Secondary milia are known as a localized form of milia that may be associated with disease states, medications, or trauma. They are believed to be the result of overlying epidermis, hair follicles, or sebaceous ducts (Berk & Bayliss, 2008).

Primary milia are described as white or yellow-white papules found primarily on the cheeks, forehead, and nose (Berk & Bayliss, 2008; Eichenfield et al., 2015; Tappero & Honeyfield, 2014). The differential diagnosis is limited to congenital milia versus sebaceous hyperplasia (Berk & Bayliss, 2008). Diagnostic confirmation is typically based on clinical assessment. In rare situations, laboratory analysis of the keratinous contents of the milia itself can be pursued. Management and treatment are limited to clinical observation, as these milia will spontaneously resolve.

The oral counterparts to congenital milia are known as Epstein's pearls or Bohn's cysts (Eichenfield et al., 2015). Epstein pears are small (< 3 mm) firm epidermal cysts. The etiology is the result of trapped epidermal tissue that occurs with fusion of the palate during fetal development (Berk & Bayliss, 2008). A 50% to 85% incidence of Epstein pearls is reported with predominance in Caucasian infants (Berk & Bayliss, 2008; Eichenfield et al., 2015). When these oral milia present in the alveolar margins they are referred to as *Bohn cysts* and follow the same benign course as Epstein pearls. Both Epstein pearls and Bohn cysts resolve spontaneously within weeks to months and without treatment.

Similar to primary milia, secondary milia also resolve spontaneously. They appear in conjunction with certain disease states, as a result of medication administration, or from localized trauma to the epidermal layer of the skin. Common examples of disease states associated with milia are EB, HSV, contact dermatitis, congenital syphilis, and staphylococcal scalded skin syndrome (Berk & Bayliss, 2008). Common examples of medications that may invoke the development of milia include topical corticosteroids. Repeated heel sticks, skin grafts, radiotherapy, and skin burns are common causes for the development of secondary milia in infants and older children.

MILIARIA

Obstruction of the sweat ducts, often the result of overheating, can invoke miliaria, a rash of variable severity found primarily on the forehead, scalp, neck, trunk, or groin (Eichenfield et al., 2015; Tappero & Honeyfield, 2014). In the presence of excess heat or humidity, sweat glands may become obstructed, which causes leakage of eccrine sweat into the epidermal or dermal layer and a resultant miliaria rash of variable severity.

The miliaria rash is differentiated by clinical presentation and classified within three categories: miliaria crystallina, miliaria rubra, or miliaria profunda (Tappero & Honeyfield, 2014). Small clear vesicles located directly under the stratum corneum characterize *miliaria crystallina*, neutrophil-filled lesions that look similar to small drops of water (Eichenfield et al., 2015). These papules are rarely congenital, however, cases of congenital miliaria crystallina associated with chorioamnionitis have been reported (Babu & Sharmila, 2008).

In cases of prolonged sweat gland obstruction caused by overheating or a febrile state, *miliaria rubra* may develop (Tappero & Honeyfield, 2014). The anatomic location of the obstruction is deep within the epidermal skin layer. The papules are slightly larger than miliaria crystallina (2–4 mm in diameter), are erythematous, pruritic, and can be easily mistaken for infectious skin lesions or infantile acne (Tappero & Honeyfield, 2014).

The most significant classification of sweat gland obstruction is referred to as *miliaria profunda*, a condition rarely observed in the newborn period (Eichenfield et al., 2015). Glandular obstruction is deep, often at or below the dermal–epidermal junction, producing an obstruction at the junction of the dermis and epidermis and resultant flesh-colored papules (Babu & Sharmila, 2012; Eichenfield et al., 2015). Diagnosis is by clinical observation and treatment for all classifications of miliaria involves mitigating the iatrogenic or physiologic cause(s) for overheating.

MONGOLIAN SPOTS

Mongolian spots (Figure 11.3) are common, often benign cutaneous pigmented lesions observed in 70% to 90% of all African American, Asian, and Hispanic infants (Eichenfield et al., 2015; Snow, 2005; Tappero & Honeyfield, 2014). They present as a result of arrested migration of melanocytes from the neural crest to the epidermis (Snow, 2005).

These lesions are typically brown, blue-black, or blue-gray in hue and are located over the shoulders, lower back, or sacral region (Eichenfield et al., 2015; Tappero & Honeyfield, 2014). The color typically regresses over the first 3 years of life (Eichenfield et al., 2015; Tappero & Honeyfield, 2014). Although rare, excessive Mongolian spots have been reported to be associated with inborn errors of metabolism, such as mucopolysaccharidosis and GM1 gangliosidosis (Snow, 2005). Diagnosis is by clinical observation and management and treatment are guided by any clinical association (i.e., inborn error of metabolism) and not the Mongolian spot itself.

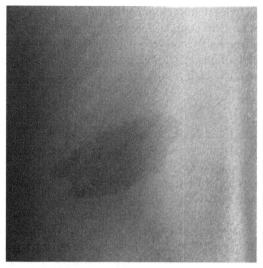

***Figure* 11.3** Mongolian Spot

NEONATAL ACNE

Neonatal acne, also known as neonatal cephalic pustulosis, typically occurs in the first 2 to 3 weeks of life and is a benign skin lesion (Eichenfield et al., 2015). *Malassezia* species have been hypothesized as one possible etiology for this rash, although these organisms are commonly found on the skin surface even in the absence of neonatal acne (Eichenfield et al., 2015).

The rash is classified by erythematous papules and pustules scattered at random or in clusters over the cheeks and face (Eichenfield et al., 2015). The differential diagnosis should include miliaria rubra and SD.

Diagnosis is by clinical examination, however, Giemsa staining can identify fungal spores, neutrophils, and inflammatory cells (Eichenfield et al., 2015). The condition is benign and resolves spontaneously without treatment (Eichenfield et al., 2015). Of note, *infantile acne*, which presents after 2 months of age, is a condition that does not resolve and may require treatment with topical corticosteroids or erythromycin to prevent scarring (Eichenfield et al., 2015).

SEBORRHEIC DERMATITIS

SD is also referred to as "cradle cap." It is often recognized within the first 3 to 5 weeks of life and typically peaks during the first 4 to 6 months of life (Eichenfield et al., 2015; Poindexter, Burkhardt, & Morrell, 2012). *Malassezia furfur* has been hypothesized as the etiology for SD with two studies showing the detection of this organism in most infants with SD and in none of the control infants (Eichenfield et al., 2015).

SD is characterized by greasy, scaly, yellow plaques primarily found on the scalp and in the absence of alopecia (Poindexter et al., 2009). The differential diagnosis should include erythroderma, erythema desquamativum, psoriasis, atopic dermatitis, and neonatal immunodeficiencies. Of note, diaper dermatitis should be included as an adjunct to the differential diagnosis list, as SD has been known to present within the skin folds of the axillae and perianal regions (Poindexter et al., 2009).

Treatment for SD includes shampooing with a mild tar solution daily and oatmeal baths once or twice a day (Eichenfield et al., 2015). In addition, 1% hydrocortisone can be used three times per day and frequently recovery will be noted within a few weeks (Eichenfield et al., 2015). Dark-skinned infants may develop hypopigmentation in the postinflammatory phase, but this improves as the rash resolves (Eichenfield et al., 2015).

SUCKING BLISTERS

Sucking blisters are considered benign and the result of self-inflicted trauma, often in utero suckling of a lip or extremity, and are commonly observed yet infrequently reported in the literature (Aydin, Hakan, Zenciroglu, & Demirol, 2013). The last known systematic review, published by Murphy and Langley (1963), estimated the incidence of sucking blisters at one in every 250 live births. Bullous lesions appear on the mucosa of the mouth, lips, or arms.

Clinical manifestations include the appearance of flaccid bullae on the arm, wrist, hand, or mouth (Libow & Reinmann, 1998). The bullae may have defined or scalloped edges with a denuded base. Size varies from 0.5 to 1.5 cm in diameter. The differential diagnosis includes infectious lesions such as HSV, varicella, congenital syphilis, congenital candidiasis, and group B streptococcal infection. The presence or absence of sepsis, congenital malformations, or other clinical manifestations associated with infectious etiologies aid in narrowing the differential diagnosis. Diagnosis is made primarily by clinical observation. In rare circumstances, confirmation by Tzank smear, Gram's stain, or culture can be pursued. These lesions resolve spontaneously without intervention.

TRANSIENT NEONATAL PUSTULAR MELANOSIS

Transient neonatal pustular melanosis (TNPM) is one of the more common, benign skin conditions observed with term newborns. The presentation begins with erythemous pustules, elevated secondary lesions typically filled with a clear or purulent fluid, that rupture within 24 to 48 hours of presentation. Once ruptured, the pustules dissipate into small hyperpigmented macules occasionally surrounded by white scales and lasting up to 3 months (Eichenfield et al., 2015; Tappero & Honeyfield, 2014). The most common locations for the macules include the forehead, chin, neck, back, hands, and feet. The etiology is unknown. Diagnosis is primarily by clinical examination; if ruptured and analyzed, the contents of the pustules will contain few neutrophils and no eosinophils (Laude, 1995). No further evaluation or treatment is indicated in an otherwise healthy infant and the macules typically resolve spontaneously after approximately 3 months.

INFECTIOUS SKIN LESIONS

Infectious skin lesions differ from benign skin lesions. They are considered primary lesions, carry clinical and diagnostic significance, and are often a first indicator of a more serious infectious etiology. The lesions themselves are often not subjected to specific treatment(s); however, the primary infection often requires prompt, evidence-based diagnosis and treatment. Therefore, differentiating these lesions from benign lesions, initiating an interprofessional approach to diagnosis and treatment, and providing appropriate education and support to the family are critical. Prominent congenital viral infections, including congenital cytomegalovirus (CMV), congenital rubella, toxoplasmosis, congenital syphilis, and congenital herpes infections, can present with the classic "blueberry muffin rash," making a thorough history, physical exam, and further diagnostic acumen essential. Congenital rubella is considered eradicated in the United States and therefore will not be a focus of this chapter. This section of the chapter provides an overview of common infectious skin lesions.

CANDIDIASIS

Candidiasis is a common fungal infection observed in NICUs, either transmitted vertically from mother to fetus or via nosocomial transmission (Eichenfield et al., 2015). It may be classified as congenital, systemic, invasive, or localized. The etiology is infectious in origin and can involve a variety of fungal pathogens, some of which are described next.

Congenital candidiasis presents within the first days after birth, appearing as a severely erythematous papulovesicular rash affecting the face, palms, or soles of the feet and often limited to the stratum corneum (Eichenfield et al., 2015). The rash quickly progresses to pustules that rupture, crust, and desquamate (Eichenfield et al., 2015).

Systemic candidiasis affects the urine, bloodstream, or cerebrospinal fluid and most often involves perinatal transmission of the virus from mother to fetus. Clinical manifestations include diffuse, severe erythema resembling a scalded appearance, papules, pustules, diaper rash, cutaneous abscesses, and occasional oral thrush (Eichenfield et al., 2015).

Invasive candidiasis, involving the species *Candida albicans*, is regarded as the fourth most common bloodstream infection and second highest mortality risk in the face of a bloodstream infection (Roilides, 2011). The incidence of invasive candidiasis is estimated to be 150 per 100,000 live births and the risk is inversely proportional to gestational age at birth (Roilides, 2011). Clinical manifestations include crusting lesions with fungal invasion well into the epidermis (Eichenfield et al., 2015). Diagnosis is confirmed through fungal culture of the blood, urine, or cerebrospinal fluid or through tissue biopsy (American Academy of Pediatrics [AAP] Committee on Infectious Diseases, 2012).

Localized candidiasis is considered to be of mucotaneous origin. Clinical manifestations of oral mucotaneous thrush include fixed white plaque(s) located on the tongue or mucous membranes that appear similar to cow's milk yet are unable to be easily scraped away (Eichenfield et al., 2015). Erythematous plaques, papules, and pustules describe candida diaper dermatitis (Eichenfield et al., 2015). Diagnosis is made by clinical assessment.

The drug of choice for the treatment of congenital, systemic, and invasive candidiasis is amphotericin B, a potent fungicidal and fungistatic agent. Alternative medications may include fluconazole or micafungin (Tripathi, Watt, & Benjamin, 2012). Prompt removal of any invasive catheters is indicated with invasive candidiasis (AAP Committee on Infectious Diseases, 2012). An oral or topical antifungal agent, such as nystatin or fluconazole, can be used with mucotaneous candidiasis.

CONGENITAL CYTOMEGALOVIRUS

CMV afflicts approximately 0.5% to 2% of all pregnancies in the United States and Europe and is regarded as the most common congenital viral infection (AAP Committee on Infectious Diseases, 2012; Schleiss, 2013). It is classified as either congenital or postnatally acquired (AAP Committee on Infectious Diseases, 2012). Vertical transmission of CMV can occur transplacentally via direct contact with the vaginal canal during birth or through the ingestion of infected maternal breast milk (AAP Committee on Infectious Diseases, 2012).

Congenital CMV is the leading cause for sensorineural hearing loss in infants through the first year of life (AAP Committee on Infectious Diseases, 2012). Additional common clinical manifestations of congenital CMV include intrauterine growth restriction, microcephaly, jaundice, retinitis, and neurodevelopmental delays. The differential diagnosis includes other congenital infections (rubella, toxoplasmosis, syphilis, herpes, and varicella), sepsis, and metabolic disorders that may produce cerebral calcifications similar to CMV.

Definitive diagnosis of CMV can be made through urinary polymerase chain reaction (PCR) testing or serum antibody titers (CMV IgM ELISA testing; Albanna, El-Iatif, Sharaf, Gohar, & Ibrahim, 2013). Additional diagnostic testing may include liver function testing, imaging studies, TORCH screen (toxoplasmosis, other agents, rubella, CMV, HSV), or other viral studies. Treatment of CMV with term infants includes intravenous or oral antiviral therapy of ganciclovir or valganciclovir, respectively (AAP Committee on Infectious Diseases, 2012). Careful consideration with close, frequent monitoring is indicated if antiviral therapy is pursued with a premature infant diagnosed with congenital CMV (AAP Committee on Infectious Diseases, 2012).

Congenital HSV

Neonatal HSV infection is associated with herpes type 1 or type 2 infection, with approximately 1,500 cases reported per year (Tian, Ali, & Weitkamp, 2010). Vertical transmission from mother to fetus or neonate can occur during active outbreaks or with passive shedding of the virus, before, during, or after delivery of the neonate. Transmission risk varies, with a 2% risk reported during pregnancy, 88% to 93% risk during the intrapartum period, and 50% to 100% risk after birth (Tian et al., 2010). Because clinicians may or may not know whether a pregnant female has been previously or recently infected, or whether she is shedding the virus at the time of delivery, careful and accurate neonatal assessments are critical to ensure prompt recognition of clinical manifestations that raise the index of suspicion for HSV.

Congenital or acquired HSV typically presents within the first 24 hours to 2 weeks following birth, respectively, with up to 33% of neonates displaying no skin lesions whatsoever. With intrauterine transmission, dermatologic findings may include active lesions observed immediately after birth to scarring or calcifications (Tian et al., 2010). With intrapartum transmission, lesions may be limited to the skin/eyes/mouth or considered disseminated (Berardi et al., 2011; Caviness, 2013). Vesicles or zoster-like eruptions (Figures 11.4 and 11.5), most commonly found at the vertex of the scalp, first appear. After 1 to 3 days, the vesicles convert to pustules and rupture either mechanically or spontaneously over time. This is followed by superficial sloughing and eschar formation (Berardi et al., 2011; Eichenfield et al., 2015; Yasmeen & Ibhanesebhor, 2014).

If left undiagnosed, 70% of skin–mouth HSV outbreaks will become disseminated, thereby imposing a mortality risk of 50% (HSV-2) to 70% (HSV-1) on the vulnerable neonate (Tian et al., 2010). Diagnosis of HSV involves the following steps: (a) obtain oral, nasopharyngeal, conjunctival, and anal surface cultures in the order listed (clinicians may use one swab stick but must end with the anal sample); (b) skin vesicle and cerebrospinal fluid (CSF) for HSV culture and PCR; (c) serum for HSV PCR; (d) serum for alanine aminotransferase (ALT) analysis (AAP Committee on Infectious Diseases, 2012).

The gold standard for the treatment of HSV infection in the neonate is intravenous administration of acyclovir (AAP Committee on Infectious Diseases, 2012). Recommended dosing is 20 mg/kg three times daily for a total of 14 days for skin–mouth disease. An extended treatment window of 21 days is indicated with disseminated (central nervous system [CNS]) disease. The provision of 6 months of suppressive therapy with oral acyclovir after initial intravenous treatment may prevent recurrence as well as optimize neurodevelopmental outcomes (AAP Committee on Infectious Diseases, 2012). Ocular involvement may require additional treatment with topical ophthalmic agent(s).

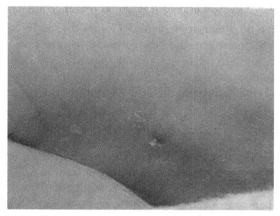

Figure 11.4 Crusted HSV Lesions (After Spontaneous Eruption)
HSV, herpes simplex virus.

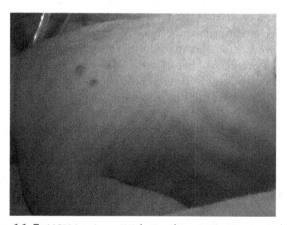

Figure 11.5 HSV Lesions With Erythematous Base and Crust
HSV, herpes simplex virus.

CONGENITAL SYPHILIS

The incidence of congenital syphilis has risen over 20% from 2004, to 8.2 to 10.1 per 100,000 live births (Centers for Disease Control and Prevention [CDC], 2016; Weintrub, 2010). The etiology for congenital syphilis is acquisition of the spirochete bacterium *Treponema pallidum*, passed from a mother to her fetus or newborn.

Clinical manifestations associated with congenital syphilis include the presence of oval-shaped "ham-colored" macules. These macules progressively transition to a hyperpigmented, copper-brown color over time (Eichenfield et al., 2015). Additional clinical manifestations include petechiae, bullae, annular or polymorphous eruptions, populosquamous eruptions or rashes, nail deformities, paronchyia, or alopecia (Eichenfield et al., 2015).

Diagnosis is dependent on (a) identification and confirmation of maternal syphilis; (b) assessment of maternal therapy (if any) and response; (c) comparison of maternal and neonatal serologic titers; (d) assessment of the neonate's nontreponemal testing, physical examination, ophthalmologic examination, long-bone and chest radiographs, liver function tests, complete blood count, platelet count, cerebrospinal fluid cell count, protein and quantitative Venereal Disease Research Laboratory test (AAP Committee on Infectious Diseases, 2012).

Management and treatment are based on maternal treatment prior to and during pregnancy as well as her response to treatment, or lack thereof (AAP Committee on Infectious Diseases, 2012). Intravenous aqueous penicillin G is the gold standard for treatment of confirmed or suspected congenital syphilis (AAP Committee on Infectious Diseases, 2012).

CONGENITAL VARICELLA ZOSTER VIRUS

Congenital varicella zoster virus (VZV), first recognized in 1947, involves transplacental transmission of the virus from a pregnant mother to her fetus(es) (CDC, 2016; Satti, Ali, & Weitkamp, 2010). VZV is an adjunct of the herpes family of viruses, is considered highly communicable, and when contracted during the first 20 to 24 weeks of pregnancy imposes significant mortality (30%) and mortality risks on the developing fetus (Lamont et al., 2011). The incidence within the United States is approximately 1.6 to 4.6 per 1,000 pregnancies (Satti et al., 2010).

Clinical presentation of VZV in the neonate is dependent on the timing of infection; a typical incubation period of 10 to 23 days is reported (Bhardwaj, Sharma, & Sharma, 2011). Fetal infection is known as varicella embryopathy, which is rarely reported in the literature as a result of the vast prevalence of maternal immunity in today's society. A *perinatal VZV infection* is defined in the presence of two criteria: (a) mother is infected 5 days prior to delivery to 2 days after the birth of her child and (b) the neonate presents with clinical manifestations within the first 10 days after birth. A 30% mortality rate is reported with symptomatic neonates.

Clinical manifestations of VZV include observable congenital anomalies (12%), intrauterine growth restriction (23%), skin lesions and cicatricial scarring (70%), limb hypoplasia (46%–72%), muscular atrophy (7%–22%), encephalitis or other neurologic deficits (48%–62%), chorioretinitis, microopthalmia or cataracts (44%–52%), and microcephaly (CDC, 2016; Lamont et al., 2011). Skin lesions may present as shiny papules or vesicles surrounded by a small erythematous base, most often on the forehead, face, trunk, or limbs. These lesions can be easily mistaken for HSV, therefore, confirmatory diagnostic testing is indicated despite similarities in treatment regimens.

Diagnosis is first suspected with the clinical assessment, visual and physical examination of the neonate. Serological testing is thereby ordered as confirmatory testing, and includes neonatal immunoglobulin M (IgM) and immunoglobulin G (IgG) antibody testing as well as VZV PCR testing. Surface cultures of fluid originating from within the pustules or vesicles, as well as skin scrapings, are also helpful in confirming the diagnosis of VZV. The management and treatment of VZV includes intravenous administration of acyclovir, the first-line drug of choice for VZV treatment, preferably initiated within 24 hours of onset of symptoms (AAP Committee on Infectious Diseases, 2012).

IMPETIGO

Impetigo is a highly contagious, common bacterial infection that afflicts neonates, which is caused by invasion of *Staphylococcus aureus* (Eichenfield et al., 2015). Unlike staphylococcal scalded skin syndrome (SSSS), in which toxin circulates throughout the body provoking blisters in areas distant from the site of infection, the toxin involved with bullous impetigo invokes the production of localized lesions at the site of infection, often in the abdominal region near the umbilicus or pelvis.

The fluid-filled bullous lesions, often referred to as "blisters," rapidly proliferate (Calabresi, 2010). The blisters are incredibly fragile and may be singular, appear in groups, or contain purulent or semipurulent fluid (Eichenfield et al., 2015; Tappero & Honeyfield, 2014). If ruptured, the bullae are reduced to scales that resolve without permanent scarring; however, alterations in skin pigmentation in these localized areas have been reported to persist for up to several months after resolution of the infectious process (Eichenfield et al., 2015). With nonbullous impetigo, the condition presents with honey-colored crusts and mild systemic clinical manifestations.

Diagnosis of impetigo is confirmed by culture and sensitivity of suspected skin lesions or by skin biopsy. Superficial epidermal blisters are seen with bullous impetigo (Stanley & Amagai, 2006). Management and treatment involves antibiotic therapy, which may be complicated in the presence of methicillin resistance.

Periumbilical Erythema (Funisitis/Omphalitis)

Periumbilical infections are limited to funisitis or omphalitis. Funisitis is a prenatally diagnosed acute inflammatory process occurring within the umbilical cord vessels or Wharton jelly (Reilly & Faye-Peterson, 2008). Funisitis is tightly associated with chorioamnionitis, which affects approximately 1% to 4% of births in the United States (Tita & Andrews, 2011). Omphalitis is a rare postnatal periumbilical infection of the umbilical region with a reported incidence of less than 1% (Broom & Smith, 2013). The etiology is infectious in nature.

Cranial ultrasound findings associated with funisitis include white matter lesions and periventricular leukomalacia, suspected to occur secondary to elevated concentrations of cytokines within the amniotic fluid (Reilly & Faye-Peterson, 2008). Postnatal clinical manifestations associated with periumbilical erythema (PE) are described as streaking erythema or erythema that extends in a lateral or horizontal direction from the umbilical area (Henbest & Steele, 2013). PE associated with funisitis refers to early, intra-amniotic inflammation, which is most often associated with chorioamnionitis and postnatally treated with broad-spectrum antibiotics. Omphalitis involves erythema with inflammation, edema, and tenderness around the umbilicus (Blackburn, 2013; Henbest & Steele, 2013). Severity is based on the presence of all or some of the following characteristics: purulent discharge only, cellulitis and lymphangitis of the abdominal wall, and inflammation extending into the subcutaneous fat and deeper facia (Fraser, Davies, & Cusack, 2006). Affected neonates may present with septicemia, necrotizing fasciitis, peritonitis, superficial cutaneous or intra-abdominal abscesses, hepatic obstruction, or eviscerated bowel (Fraser et al., 2006).

Diagnosis involves obtaining a Gram stain and culture of the fluid discharge from the umbilical region. Systemic antibiotics are thereby indicated, in addition to physiologic supportive measures.

Staphylococcal Scalded Skin Syndrome

SSSS is a serious, life-threatening disease caused by toxin produced by *Staphylococcus aureus* infection (Tappero & Honeyfield, 2014). It most often presents within the first 7 days after birth (Eichenfield et al., 2015). The incidence is approximately 0.09 to 0.13 per 1 million live births.

The clinical presentation associated with SSSS involves the onset of generalized erythema, often beginning with the face and mouth followed by epidermal stripping (Eichenfield et al., 2015; Tappero & Honeyfield, 2014). Within the next 24 hours, bullae appear, most often in regions experiencing frequent friction, including shoulders, buttocks, feet, and hands

(Eichenfield et al., 2015). The bullae quickly rupture and leave behind large areas of epidermal peeling (Eichenfield et al., 2015; Tappero & Honeyfield, 2014).

Clinical diagnosis begins with prompt recognition upon physical assessment of the skin. When SSSS is suspected, a light application of pressure on the skin may provoke separation of the superficial and deeper layers of the skin. This is known as a positive Nikolsky sign and is one positive diagnostic indicator of SSSS (Baartmans, Mass, & Dokter, 2006). Blood culture analysis is indicated to confirm the organism and obtain sensitivities. Skin biopsy will show a subepidermal blister with necrotic keratinocytes in toxic epidermal necrolysis (Stanley & Amagai, 2006). Pharyngeal swab and gastric aspirate culture can be used to identify staphylococcal species (Kadam, Tagare, Deodhar, Tawade, & Pandit, 2009).

Management and treatment are thereby based on sensitivity testing from the blood culture. Some infants require topical application of antibiotic cream in addition to intravenous antibiotic administration. Corticosteroid application is contraindicated and most case reports indicate successful healing without scarring within 10 to 14 days of diagnosis (Eichenfield et al., 2015).

VASCULAR SKIN ANOMALIES

Vascular skin anomalies are common in newborns and are usually benign and self-limiting. Vascular tumors, such as hemangiomas, are characterized by endothelial hyperplasia, whereas vascular malformations have normal endothelial cell turnover. Occasionally, vascular skin anomalies are signs of systemic disorders or are associated with other complications.

CUTIS MARMORATA

Cutis marmorata is a condition in which the infant's skin color may be bluish, mottled, or marbled (Eichenfield et al., 2015; Tappero & Honeyfield, 2014). This color pattern is caused by capillary vasoconstriction as a response to cold, stress, or overstimulation (Eichenfield et al., 2015; Tappero & Honeyfield, 2014). Infants with trisomy 21, trisomy 18, or Cornelia de Lange syndrome may exhibit persistent episodes of cutis marmorata (Tappero & Honeyfield, 2014). The differential diagnosis includes cutis marmorata telangiectatica, port wine stain, or infantile proliferative hemangioma. The condition generally resolves with rewarming of the skin; no further treatment is indicated (O'Conner & McLaughlin, 2008).

HARLEQUIN SIGN

Harlequin sign refers to a condition in which the infant displays a reddened color on the dependent part of the body when lying on his or her side (Eichenfield et al., 2015; Tappero & Honeyfield, 2014). This condition is reported in up to 10% of term newborns and most often occurs within the first 2 to 5 days of life (Tappero & Honeyfield, 2014). The phenomenon has no pathologic significance and is suggested to be a result of autonomic vasomotor control immaturity (Eichenfield et al., 2015; Tappero & Honeyfield, 2014).

Clinical manifestations make the Harlequin sign unique and easy to diagnose. A sharp vertical line of demarcation extending down the midsternum appears as a result of discordance in blood flow secondary to vasodilation, with half of the body displaying erythema and the other half displaying pallor (Eichenfield et al., 2015). The duration of color change is typically less than 30 minutes and has been reported to rapidly resolve with position change (Eichenfield et al., 2015; Tappero & Honeyfield, 2014).

Management and treatment are limited to observation and position change. No invasive therapies or treatments are required.

HEMANGIOMA

In the newborn, the most common vascular tumor is the hemangioma. The incidence of hemangioma formation is estimated to be 1% to 2.6% of healthy term infants and 15% to 30% in preterm infants with birth weight less than 1,500 g (Eichenfield et al., 2015). Females tend to have a higher incidence than males with a ratio of 2:1 to 9:1 (Gleason & Devaskar, 2012). Two etiologies have been proposed: failure of angioblastic cells to connect to the normal vascular system or primitive tumor development capable of differentiation into varying cell types (Bauland, van Steensel, Steijlen, Reiu, & Spauwen, 2006).

The clinical appearance of a hemangioma is dependent on anatomic location, although most are observed in the head and neck region. The first clinical indicator may be a precursor lesion, described as areas of telangiectases, erythematous macules, or bruising (Gleason & Devaskar, 2012). Hemagiomas occur as superficial, deep, or mixed lesions that are bright red in color, soft, spongy, raised, and lobulated (Figure 11.6). They may present at birth (congenital) or present within the first month of life (infantile; Tappero & Honeyfield, 2014). A rare form of hemangioma, called the *cavernous hemangioma*, is a vascular malformation located within the brain or orbital region that is only identified by imaging studies. Hemangiomas proliferate because of endothelia cell hyperplasia and do so during the first 6 to 12 months of life (Figure 11.7). Growth plateaus after this time frame and slow involution often begins. The differential diagnosis includes Kaposiform hemangioendotheliomas, tufted angiomas, pyogenic granulomas, capillary malformations, cutis marmorata, or venous/glomuvenous/lymphatic/arteriovenous malformations (Perman, Castelo-Soccio, & Jen, 2012).

Comprehensive review of the family history and physical examination are essential for diagnostic accuracy. Imaging studies and skin biopsy with cytogegnic markers are a helpful adjunct (Perman et al., 2012). Referral to a pediatric vascular specialist is indicated to ensure prompt assessment and treatment.

Management and treatment regimens are customized to the evolution and degree of involution of the hemangioma as well as its location. Close monitoring is required with spontaneous and uncomplicated regression (Eichenfield et al., 2015). When the lesion threatens to implicate the airway or vision, corticosteroid therapy may be indicated (Tappero & Honeyfield, 2014). Propranolol has also been recently suggested as a promising treatment modality (Tappero & Honeyfield, 2014). Plastic surgery has been reported with cases involving cutaneous atrophy after involution (Perman et al., 2012).

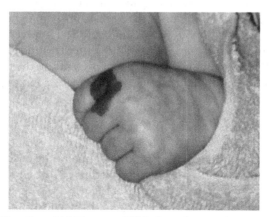

Figure 11.6 Ten-Day-Old Neonate With Strawberry Hemangioma on Hand

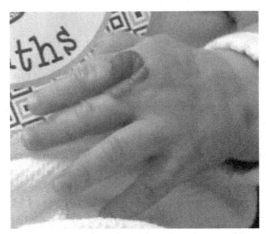

Figure 11.7 Evolution of Strawberry Hemangioma on Same Infant at 5 Months of Age

PORT WINE STAIN

Port wine stains (PWS) are the most common vascular malformation of infancy, occurring most commonly on the head and neck (Iljin, Siewiera, & Kruk-Jeromin, 2010). Frequently evident immediately at birth, PWS are the result of dilated congested capillaries (Eichenfield et al., 2015; Tappero & Honeyfield, 2014). They are reported to affect three of every 1,000 live births (Mermod, El Ezzi, Raffoul, Erba, & de Buys Roessingh, 2015). Approximately 10% of all PWS involve the trigeminal nerve and are associated with Sturge–Weber syndrome (Gleason & Devaskar, 2012). The etiology is due to a mutation with the guanine nucleotide binding protein, Gq class (GNAQ) gene.

Clinical manifestations are influenced by ethnicity. PWS are reported to be jet black with African American infants and pink or reddish-purple with other ethnicities (Eichenfield et al., 2015; Tappero & Honeyfield, 2014). The lesion has sharp edges and does not blanch with application of light pressure (Tappero & Honeyfield, 2014). In facial lesions, the thickness of the defect will increase with time and the color may change to a deep-purple hue or crimson red from the original pink red (Eichenfield et al., 2015). The differential diagnosis may include Sturge–Weber syndrome, spinal or cranial dyraphism, infantile hemangioma, or a tufted angioma.

A PWS does not resolve without management and treatment (Eichenfield et al., 2015). The treatment of choice for PWS lesion is the flash-lamp-pumped pulsed dye laser (Mermod, El Ezzi, Raffoul, Erba, & de Buys Roessingh, 2015). However, even with treatment, up to 10% of PWS will recur, some several months after treatment to 15 years later (Tappero & Honeyfield, 2014). In addition, any PWS that presents on the face or forehead should prompt the clinician to order an ophthalmologic consult as soon as possible. In addition, brain MRI may be indicated.

SALMON PATCHES

Salmon patches (Figures 11.8 and 11.9), the most common of neonatal capillary malformations, occur with 40% to 50% of live births. The birthmarks, often termed "fading macular stains," are most frequently located on the nape of the neck, the upper eyelids, bridge of the nose, or upper lip (Eichenfield et al., 2015; Tappero & Honeyfield, 2014). The etiology is suggested to be an excess of remnants of an unmodified primitive capillary plexus (Turkoglu, Kuru, Kavala, & Turkoglu, 2010).

Salmon patches, or nevus simplex, are described as flat, pink capillary malformations that can create a flushed facial appearance when multiple patches are present. The nomenclature associated with salmon patches is based on the anatomic location of the lesion. Patches located on the forehead are referred to as "angel kisses" and those present on the nape of the neck are termed "stork bites" (Eichenfield et al., 2015). Pigment-based patches are termed *congenital melanocytic nevi* and comprise nevomelanocytes, or melanin-producing cells.

Salmon patches that do not involute within the first 5 years of life are thereby termed *medial telangiectatic nevi* (MTN). MTNs may be associated with hamartomas, intracranial malformations, spinal dysraphism, meningomyelocele, meningoencephalocele, trisomy 13 to 15 and 21, Beckwith–Wiedemann syndrome, or craniofacial synostosis (Turkoglu et al., 2010).

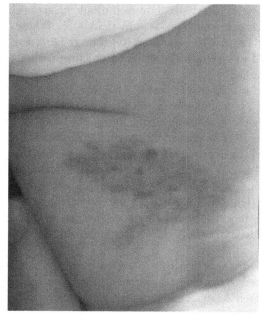

Figure 11.8 Six-Month-Old Neonate With Salmon Patch, Nevus Simplex on Right Leg

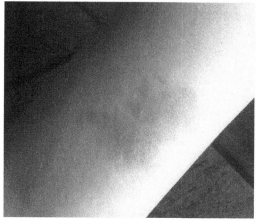

Figure 11.9 Four-Year-Old Child With Fading Salmon Patch on Left Forearm

Management and treatment are mainly limited to clinical observation. Most salmon patches fade and disappear within the first 1 to 2 years of life, whereas some persist into adulthood (Eichenfield et al., 2015; Tappero & Honeyfield, 2014). Treatment is directed toward any associated malformations or cosmetic removal.

OTHER SKIN ANOMALIES

CAL SPOTS

CAL spots are a type of pigmented lesion present in up to 1.8% of newborns and 25% to 40% of infants and children (Eichenfield et al., 2015). Clinical significance is based on the number of lesions found on the body. Three or more CAL lesions have been associated with genetic disorders in 0.2% to 0.3% of school-age children (Tekin, Bodurtha, & Riccardi, 2001). Six or more CAL spots of any size, however, should raise the clinician's index of suspicion for an underlying genetic condition, as more than 90% of these cases are significant for neurofibromatosis or other genetic syndromes (Gleason & Devaskar, 2012). The etiology of CAL spots is attributed to aggregation of excess melanin with the presence of enlarged melanosomes (Tekin et al., 2001).

Clinical manifestations consistent with CAL spots include the presence of pigmented lesion(s), often described as macules or patches, with a light- to dark-brown hue, round to oval in shape, and with a smooth to irregular border (Figure 11.10) (Tekin et al., 2001). Axillary or inguinal freckling in conjunction with CAL spots is a significant indicator for neurofibromatosis type I. Lesions may begin small during infancy and increase in size after puberty (Tekin et al., 2001). When six or more lesions are identified, the differential diagnosis may include neurofibromatosis, legius syndrome, tuberous sclerosis, McCune-Albright syndrome, LEOPARD (lentigines, electrocardiographic conduction anomalies, ocular hypertelorism, pulmonary stenosis, abnormalities of genitalia, retardation of growth, deafness) syndrome, Noonan syndrome, and Russell–Silver syndrome (Eichenfield et al., 2015; Gleason & Devaskar, 2012).

Diagnosis of the CAL spot itself is based on clinical assessment and observation. Further studies are aimed to confirm a suspected genetic disorder or syndrome, not to diagnose the skin lesion itself. Management and treatment are therefore disease or syndrome specific.

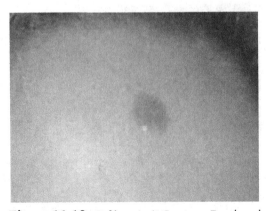

***Figure* 11.10** Café au Lait Spot on Forehead

CYSTIC HYGROMA

Cystic hygroma is regarded as the most common lateral neck mass diagnosed in infancy (Gleason & Devaskar, 2012). It is a tumor of lympatic origin with a reported incidence of 6% that is equally prevalent in males and females (Kumar, Kohli, Pandey, & Tulski, 2010). Half of all tumors are present at birth; the remaining 50% evolve over the first year of life. When diagnosed prenatally, a correlation with hydrops is reported and prognosis is typically poor (Gallagher, Mahoney, & Gosche, 1999). The etiology is attributed to sequestration of primitive lymphatic tissue or a congenital obstruction of lymphatic drainage causing progressively worsening lymphedema and dilation of the surrounding tissues (Kumar et al., 2010).

Clinical manifestations begin with the presence of a translucent, serous or chylous fluid-filled structure often located at the lateral neck region (Figure 11.11) (75%) or axilla (20%) that is covered by a thin layer of endothelium. The tumor is fluctuant and will swell with crying. The differential diagnosis may include cystic hygroma, hemangioma, lipoma, lymphoma, dermoid, chondroma, chordoma, craniopharyngioma, encephalomeningocoele, glioma, rhabdosarcoma, lymphoma, Rathke's pouch, congenital goiter, laryngocoele, branchial cleft cyst, thyroglossal cyst, and teratoma (Clifton, Ross, Gupta, & Gibbin, 2007).

Pre- and postnatal diagnostic imaging studies, specifically ultrasound, MRI, and/or CT scan, are useful tools (Gleason & Devaskar, 2012). Serial monitoring of alpha-fetoprotein levels is useful in determining whether the mass is consistent with a teratoma versus a cystic hygroma. Fine-needle aspiration can be pursued to confirm the absence of tumor cells.

Prenatal management strategies may involve a careful assessment of mass size to determine feasibility and safety of vaginal versus cesarean delivery method as well as strategies needed to protect the infant's airway after birth. Fluid aspiration is an effective emergency modality for rapid decompression when airway obstruction is evident and immediate surgical excision is not feasible. Emergency tracheostomy may be required with large obstructive masses. After birth, the treatment of choice is surgical excision, with an estimated recurrence risk of 17%. Additional management and treatment strategies include sclerosing agents, radiotherapy, enucleation, or close monitoring of spontaneous regression.

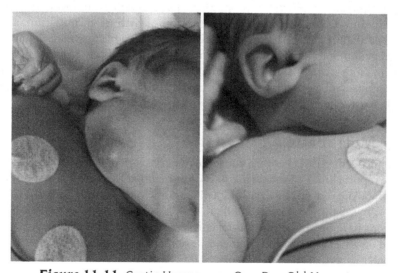

***Figure* 11.11** Cystic Hygroma on One-Day-Old Neonate

EPIDERMOLYSIS BULLOSA

The term *epidermolysis bullosa* describes a group of inherited disorders that afflict the basement layer of skin or the junction between the epidermis and dermis. The incidence of EB is estimated at 20 per 1 million live births in the United States (Fine, 2010). Friction or trauma of any degree induce painful blistering of the skin. EB is classified by location of blistering as either simplex (blisters originate at the epidermal layer), junctional (blisters originate at the junction between the epidermis and dermis), dystrophic (blisters arise at the superficial dermal layer), or Kindler syndrome (blisters arise from multiple locations).

EB is primarily an inherited disorder (National Institute of Health [NIH], 2013). Autosomal dominant EB involves inheritance of the EB gene from one parent with a 50% risk that offspring will display the disorder. Autosomal recessive inheritance involves acquisition of the EB gene from both parents, with a 25% risk that offspring will display the disorder. Rarely, EB is an acquired disorder through abnormal gene mutation (NIH, 2013).

Clinical manifestations of EB in neonates are consistent regardless of classification of the disorder. For all infants with EB, friction of any kind induces prompt erythema, blistering, and erosion of the skin or mucous membranes. The severity and distribution of blistering, however, aid clinicians in classifying the disorder. EB simplex is considered the mildest of all forms of EB, with blisters that are small, mild, and localized. Junctional and dystrophic EB involve a more severe presentation with blistering encompassing a more generalized proportion of skin surface area (Eichenfield et al., 2015). The differential diagnosis for EB may include erythroderma, congenital prophyrias, aplasia cutis, immunobullous diseases, congenital or acquired viral infections, bullous impetigo, SSSS, or lichen planus.

The initial diagnosis of EB is made through clinical observation because of the classic presentation of blistering lesions found in high-friction areas, such as the extremities, mouth or face, and groin. EB can present at birth or into infancy; therefore, clinical acumen with all physical assessments is imperative. A positive Nikolsky's sign is observed with the more severe or lethal types of EB. Confirmatory diagnosis of classification/type of EB is indicated and requires skin biopsy of fresh blister(s) (Eichenfield et al., 2015).

The management and treatment of EB extends across the life span as it is considered an incurable disorder. Goals for the interprofessional health care team and family include parental education and support; the promotion of skin integrity and wound healing; mitigation of pain and discomfort; and the promotion of hydration, nutrition, and growth (Eichenfield et al., 2015). Management of existing and new blisters may require extensive wound care, including lysing of new or existing blisters to facilitate emptying of fluid. Bandaging, use of cloth diapers and soft clothing, careful lifting that avoids creating friction under the armpits, and meticulous dressing-change procedures are essential. All interventions must be customized to the needs of the infant and family.

ERYTHEMA MULTIFORME

Erythema multiforme (EM) is a rare but acute hypersensitivity (Ang-Tui & Nicolas, 2013). Limited case reports link EM to vaccination administration (hepatitis B), parainfluenza, and acquired CMV (Ang-Tiu & Nicolas, 2013; Cho, Huh, Hong, Jung, & Suh, 2011; Cieza-Diaz et al., 2013; Wine, Ballin, & Dallal, 2006).

EM lesions have been described as macules, papules, patches, plaques, or wheals, with a centralized dusky erythematous cutaneous lesion encircled by a white ring and two erythematous outer rings (Ang-Tui & Nicholas, 2013). Atypical presentations involve two zones, the cutaneous lesion and outer single ring (Eichenfield et al., 2015). Less severe cases involve only the mouth or skin, whereas more severe cases can be associated with Stevens–Johnson syndrome (SJS) and involve two or more mucous membranes plus the skin (Eichenfield et al., 2015). The differential diagnosis list may include irritant and allergic dermatitis, staphylococcal scalded skin syndrome, SJS, and drug eruptions, including hypersensitivities to hepatitis B administration in the neonatal period. Diagnosis is made by clinical observation as well as by skin punch biopsy in some cases.

Diagnosis can be made through histological studies. Findings include hyperkeratosis, vacuolar changes, inter- and intracellular edema, and dysmorphic or necrotic keratinocytes within the epidermis (Ang-Tui & Nicolas, 2013). Management and treatment may include supportive care with no invasive intervention to corticosteroid administration.

Harlequin Ichthyosis

Ichthyoses are autosomal recessive inherited or acquired disorders of skin cornification or keratinization. Mutations in the ATP-binding cassette subfamily A_{12} (ABCA$_{12}$) genes cause insufficient lipid transport and thereby induce abnormal development of the skin (Gleason & Devaskar, 2012).

Clinical manifestations include thick, cracked skin with ridges and horny plates that can cover large amounts of surface area over the entire body. Other clinical features include flattened nares and ears, everted and gaping lips, absence of nails, restricted joint movement, and ischemia of the hands and feet (Gleason & Devaskar, 2012). The differential diagnosis may include restrictive dermopathy, lamellar ichthyosis, self-healing lamellar ichthyosis of the newborn, Conradi disease, trichothiodystrophy, Gaucher syndrome, or Neu–Laxova syndrome.

Accurate diagnosis is essential to provide a realistic management and treatment plan, as ichthyoses range from mild to life-threatening. Noting age of onset; integrity or absence of the collodian membrane; blistering; erythroderma; type, color, and distribution of scaling is essential (Lebwohl, 2014). Management and treatment are limited to supportive care only as these infants typically die shortly after birth. Mortality risk is associated with severe cutaneous infection (Gleason & Devaskar, 2012).

Subcutaneous Fat Necrosis

Subcutaneous fat necrosis (SFN) is a subcutaneous lesion found mainly in term newborns with a coexisting diagnosis of perinatal asphyxia and hypoxic ischemic encephalopathy. Perinatal hypoxia starves subcutaneous fat layers (comprised mainly of saturated fats) of oxygen, causing the crystallization and the subsequent formation of necrotic nodules. In infants with no history of perinatal asphyxia, experts posit that the etiology is caused by a defect in fat composition or metabolism (Eichenfield et al., 2015).

Lesions typically present within the first 2 weeks of life and are located in fatty areas such as the buttocks, back, arms, and legs (Gleason & Devaskar, 2012). Clinical manifestations often start with an erythematous firm but mobile nodule located in the subcutaneous tissue. The nodule may be tender to palpation. Associated findings include irritability, vomiting, nephrocalcinosis, feeding intolerance, hypoglycemia, and poor linear growth (Eichenfield et al., 2015; Gleason & Devaskar, 2012). The differential diagnosis may include sclerema neonatorum, scleroderma, lipogranulomatosis, or infectious or nodular panniculitis (Eichenfield et al., 2015).

Diagnosis is first made by clinical examination and assessment. Additional tools may include skin biopsy or fine-needle aspiration biopsy (Eichenfield et al., 2015). Hypercalcemia is often associated with SFN and warrants close monitoring. The presence of actual hypercalcemia may prompt clinicians to pursue radiographic imaging of the suspected lesions, which may show areas of soft tissue calcification (Eichenfield et al., 2015).

Management should involve monitoring of serum calcium levels and renal function. Treatment of the lesions is typically limited to supportive care. Topical antibiotics and occlusive hydrocolloid dressings may be indicated with ulcerated lesions.

Case 11.1

A 24-week male infant is born to a 19-year-old G2P0 female with history of inadequate prenatal care, unknown prenatal labs, and preterm labor. He is intubated at birth because of poor respiratory effort and the inability to increase heart rate with mask positive pressure ventilation. His clinical status improves after intubation and he is taken to the neonatal intensive care unit (NICU) for further management. An umbilical arterial and venous line are placed and securely sutured to the umbilical cord stump. After radiographic confirmation of appropriate placement, the lines are further secured with an occlusive dressing placed over a hydrocolloid protective layer to the abdominal skin.

1. **Risk factors that increase the risk of skin breakdown in this infant include all of the following except:**

   A. Gestational age less than 32 weeks
   B. Use of a hydrocolloid barrier
   C. Use of lead pads and electrodes

   ANSWER: B. *The integumentary system comprises the skin, appendages, eccrine, apocrine, apoeccrine, and sebaceous glands, hair, and nails (Blackburn, 2013). The skin is the largest major organ of the premature infant and provides a barrier against infection, helps facilitate temperature regulation and minimize insensible water loss, stores fats, and excretes electrolytes and water (Blackburn, 2013). The epidermis, the outermost layer of the skin, acts as a barrier from outside penetration but is weakened with premature infants because of incomplete maturation (Verklan & Walden, 2015). Common causes of tissue injury with the premature neonate include the use of tape, electrodes, probes, adhesive solvents, and adhesive removal products.*

2. **At birth, this infant's skin will be initially _____ and with the help of the vernix caseosa will eventually become _____ to protect against bacterial invasion.**

   A. Alkalotic/acidic
   B. Acidic/neutral
   C. Neutral/acidic

   ANSWER: A. *Vernix caseosa is regarded as a mixture of desquamating cells and sebum, is white or yellow in color, and comprises sebaceous gland secretions and exfoliated skin cells (Verklan & Walden, 2015). Vernix presents during the third trimester, increases the acidity of the epidermal layer of the skin, and the amount present is proportional to increasing*

(continued)

Case 11.1 (*continued*)

gestational age. The normal pH of the skin at term is 5 to 6, providing an effective barrier against bacterial invasion (Verklan & Walden, 2015).

3. **Strategies to prevent skin breakdown in the premature infant include:**

   A. Providing frequent bathing to decrease bacterial colonization
   B. The use of isopropyl alcohol in sterile procedures
   C. Bathing infrequently with warm water only

   ANSWER: C. *Effective strategies to prevent skin breakdown with premature neonates include gentle handling, infrequent bathing, the use of warmed sterile water for cleansing after sterile procedures, and humidification (AWHONN, 2013).*

Case 11.2

You are called to the newborn nursery to evaluate a 36-hour-old, full-term infant with a "rash." Review of the history reveals a 22-year-old primigravida mother of baby with no documented prenatal care. She reports no problems during the pregnancy and no significant medical history. The infant was born precipitously in the hallway of the emergency room via spontaneous vaginal delivery.

The physical examination is significant for small, clear, fluid-filled vesicles on the scalp. Over the next several days, the vesicles spread over the entire body, including the hands, feet, and below the scapula. Fresh lesions evolve into pustules that subsequently and spontaneously erupt and form crusts.

1. **The most likely diagnosis for this infant is:**

   A. Erythema toxicum
   B. Herpes simplex virus (HSV)
   C. Epidermolysis bullosa

   ANSWER: B. *HSV-1 is most commonly transmitted from mother to fetus during delivery. The virus multiplies within the maternal genital tract and transfers to the baby with direct contact. Rarely (< 5% of cases) does the virus cross the placenta and cause congenital HSV. HSV can also be transmitted through close maternal contact, primarily kissing (Blackburn, 2013). Infants can also be infected with HSV-1 if a mother has primary active HSV-1 infection, usually in the throat and mouth at delivery. Presumably in this case, infection of the infant occurs from close maternal contact. Hallmark clinical manifestations include a widespread rash with small, round, elevated, and fluid-filled lesions, typically less than 1 mm in diameter (Blackburn, 2013; Tappero & Honeyfield, 2014).*

(continued)

Case 11.2 (*continued*)

2. *To confirm your diagnosis, which of the following tests should be ordered?*

   A. Wright stain

   B. Oral, nasopharyngeal, conjunctival, and anal cultures

   C. IgM and IgG antibody testing

   ANSWER: B. *HSV polymerase chain reaction (PCR) of cerebrospinal fluid and blood, as well as oral, nasopharyngeal, anal skin surface cultures are used to confirm diagnosis and aid in the determination of length of treatment.*

3. *The gold standard for treatment of this infection is:*

   A. None; vesicles will resolve spontaneously in a few days

   B. Intravenous acyclovir

   C. Intravenous aqueous penicillin G

   ANSWER: B. *Acyclovir is the recommended treatment of choice for skin, eye, mouth, and disseminated HSV infection. Clinicians are encouraged to refer to the most current edition of the AAP Red Book (American Academy of Pediatrics Committee on Infectious Diseases, 2012) when determining the most optimal diagnostic and treatment regimen for HSV infection.*

Case 11.3

An infant was delivered via spontaneous vaginal delivery with vacuum extraction assist at 39 weeks gestational age. On examination, a flat, pink, V-shaped lesion in the center of her forehead as well as over the left eyelid are noted. Borders are irregular and the lesion blanches when gentle pressure is applied. Review of the maternal history is insignificant with all negative prenatal labs, adequate prenatal care, and no reported complications during pregnancy.

1. *Based on the photo, the lesion is most consistent with a:*

   A. Nevus simplex

   B. Port wine stain (PWS)

   C. Strawberry hemangioma

   ANSWER: A. *The three most common vascular lesions found in neonates include salmon patches, PWS, and strawberry hemangiomas, respectively. The nevus simplex is a type of salmon patch found in 30% to 50% of neonates at birth and is considered a benign macular lesion comprising distended capillaries (Verklan & Walden, 2015).*

(*continued*)

Case 11.3 *(continued)*

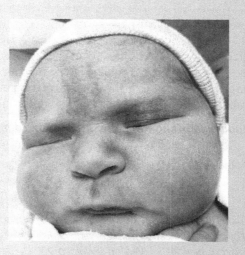

2. *The parents are worried about cosmetic aspects and long-term problems. What would be the best advice to provide to this family?*

   A. The infant will need follow-up with a dermatologist for possible surgical removal
   B. The infant will need to have a topical medication for resolution
   C. Most of these defects will resolve spontaneously in the first 1 to 2 years of life

   ANSWER: C. *This lesion will become darker in color with crying and blanch when soft pressure is applied. The nevus simplex typically involutes within the first 2 years of life.*

3. *The father is worried that this is a genetic condition that will recur with future offspring. He asks whether further genetic testing should be pursued to determine the absolute risk with future pregnancies. Your response should include which of the following statements?*

   A. This is a common lesion found in up to 50% of healthy infants
   B. This lesion is associated with chromosomal anomalies and no genetic counseling is indicated
   C. The lesion is most likely inherited from the mother and will recur with future pregnancies

   ANSWER: A. *Most salmon patches fade and disappear within the first 1 to 2 years of life, whereas some persist into adulthood (Eichenfield et al., 2015; Tappero & Honeyfield, 2014). Salmon patches that do not involute within the first 5 years of life are thereby termed medial telangiectatic nevi (MTN). MTNs may be associated with hamartomas, intracranial malformations, spinal dysraphism, meningomyelocele, meningoencephalocele, trisomy 13 to 15 and 21, Beckwith–Wiedemann syndrome, or craniofacial synostosis (Turkoglu et al., 2010).*

Case 11.4

You are asked to assess a full-term infant, now day of life (DOL) 5, who is in the neonatal intensive care unit (NICU) and is currently being treated with a 7-day course of antibiotics because of suspected pneumonia with a history of mild respiratory distress at birth. The nurse is concerned because the infant has erythematous eruptions, including white and yellow pustules in the diaper area, mostly in the skin folds of the groin. The infant exhibits discomfort during diaper changes and with cleansing of the genital area.

1. *Based on your readings, you know that the second most common cause of diaper dermatitis is:*

    A. *Staphylococcus aureus*
    B. *E. coli*
    C. *Candida*

    ANSWER: C. *Candida diaper dermatitis is the second most common cause of diaper dermatitis. It is caused by a fungal infection from Candida albicans. The groin, buttocks, thighs, and lower abdomen may be affected (Verklan & Walden, 2015).*

2. *The diagnosis of Candida diaper rash is based on:*

    A. Clinical assessment
    B. Wright stain
    C. Skin swab for Gram stain and culture

    ANSWER: A. *The presence of white or yellow pustules comingled with an erythematous rash is confirmatory for this diagnosis.*

3. *Pharmacologic treatment of Candida diaper rash includes:*

    A. Penicillin G
    B. Intravenous amphotericin B
    C. Topical nystatin

    ANSWER: C. *Treatment is indicated and antifungal creams, such as nystatin topical cream, are typically effective when applied several times daily. The differential diagnosis for infants who present beyond the neonatal period with a Candida-type rash should include zinc deficiency, malabsorption syndrome, cellulitis, or atopic dermatitis. Staphylococcus aureus is not associated with diaper dermatitis, but rather is a skin infection that produces a severe erythematous epidermolysis with lesions that spread rapidly over the body and exfoliate.*

Case 11.5

You admit an infant to a neonatal intensive care unit (NICU) within the United States who was delivered at 34 weeks gestation secondary to preterm labor. Mother is an 18-year-old primigravida with limited prenatal care. The mother is a U.S. citizen who has not traveled outside the country. She received one prenatal visit at 24 weeks gestation in the emergency department but did not follow up as prescribed. The infant was delivered via spontaneous vaginal delivery after a precipitous labor. The mother had an unknown group B *Streptococcus* (GBS) status and received no antibiotic prophylaxis because of the precipitous delivery. Maternal lab work obtained included HIV (negative), hepatitis B (negative), rapid plasma reagin (RPR) nonreactive, gonorrhea negative, and chlamydia positive.

The infant's growth parameters included a birth weight of 1,825 g, length of 39 cm, and head circumference of 26 cm. The infant presents with a "wasted" appearance, microcephaly, enlarged liver and spleen, jaundice to upper chest, profuse scattered petechiae that look similar to a "blueberry muffin rash." A blood culture and complete blood count are obtained, initially significant for a platelet count of 22,000 k/mcL. As a result of jaundice, a total serum bilirubin is obtained shortly after birth and resulted as 9.6 mg/dL.

1. ***What would be the most likely viral infection based on the maternal history, infant's presentation, and reported lab values?***

    A. Herpes zoster virus

    B. Congenital rubella

    C. Cytomegalovirus (CMV)

    ANSWER: C. *Congenital rubella has been considered eradicated in the United States, making it unlikely within this scenario. Common clinical manifestations of congenital rubella do include intrauterine growth retardation, jaundice, petechiae, and a blueberry muffin rash (CDC, 2014; Verklan & Walden, 2015). Congenital herpes virus presents as a vesicular or pustular rash; pustules subsequently rupture and crust over, making this diagnosis unlikely in the scenario provided. CMV is the most common congenital viral infection. It can be transmitted in one of three ways: horizontally through sharing of secretions, vertically from mother to infant during pregnancy, perinatally, postnatally, or by transfusion or transplantation from host to recipient (Verklan & Walden, 2015). Classic clinical manifestations include the absence of obvious abnormal findings to jaundice, hepatosplenomegaly, intrauterine growth retardation, microcephaly, and/or a blueberry muffin rash.*

2. ***What would be the most appropriate diagnostic test to utilize in this case?***

    A. Urine polymerase chain reaction (PCR) and IgM titer

    B. Lumbar puncture and IgG titer

    C. Surface and blood cultures

    ANSWER: A. *When CMV is suspected, diagnosis should be confirmed by testing the urine or blood. The high anti-CMV IgM titer is the correct blood test for suspected CMV (Verklan & Walden, 2015).*

(continued)

Case 11.5 (continued)

3. The recommended treatment regimen for this disease includes:

A. Acyclovir

B. Ganciclovir

C. Fluconazole

ANSWER: B. *Intravenous ganciclovir is the gold standard treatment.*

4. What is one of the most common long-term complications associated with congenital viral infections?

A. Blindness

B. Sensorineural hearing loss

C. Cerebral palsy

ANSWER: B. *All infants with suspected congenital viral infections should be closely followed after discharge, to include follow-up hearing testing, as sensorineural hearing loss is reported with all congenital viral infections. Up to 21% of all hearing loss at birth is attributed to congenital CMV infection (Verklan & Walden, 2015).*

Case 11.6

A 38-week-old female infant is born to a 26-year-old primigravida female with an appropriately supervised and unremarkable prenatal history. On admission to the nursery, the infant weighs 3.7 kg, is 21cm in length, and has a head circumference of 35 cm. Vital signs are as follows: temperature 37°C (98.6°F), heart rate 153 beats per minute, respirations 44 breaths per minute.

The physical examination is significant for blisters on the lower extremities, elbows, lips, and dorsum of both hands. A few small, denuded areas are noted at the base of the toes and both great toenails are visibly dystrophic. Shortly after application of the diaper, erythema and blistering are noted on friction points around the edges of the diaper and groin. No family member of the patient reports a similar dermatologic history.

1. The features of this neonate's physical examination are associated with which of the following categories of skin lesions?

A. Benign lesions

B. Infectious lesions

C. Other lesions

ANSWER: C. *Skin lesions are commonly divided into three distinct categories: benign, infectious, and "other." Benign skin conditions involve those diagnosed based on clinical characteristics and history. Newborns can present with benign skin lesions or individuals may de-*

(continued)

Case 11.6 (*continued*)

velop them over the course of the life span. These lesions are harmless, yet some may cause altered self-image and are electively removed. Infectious skin conditions are more serious and require prompt identification, diagnosis, and treatment as lifelong complications may emerge. Other lesions encompass a wide range of skin lesions that have genetic correlations or can be the result of pathologies, such as hypoxic ischemic encephalopathy.

2. **The differential diagnosis for the infant should include which of the following?**

   A. Transient neonatal pustular melanosis
   B. Erythema toxicum
   C. Epidermolysis bullosa (EB)

   ANSWER: C. *EB is one example of a skin lesion categorized as "other" that is associated with fragile, easily traumatized, and blistering skin that can lead to infection, dehydration, and other significant physiologic aberrations. Four types of EB have been identified in the literature with the mildest termed EB simplex and the most severe termed Dowling-Meara EB.*

3. **Confirmatory diagnostic testing for this skin lesion should include:**

   A. Perilesional skin biopsy
   B. Polymerase chain reaction (PCR) testing
   C. Gram stain and culture of aspirated fluid

   ANSWER: A. *Skin biopsy is necessary for diagnosis and careful handling, lifting, and wrapping of exposed skin is often necessary to maintain the most optimal skin integrity for the individual.*

4. **Management plans extending across the infant's life span may include all of the following except:**

   A. Lancing of blisters to facilitate emptying of fluid
   B. Lifting of the patient from under the armpits
   C. Use of cloth diapers

   ANSWER: B. *Skin blistering can begin shortly after birth and extend throughout the individual's life span. Careful lifting from the armpits reduces friction and the likelihood of additional blisters.*

Case 11.7

A male newborn weighing 2.910 kg is delivered by emergency cesarean section as a result of persistent fetal bradycardia and suspected placental abruption. The infant is pale, bradycardic, and nonvigorous at birth and does not respond to drying and vigorous stimulation. Endotracheal intubation, chest compressions, and fluid resuscitation via an

(*continued*)

Case 11.7 *(continued)*

emergency umbilical venous catheter are required. Apgar scores assigned are 1, 3, and 5 for 1, 5, and 10 minutes, respectively.

No spontaneous activity and decerebrate posturing are noted with admission to the neonatal intensive care unit (NICU). The infant's tone is flaccid, primitive reflexes are absent, and pupils are constricted. Vital signs are as follows: temperature 36.1°C, heart rate 85 beats per minute, respirations 40 breaths per minute (provided per the mechanical ventilator's backup rate). Therapeutic body cooling for suspected hypoxic ischemic encephalopathy is initiated.

Approximately 96 hours after birth and after body cooling therapy was completed, multiple firm, reddened, indurated, and slightly edematous nodules are noted on the infant's back and buttocks. The largest mass was noted on the deltoid region and measured 1.5 × 2 cm. A serum calcium level is ordered and reported at 2.96 mmol/L. Palpation of the affected area confirms firm, mobile nodules under the cutaneous layer of skin. The infant grimaces with palpation of the nodules.

1. **Based on the information available, what is the most likely skin-related diagnosis?**

   A. Scleroderma
   B. Systemic lupus erythematosus
   C. Subcutaneous fat necrosis (SFN)

   ANSWER: C. *Neonatal scleroderma (NS) is a rare disease of the neonate often observed in premature infants suffering from hypothermia and hypoalbuminemia. It can present with similar manifestations as SFN, however, hallmark differences in appearance and presentation are observed. NS presents as pale, shiny, and firm skin to palpation that cannot be pinched because of its tight adhesion to the subcutaneous tissues (Martin et al., 2015). SFN first appears on the thighs and buttocks and then becomes generalized. The clinical manifestations of SFN include erythematous indurations found under the dermal skin layer that are tender with palpation, occurring mainly on the trunk, extremities, and face (Verklan & Walden, 2015). These nodules typically appear within the first 2 weeks of life and are caused by the crystallization of fat cells.*

2. **Which of the following evaluations should be obtained immediately after diagnosis of this skin lesion?**

   A. Head ultrasound
   B. Serum electrolyte panel
   C. Complete blood count

   ANSWER: B. *SFN often occurs secondary to perinatal asphyxia, however, associations with maternal smoking, high blood pressure and diabetes, familial history of thrombosis, operative vaginal delivery, neonatal cold stress, and shock have also been reported (Martin et al., 2015; Verklan & Walden, 2015). Hypercalcemia is a significant risk factor that requires prompt evaluation through interval monitoring of serum electrolyte panels.*

(continued)

Case 11.7 (continued)

3. Confirmatory diagnostic testing should include which of the following?

A. Histopathology
B. Aspiration cytology
C. All of the above

ANSWER: C. *Histological findings that confirm SFN include fat lobule necrosis, crystallization of fat, and lipocytes present in a radial arrangement. Surrounding skin often contains granular infiltrates of lymphocytes, macrophages, and giant cells. Fine-needle aspiration can confirm the stage of evolution of the SFN. Early stages are associated with minimal inflammation and necrosis. Fat cells reflect a crystalline shape. Later stages are associated with advanced necrosis, inflammation, and crystallization.*

4. Appropriate management for this pathology includes:

A. Interval monitoring of serum calcium levels
B. Supportive care
C. Y-excision with skin grafting

ANSWER: A. *Because small areas of calcium deposition are scattered throughout the necrotic areas and calcifications may be present, serial monitoring of serum calcium levels is indicated. Spontaneous resolution is observed but may take several weeks.*

Case 11.8

You are called to attend a delivery of an infant who is estimated 37 5/7 weeks gestation. Mother has received appropriate prenatal care and all of her labs are negative. Her pregnancy was complicated by gestational diabetes controlled with diet changes. Her labor and delivery are complicated by rupture of membranes × 12 hours with meconium-stained fluid. The infant is delivered via forceps-assisted operative vaginal delivery. The infant's birth weight is 3.54 kg, head circumference 34 cm, and length 51 cm. The infant exhibits no respiratory distress, has a noted ruddy complexion, and a flat red lesion measuring 2 × 4 cm located on the glabella. The lesion grows over the next 3 weeks of life, becoming raised, lobulated, and spongy. Edges intrude into the space of the inner canthus of the eyes bilaterally. In addition, the inner portion of the lesion begins to show signs of ulceration.

1. The clinical presentation and evolution of this lesion are most consistent with which of the following diagnoses?

A. Port wine stain (PWS)
B. Cystic hygroma
C. Hemangioma

(continued)

Case 11.8 *(continued)*

ANSWER: C. *The PWS is a flat skin lesion that takes on a red to purple hue. This particular type of nevus ranges widely in size, from small lesions to lesions encompassing a vast surface area (Verklan & Walden, 2015). Unlike the cystic hygroma or hemangioma, PWS do not change in size. The cystic hygroma is a congenital malformation of the lymphatic system and the most commonly diagnosed lateral neck mass. Progressive swelling of the lymphatic region and surrounding tissues account for the visible mass observed after birth. Cystic hygromas can grow in size over the first 2 years of life and rarely spontaneously regress, with surgical excision noted as the treatment of choice (Martin et al., 2015). The hemangioma, on the other hand, is less likely to present at the lateral neck and is not a flat lesion like the PWS. This skin lesion may present externally on the head, neck, trunk, or extremities (including the digits) as well as internally in the throat or inner cheek and, when observed externally, takes on a bluish-red to strawberry hue (Verklan & Walden, 2015).*

2. **What would be the best treatment choice for this infant based on the progression of the lesion?**
   A. Close monitoring of the site
   B. Systemic corticosteroids
   C. Surgical debridement

   ANSWER: B. *The hemangioma will often increase in size over the first 6 to 12 months of life and then slowly and spontaneously regress (Verklan & Walden, 2015). The cases in which the location of the hemangioma and its expected growth will compromise vital organ function, systemic corticosteroids are recommended as a first-line treatment agent (Verklan & Walden, 2015).*

3. **The parents have been researching on the Internet and tell you that they would prefer not to begin medical treatment and would rather allow time for the lesion to involute spontaneously, your advice would be:**
   A. "That is a reasonable plan; let's schedule a follow-up appointment in 6 months."
   B. "Based on the location, concern for visual involvement, and risk for infection secondary to ulceration, we should administer corticosteroid treatment at this time."
   C. "Based on the location and potential interference with vision, I recommend surgical excision."

   ANSWER: B. *As previously stated, the cases in which the location of the hemangioma and its expected growth will compromise vital organ function, systemic corticosteroids are recommended as a first-line treatment agent (Verklan & Walden, 2015). Information should be shared in a manner that is understood by both parents, with opportunity for clarifying questions and follow-up to ensure knowledge transfer has occurred.*

CONCLUSIONS

A comprehensive, systematic head-to-toe physical examination of the neonate is essential. The ability to differentiate benign from infectious or other lesions, ensures the accurate, effective identification of lesions and an appropriate diagnosis. The utilization of proper descriptive terminology facilitates accurate communication of findings with interprofessional team members, including pediatric dermatology subspecialists. This aids in the initiation of a timely management and treatment regimen, as well as consistent counseling and education for the family unit.

ACKNOWLEDGMENTS

The authors would like to thank their husbands, Eric, Jason, and Victor, and children, Mya, Ryan, Piper, Anika, Luke, William, and Andre, for their patience and understanding during the creation of this chapter.

REFERENCES

Albanna, E. A., El-Iatif, R. S., Sharaf, H. A., Gohar, M. K., & Ibrahim, B. M. (2013). Diagnosis of congenital cytomegalovirus infection in high risk neonates. *Mediterranean Journal of Hematology and Infectious Diseases, 5*(1), e2013049. doi:10.4084/MJHID.2013.049

Alikhan, A., Ibrahimi, O. A., & Eisen, D. B. (2012). Congenital melanocytic nevi: Where are we now? Part I. Clinical presentation, epidemiology, pathogenesis, histology, malignant transformation, and neurocutaneous melanosis. *Journal of the American Academy of Dermatology, 67*(4), 495.e1–495.e17.

American Academy of Pediatrics (AAP) Committee on Infectious Diseases. (2012). *Red book* (29th ed.). Elk Grove Village, IL: American Academy of Pediatrics.

Ang-Tiu, C. U., & Nicolas, M. E. (2013). Erythema multiforme in a 25-day old neonate. *Pediatric Dermatology, 30*(6), e118–e120. doi:10.1111/j.1525-1470.2012.01873.x

Association of Women's Health, Obstetric and Neonatal Nurses. (2013). *Neonatal skin care* (3rd ed.). Washington, DC: Author.

Aydin, M., Hakan, N., Zenciroglu, A. & Demirol, H. A. (2013). A rare location of sucking blister in newborn: The lips. *European Journal of Pediatrics, 172,* 1423–1424. doi:10.1007/s00431-013-2055-y

Babu, T. A., & Sharmila, V. (2012). Congenital miliaria crystalline in a term neonate born to a mother with chorioamnionitis. *Pediatric Dermatology, 29*(3), 306–307. doi:10.1111/j.1525-1470.2011.01435.x

Bauland, C. G., van Steensel, M. A., Steijlen, P. M., Reiu, P. N., & Spauwen, P. H. (2006). The pathogenesis of hemangiomas: A review. *Plastic and Reconstructive Surgery, 117,* 29e–35e. doi:10.1097/01.prs.0000197134.72984.cb

Beeram, M., Olvera, R., Krauss, D., Loughran, C., & Petty, M. (2006). Effects of topical emollient therapy on infants at or less than 27 weeks' gestation. *Journal of the National Medical Association, 98*(2), 261–264.

Berardi, A., Lugli, L., Rossi, C., Maria, C. L., Guidotti, I., Gallo, C., & Ferrari, F. (2011). Neonatal herpes simplex virus. *Journal of Maternal–Fetal & Neonatal Medicine, 24*(5), 88–90. doi:10.3109/14767058.2011.607560

Berk, D., & Bayliss, S. J. (2008). Milia: A review and classification. *Journal of the American Academy of Dermatology, 59*(6), 1050–1062. doi:10.1016/j.jaad.2008.07.034

Bhandari, V., Brodsky, N., & Porat, R. (2005). Improved outcome of extremely low birth weight infants with Tegaderm application to skin. *Journal of Perinatology, 25*(4), 276–281. doi:10.1038/sj.jp.7211260

Bhardwaj, A., Sharma, P., & Sharma, A. (2011). Neonatal varicella: A case report. *Australasian Medical Journal, 4*(6), 291–293. doi:10.4066/AMJ.2011.682

Bhatia, J. (2006). Fluid and electrolyte management in the very low birth weight neonate. *Journal of Perinatology, 26*(Suppl. 1), S19–S21. doi:10.1038/sj.jp.7211466

Bissinger, R. L., & Annibale, D. J. (2010). Thermoregulation in very low-birthweight infants during the golden hour: Results and implications. *Advances in Neonatal Care, 10*(5), 230–238. doi:10.1097/ANC.0b013e3181f0ae63

Blackburn, S. T. (2013). *Maternal, fetal & neonatal physiology: A clinical perspective.* (4th ed.). Maryland Heights, MO: Elsevier Saunders.

Broom, M. A., & Smith, S. L. (2013). Late presentation of neonatal omphalitis following dry cord care. *Clinical Pediatrics, 52*(7), 675–677. doi:10.1177/0009922812446745

Caviness, A. C. (2013). Neonatal herpes simplex virus infection. *Clinical Pediatric Emergency Medicine, 14*(2), 135–145. doi:10.1016/j.cpem.2013.04.002

Centers for Disease Control and Prevention. (2016). Chickenpox (Varicella): People at high risk for complications. Retrieved from http://www.cdc.gov/chickenpox/hcp/high-risk.html

Cho, Y. J., Huh, S. Y., Hong, J. S., Jung, J. Y., & Suh, D. H. (2011). Neonatal erythema multiforme: A case report. *Annals of Dermatology, 23*(3), 382–385. doi:10.5021/ad.2011.23.3.382

Cieza-Diaz, D. E., Campos-Dominguez, M., Santos-Sebastian, M. M., Martinez, M., Ceballos-Rodriguez, M., Navarro-Gomez, M. L., & Suarez-Fernandez, R. (2013). Erythema multiforme in a newborn associated with acute acquired cytomegalovirus infection. *Pediatric Dermatology, 30*(6), e161–e163. doi:10.1111/j.1525-1470.2012.01755.x

Clifton, N. J., Ross, S. K., Gupta, B., & Gibbin, K. P. (2007). Hygroma or teratoma? *International Journal of Pediatric Otorhinolaryngology, 2*(1), 61–64. doi:10.1016/j.pedex.2006.12.009

Dasgupta, R. (2014). Surgical management of vascular anomalies. *Current Otorhinolaryngology Reports, 2*, 285–291. doi:10.1077/s40136-014-0066-5

Eichenfield, L., Frieden, E., Zaenglein, A. L, & Mathes, E. F. (2015). *Neonatal and infant dermatology* (3rd ed.). Philadelphia, PA: Elsevier Saunders.

Fine, J. D. (2010). Inherited epidermolysis bullosa. *Orphanet Journal of Rare Diseases, 5*, 12. doi:10.1186/1750-1172-5-12

Fraser, N., Davies, W., & Cusack, J. (2006). Neonatal omphalitis: A review of its serious complications. *Acta Pediatrica, 95*, 519–522. doi:10.1080/08035250600640422

Gallagher, P. G., Mahoney, M. J., & Gosche, J. R. (1999). Cystic hygroma in the fetus and newborn. *Seminars in Perinatology, 23*(4), 341–356. doi:10.1016/S0146-0005(99)80042-1

Gaylord, M. S., Wright, K., Lorch, V., Lorch, E., & Walker, E. (2001). Improved fluid management utilizing humidified incubators in extremely low birth weight infants. *Journal of Perinatology, 21*(7), 438–443. doi:10.1038/sj.jp.7210561

Gleason, C. A., & Devaskar, S. U. (2012). *Avery's diseases of the newborn* (9th ed.). Philadelphia, PA: Elsevier Saunders.

Henbest, D. M., & Steele, R. W. (2013). Periumbilical erythema in a neonate. *Clinical Pediatrics, 52*(4), 374–377. doi:10.1177/0009922813479167

Hoath, S. B., & Narendran, V. (2001). Development of the epidermal barrier. *Neoreviews, 2*(12), e269–e281.

Iljin, A., Siewiera, I., & Kruk-Jeromin, J. (2010). Port wine stains. *Advances in Dermatology and Allergology, 27*, 460–466.

Kadam, S., Tagare, A., Deodhar, J. Tawade, Y., & Pandit, A. (2009). Staphylococcal scalded skin syndrome in a neonate. *Indian Journal of Pediatrics, 76*, 1074.

Kim, S. M., Lee, E. Y., Chen, J., & Ringer, S. A. (2010). Improved care and growth outcomes by using hybrid humidified incubators in very preterm infants. *Pediatrics, 125*(1), e137–e145. doi:10.1542/peds.2008-2997

Klunk, C., Domingues, E., & Wiss, K. (2014). An update on diaper dermatitis. *Clinics in Dermatology, 32*, 477–487. doi:10.1016/j.clindermatol.2014/02.003

Knobel, R. B., Wimmer, J. E., & Holbert, D. (2005). Heat loss prevention for preterm infants in the delivery room. *Journal of Perinatology, 25*(5), 304–308. doi:10.1038/sj.jp.7211289

Kumar, N., Kohli, M., Pandey, S., & Tulsi, S. P. S. (2010). Cystic hygroma. *National Journal of Maxillofacial Surgery, 1*(1), 81–85. doi:10.4103/0975-5950.69152

Lamont, R. F., Sobel, J. D., Carrington, D., Mazaki-Tovi, S., Kusanovic, J. P., Vaisbuch, E., & Romero, R. (2011). Varicella-zoster virus (chickenpox) infection in pregnancy. *International Journal of Obstetrics and Gynecology, 118*, 1155–1162. doi:10.1111/j.1471-0528.2011.02983.x

Larson, A. A., & Dinulos, J. G. (2005). Cutaneous bacterial infections in the newborn. *Current Opinion in Pediatrics, 17*(4), 481–485. doi:10.1097/01.mop.0000171321.68806.bd

Laude, T. A. (1995). Approach to dermatologic disorders in black children. *Seminars in Dermatology, 14*(1),15–20.

Lebwohl, M. (2014). *Treatment of skin disease: Comprehensive therapeutic strategies* (4th ed.). Elsevier Saunders.

Libow, L. F., & Reimann, J. G. (1998). Symmetrical erosions in a neonate: A case of neonatal sucking blisters. *Cutis, 62*(1), 16–17.

Lund, C. H., & Keller, J. M. (2007). Integumentary system. In C. Kenner & J. W. Lott (Eds.), *Comprehensive neonatal care: An interdisciplinary approach* (4th ed., pp. 65–91). St. Louis, MO: Saunders Elsevier.

Mancini, A. J., Sookdeo-Drost, S., Madison, K., Smoller, B. R., & Lane, A. T. (1994). Semipermeable dressings improve epidermal barrier function in premature infants. *Pediatric Research, 36*(3), 306–314. doi:10.1203/00006450-199409000-00007

Martin, R., Fanaroff, A. A., & Walsh, M. C. (2015). *Fanaroff and Martin's neonatal-perinatal medicine: Diseases of the fetus and infant* (10th ed.). Philadelphia, PA: Saunders.

Mermod, T., El Ezzi, O., Raffoul, W., Erba, P., & de Buys Roessingh, A. (2015). Assessment of the role of LASER-Doppler in the treatment of port wine stains in infants. *Journal of Pediatric Surgery, 50*(8), 1388–1392. doi:10.1016/j.jpedsurg.2014.12.022

Monteagudo, B., Labandeira, J., Cabanillas, M., Acevedo, A., & Toribio, J. (2012). Prospective study of erythema toxicum neonatorum: Epidemiology and predisposing factors. *Pediatric Dermatology, 29*(2), 166–168. doi:10.1111/j.1525-1470.2011.01.536.x

National Institute of Health. (2013). *Questions and answers about epidermolysis bullosa* (DHHS Publication No. 13-7038). Washington, DC: U.S. Government Printing Office.

O'Conner, N., & McLaughlin, M. (2008). Newborn skin: Part 1. Common rashes. *American Family Physician, 77*(1), 47–52.

Perman, M. J., Castelo-Soccio, L., & Jen, M. (2012). Differential diagnosis of infantile hemangiomas. *Pediatric Annals, 41*(8), 1–7. doi:10.3928/00904481-20120727-09

Poindexter, G. B., Burkhart, C. N., & Morrell, D. S. (2009). Therapies for pediatric soberrheic dermatitis. *Pediatric Annals, 38*(6), 333–338. doi:10.3928/00904481-20090521-01

Reilly, S. D., & Faye-Peterson, O. M. (2008). Chorioamnionitis and funisitis: Their implications for the neonate. *Neoreviews, 9*(9), e411–e417.

Roilides, E. (2011). Invasive candidiasis in neonates and children. *Early Human Development, 87*S, S75–S76. doi:10.1016/j.earlhumdev.2011.01.017

Satti, K. F., Ali, S. A., & Weitkamp, J. H. (2010). Congenital infections, part 2: Parvovirus, listeria, tuberculosis, syphilis, and varicella. *Neoreviews, 11*(12), e681–e695.

Schleiss, M. R. (2013). Cytomegalovirus in the neonate: Immune correlates of infection and protection. *Clinical and Developmental Immunology, 2013*, 1–14. doi:10.1155/2013/501801

Snow, T. (2005). Mongolian spots in the newborn: Do they mean anything? *Neonatal Network, 24*(1), 31–33.

Stanley, J. R., & Amagai, M. (2006). Pemphigus, bullous impetigo, and the staphylococcal scalded-skin syndrome. *New England Journal of Medicine, 355*(17), 1800–1810. doi:10.1056/NEJMra061111

Steinhorn, R. H. (2008). Evaluation and management of the cyanotic neonate. *Clinical Pediatric Emergency Medicine, 9*(3), 169–175. doi:10.1016/j.cpem.2008.06.006

Tappero, E., & Honeyfield, M. (2014). *Physical assessment of the newborn: A comprehensive approach to the art of physical examination* (5th ed.). Petaluma, CA: NICU Ink.

Tekin, M., Bodurtha, J. N., & Riccardi, V. M. (2001). Café au lait spots: The pediatrician's perspective. *Pediatrics in Review, 22*(3), 82–90.

Tian, C., Ali, S. A., & Weitkamp, J. H. (2010). Congenital infections, part 1: Cytomegalovirus, toxoplasma, rubella, and herpes simplex. *Neoreviews, 11*(8), e436–e446.

Tita, A. T., & Andrews, W. W. (2010). Diagnosis and management of clinical chorioamnionitis. *Clinics in Perinatology, 37*(2), 339–354. doi:10.1016/j.clp.2010.02.003

Tollin, M., Bergsson, G., Kai-Larson, Y., Lengqvist, J., Sjovall, J., Griffiths, W., . . . Agerberth, B. (2005). Vernix caseosa as a multi-component defence system based on polypeptides, lipids and their interactions. *Cellular and Molecular Life Sciences, 62*(19), 2390–2399. doi:10.1007/s00018-005-5260-7

Tripathi, N., Watt, K., & Benjamin, D. K. (2012). Treatment and prophylaxis of invasive candidiasis. *Seminars in Perinatology, 36*(6), 416–423. doi:10.1053/j.semperi.2012.06.003

Turkoglu, Z., Kuru, B. C., Kavala, M., & Turkoglu, O. (2010). Angel's kiss in three generations. *Indian Journal of Dermatology, Venereology and Leprology. 76*(5), 592. doi:10.4103/0378-6323.69098

Verklan, M. T., & Walden, M. (2015). *Core curriculum for neonatal intensive care nursing* (5th ed.). St. Louis, MO: Elsevier Saunders.

Visscher, M. O., Narendran, V., Pickens, W. L., LaRuffa, A. A., Meinzen-Derr, J., Allen, K., & Hoath, S. B. (2005). Vernix caseosa in neonatal adaptation. *Journal of Perinatology, 25*(7), 440–446. doi:10.1038/sj.jp.7211305

Vohra, S., Roberts, R. S., Zhang, B., Janes, M., & Schmidt, B. (2004). Heat loss prevention (HeLP) in the delivery room: A randomized controlled trial of polyethylene occlusive skin wrapping in very preterm infants. *Journal of Pediatrics, 145*(6), 750–753. doi:10.1016/j.jpeds.2004.07.036

Wine, E., Ballin, A., & Dalal, I. (2005). Infantile erythema multiforme following hepatitis B vaccine. *Acta Paediatrica, 95,* 890–891. doi:10.1080/08035250500462109

Wolf, R., Wolf, D., Tuzun, B., & Tuzun, Y. (2000). Diaper dermatitis. *Clinics in Dermatology, 18,* 657–660.

Yasmeen, A., & Ibhanesebhor, S. E. (2014). Severe congenital herpes simplex virus infection. *Archives of Disease in Childhood—Fetal and Neonatal Edition, 99,* F153–F157. doi:10.1136/archdischild-2013-304682

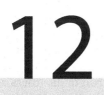

Fluids, Electrolytes, and Nutrition Cases

Patricia J. Johnson

Chapter Objectives

1. Interpret laboratory findings reflecting fluid and electrolyte homeostasis in the neonate
2. Identify the underlying deficiencies of fluid and electrolyte homeostasis that increase with decreasing gestational age
3. Calculate fluid and calorie intake in the neonate
4. Assess fluid and calorie intake for adequacy or deficiencies in the neonate
5. List the etiologies or differential diagnoses for common electrolyte imbalances in the neonate
6. List the alterations in fluid needs for neonates with various conditions and diseases
7. Define *maintenance fluid* and electrolyte needs by gestational and postnatal age
8. Apply understanding of fluid and electrolyte needs in the neonate with fluid and/or electrolyte imbalance to calculations of supplemental fluid and electrolyte orders
9. Compare and contrast parenteral and enteral sources that provide adequate nutrition for the neonate based on gestational and postnatal age
10. Define the essential components in parenteral nutrition (PN) for the neonate
11. Demonstrate the ability to order PN
12. Recognize complications of PN infusions

This chapter reviews principles and methods of fluid, electrolyte, and nutrition (FEN) management in the neonate. It addresses special needs of neonates with complex fluid and electrolyte requirements, including premature newborns, low-birth-weight (LBW) newborns, infants with unique fluid and electrolyte alterations, and infants with respiratory and cardiovascular abnormalities affecting fluid and electrolyte homeostasis. The chapter reviews FEN management of neonates with primary fluid and electrolyte disorders as apparent from acid–base imbalances, mineral imbalances, and metabolic disorders. It reviews the common fluid shifts with their underlying complications and discusses complications of inadequate nutrition.

ASSESSMENT OF FLUID AND ELECTROLYTE STATUS IN THE NEWBORN

Fluid and electrolyte assessment and management are an essential part in the comprehensive management of the newborn. Because of the physiologic immaturity of the newborn, the internal compartments are especially susceptible to acute and chronic alterations in fluid and electrolyte stability. As with other systems, the degree of immaturity increases potential for fluid and electrolyte alterations with decreasing gestation and postnatal age. The less mature the infant, the greater the total body, especially extracellular water content. For example, a 23-week premature infant has 90% water content with 60% extracellular fluid and 30% intracellular fluid. Extracellular fluid is more accessible to loss. The term newborn has 75% water content with 40% extracellular fluid (Ambalavanan, 2014).

Assessment of fluid and electrolyte needs should be individualized in the newborn and will be dependent on indicators of insensible and sensible water loss. The sensible losses, including urine, stool, gastric drainage, and other compartment fluid losses, such as central nervous system, peritoneal, and pleural losses, can be measured and are easily quantified. Insensible losses are not easily measured (Ambalavanan, 2014). Most insensible losses are from the skin through evaporation (two thirds) or the respiratory system (one third). Losses from the respiratory system can be virtually eliminated if heated humidity is used with the delivery of gases or ventilation. Skin losses are gestation dependent and relative to the maturity of the skin. Insensible water loss from skin can be minimized by providing a heated, humidified environment, especially for infants less than 1,250 g. The extremely low-birth-weight infant (ELBW) can lose in excess of 150 mL/kg/d from insensible water loss, whereas the term newborn is at risk for losing approximately 30 to 40 mL/kg/d from insensible losses. The difference is caused by characteristic maturation, including keratinization of the skin, increased water content, and increased ratio of surface area to mass (Dell, 2015; Profit, 2015).

Clinical indicators of hydration status in the newborn include heart rate, blood pressure, skin turgor, capillary refill, oral mucosal moisture, and anterior fontanel fullness or depression (Dell, 2015). Careful assessment of fluid intake and output is essential in the fluid management of newborns with the expectation that intake should exceed output by 50% to 67%. Weight is a useful measure of water weight in the first week of life (Ambalavanan, 2014). Weight losses of 5% to 15% are expected in the newborn as a result of total body losses but excess weight loss is an indication that the fluid intake is not adequate and newborns, especially premature newborns, are at increased risk of developing dehydration (Dell, 2015). Fluid needs must be addressed daily and fluid intake adjusted daily in the sick and premature newborn to minimize iatrogenic fluid alterations, especially dehydration. In addition, early weight gain may indicate inadequate output in infants with cardiorespiratory or neurologic pathology and those infants are at risk of fluid overload with daily weight being a useful gross indicator of total body water in the first week of life. Excessive fluid overload in the newborn may present with congestive heart failure and increased respiratory distress, especially tachypnea and tachycardia.

Serum electrolytes are essential in evaluating fluid balance when physical signs of fluid imbalance are present in the newborn. Alterations in sodium are especially important given that sodium is the primary cation in extracellular fluid. Serum sodium reflects sodium concentration and not total body sodium levels, which are related to total body volume as well as sodium concentration (Dell, 2015). Elevated sodium, hypernatremia, is often seen in LBW infants with inadequate volume intake. Low serum sodium, hyponatremia, may be seen in newborns who are retaining fluid or receiving excess free water without electrolytes. Other electrolyte abnormalities may be seen in fluid alterations, including elevated chloride, or hyperchloremia. Chloride is the most plentiful anion in extracellular fluid and chloride concentrations may increase with intravascular volume depletion or decrease to hypochloremia with intravascular hypervolemia. Elevations in blood urea nitrogen (BUN) levels may also be seen with various states of intravascular hypovolemia or dehydration (Dell, 2015). Infants with midline defects and exposed organs may need excessive fluid replacement for excess losses until closure or temporary barriers are established to prevent excess heat and fluid losses.

FLUID AND ELECTROLYTE MANAGEMENT GOALS

Total fluid requirements vary by postnatal age and range between 60 mL/kg/d and 200 mL/kg/d. In general, infants on parenteral fluid intake require 80 to 150 mL/kg/d starting on the first day at 80 mL/kg/d and advancing to 150 mL/kg/d by 5 to 6 days of age. All newborns, and especially very low-birth-weight (VLBW) infants, have a loss of extracellular fluid in the first 5 to 7 days associated with a 10% to 15% weight loss. When there is extracellular fluid (ECF) fluid loss, neonates also lose sodium (Oh, 2012).

Constitutional or disease-related alterations in fluid balance must be considered when managing fluids in the newborn. If the newborn is extremely immature and has excess insensible losses, fluid requirements will need to be evaluated every 8 to 12 hours and fluid intake appropriately adjusted. Infants with respiratory distress and inadequate output require less fluid intake until they have natural diuresis. Newborns with hydrops may need to have an estimated dry weight for fluid management given they have added compartment fluid overload that contributes erroneously to their measured weight. Newborns with risk for or with confirmed cardiac lesions may require fluid restriction, as will infants with underlying renal disease. Infants with hypoxic ischemic encephalopathy (HIE) or perinatal asphyxia often develop syndrome of inappropriate antidiuretic hormone (SIADH) secretion and require fluids restricted to insensible water loss plus urine output to minimize cerebral edema. Insensible water loss in the term newborn is 30 mL/kg/d (Dell, 2015).

Once the infant is growing, water must be considered an essential nutrient and adequate fluid intake must be maintained to support growth and promote excretion of metabolic by-products of growth in urine (see Table 12.1 for fluids per kilogram per day based on age).

Calculating fluids in the newborn (weight in kilograms to be used is birth weight unless weight above birth weight is due to growth):

$$\frac{\text{Weight} \times \text{desired mL/kg/d}}{24 \text{ hr}} = \text{milliliters (mL) per hour for infusion}$$

Fluid balance and needs should be evaluated daily and more frequently if there is concern for excess loss or unexpected gain.

Evaluate urine output:

$$\frac{\text{Urine (mL) for a period of time (usually 24 hr)/kg}}{\text{Total number of hours (24 hr)}} = \text{mL/kg/hr (Table 12.2)}.$$

Table 12.1 Maintenance Fluids per Kilogram per Day Based on Day of Life

Weight (g)	Range of H_2O Loss (mL)	Day 1–2	Day 3–7	Day 8–30
<750	100–200	100–200+	150–200+	120–180
750–1,000	60–70	80–150	100–150	120–180
1001–1,500	30–65	60–100	80–150	120–180
>1,500	15–30	60–80	100–150	120–180

Source: Dell (2015).

Table 12.2 Expected Urine Output

Age	UOP (mL/kg/hr)
First 24 hours	0.7–2.5
Day 2–3	1.5–6
Average after day 3	2–4
Oliguria	<1
Diuresis	>6

UOP, urine output.

Sources: Bidiwala, Lorenz, and Kleinman (1988), Devarajan (2014).

COMMON ELECTROLYTE ABNORMALITIES

Electrolyte management in the newborn is as important as fluid management and directly related to fluid management. Medications administered to both mother and newborn increase the risk for renal injury and impaired renal development and, therefore, impaired renal function in the first few weeks (Girardi et al., 2015). Electrolyte imbalance is a common risk for high-risk and premature newborns, especially VLBW and ELBW newborns. Hyponatremia is the most common electrolyte abnormality in the premature newborn because of developmental renal sodium wasting. ELBW and VLBW infants will often exhibit hypernatremia in the first few days of life; this is most likely caused by extracellular water loss exceeding sodium loss. Once the total body water loss is partially or completely compensated, the total body sodium loss is difficult to resolve acutely, and may become a chronic issue. *Hypernatremia* is defined as serum sodium (Na^+) greater than 150 mEq/L and *hyponatremia* is serum sodium (Na^+) less than 130 mEq/kg. Initial electrolytes obtained at 12 to 24 hours of life likely reflect maternal electrolytes, but with adequate urine output, after 24 hours the electrolytes will reflect the newborn's true levels and should be addressed early in the management plan with appropriate supplementation (Ambalavanan, 2014; Dell, 2015).

Potassium (K^+) abnormalities are likely caused by inadequate renal function and less likely the result of minor fluid management alterations. Obviously, alterations in primary renal function will result in elevated potassium levels, but for infants who are voiding with elevated K^+, one must consider the source of the specimen (heel stick or venipuncture). Heel-stick levels will often yield elevated K^+ levels and may need to be rechecked by venipuncture. In addition, whole-blood specimens obtained with blood gases may have alterations that warrant verification to optimize treatment accuracy. Low K^+ levels are unlikely with adequate maintenance of K^+ in intravenous (IV) or enteral intake unless there is a metabolic/endocrine abnormality. Infants receiving diuretic therapy may develop hypokalemia despite routine K+ supplement because of renal losses. Elevated K^+ may be seen in VLBW and ELBW infants in the first 24 hours as a result of nonoliguric hyperkalemia associated with a K^+ ion shift from intracellular to extracellular fluid. Extensive tissue damage may be another cause of elevated K^+ as seen with severe bruising, shock, ischemia, and renal injury. Finally, acid–base alterations may result in alterations in serum K+ with acidosis shifting K+ to extracellular fluid causing hyperkalemia, and alkalosis reducing K+ in extracellular fluid spaces causing hypokalemia (Bochenhour & Zieg, 2004; Nash, 2007). *Hypokalemia* is defined as potassium less than 3 mEq/L and *hyperkalemia* is potassium greater than 6 mEq/L (Ambalavanan, 2014). The goal of treatment for K+ alterations is to redistribute the K+ if the alterations are associated with myocardial dysfunction.

Acid–base balance is important in the newborn. Chloride levels relate to metabolic acid load and serum CO_2 levels relate to base levels. Newborns, especially VLBW and ELBW newborns, tend to excrete bicarbonate and have deficient renal production of bicarbonate, rendering them prone to metabolic acidosis. In addition, high-risk and preterm newborns often present with respiratory impairment and are unable to buffer metabolic acid loads. Managing the acid–base balance is important and often requires daily adjustment of the chloride-to-acetate ratio in salt infusions. In the first week, newborns on parenteral fluids may require maximum acetate. After about 1 week, excess acetate will increase the carbon dioxide that needs to be excreted to prevent progressive acidosis. The chloride-to-acetate ratio is individualized and may need daily titrating up or down to provide the ideal intake of chloride to minimize acid–base alterations. It is important to consider all sources of chloride and the potential acid load from the excess hydrogen ion produced with metabolism of the cationic amino acids (AAs) in PN (Richards, Drayton, Jenkins, & Peters, 1993; Thomas & Udall, 2007). Infants with metabolic acidosis should receive acetate primarily in PN and flush solutions. Infants with compensated respiratory acidosis should receive chloride primarily in PN and flush solutions. Infants with chronic lung disease may require an oral supplement with 1 to 2 mEq/kg/d of sodium chloride because of their hypercarbia and compensated respiratory acidosis, which leads to low chloride levels and associated low sodium levels, which will impede growth. These newborns will require follow-up of their serum electrolytes at least weekly. Similarly, infants on chronic diuretic therapy may have Na, K, Cl, and Ca alterations because of excess urinary losses and may need an oral supplement and close serum electrolyte monitoring (Dell, 2015). Sodium bicarbonate replacement is seldom required because there is no bicarbonate deficit, and attempting to correct an acid–base imbalance with sodium bicarbonate will merely require excessive ventilation (Johnson, 2011).

Additional electrolytes that need specific attention include calcium, phosphorus, and magnesium. Calcium is commonly deficient in the preterm newborn because the transfer of calcium across the placenta occurs in the last 4 to 6 weeks of pregnancy. Serum phosphorus levels are affected by gestational age and dependent on appropriate calcium phosphorus ratio in parenteral and enteral intake. In addition, magnesium levels and need for magnesium supplementation in PN also require specific attention. Some newborns receive excess magnesium when mothers are treated for seizure prophylaxis with hypertensive disorders and others for neuroprotection. Magnesium is excreted in the urine and, after 3 days of urine output, newborns with maternal exposure of magnesium should receive magnesium maintenance (Ambalavanan, 2014; see Table 12.3 for electrolyte requirements in the newborn).

Newborns who are receiving primarily enteral intake with breast milk or formula require minimal, if any, electrolyte supplementation in additional IV fluids. However, the more IV fluids needed to supplement feedings, the more electrolytes need to be added to IV fluids to meet the daily requirements not received in the enteral intake for the day. Calculate the daily requirement of electrolytes and the total fluids required for the day. Add the electrolytes into the volume of IV solution that would be required if the infant were not receiving any enteral intake. For example, if the infant receives 50% enteral intake, and is receiving 50% of his or her electrolyte requirements orally, then the infant will receive 50% of his or her electrolyte requirements in the IV fluids and the other 50% in the enteral intake. If the full electrolytes are ordered in only 50% of the daily fluids because the infant is expected to take 50% of his or her total fluids from enteral feedings, the parenteral solution will deliver

Table 12.3 **Electrolyte Needs in the Newborn**

Electrolyte	Initial	Prediuretic	Postdiuretic	Low serum level (mEq/L)	High serum level (mEq/L)
Sodium	0–1 mEq/kg/d	2–3 mEq/kg/d	3–5 mEq/kg/d	< 130	> 150
Potassium	None	1–2 mEq/kg/d	2–3 mEq/kg/d	< 3	> 6.5
Chloride	0%–30%	30%–50%	70%–100%	< 98	> 110
Calcium	3 mEq/kg/d	3 mEq/kg/d	2–2.5 mEq/kg/d	< 7	> 11
Phosphorus	50% of Ca	50% of Ca	50% of Ca	< 4	> 7
Magnesium	0	0.3 mEq/k/d	0.4–0.5	< 1	> 3

Source: Johnson (2014b).

excess electrolytes in a concentrated volume of fluid. If the infant suddenly does not tolerate the feedings, the residual total parenteral nutrition (TPN) will not be an adequate volume for the remainder of the daily infusion; it will not provide adequate free water.

Example of Calculating IV Electrolytes for Total Parenteral Nutrition (TPN)		
Birth weight*: 1,733 g	Day 3 weight 1,610 g	Serum: Na 145, K 4.9, Cl 112, CO_2 18, Ca 7.8

*Use birth weight for 7 days until growth weight is greater than birth weight. Normal newborns are not expected to lose weight and weight generally is not greater than birth weight before 7 days.

Weight in kg x electrolyte in mEq/k/d (or mg/k/d or mmol/k/d)
Na 2 mEq/kg/d $1.733 \times 2 = 3.466$ mEq (OK to order 3.5 mEq/kg/d)
K 1.5 mEq/kg/d $1.733 \times 1.5 = 2.5995$ or 2.6 mEq/kg/d
Cl::Acetate   0::100
Ca   3 mEq or 300 mg/kg/d
P   1.5 mmol/kg/d
Mg   0.25 or 0.3 mEq/k/d

Fluid calculations:

Enteral feeds by day 3 are likely 40–50 mL/kg/d = or 8–10 mL every 3 hours plus intravenous fluids (IVF) with TPN and 20% intralipids (IL)

Order total IVF at full fluid needs for the day: approximately 120 mL/kg/d = 1.733×120 mL/kg/d = 208 mL/24 hr = 8.7 mL/hr

This total fluid order would include IV and tolerated feedings; therefore, if tolerating 9 mL every 3 hours, then the IV would infuse at 5.7 mL/hr (8.7–3 mL = 5.7 mL).

NUTRITIONAL REQUIREMENTS OF THE NEWBORN

The goal of nutrition in the newborn is to approximate the age-appropriate continuum of composition (lean body mass with age appropriate accretion) and rate of weight gain attained in utero. This goal is possible in the normal-term breastfed newborn after about 1 week, but is merely an ambitious target in the preterm and sick newborn requiring PN with or without enteral intake. The required nutrition for growth is dependent on the infant's ability to tolerate the composition and rate of parenteral and enteral intake, which is often limited by the infant's complicating disease process or degree of immaturity (Poindexter & Ehrenkranz, 2015). Nutritional needs are optimally met by providing enteral feedings but it may take days or weeks before a compromised newborn can tolerate the enteral intake needed for weight gain and growth. Therefore, it is important to understand the administration of PN that will be needed to minimize the risk of postnatal growth failure until full enteral feedings can be achieved.

Energy needs are met with the adequate administration of carbohydrates and fat. Carbohydrates provide a quick energy source, whereas fat requires energy and time to metabolize but provides more energy gram for gram compared to carbohydrates. Both are important in a balanced diet. Protein is a building block and essential for growth. Protein can be metabolized to an energy source but that is not the goal. The goal is to provide adequate energy to support the base functions and energy needs while providing adequate protein for growth. Carbohydrates, fat, and protein are the three macronutrients in enteral and PN and water can be considered the fourth important nutrient required to sustain functions and support growth. Micronutrients required include electrolytes, trace elements, and vitamins (Johnson, 2014b).

PN with AA hydrolysate (a 10% TrophAmine solution) needs to be individualized in the newborn and is initiated early on the first day of life to minimize the development of negative nitrogen balance, which may be difficult to reverse even after 1 or 2 days of inadequate protein intake in the ELBW and LBW infant. AA hydrolysate is ordered in grams per kilogram per day starting with 3 g/kg/d and advancing to the maximum amount of 3.5 g/kg/d in the term newborn and 4 g/kg/d in the preterm newborn (Johnson, 2014). Most "starter" PN has 6.25% AA and, if administered at 2 mL/kg/hr, will provide 3 g/kg/d. Newborns generally tolerate advancing AA to the maximum amount by the second day of life (Poindexter & Ehrenkranz, 2015). Including additional cysteine in the PN may improve glutathione synthesis and does augment the solubility of calcium and phosphorus but may increase metabolic acidosis and is often on the drug shortage list (Johnson, 2012; Schanler, 2015). In addition to optimal protein infusion, energy needs must be met with carbohydrates and fat infusion. Carbohydrate infusion is provided with 5% to 15% dextrose to provide 3 to 12 mg/kg/min of glucose. Glucose is utilized at a rate of 6 to 8 mg/kg/min in the preterm newborn and 3 to 5 mg/kg/min in the term newborn (Lucas, Morley, & Cole, 1998). Calculating the glucose infusion rate (GIR) is important in the newborn. Chowning and Adamkin (2015) have published a table to allow quick calculation of GIR. Otherwise, the formula is:

$$GIR = [IV \text{ rate (mL/hr)} \times \text{dextrose (g/dL)}] \div [\text{Weight (kg)} \times 6]$$

ELBW and VLBW infants may have glucose intolerance because of ineffective insulin secretion, end organ insulin resistance, decreased glucose intracellular transporters, elevated catecholamines and glucocorticoids, which alter glucose metabolism and limit glucose utilization (Schanler, 2015). Limiting glucose infusion and ensuring adequate protein infusion as well as introduction of enteral stimulus for insulin secretion will usually minimize hyperglycemia, or serum glucose greater than 150 mg/dL, until the infant gradually develops tolerance of glucose infusion. When the infant exhibits hyperglycemia, the fat infusion must also be limited to avoid increased free fatty acid concentrations in plasma, which further decreases peripheral glucose utilization and inhibits the insulin effect. Reduction of GIR is generally preferred to insulin infusions, which may increase the risk of hypoglycemia, reduced protein synthesis, reduced growth, and lead to potential lactic acidosis. The infusion rate of insulin for infants with refractory serum glucose of greater than 200 to 250 mg/dL is 0.01 to 0.1 units/kg/min, which can be added to a second 50-mL bag of TPN. The dose in a 50-mL bag would be:

$$[\text{Weight in kg}] \times 10 = 0.02 \text{ units insulin}/0.1 \text{ mL/hr}$$

This requires frequent glucose monitoring and can usually be avoided by infusing PN with 4% to 5% dextrose until the problem resolves (Johnson, 2014).

Fat is provided as a 20% lipid emulsion, which is required to provide a high-energy source, sparing dietary enteral or parenteral protein for growth and preventing essential fatty acid deficiency (EFAD). EFAD can occur as early as the second day of life in the premature infant in the absence of supplemental essential fatty acids and will manifest as scaly skin lesions, thrombocytopenia, and poor growth within 1 week without essential fatty acid supplement (ElHassan & Kaiser, 2011; Schanler, 2015). Lipid infusions are usually started on the second day of life (after 24 hours) when standard customized PN is infusing. Infants tolerate starting at 1 g/kg/d advancing fairly rapidly to 3 g/kg/d as total fluids are advanced. When enteral feedings are advanced to 80 mL/kg/d, the fat infusion should be reduced 50% and then discontinued when the enteral intake reaches 100 mL/kg/d to maximize the protein infusion in PN. Remember the enteral nutrition has fat; and if breast milk is the enteral intake, the fat content is ideal for the infant. Fat infusions are deducted from the desired total fluids and the daily PN infusion volume is the total fluid minus the fat infusion.

[Total fluids = 150 mL/kg/d] – [Fat at 1–3 g/kg/d (5–15 mL/kg/d)] =
PN 135–145 mL/kg/d, including 4 g/kg/d of AA

Micronutrients are required for adequate PN and they include electrolytes, trace elements, and vitamins. Calcium is the only electrolyte commonly added to "starter" PN on the first day as calcium gluconate at approximately 300 to 350 mg/kg/d or 3 to 3.5 mEq/kg/d and the other electrolytes are added as needed once the infant is losing electrolytes in urine, as evidenced by serum electrolytes. Commonly, the major cations, sodium and potassium, are ordered as ions in mEq/kg/d and the anions, chloride acetate, are ordered as a ratio, often maximizing acetate at 100% initially and gradually increasing chloride to 70% to 100% by 7 to 10 days. The systems that require providers to order the salts result in more complex calculations. Phosphorus is ordered as an ion in mmol/kg/d to provide a calcium-to-phosphorus ratio of approximately 2:1. Phosphorus must be added by day 2 to 3 to minimize the potential of developing hypercalcemia. Magnesium is added as an ion but should be withheld for 2 to 3 days until adequate urine output is established in infants whose mothers received magnesium in labor (Johnson, 2014).

Vitamin supplementation in PN is inadequate for vitamin A, and adequate for vitamins K and E with likely excess amounts of vitamins C and B_2. Fat-soluble vitamins are also found in lipid infusions (Schanler, 2015). Parenteral vitamin preparations are often affected by drug shortages of PN additives in the United States (Johnson, 2012). Trace element preparations for PN in the newborn include zinc, copper, manganese, chromium, and selenium. These parenteral additives are also affected by drug-shortage issues in the United States. Standard trace element preparations are commonly adequate for short-term PN but may be inadequate for infants receiving long-term, greater than 1 month, TPN without enteral nutrition. Copper and manganese are generally withheld in infants with cholestasis, and chromium and selenium are withheld in infants with renal failure. Monitoring trace elements and vitamin levels is recommended at 3 months for infants receiving long-term TPN (Buchman et al., 2009; Johnson, 2014). Iron deficiency is generally addressed when the infant is able to receive an iron supplement orally but can be added to PN as iron dextran in special circumstances.

Enteral feedings should be initiated early to minimize gut atrophy, and advanced slowly using a defined weight-based feeding protocol. There is no one protocol that is better than another but consistency of feeding advancement is recommended to promote tolerance of enteral intake (McCallie et al., 2011). In newborns who are receiving PN+IL+enteral feedings, order the PN+IL as if the infant was on NPO (nothing by mouth) restriction and direct the nurse to deduct one third of the tolerated every-3-hour feeding from the hourly rate of the PN infusion.

For example, if the infant was 1,200 g on 150 mL/kg/d with PN+3 g IL/kg/d and 40 mL/kg/d of enteral feeding, order the following:

PN (150 mL × 1.2 kg) 180 – (3 g × 1.2 kg) 18 mL of IL = 162 mL/d of PN
and tolerated enteral feedings
Therefore, the PN would infuse at (6.8 – 2 mL) = 4.8 mL/hr with IL at 0.75 mL/hr
if the infant tolerates 6 mL every 3 hours of enteral feeding.

If PN is ordered with all the desired adds, including AA/kg/d in the volume less IL *and* less the presumed feeding volume for the day (48 mL), you will have a very concentrated solution that will provide more additive, including protein, and may risk having less PN volume for the 24 hours if the infant does not tolerate the feedings. Order the full volume of TPN as if the infant were NPO and deduct the tolerated feedings after each feeding to maintain the desired total fluids ordered.

ENTERAL FEEDINGS

The nutritional goals of enteral feedings are to provide energy and support growth velocity at a rate that is appropriate for the infant's postnatal and gestational age. In the newborn, desired growth velocity between 7 and 28 days is approximately 15 g/kg/d (Martin et al., 2009). This growth velocity can usually be met by ad lib breastfeeding in the normal term newborn after the mother's milk supply is established and after birth weight is regained at 7 to 10 days of age. The growth-restricted and VLBW newborn will likely have a growth velocity equivalent to or exceeding that of the third trimester in utero weight gain of 14 to 18 g/kg/d (Poindexter & Ehrenkranz, 2015). In both sick and well newborns, the first week after birth is usually not associated with growth because of less than optimal fluid and caloric intake resulting from obvious limits in availability and tolerance. Full enteral intake is often delayed in the infant born prematurely or with problems, and nutritional goals are met by a combination of parenteral and enteral intake as tolerated. Once enteral feedings are tolerated in the neonatal intensive care unit (NICU) infant, volume per feeding; type of feeding, including fortification; and route of feeding must be ordered. Most NICU infants are fed by nipple, gavage, or gastrostomy bolus every 3 hours. Occasionally, infants with feeding intolerance will need slow infusion of feedings or continuous infusion of feedings or alternative feeding compositions if there are single nutrient absorption abnormalities.

Enteral feeding orders need to be individualized but will usually be 150 to 180 mL/kg/d to provide adequate calories for growth at approximately 120 kcal/kg/d. Newborns require more enteral calories than parenteral calories to make up for inadequate absorption and the energy required for digestion. However, enteral feedings are more ideal for growth than parenteral intake. The ideal enteral feeding for all newborns is mother's milk. Mothers should be encouraged to breastfeed or pump to provide adequate milk for their infant unless restricted by obligated separation such as incarceration or continuing restricted drug use. The nutritional adequacy of mother's milk may not be presumed until the infant is taking full-volume feedings but that is also true of infants taking full-volume commercial formulas.

Each NICU infant must be evaluated at least weekly for growth velocity and appropriate consideration should be given to the need to fortify mother's milk, the alternative donor breast milk, or commercial formula. The recommended calculation for growth velocity is (Patel, Engstrom, Meier, Jegier, & Kiura, 2009):

$$[\text{Current weight} - 7 \text{ days past weight} \times 1{,}000] \div$$
$$[\text{Current weight} + 7 \text{ days past weight}/2 \times 7]$$

Adequate protein intake as well as adequate energy intake in the form of fat and carbohydrate must be established to optimize growth. Monitoring BUN and albumin levels may help with assessment of adequate protein. If the BUN level is less than 10, the protein intake may be inadequate. Sources of fortification available include additional protein, and a single-nutrient source of protein is also commercially available. In addition, there are high-protein commercial formulas for premature newborns. Mother's milk has been shown to reduce the incidence of necrotizing enterocolitis (NEC) in the high-risk premature newborn. The risk of NEC or feeding intolerance associated with fortification of breast milk with bovine-based fortifiers is a possibility that may be reduced with the use of a human milk fortifier but with a reduction in nutrition delivery (Parker, Neu, Torrazza, & Li, 2013). The goal for the VLBW infant is to provide 4 g/kg/d of protein, and approximately 80 kcal of energy nutrients per kilogram per day with the addition of added sodium, and a Ca/Phos ratio of 2/1.

The ongoing question when fortifying breast milk or commercial formula for the preterm newborn born at 2 kg or more with a gestation greater than 34 weeks, is how much fortification is needed and how much is too much? This remains a topic of ongoing study (Meier, Patel, Wright, & Engstrom, 2013; Simmer, 2015).

SUMMARY

This chapter has provided an evidence-based basic principle of FEN management in the newborn and especially in the newborn born prematurely and with risk for alterations. Individual considerations have been addressed but specific abnormalities will require more in-depth review of the literature.

Case 12.1

A late preterm 36-week male newborn who has a birth weight of 2,650 g and is breastfeeding only has weight of 2,210 on day 2 of his life.

1. *What weight would you use for calculating fluids?*

   ANSWER: 2,650 g. *Use the birth weight for calculating fluids for the first 7 days and until the weight is more than birth weight due to growth and not just fluid retention.*

Case 12.2

An extremely low-birth-weight (ELBW) 26-week newborn weighed 960 g at birth and is now on day 3 with the following serum lab results: glucose 140 mg/dL; Na 149 mEq/L, K 3.8 mEq/L, Cl 114 mEq/L, CO_2 18 mEq/L, Ca 7.9 mg/dL, blood urea nitrogen 42, creatinine 0.89. The newborn is receiving expressed breast milk of 1.5 mL every 6 hours, total parenteral nutrition (TPN) with D10W, AA 4 g/kg/d, Na 2 mEq/kg/d, K 1.5 mEq/kg/d, 50% Cl and 50% acetate, calcium gluconate of 3 mEq/kg/d, phosphorus of 0.5 mmol/kg/d, zinc, trace elements, and MVI (Multi-Vitamin for Infusion) Pediatric as standard for gestation and age.

1. *What alterations in fluid and electrolytes would you make?*

   ANSWER: Increase K to 2.5 mEq, change Cl to 20% and acetate to 80%, increase Ca to 3.5 mEq/kg/d, and increase Phos to 1.5 mm/kg/d. Increase the total fluids, but there is possibly a need to reduce dextrose to D9W. *The serum K is low at 3.8 mEq/L and the K*

(continued)

Case 12.2 (continued)

can be increased in the TPN to 2.5 mEq/k/d. The serum Cl is elevated at 114 mEq/L and the serum CO_2 is low at 18 mEq/L. Therefore, increasing the acetate to 80% and decreasing the Cl to 20% will add more buffer. The serum Ca is low at 7.9 mg/dL and increasing the Ca gluconate from 3 to 3.5 mEq/k/d improves supplement of Ca. With increase in Ca, the Phos should be increased to 1.5 mmol/k/d to optimize the 2::1 ratio of Ca::P. On day 3 of life, the total fluids can be increased daily; but given the borderline high serum glucose at 140 mg/dL, the dextrose should be reduced to avoid increasing the glucose infusion rate (GIR).

Case 12.3

An oxygen-dependent premature infant, now 43 days old and corrected gestational age of 32 weeks 0/7 days on full feedings of 24 cal/oz donor milk with high-protein human milk fortifier (HP HMF) at 160 mL/kg/d with nutrition labs with Na 130 mEq/L, K 4.5 mEq/L, Cl 93 mEq/L, CO_2 30 mEq/L, Ca 10.4 mg/dL and phosphorus 6.5 mg/dL, Mg 1.4 mg/dL, blood urea nitrogen (BUN) 8, and creatinine 0.3. The infant's "average" weight gain in the past week is 12 g/kg/d.

1. *What macronutrient is likely deficient? Would the infant benefit from an electrolyte supplement?*

   ANSWER: The macronutrient that is likely deficient is protein because donor milk usually has a lower protein content than expressed breast milk. The infant would benefit from an oral NaCl supplement. *Adequate protein and sodium are required for optimal weight gain and growth. The BUN is less than 10 indicating suboptimal protein intake and the serum Na and Cl are low.*

Case 12.4

A 4.2-kg infant with hypoxic ischemic encephalopathy (HIE) and a history of a seizure at 4 hours of age is now 24 hours of age and needs maintenance fluid orders. Urine output has been 0.7 mL/kg/hr over the past 24 hours.

1. *What insensible fluid rate would you order?*

   ANSWER: 4.2 kg × 30 mL/kg/d = 126 mL/d or 5.25 mL/hr. *This newborn with HIE has reduced urine output likely due to inappropriate antidiuretic hormone related fluid retention or renal failure due to hypoxic insult. Therefore, the newborn needs only insensible losses for maintenance hydration = 30 mL/k/d.*

Case 12.5

An infant presents with gastroschisis at birth and requires intravenous fluids prior to and after surgery applies a silo.

1. *Would you order different fluid rate prior to application of the silo versus after application of the silo?*

   ANSWER: Yes, the fluid rate before the silo is applied could be as high as 150 to 200 mL/kg/d but once the silo is placed, the fluid rate can be reduced to standard fluid management for gestation and weight with replacement of any fluid losses from the site of the defect and excessive gastric output. *Insensible loss before the silo is placed is excessive. The silo actually prevents added insensible loss once it is applied and intact.*

Case 12.6

A 4-day-old infant transferred from community hospital for feeding intolerance and possible necrotizing enterocolitis needs orders for total parenteral nutrition (TPN) and intralipids. Birth weight is 1, 610 g and the admission weight is 1,500 g.

1. *If you are planning to order 140 mL/kg/d with TPN and IL at 2 g/kg/d, what TPN rate would you order?*

   ANSWER: $140 \times 1.61 = 225.4 - 16.1$ (IL) $= 209$ mL TPN $= 8.7$ mL/hr

Case 12.7

A 42-day-old, former 26-week preterm infant, now 1,440 g, received 140 mL/kg/d of unfortified breast milk.

1. *What feeding adjustment would you order to maintain optimal growth, if the infant has an adequate amount of mother's milk available?*

   ANSWER: Add high-protein human milk fortifier to increase the protein intake to enhance growth. *Mother's expressed breast milk after 2 to 3 weeks has reduced protein and breast milk is deficient in sodium for premature infants. Both protein and Na are added to high-protein human milk fortifier (HP HMF) and the newborn will need the added components in breast milk to optimize growth.*

REFERENCES

Ambalavanan, N. (2014). Fluid, electrolyte, and nutrition management of the newborn. Retrieved from http://emedicine.medscape.com/article/976386-overview

Bidiwala, K. S., Lorenz, J. M., & Kleinman, L. I. (1988). Renal function correlates of postnatal diuresis in preterm infants. *Pediatrics, 82*(1), 50–58.

Bochenhour, D., & Zieg, J. (2014). Electrolyte disorders. *Clinics in Perinatology, 41,* 575–590. doi:10.1016/k/clp.2014.05.007

Buchman, A. L., Howard, L. J., Guenter, P., Nishikawa, R. A., Compher, C. W., & Tappenden, K. A. (2009). Micronutrients in parenteral nutrition: Too little or too much: The past, present and recommendations for the future. *Gastroenterology, 137,* S1–S6.

Chowning, R., & Adamkin, D. H. (2015). Table to quickly calculate glucose infusion rates in neonates. *Journal of Perinatology, 35,* 463. doi:10.1038/jp.2015.42

Dell, K. M. (2015). Fluid, electrolytes, and acid-base homeostasis. In R. J. Martin, A. A. Fanaroff, & M. C. Walsh (Eds.), *Fanaroff and Martin's neonatal-perinatal medicine: Diseases of the fetus and infant* (10th ed., pp. 613–629). Philadelphia, PA: Saunders.

Devarajan, P. (2014). Oliguria. Retrieved from http://emedicine.medscape.com

ElHassan, N. O., & Kaiser, J. R. (2011). Parenteral nutrition in the neonatal intensive care unit. *Neo-Reviews, 12,* c130–c140.

Girardi, A., Rachi, E., Galleti, S., Poluzzi, E., Faldella, G., Allegaert, K., & De Ponti, F. (2015). Drug-induced renal damage in preterm neonate: State of the art and early detection. *Drug Safety, 38,* 535–551.

Johnson, P. J. (2011). Sodium bicarbonate in the treatment of acute neonatal lactic acidosis: Benefit or harm? *Neonatal Network, 30*(3), 199–205. doi:10.1891/0730-0730-0832

Johnson, P. J. (2012). The ongoing drug shortage problem affecting the NICU. *Neonatal Network, 31*(5), 323–327. doi:10.1891/0730-0832.31.5.323

Johnson, P. J. (2014a). Review of macronutrients in parenteral nutrition for neonatal intensive care population. *Neonatal Network, 33*(1), 29–34. doi:10.1891/0730-832.33.1.29

Johnson, P. J. (2014b). Review of micronutrients in parenteral nutrition for the NICU population. *Neonatal Network, 33*(3), 155–161. doi:10.1891/0730-0832.33.3.155

Lucas, A., Morely, R., & Cole, T. J. (1998). Randomized trial of early diet in preterm babies and later intelligence quotient. *British Medical Journal, 317*(7171), 1481–1487.

Martin, C. R., Brown, Y. F., Ehrenkranz, R. A., O'Shea, T. M., Allred, E. N., Belfort, M. B., . . . Extremely Low Gestational Age Newborns Study Investigators. (2009). Nutritional practices and growth velocity in the first month of life in extremely premature infants. *Pediatrics, 124*(2), 649–657. doi:10.1542/peds.2008-3258

McCallie, K. R., Lee, H. C., Mayer, O., Cohen, R. S., Hintz, S. R., & Rhine, W. D. (2011). Improved outcomes with a standardized feeding protocol for very low birth weight infants. *Journal of Perinatology, 31,* S61–S67. doi:10.1038/jp.2010.185

Meier, P., Patel, A. L., Wright, K., & Engstrom, J. L. (2013). Management of breastfeeding during and after the maternity hospitalization for late preterm infants. *Clinics in Perinatology, 40,* 689–705. doi:10.1016/j.clp.2013.07.014

Nash, P. L. (2007). Potassium and sodium homeostasis in the neonate. *Neonatal Network, 26*(2), 125–128.

Oh, W. (2012). Fluid and electrolyte management of very low birth weight infants. *Pediatrics and Neonatology, 53,* 329–333. doi:10.1016/j.pedneo.2012.08.010

Parker, L. A., Neu, J., Torrazza, R. M., & Li, Y. (2013). Scientifically based strategies for enteral feeding in premature infants. *NeoReviews, 14*(7), e350–e359. Retrieved from http://neoreviews.aappublications.org

Patel, A. L., Engstrom, J. L., Meier, P. P., Jegier, B. J., & Kiura, R. E. (2009). Calculating postnatal growth velocity in very low birth weight (VLBW) premature infants. *Journal of Perinatology, 29*(9), 618–622. doi:10.1038/jp.2009.55

Poindexter, B. B., & Ehrenkranz, R. A. (2015). Nutrient requirements and provision of nutritional support in the premature newborn. In R. J. Martin, A. A. Fanaroff, & M. C. Walsh (Eds.), *Fanaroff and Martin's neonatal-perinatal medicine: Diseases of the fetus and infant* (10th ed., pp. 592–612). Philadelphia, PA: Saunders.

Profit, J. (2015). Fluid and electrolyte therapy in newborns. *UpToDate*. Retrieved from www.upto date.com

Richards, C. E., Drayton, M., Jenkins, H., & Peters, T. J. (1993). Effect of different chloride infusion rates on plasma base excess during neonatal parenteral nutrition. *Acta Pediatrica, 82*(8), 678–682.

Schanler, R. J. (2015). Parenteral nutrition in premature infants. *UpToDate*. Retrieved from www.up todate.com

Simmer, K. (2015). Human milk fortification. In N. D. Embleton, J. Katz, & E. E. Ziegler (Eds.), *Nestle Nutrition Institute Workshop Series: Low-birthweight baby: Born too soon or too small*. (Vol. 81, pp. 111–121). Basel, Switzerland: S. Karger. doi:10.1159/000365808

Thomas, M. P., & Udall, J. N., Jr. (2007). Parenteral fluids and electrolytes. In S. S. Baker, R. D. Baker, & A. M. Davis (Eds.), *Pediatric nutrition support* (pp. 290–298). Sudbury, MA: Jones & Bartlett.

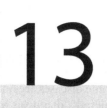

13

Gastrointestinal Cases

Mary Beth Whalen

Chapter Objectives

1. Review embryology of the gastrointestinal (GI) tract and understand how disruptions contribute to disease
2. Review obstructive pathology of the GI system
3. Recognize the classic presenting sign(s) or symptom(s) for (a) duodenal atresia, (b) malrotation and midgut volvulus, (c) necrotizing enterocolitis (NEC), (d) short bowel syndrome (SBS), (e) meconium ileus, and (f) Hirschsprung's disease
4. Apply the radiologic findings in an infant with duodenal atresia to the corresponding physiology
5. Apply the embryology of the GI tract (foregut, midgut, and hindgut) to understand the pathophysiology that makes the midgut volvulus a surgical emergency
6. Discuss the association between meconium ileus and cystic fibrosis (CF)
7. Describe the clinical symptoms associated with NEC
8. Apply the radiographic findings described as the transition zone to the infant with Hirschsprung's disease
9. Differentiate between gastroschisis and omphalocele

This chapter presents some of the more common GI diseases and highlights the importance of recognizing classic symptoms in the infant as they relate to illness. Each of the disturbances is presented initially as a case study. From each of the case studies the learner will be expected to identify key elements from the maternal and infant history along with signs and/or symptoms that are of concern for disease. From the key elements, a differential diagnostic list of potential disease is generated that will guide testing and treatment. This list is placed in order of importance from most to least likely to further prioritize and tailor tests and treatment. In addition, the reader will note that there is much overlap of the diagnostic testing required as many diseases present with multiple symptoms, making ongoing evaluation a must throughout the process of treatment.

It is important to keep in mind that if untreated certain diseases can lead to devastating outcomes. Therefore, testing and treatments for multiple possible diagnoses are instituted simultaneously. As the more likely diagnosis is elucidated, treatments are then tailored for the most likely or known diagnosis. It is important to understand that some diseases are not truly identified at all or not until treatment is complete, which is considered a diagnosis of exclusion. In other words, not all diagnoses are clear cut and easily defined. One example would be the treatment for feeding intolerance caused by distention, radiographic findings suggestive of an ileus, and the question of pneumatosis. These findings would require treatment for possible infection, NEC, and feeding intolerance. The infant recovers and 2 weeks later presents with the same symptoms and the final diagnosis is Hirschsprung's disease. Because signs and symptoms can mimic more than one disease, such as NEC, a devastating disease if untreated, treatment is provided, and only when the infant presents with repeat symptoms is the true diagnosis discovered.

The GI diseases discussed in this chapter appear in a cephalocaudal progression and include duodenal atresia, midgut volvulus, NEC, SBS, meconium ileus, and Hirschsprung's disease. The embryology of these congenital anomalies is presented, including the relationship to the presenting sign or symptom. Also included in this chapter are (a) the symptoms associated with NEC, (b) discussion of the normal absorption and digestion of both macro- and micronutrients, (c) the complications of disruption for the infant with short gut, and (d) the classic radiologic findings related to these anomalies or disease.

EMBRYOLOGY OF THE GI TRACT

FOREGUT

Knowing how and when the GI tract develops in the fetus is very helpful to understanding the development of disruptions. This section covers a basic review of the embryology of the GI tract in the developing fetus. The embryology of the GI tract begins during the fourth week of gestation with the development of the foregut. The pharyngeal arches, which will give rise to the oral cavity, pharynx, tongue, tonsils, salivary glands, and the upper respiratory tract, are beginning to develop. At the same time the lower respiratory tract, esophagus, stomach, duodenum, liver, biliary apparatus, and the pancreas are forming simultaneously. The esophagus begins with the laryngotracheal groove, which elongates to form a pouch called the *laryngotracheal diverticulum*. Longitudinally, ridges known as *tracheoesophageal folds* form in the diverticulum and grow toward each other to fuse, forming a partition known as the *tracheal esophageal septum*. It is during this period that incomplete fusion of the tracheal esophageal folds leads to defects in the septum and abnormal communication between the trachea and the esophagus (Moore, Persaud, & Torchia, 2016). The esophagus is initially short, but elongates rapidly, reaching its full length at 7 weeks gestation. The epithelial cell lining grows to obliterate the lumen, either partially or completely. By 8 weeks gestation recanalization occurs. Failure to recannulate leads to isolated esophageal atresia (Moore et al., 2016).

During the fourth week, the stomach begins to form out of the distal foregut. During weeks 5 and 6, the dorsal border of the primordial stomach grows faster than the ventral border, creating the greater curvature of the stomach. As the stomach enlarges, it rotates 90° clockwise. This rotation places the ventral, or lesser curvature of the stomach, to the right, the dorsal or greater curvature of the stomach to the left, as the long axis of the stomach takes a transverse position to the long axis of the body. Also during the fourth week, the duodenum develops out of the caudal portion of the foregut and cranial portion of the midgut. The junction of these two parts of the duodenum is just distal to the origin of the common bile duct. This distinction is important because obstruction with or without bilious vomiting helps the practitioner identify approximately where the obstruction occurs. Bile production occurs by the 12th week of gestation and enters the duodenum by the 13th week, giving meconium its dark-green color. The rapid growth of the duodenum causes a C-shaped loop that crosses the midline of the spine and then returns. This positioning is very distinct and used as a clinical marker in identifying malrotation of the intestine. During weeks 5 and 6, the epithelial cell lining grows to obliterate the lumen either partially or completely, with recanalization occurring by the end of the eighth week (Moore et al., 2016).

Early in the fourth week, the hepatic diverticulum or liver bud develops from the foregut, giving rise to the liver, biliary duct, and gallbladder. A small portion of the hepatic diverticulum gives rise to the gallbladder, cystic duct, and bile duct. Between weeks 5 and 10, the liver grows rapidly, taking up most of the abdominal cavity (Moore et al., 2016).

MIDGUT

Most of the duodenum, jejunum, ileum, cecum, vermiform appendix, ascending colon, and a portion of the transverse colon to the right side develop from the midgut. As a result of the lack of space in the abdomen during the sixth week of gestation, the midgut forms a U-shaped loop, and the intestine herniates out into the proximal portion of the umbilical cord. The cranial limb grows rapidly, forming the jejunum and the ileum, while the caudal limb grows slowly allowing for the formation of the cecal diverticulum. While the intestine is herniated, it undergoes a 90° counterclockwise turn, positioning the cranial limb to the right and the caudal limb to the left. During the 10th week of gestation, the intestine returns to the abdomen. The small intestine returns first to occupy the center of the abdomen. The large intestine follows, making a 180° counterclockwise turn and rests on the right side of the abdomen. The large intestine pushes the duodenum against the posterior wall, allowing most of the duodenal mesentery to be absorbed. The mesentery of the ascending colon also disappears, leaving the fan-shaped mesentery of the jejunum and ileum. The remaining mesentery forms a new line of attachment passing through the duodenal–jejunal junction inferior laterally to the ileocecal junction (Moore et al., 2016). The importance of this attachment and the proper rotation of the bowel prevent the bowel from rotating on itself and creating a volvulus, which is the cutting off blood supply to the intestine, and leads to bowel death.

HINDGUT

The hindgut development is responsible for the later one third to half of the transverse colon, descending and sigmoid colon, rectum, and superior part of the anal canal. The hindgut is also responsible for the epithelium of the urinary bladder and most of the urethra. By the seventh week of gestation, the cloacae are separated by a wedge of mesenchyme known as the *urorectal septum*. One portion forms the rectum and cranial part of the anal canal dorsally and the other forms the urogenital sinus ventrally. This becomes the perineum of the adult. The inferior one third of the anal canal is derived from the anal pit. The anorectal lumen is blocked by an epithelial plug. By the eighth week apoptosis occurs, allowing recanalization to occur thereby forming the anal pit and the anal opening (Moore et al., 2016).

DUODENAL ATRESIA

Case 13.1

A 39 6/7-week-gestation male infant who is now 1 day old presents with vomiting, poor feeding, and generalized low tone in a level-one nursery. This infant is noted to have phenotypical findings consistent with trisomy 21, for which chromosomes have been sent for testing. All prenatal testing for trisomy 21 was negative. Given this presentation, the pediatrician consulted the neonatal intensive care unit for further recommendations and a request for transfer. The transferring pediatrician was instructed to obtain an anterior–posterior (AP) and lateral x-ray of the abdomen, to stop feeding, and start a peripheral intravenous (IV) line while waiting for the neonatal intensive care unit (NICU) team to arrive.

The maternal history was significant for gravida 2, now para 2 and advanced maternal age at 36 years, polyhydramnios with an amniotic fluid index (AFI) of 28 cm, and gestational diabetes that was diet controlled. Prenatal labs were unremarkable, both triple and quad screens were negative for trisomy 21. The infant was born by way of spontaneous vaginal delivery under epidural anesthesia, after artificial rupture of membranes 9 hours prior to delivery for clear fluid. The Apgar scores were 8 and 9 at 1 and 5 minutes, respectively. The infant reportedly went to the newborn nursery and, after having chromosomes drawn, received well-child care. The infant was reported to have voided and stooled since birth. He had attempted to breastfeed four times over the past 24 hours. For the past 4 hours he has shown no interest in feeding, is vomiting, and presents with abdominal distention.

1. **Given this history, what diagnosis would you consider placing first in your differential diagnostic list?**

   ANSWER: Duodenal atresia would be considered, since the infant is suspected of having trisomy 21. *This anomaly occurs 33% with trisomy 21 and up to 50% with other anomalies. In addition, the infant is not reported as having bilious vomiting and therefore is more likely to have a high obstruction.*

2. **As the advanced practice nurse (APN) you are requested to attend a delivery of a full-term infant, because this infant is delivered by vaginal birth after cesarean (VBAC). You examine the maternal record for any complications of the pregnancy and labor. Which of the findings from the maternal history listed here is a concern for bowel obstruction?**

   ANSWER: Polyhydramnios, *normal AFI is greater than 8 cm and less than 25 cm.*

DIFFERENTIAL

Listing the presenting symptoms, history, and available study results with corresponding potential diagnoses for each helps the clinician develop a list of tests to help guide further testing in an attempt to determine the cause of the infant's new-onset symptoms. The classic study for this presentation is a two-view abdominal x-ray in addition to other studies performed concurrently, as listed in Table 13.1.

Table 13.1 Concerning Symptoms, Differential Diagnoses, and Corresponding Testing for Case 13.1

Symptom	Differential	Testing
Poor tone	Chromosomal abnormality, sepsis, neurologic abnormality	Chromosome analysis, full diagnostic workup, and antibiotics (Committee on Infectious Diseases and Committee on Fetus and Newborn [CIDCFN], 2011), full neurologic and physical examination
Abdominal distention	GI obstruction, abdominal mass, sepsis presenting with ileus	Abdominal x-ray both AP and lateral, abdominal examination, note stooling pattern and feeding history, CBC with differential
Poor feeding/ vomiting	GI obstruction, sepsis, neurologic abnormality, structural abnormality of the oral pharynx	Full diagnostic workup and antibiotics (CIDCFN, 2011), full neurologic and physical examination, abdominal x-ray both AP and lateral
Polyhydramnios	GI obstruction, gestational diabetes, neurologic compromise inhibiting the ability to suck and swallow	Abdominal x-ray both AP and lateral, full neurologic examination with attention to root, suck, Moro and gag, reflexes and tone, and the mechanics of swallowing
Advanced maternal age/phenotypic findings for trisomy 21	Chromosomal abnormalities, trisomy 21	Chromosomal analysis

AP, anterior–posterior; CBC, complete blood count; GI, gastrointestinal.

DIFFERENTIAL DIAGNOSES

To evaluate the potential causes for the vomiting, abdominal distention, and poor tone of the infant presented in Case 13.1, a differential diagnostic list is compiled. Potential diagnoses are placed in order of most to least likely. A list of diagnoses can be found in Box 13.1.

Consider once again the infant in Case 13.1: The x-ray obtained at the outlying hospital was significant for signs of obstruction with a largely distended stomach and proximal duodenum with no bowel gas noted beyond the duodenum. These findings, known as the

---

Box 13.1 *Differential Diagnoses for Case 13.1*

- GI obstruction
  - Duodenal atresia
  - Duodenal stenosis
  - Pyloric stenosis
  - Annular pancreas
  - Malrotation
  - Abdominal mass
- Sepsis
- Neurologic abnormality

---

double bubble, are consistent with duodenal atresia. The double bubble results from the large dilated stomach with a narrowing at the pylorus and a large dilated duodenum proximal to the obstruction. The infant with a complete atresia will have no distal gas (deSilva, Young, & Wales, 2006; Trotter, 2011). deSilva et al. (2006) is recommended reading for more detailed description and visual of the radiographic findings.

Evaluating Radiographic Studies

When evaluating a two-view abdominal film, it is important to note the amount of bowel gas seen. Ask the question, is the gas isolated to the stomach and a small portion of the small bowel (proximal, isolated to the duodenum), is a good portion of the small bowel filled with gas (mid to distal small bowel, jejunum, or ileum), or is there bowel gas all the way to the rectum? Determining these answers requires that you obtain both an anterior–posterior (AP) view and a lateral or left lateral decubitus film to evaluate. The amount of bowel gas present should help guide your assessment as to the position of the bowel obstruction, in other words, where the obstruction lies. Examine the films for bowel distention. The more distended bowel is found proximal to the obstruction. A large amount of distention followed by a small amount of distal gas can indicate stenosis rather than atresia. The number of distended bowel loops is an important clue about where the obstruction lies, as the more distended the loops the more distal the obstruction. The presence or absence of air fluid levels implies obstruction caused by a lack of peristalsis, as bowel contents are not moving. This could be caused either by a mechanical obstruction, as with an atresia, or a functional obstruction, as with an ileus. Following the abdominal films with a contrast study helps outline the anatomy for size, shape, and position. The abdominal films along with the history will provide important information used to determine whether to introduce contrast from above as an upper gastrointestinal (UGI) series or from below as a barium enema (BE) (Trotter, 2011).

Pathophysiology

Duodenal atresia is not a common anomaly. However, if present, 50% of the time it occurs with other anomalies such as trisomy 21 (33%), imperforate anus, Cornelia de Lange, VATER, or VACTERAL sequence (vertebrae, anal atresia, cardiac anomalies, tracheoesophageal fistula, renal or kidney anomalies, and limb anomalies). The intrinsic cause of this congenital anomaly results from the lack of recanalization of a small segment of the duodenum at the end of the eighth week of gestation and has an incidence of one in 7,000 live births (Parry,

2015). Eighty percent involve the descending second and horizontal third portions of the duodenum. This section of bowel is just distal to the ampulla of Vater, where the bile duct enters the duodenum. Infants with duodenal atresia will most likely have bilious vomiting without abdominal distention (Gomella, 2013). If the obstruction occurs proximal to the ampulla of Vater, the infant will not have bilious vomiting and the abdomen is distended because of large dilation of the epigastric area. Extrinsic causes include vascular accident, malrotation with Ladd's bands (see Case 13.2 on malrotation), and annular pancreas. Annular pancreas is an abnormal ring of pancreatic tissue encircling the duodenum that results from malrotation during development (Trotter, 2011). Other related anomalies associated with duodenal atresia are trisomy 21, imperforate anus, esophageal atresias, and cardiovascular anomalies (Moore et al., 2016).

Duodenal stenosis results from incomplete recanalization of the bowel lumen resulting from faulty vascularization slightly distal to where duodenal atresia commonly occurs. Because of the incomplete obstruction seen in duodenal stenosis, distal bowel gas may be noted on x-ray. However, this diagnosis requires further testing to make the diagnosis and rule out more devastating diseases such as malrotation with volvulus (Moore et al., 2015; Trotter, 2011). Symptoms associated with duodenal atresia or stenosis include (a) bilious vomiting, (b) polyhydramnios, (c) bile-colored amniotic fluid often mistaken for meconium, (d) epigastric distention, and (e) double bubble sign on x-ray.

TREATMENT

Treatment for this anomaly requires that the infant be allowed nothing by mouth (NPO). Placement of a gastric tube to decompress the stomach and proximal duodenum is imperative to prevent further distention that may compromise the infant's respiratory status and to prevent potential perforation. Decompression of the bowel will also allow time to plan for surgical exploration when the infant is stable. A full physical examination to rule out other potential anomalies, including skeletal x-rays to evaluate for vertebral anomalies, is needed. Given the likelihood of other associated congenital anomalies, a genetics consultation and chromosomal analysis should be considered even if the infant does not have other phenotypical findings consistent with trisomy 21. Given the potential for cardiac abnormalities, a cardiology consult and echocardiogram to evaluate for other anomalies before performing surgery are usually considered as they could present a surgical risk. Surgical repair most commonly involves an end-to-end anastomosis known as the *diamond duodenoduodenostomy*. This technique allows the anastomosis to stent itself open to help prevent obstruction caused by the large-caliber proximal duodenum entering the narrow, small-caliber distal bowel (Barksdale, Chwals, Magnuson, & Parry, 2011).

RELATED COMPLICATIONS

The degree of morbidity and mortality associated with duodenal atresia is related to infants who also have congenital heart disease or trisomy 21. A genetics consult to evaluate for other related anomalies is important for the care of this infant and consideration of possible future pregnancies. Rapid treatment to relieve bowel distention is equally important, because bowel rupture presents a true morbidity risk. Following surgery, the infant may have an ileus, which prolongs the ability to start enteral intake for as long as 5 to 7 days. Because of the large dilated proximal duodenum resulting from prolonged obstruction in utero, these infants can have very slow transit times and dyskinetic bowel, making the establishment of enteral feedings difficult (Parry, 2015). Infants may require central access that puts them at potential risk for infection. Those infants who have other congenital anomalies, such as imperforate anus, may require a colostomy in addition to repair of the obstruction. Potential surgical complications, including obstruction secondary to adhesions or infection, require monitoring. Prolonged hospital stay, the need for family education, and genetic counseling also need to be considered.

MALROTATION AND MIDGUT VOLVULUS

Case 13.2

The pediatrician calls the nurse practitioner to request a consult for a 1-day-old full-term infant in the newborn nursery who presents with bilious vomiting and abdominal disten-tion. The pediatrician describes the emesis as dark green in color and of large volume. The infant is otherwise looking well, active, and alert.

This full-term female infant, birth weight 3.2 kg, was born to a 32-year-old, gravida 3, now para 3 mother who spontaneously ruptured her membranes at home with clear fluid. Membranes were ruptured for a total of 21 hours prior to delivery; however, given the time it took to get to the hospital for delivery only one dose of penicillin (PCN) was admin-istered less than 1 hour before delivery. There were no concerns for maternal temperature or clinical chorioamnionitis at the time of delivery. Maternal lab work was remarkable for positive group B *Streptococcus* (GBS). The infant was born by normal spontaneous vaginal delivery without anesthesia. Apgar scores were 9 and 9 at 1 and 5 minutes, respectively.

In the newborn nursery, this infant had been latching well at the breast and feeding every 2 to 3 hours. She voided and had two meconium stools.

1. *From this history, what symptom tells you the infant requires an immediate intervention?*

   ANSWER: Bilious vomiting. *This symptom may indicate malrotation and volvulus, which is a surgical emergency.*

2. *What intervention is the gold standard for this infant's presentation?*

   ANSWER: Upper gastrointestinal (UGI) series, examination for proper bowel rotation.

DIFFERENTIAL

Listing the presenting symptoms, history, and available study results with corresponding potential diagnoses for each helps the clinician to develop a list of tests to help guide fur-ther testing in an attempt to determine the cause of the infant's new-onset symptoms. Im-mediate study for this case presentation is a two-view abdominal x-ray in addition to other studies performed concurrently, as listed in Table 13.2.

DIFFERENTIAL DIAGNOSES

To evaluate the potential causes for the bilious vomiting and abdominal distention evident in the infant described in Case 13.2, a differential diagnostic list is compiled using the di-agnoses identified in Table 13.2. Potential diagnoses are placed in order of most to least likely. A list of diagnoses can be found in Box 13.2.

***Table* 13.2 Concerning Symptoms, Differential Diagnoses, and Corresponding Testing for Case 13.2**

Symptom/History	Differential	Testing
Membranes ruptured for 21 hours GBS (+) Abdominal distention with bilious vomiting Inadequate PCN treatment	Sepsis	Full diagnostic workup and antibiotics (CIDCFN, 2011)
Bilious vomiting Abdominal distention	Malrotation with or without volvulus until proven otherwise Small bowel obstruction distal to the ampulla of Vater Ileus Meconium plug/ileus Reflux Idiopathic Hirschsprung's disease	UGI gold standard, two-view KUB required if UGI is not immediately available Barium enema may be necessary if symptoms persist and previous studies are not diagnostic Unlikely given the infant has stooled

GBS, group B *Streptococcus*; KUB, kidney, ureters, and bladder; PCN, penicillin; UGI, upper gastrointestinal.

Box 13.2 *Differential Diagnoses for Case 13.2*

- Malrotation with or without volvulus
- Sepsis
- Small bowel obstruction distal to the ampulla of Vater
- Ileus
- Meconium plug/ileus
- Reflux
- Idiopathic

PATHOPHYSIOLOGY

Malrotation by itself is a rather common anomaly and is most often asymptomatic. With this anomaly, the midgut loop does not rotate upon reentering the abdomen during the 10th week of gestation. The caudal portion of the small bowel returns first, moving to the right side and the colon to the left, also known as *left-sided colon*. Because the large intestine is malpositioned, the duodenum remains to the right rather than being pushed against the posterior wall by the large intestine. This allows for the formation of Ladd's bands that extend from the ascending colon across the duodenum to the posterior wall (Moore et al., 2016). This position sets the bowel up for injury if the small bowel should twist on itself, cutting off blood supply from the superior mesenteric artery, leading to infarction and bowel death without immediate treatment (Trotter, 2011).

Only one in 6,000 individuals with malrotation is discovered, either by accident as a result of studies performed for an unrelated problem or as a result of obstruction. It is obstruction that leads to the infant's symptoms, 80% of the time the infant will have bilious vomiting. Abdominal distention may be present, but is not always seen if the obstruction is incomplete. Often the infants' abdomen will be tender on examination, with or without bowel sounds. This anomaly is truly a surgical emergency, as irreversible ischemia and bowel death can occur rapidly. It is for this reason that any infant under 1 year of age who presents with bilious vomiting must immediately obtain a UGI study to determine whether the infant's intestine is malrotated and, if so, whether there is a midgut volvulus (Parry, 2015; Trotter, 2011).

Gastroschisis and Omphalocele

The two other midgut anomalies important to mention briefly here are gastroschisis and omphalocele, as both of these anomalies result in malrotation. Gastroschisis is not usually associated with any other anomalies or syndromes. This anomaly occurs early in gestation with failure of the lateral folds to complete formation during the fourth week of gestation. Herniation of the abdominal contents through the abdominal wall usually occurs to the right of a normally positioned umbilicus. The viscera of the abdominal contents are exposed to the amniotic fluid, which causes irritation and edema of the bowel wall (Gomella, 2013; Parry, 2015). This defect requires surgical repair, and the timing is dependent on the size of the defect. The degree of morbidity and mortality is dependent on bowel integrity, as these infants can have atresia or prenatal bowel perforation, which complicates repair and recovery (Parry, 2015).

The second lesion to consider is an omphalocele. This occurs when the abdominal contents herniate naturally at 6 weeks gestation. The herniated contents does not return to the abdominal cavity resulting in no bowel rotation and a persistent hernia seen in the proximal part of the umbilical cord. Therefore, the contents have an epithelial covering. Occasionally the covering will rupture, making this lesion difficult to distinguish from gastroschisis (Ross, 2004). One major difference between these two anomalies is that omphalocele can be associated with other anomalies or syndromes as often as 80% of the time. The most common associations are (a) congenital heart disease, (b) trisomies, (c) Beckwith–Wiedemann syndrome, (d) pentalogy of Cantrell, (e) prune-belly syndrome, and (f) lower midline syndrome (Cooney, 1998). Morbidity and mortality are dependent on other associated anomalies rather than the omphalocele itself (Parry, 2015).

TESTING

Often an AP and lateral view abdominal x-ray is performed to examine the bowel gas pattern unless a UGI can be performed immediately. From the x-ray it can be determined whether the infant has an intrinsic duodenal obstruction by examining the x-ray for the double bubble sign. If the infant's stomach is dilated, but the duodenum is of normal caliber, it is possible that the infant has duodenal obstruction caused by Ladd's bands from malrotation and possibly volvulus (Parry, 2015; Trotter, 2011). To make this diagnosis, the UGI is the gold standard. During normal rotation and fixation, the duodenum moves under the superior mesenteric artery, forming a C shape that extends to the right of the abdomen from the pylorus, then back to the left toward the ligament of Treitz. The recommended reading for a visual description of the normal rotation can be found in Filston and Kirks (1981). It is this C shape of the duodenum that the radiologist is looking for to determine normal rotation and fixation of the bowel. Typically, the small bowel rests predominantly to the left in the abdomen, whereas the large intestine lies to the right (Trotter, 2011). In an infant with malrotation, during UGI the radiologist will find the duodenojejunal junction positioned anteriorly, low and mostly midline, and the cecum and terminal ileum will be pointing upward toward midline. This midline positioning is concerning for malrotation. In the infant with bilious vomiting and malrotation or a critically ill infant with suspected malrotation, immediate surgery is required (Parry, 2015; Trotter, 2011).

TREATMENT

Infants with a concerning abdominal radiograph will require a gastric tube to decompress the stomach and proximal bowel. All infants with confirmed malrotation by UGI will require exploratory laparotomy. For these infants the gastric tube will remain in place postoperatively until the ileus is resolved. Intravenous fluids and broad-spectrum antibiotics will be initiated. These infants are at risk of shock resulting from a lack of blood supply, poor lymphatic drainage, bowel swelling, and necrosis. Intraoperative blood products must be available. Immediate surgery to relieve torsion is required, Ladd's bands are divided, and an appendectomy is performed. The bowel is returned to the abdomen in a fully nonrotated position. This would potentially position the appendix in the left upper quadrant. Therefore, to avoid any complications associated with a missed diagnosis in the future, the appendix is removed at this time (Barksdale et al., 2011; Trotter, 2011). Any necrotic bowel will be resected; sometimes this will require an ostomy, depending on the degree of injury. The degree of bowel loss will affect related complications and long-term outcome.

RELATED COMPLICATIONS

Mortality in infants with malrotation is approximately 3% to 9% because of significant bowel necrosis, shock, prematurity, or other related anomalies. The degree of injury will determine the need for a colostomy and associated complications. Infants requiring an ostomy will need follow-up ostomy care and eventual reanastomosis. Slow transit times and dyskinetic bowel are always a concern given the potential for ileus and bowel disruption, which can make the establishment of enteral feedings difficult. Potential surgical complications, including obstruction secondary to adhesions or wound infection, require close monitoring (Parry, 2015). Infants may require a central-access line, which puts them at additional risk for infection. Those infants who require the removal of large amounts of bowel because of necrosis are at risk of SBS and associated complications (see Case 13.4 on SBS). Prolonged hospital stay, the need for family education, support, and counseling also must be considered.

NECROTIZING ENTEROCOLITIS

Case 13.3

A former 25-week-gestation male infant now on day of life (DOL) 28 presents with abdominal distention, loopy bowel, and abdominal tenderness. The infant has been on continuous positive airway pressure (CPAP) with a peek end-expiratory pressure (PEEP)

(continued)

Case 13.3 *(continued)*

of 4 and room air for the past 3 days. He has had increased apnea and bradycardic episodes that require vigorous stimulation over the past 12 hours and an increase oxygen requirement to 34%. Upon further examination, the nurse practitioner finds the infant to have decreased tone overall. The infant was due for a feeding at this time and was found to have no gastric aspirate.

Further examination of the medical record reveals that the infant had been treated for the first 7 days of life with antibiotics for presumed sepsis as a result of persistent abnormal complete blood counts (CBCs) that normalized on DOL 4, an elevated C-reactive protein of 136 mg/L on DOL 3, although the blood culture remained negative.

The maternal history was significant for maternal fever at 38.3°C and clinical chorioamnionitis at the time of delivery and was treated adequately with ampicillin and gentamicin prior to delivery. The infant was started on enteral feedings on DOL 2 and progressed to full feedings of 24 cal/oz of maternal breast milk on DOL 16.

1. **Given this clinical presentation, what test should you plan to immediately consider?**

    ANSWER: Two-view abdominal x-ray. *Given the abdominal distention, tenderness, and lethargy close observation for necrotizing enterocolitis (NEC) is imperative. Second, blood work including a complete blood count (CBC), and blood gas will help to determine if the symptoms are respiratory or infectious in origin. Keep in mind much of the diagnostic workup occurs concurrently.*

2. **Which of the presenting symptoms is most concerning for NEC?**

    ANSWER: Abdominal tenderness, as well as a change in the infants overall clinical status with increased apnea, bradycardia, and lethargy. *Abdominal distention and loopy bowel can also be signs of NEC, but may be signs of air trapping from continuous positive airway pressure (CPAP) and/or constipation. All potential diagnoses must be considered while concurrent testing is performed.*

DIFFERENTIAL

Listing the presenting symptoms, history, and available study results with corresponding potential diagnoses for each helps the clinician develop a list of tests to help guide further testing in an attempt to determine the cause of the infant's new-onset symptoms. Immediate study for this case presentation is a two-view abdominal x-ray in addition to other studies performed concurrently, as listed in Table 13.3.

DIFFERENTIAL DIAGNOSES

To evaluate the potential causes for the abdominal distention, loopy bowel, abdominal tenderness, and lethargy indicated in Case 13.3, a differential diagnostic list is compiled using the diagnoses identified in Table 13.3. Potential diagnoses are placed in order of most to least likely. A list of diagnoses can be found in Box 13.3.

Table 13.3 Concerning Symptoms, Differential Diagnoses, and Corresponding Testing for Case 13.3

Symptom/History	Differential	Testing	Rationale
Abdominal distention, loopy bowel, abdominal tenderness, full feedings of 24 cal/oz	NEC, sepsis, distention caused by CPAP increasing bowel gas, constipation	Two-view abdominal x-ray, CBC with differential (Kimberlin, Brady, Jackson, & Long, 2015), test results will determine further studies and treatment, examine the medical record for stooling pattern and other medications or treatments that may alter feeding tolerance (i.e., PDA treatment, caffeine)	X-ray will determine obstruction, ileus, or specific signs for NEC such as pneumatosis; CBC will guide concerns for infection (Henry & Moss, 2009); early antimicrobial treatment prevents gut colonization with beneficial bacteria (Gephart, McGrath, Effken, & Halpern, 2012)
Increased apnea and bradycardia	Sepsis, stress related to worsening respiratory distress or tiring on CPAP	Blood gas, CBC as mentioned previously, consider initiating caffeine or check level if on caffeine	Blood gas will provide adequacy of gas exchange and evaluate for metabolic acidosis seen with infection or bowel necrosis (Henry & Moss, 2009); if all other testing is negative caffeine adjustment would be indicated
Lethargy	Sepsis, NEC, stress related to worsening respiratory distress, tiring on CPAP	CBC as mentioned previously, two-view KUB Full physical examination with attention to infant tone and response to intervention	Lethargy as a sign of infection possibly just tiring of preterm infant; rationale is the same as mentioned previously.
Increased oxygen requirement	Worsening respiratory distress	Blood gas, CBC as mentioned previously, CXR	Blood gas to evaluate carbon dioxide retention and acidosis; CBC to evaluate possible infection; CXR to evaluate for lung collapse, signs of congestive heart failure seen with PDA or pneumonia
Prolonged antibiotic administration first week of life	Decreased intestinal colonization		Beneficial bacteria decrease the overgrowth of pathogenic bacteria (Gephart et al., 2012; Henry & Moss, 2009)

CBC, complete blood count; CPAP, continuous positive airway pressure; CXR, chest x-ray; KUB, kidney, ureters, bladder; NEC, necrotizing enterocolitis; PDA, patent ductus arteriosus.

PATHOPHYSIOLOGY

NEC is the leading cause of emergency surgery and mortality among premature infants in the neonatal intensive care unit (NICU) (Gephart, Poole, & Crain, 2014). Although 7% to 15% of full-term infants can develop NEC, it is primarily a disease of the preterm infant. In the full-term infant, this disease usually presents within the first few days of life and is associated with acute ischemic injury; examples include birth hypoxia, cyanotic heart disease, and congenital bowel malformations (Neu, 2014). For the premature infant, the younger the gestation, the greater the risk of developing this devastating disease, which carries a mortality risk of 20% to 30%, the greatest risk among those anomalies requiring surgical intervention (Gephart et al., 2014; Neu, 2014). This disease can be illusive because symptoms are nonspecific and mimic other problems that plague the preterm infant, such as feeding intolerance, constipation, gastric air trapping from noninvasive modes of respiratory therapy, and sepsis. Neu (2014) describes this disease as a combination of immaturity and immature gut, microbial dysbiosis, and genetics. NEC, a disease primarily of the preterm infant, is not usually the result of primary ischemic injury, but rather of a multifactorial process. Because of the vague nature of the symptoms, Gordon, Swanson, Attridge, and Clark (2007) point out the difficulty in determining which infants have feeding intolerance from those who actually have Bell's stage I criteria labeled as suspected NEC. In short, there are no really good models or criteria to clearly separate feeding intolerance from suspected NEC. As a result many infants will receive treatment for suspected NEC, which delays enteral feeding and leads to prolonged hospital stay.

The premature infant's intestine is at risk of injury as the permeability of the immature intestine is increased because of loose junctions and oversaturation of the mesenteric nodes by bacterial endotoxins, which allow bacteria to penetrate the bowel wall (de Silva et al., 2006). This is coupled with a decreased glycoprotein mucin layer, further enhancing permeability and the ability for bacteria to adhere (Henry & Moss, 2009). The overgrowth of bacteria that can be encouraged by extensive antibiotic use, antacid administration, constipation, and lack of enteral feedings further encourages the necessary milieu for bowel injury in the preterm infant (Gephart, McGrath, Effken, & Halpern, 2012; Henry & Moss, 2009; Neu, 2014). This is further complicated by the premature infant's exaggerated inflammatory response to injury, which causes ongoing bowel damage (Gephart et al., 2014). In NEC, the ileocolic region is the most commonly affected segment of the bowel, as this area is far removed from its blood supply, the superior mesenteric artery, known as the watershed area. Decreased oxygen supply from hypoxia or anemia makes the area vulnerable (Horton, 2005). However, NEC can really occur anywhere in the intestine (Gephart et al., 2014).

Keen observation skills and prompt evaluation are necessary to determine which infants require further intervention and testing. This disease can be insidious, as vague symptoms tend to smolder over a few days or symptoms can be very abrupt, presenting with rapid deterioration. Symptoms associated with NEC can include, but are not limited to, abdominal distention, visibly loopy bowel, abdominal tenderness, abdominal discoloration, grossly bloody stool, change in clinical status that may present with increase in apnea and bradycardia, poor tone, irritability, metabolic acidosis, deteriorating respiratory status, and even shock (Gephart et al., 2012; Henry & Moss, 2009; Moss et al., 2008; Neu, 2014). Many of these symptoms are vague and alone they are not as much of a concern; however, when the infant develops symptoms that indicate a change in clinical status that cannot be explained by clinical history or recent environmental events, further testing is often warranted. A list of risk factors associated with acquiring NEC can be found in Box 13.4. It is important to note that there is no direct correlation between risk and disease (Moss et al., 2008; Neu, 2014).

Symptoms that are not helpful in identifying NEC are gastric aspirate or guaiac-positive stools. As a singular symptom, gastric aspirate has not been shown to have a direct correlation to NEC. Guaiac-positive stools can be secondary to other extrinsic causes, such as suctioning, gastric tube placement, or rectal fissure (Caplan, 2015; Moore & Wilson, 2011; Neu, 2014). Furthermore, Caplan (2015) points out that although many of these symptoms mimic feeding intolerance, feeding intolerance itself is not a reliable marker of intestinal injury. Moore and Wilson (2011) performed a concept analysis to determine symptoms that have been found in the literature to support a definition of feeding intolerance. Their findings suggest that gastric residuals of the previous feeding greater than 50%, abdominal distention, and/or emesis were the only consistent symptoms to support feeding intolerance. This is an important distinction, as preterm infants do experience feeding intolerance that can be the result of the substrate, bowel dysmotility of immaturity, feeding volume, and multiple other environmental stressors that can influence digestion. Feeding intolerance may require bowel rest of varying lengths of time and often is a diagnosis of exclusion. After

---

Box 13.4 Risk Factors Associated With Acquiring NEC

- Prematurity, extremely premature at greatest risk
- Fed infant
- Rapid feeding advance
- Hypoxic ischemic encephalopathy
- Intrauterine growth restriction
- Formula fed

More controversial risks
- Polycythemia
- History of exchange transfusion
- Blood transfusion
- Gastroschisis
- Myelomeningocele
- Congenital heart disease

NEC, necrotizing enterocolitis.
Sources: Caplan (2015), Gephart et al. (2012).

monitoring abdominal x-rays, laboratory studies, and clinical examination, most clinicians are willing to consider the symptoms of feeding intolerance instead of NEC (Gordon et al., 2007).

TESTING

When an infant presents with GI symptoms and a change in clinical status that cannot be explained by clinical history or recent environmental events, further testing is warranted. As presented here in Case 13.3, abdominal tenderness with a change in clinical status is very concerning. As with most symptoms that warrant further investigation, many tests are performed concurrently, as presented in Table 13.3. However, the first test that should be performed here is a two-view (AP) abdominal x-ray. A nonspecific initial finding with early disease may be dilated bowel loops and concern for an ileus; if the pattern is stagnant on serial films, this is consistent with modified Bell's stage I (Walsh & Kliegman, 1986). The diagnosis of NEC is made by the observation of pneumatosis intestinalis, which is air in the bowel wall, Bell's stage II (Henry & Moss, 2009). This classic finding is the result of gas from gas-producing bacteria that transect the bowel wall at the site of intestinal injury. The finding of a linear or circular pattern within the bowel wall on abdominal x-ray indicates subserosal air, whereas a stagnant bubbly pattern indicates air that is submucosal. An x-ray presenting this pattern can be found in Donahue (2007). However, a bubbly pattern can also indicate stool (Neu, 2014). Other signs include bowel distention, thickened bowel wall, air fluid levels, free intraperitoneal air (pneumoperitoneum), and portal venous gas (Moss et al., 2008). If the bowel should perforate, pneumoperitoneum (free air) can be seen on the x-ray and confirmed by a left lateral decubitus x-ray, which allows the free air to transect up over the liver. Abdominal ultrasound can also be used if available and is 100% reliable in demonstrating free air and lack of blood flow to a necrotic intestine (Neu, 2014).

Although pneumatosis is a finding consistent with NEC, the determination of this finding is subjective. Bell's staging for NEC is helpful to separate cases of feeding intolerance from actual NEC and further helps in determining those cases suspected of stage II and III NEC. Furthermore, the staging of symptoms provides a framework for treating and researching this very heterogeneous disease (Bell et al., 1978). Walsh and Kliegman (1986) modified Bell's staging for ease of use and can be found in Table 13.4.

TREATMENT

The infant suspected of having NEC should have all enteral intake discontinued and will require a gastric tube to decompress the bowel, allowing for bowel rest. To assist with bowel decompression, intubation and ventilation should be considered for infants who are on non-invasive forms of respiratory support. If decompression is not achieved, troubleshooting the gastric decompression device is imperative to eliminate any mechanical problems (Neu, 2014). Intravenous fluids (consider hyperalimentation) and even fluid resuscitation may be indicated. Evaluate the need for blood products to support intravascular volume and replace blood lost to intra-abdominal bleeding. Closely monitor the need for blood pressure support. Monitoring of electrolytes and acid–base balance are critical during initial stabilization (Neu, 2014). Fluid requirements may be increased as a result of bowel wall edema and fluid loss through gastric suctioning should also be replaced. Close monitoring of electrolytes to customize fluid replacement is critical (de Silva et al., 2006). Blood, urine, and possibly sputum cultures are obtained before initiating broad-spectrum antibiotics. Stool cultures are not typically performed, as they have not been shown to identify a causative agent

Table 13.4 Modified Bell's Staging Criteria for NEC

Stage	Classification	Clinical Signs	Radiographic Signs
I	Suspected NEC	Abdominal distention, bloody stools, emesis/gastric residual, apnea/lethargy, temperature instability	Ileus/dilatation
II	Proven NEC mild/moderate	As in stage I, plus: abdominal tenderness, metabolic acidosis, thrombocytopenia	Bowel distention/ pneumatosis intestinalis, portal venous gas and/ or ascites
IIIa	Advanced NEC	As in stage II, plus: hypotension, significant acidosis, thrombocytopenia/DIC, neutropenia	As in stage II, with ascites
IIIb	Advanced NEC with bowel perforation	Same as stage IIIa	As in stage IIIa with pneumoperitoneum

DIC, disseminated intravascular coagulation; NEC, necrotizing enterocolitis.
Adapted from Walsh and Kliegman (1986).

(Gordon et al., 2007). Given the concern for bowel wall injury, close monitoring for metabolic acidosis and thrombocytopenia is indicated, as acidosis and thrombocytopenia are signs of worsening bowel necrosis (Henry & Moss, 2009; Neu, 2014).

Frequent serial x-rays are necessary to follow the bowels' response to treatment and the potential for free air, indicating bowel perforation, a surgical emergency (Gephart et al., 2012; Neu, 2014). Other signs that would indicate the need for surgical exploration other than pneumoperitoneum include persistent or worsening thrombocytopenia or metabolic acidosis, persistent fixed dilated loops of bowel unresponsive to medical management, oliguria, hypotension, portal venous gas, and overall clinical deterioration (Henry & Moss, 2009; Neu, 2014). Should surgery be indicated, any necrotic bowel is resected, sometimes this will require an ostomy depending on the degree of injury and surgeon's preference. The degree of bowel loss will impact related complications and long-term outcome. If the infant is too unstable for surgery, bedside peritoneal drain placement can be performed. Research has been unable to determine whether open laparotomy is preferable to bedside peritoneal drain. Studies favor improved outcomes for the infant undergoing the laparotomy procedure; however, those infants requiring the peritoneal drain are much more critical and usually more premature, therefore the concern for bias may underestimate the value of this bedside procedure (Henry & Moss, 2009; Neu, 2014).

Infants treated for NEC are without enteral feedings for varied amounts of time, based on Bell's staging of NEC. For example, Bell's stage II NEC patients are typically NPO for

7 to 10 days, whereas in those who require surgical intervention, an NPO status for up to 14 days is common (Good, Sodhi, & Hackam, 2014). Enteral intake should be initiated with an elemental substrate, because infants who have had NEC may experience protein intolerance and malabsorption of carbohydrates and fats. This makes human milk, preferably mother's own milk, the ideal substrate to begin with. If formula is required, a protein hydrolysate formula that is lactose free and contains medium chain triglycerides (MCT) is preferred for the term infant. For the preterm infant at increased risk for an allergic response to protein, an amino acid–based formula is preferred initially with transition to a preterm formula once feeding is well established. It is important to consider the degree of mucosal injury when initiating feedings, as this will influence the need to consider the use of bolus versus a continuous-feeding strategy (Perks & Abad-Jorge, 2008).

RELATED COMPLICATIONS

The poorest long-term outcomes are related to the infants who require surgery for this disease. Mortality is approximately 10% to 30% as a result of significant bowel necrosis, shock, and prematurity. The risk of SBS (see Case 13.4 on SBS) in patients who have surgical NEC is as much as 25% (Perks & Abad-Jorge, 2008). The degree of injury will determine the need for an ostomy, which may lead to other associated complications, such as SBS and skin breakdown.

Following surgery the infant may have an ileus, which prolongs the ability to start enteral intake. Slow transit times and dyskinetic bowel are always a concern given the potential for postoperative ileus and bowel disruption, which can make the establishment of full enteral feedings difficult, further prolonging the use of central-line access and length of hospital stay. In addition, although rare, the risk of recurrent NEC is about 4% to 6% (Good et al., 2014). Potential surgical complications, including obstruction (complete or partial) secondary to adhesions or wound infection, also require monitoring (Caplan, 2015). One third of patients treated either medically or surgically are at risk of strictures that may require further surgical intervention (Henry & Moss, 2009).

Those infants who require central-line access are at increased risk for infection and complications associated with long-term total parenteral nutrition (TPN), such as cholestasis and osteopenia (Bingham, 2012). Prolonged hospital stay can be significant for infants with NEC, and those who develop SBS may require discharge home on TPN, long-term nursing services, ostomy care, and additional surgery to reverse the ostomy. Preterm infants who experience NEC, Bell's stage greater than or equal to II, are at increased risk for poor neurodevelopmental outcomes as well, with an even greater increased risk seen in those requiring surgical treatment (Caplan, 2015; Henry & Moss, 2009). There will be a need for family education, support, and counseling by the advanced practice nurse (APN).

PREVENTATIVE MEASURES

The ultimate goal is to recognize the symptoms related to the risks for NEC and to prevent this devastating disease. Although the rates of NEC seen in the NICU have not changed much in 30 years (Caplan, 2015), studies have shown a decreased incidence in NEC within individual units that utilize feeding protocols to standardize when to begin feeding, how to advance volume and calories, and what to feed when human milk is not available (Gephart & Hanson, 2013; Patole & de Klerk, 2005). Trophic feedings begun in small amounts of 10 to 20 mL/kg/d within 1 to 4 days of life have been shown not to increase the risk of NEC (Morgan, Bombell, & McGuire, 2013). In addition, trophic feedings have been found to protect the premature intestine from atrophy, loss of villus height, and to encourage enzyme

---

Box 13.5 *Preventative Measures to Reduce* NEC

- Use of human milk
- Early enteral feeding
- Judicious advance of enteral feeding
- Use of feeding protocol
- Separation of enteral hyperosmolar medications
- Cautious feeding with pharmacologic treatment for patent ductus arteriosus (PDA)

NEC, necrotizing enterocolitis.

Sources: Caplan (2015), Gephart and Hanson (2013), Neu (2014), Patole and de Klerk (2005).

---

production and gut motility. These processes decrease the potential for bacterial overgrowth within the intestine as well as intestinal permeability (Bingham, 2012). The benefits of trophic feedings are even further enhanced when only human milk is provided (Lucas & Cole, 1990). Preventative measures are listed in Box 13.5.

SHORT BOWEL SYNDROME

Case 13.4

Our former 28-week-gestation infant who developed necrotizing enterocolitis (NEC) in Case 13.3 is now 54 days old. He has undergone surgical repair for pneumoperitoneum and bowel perforation on day of life (DOL) 31. He also had persistent thrombocytopenia with a nadir platelet count of 28,000 for which he received four platelet transfusions over the course of his treatment for NEC. His most recent platelet count was stable at 134,000 on DOL 53. He had been on triple antibiotic therapy with ampicillin, gentamicin, and Flagyl for a total of 14 days, and his blood culture was reported as negative for this final course of treatment. His surgical repair included resection of necrotic bowel, including one third of the distal jejunum and his entire ileum and the ileocecal valve with an end-to-end anastomosis. Enteral feedings were initiated at a rate of 8 mL/kg/d divided every 3 hours on DOL 43. His feedings have been increased to 5 mL/kg/d over this past week. He continues with hyperalimentation support through a percutaneous central line while increasing on feedings.

Now at DOL 54, he is 35 5/7 weeks of corrected age and is feeding maternal breast milk by mouth at 63 mL/kg/d divided every 3 hours. He has had approximately four stools per day that had been reported as loose over this past week. In addition, his weight has leveled off with no growth over the past week. Today he has had eight watery foul-smelling stools that absorb into his diaper. The nurse reports that he has been more irritable, pulling his legs up with feedings. His abdomen is round and soft with overly active bowel sounds, is nontender on examination and he remains eager to eat. He has developed tachypnea with an average respiratory rate of 80 to 100 breaths per minute, whereas

(continued)

Case 13.4 *(continued)*

oxygen saturations remain 95 to 100. He is currently in room air and has not required any respiratory support for the past 5 days. An arterial blood gas demonstrated a pH of 7.24, carbon dioxide of 32, oxygen of 112, and a base deficit of −9. Chemistries include a sodium level of 130, potassium of 3.5, chloride of 92, bicarbonate of 17, blood urea nitrogen (BUN) of 6, creatinine of 0.6, and the anion gap is 21.

1. *Which diagnosis would you place first in your differential diagnostic list and why?*

   ANSWER: Short bowel syndrome. *This complication results from a lack of absorptive surface area and leads to fluid and nutrient losses when the volume of intake exceeds the ability to absorb. Fermentation of dietary sugars into acids by colonic flora adds to the diarrhea associated with malabsorption. Lack of fat-soluble vitamin absorption with ileal loss adds to the secretory diarrhea. Malabsorption then leads to electrolyte disturbances, dehydration, and failure to thrive.*

2. *Given the blood gas results presented here, what is the most likely cause for the tachypnea?*

   ANSWER: Respiratory compensation for metabolic acidosis caused by fluid and electrolyte loss from intestinal malabsorption. *A discussion on respiratory and metabolic acidosis is beyond the scope of this chapter (refer to Shaw [2008]).*

DIFFERENTIAL

Listing the presenting symptoms, history, and available study results with corresponding potential diagnoses for each helps the clinician to develop a list of tests to help guide further testing in an attempt to determine the cause of the infant's symptoms. Immediate studies for the presentation in Case 13.4 are the recalculation of enteral fluid intake and the examination of buffer support provided in the hyperalimentation (TPN). Simultaneously, a two-view abdominal x-ray is performed in addition to other studies performed concurrently, as listed in Table 13.5.

DIFFERENTIAL DIAGNOSES

To evaluate the potential causes for the new-onset diarrhea reported in the infant in Case 13.4, a differential diagnostic list is compiled using the diagnoses identified in Table 13.5. Potential diagnoses are placed in order of most to least likely, helping the practitioner to prioritize testing. A list of diagnoses can be found in Box 13.6.

PATHOPHYSIOLOGY

Infants who undergo small bowel resection for any reason who lose a substantial amount of small bowel are at risk of SBS. The small bowel of a preterm infant at 27 weeks gestation is approximately 115 cm and grows to the full-term infant length of 250 cm (Georgeson, 1998).

Table 13.5 **Clinical History, Differential Diagnoses, and Corresponding Testing for Case 13.4**

Symptom/History	Differential	Testing
Metabolic acidosis	Sepsis, decreased cardiac output, shock, hypoxia, hemorrhage, anemia, cold stress, intestinal ischemia, lactic acidosis, SBS (Gomella, 2013)	Serum lactate, CBC with differential (American Academy of Pediatrics, 2015), test results will determine further studies and treatment, EKG to consider cardiology consult, monitor vital signs and physical examination for signs of shock and cold stress, test stool for reducing substances (measures carbohydrate), abdominal x-ray (Gomella, 2013)
Hyperventilation	Respiratory distress, CNS compensation for metabolic acidosis (Gomella, 2013)	Blood gas, monitor vital signs and respiratory status, full physical examination
Central line	Sepsis	CBC, as mentioned previously
Hyperalimentation	Examine solution for lack of buffer administration, improper mixing	Increase acetate administration; examination of the current solution for proper order and mixing
Diarrhea/poor growth	SBS, overgrowth of pathogenic bacteria, hyperosmolar feedings, rapid feeding increase, inadequate caloric administration	Stool for reducing substances, examination of feeding rate of increase, evaluate feeding substrate, examine caloric intake and optimize for growth, evaluate for any possible drug side effects
Surgical NEC with loss of distal jejunum; all of ileum including, the ileocecal valve	SBS, intestinal ischemia, recurrent NEC, bacterial overgrowth (secondary to loss of ileocecal valve)	Stool for reducing substances, x-ray, consider sepsis workup
Prolonged antibiotic use at birth and again for 14 days for NEC treatment	Overgrowth of pathogenic bacteria (leading to diarrhea and bicarbonate losses), sepsis	Decrease beneficial bacteria, and potential overgrowth of pathogenic bacteria (Gephart et al., 2012; Henry & Moss, 2009); continue to encourage human milk

(continued)

Table 13.5 **Clinical History, Differential Diagnoses, and Corresponding Testing for Case 13.4 (*continued*)**

Symptom/History	Differential	Testing
Stable thrombocytopenia	Sepsis/bone marrow suppression	CBC as mentioned previously, monitor platelet count
Enteral feedings with MBM increasing 5 mL/kg/d	SBS, inaccurate calculation, evaluate for possible increase faster than expected	Examination of feeding rate of increase, evaluate feeding substrate, consider continuous feeds (Perks & Abad-Jorge, 2008)

CBC, complete blood count; CNS, central nervous system; MBM, maternal breast milk; NEC, necrotizing enterocolitis; SBS, short bowel syndrome.

Box 13.6 *Differential Diagnoses for Case 13.4*

- SBS
- CNS compensation for metabolic acidosis
- Sepsis
- Overgrowth of pathogenic bacteria
- Lack of buffer administration, improper mixing of the solution
- Hyperosmolar feedings, rapid feeding increase, inaccurate calculation
- Intestinal ischemia
- Respiratory distress
- Decreased cardiac output, shock
- Anemia
- Cold stress
- Lactic acidosis
- Hemorrhage
- Hypoxia

CNS, central nervous system; SBS, short bowel syndrome.

In the healthy full-term infant, the bowel reaches full length around 3 to 4 years of age (Adamkin, 2009). Infants who are born with abnormalities of the GI tract or who develop injury and require resection of the bowel resulting in a remaining small bowel of 40 cm or less are at increased risk for SBS. The condition of the remaining small bowel and whether or not the infant retained the ileocecal valve impacts the infant's risk of developing symptoms of this complication. Infants who have greater than 40 cm of small bowel can also develop symptoms similar to SBS related to the condition of the remaining bowel, and can present with diarrhea and malabsorption resulting from bowel wall injury, dysmotility, and bacterial overgrowth. Therefore, any infant with malabsorption experiences interference with the ability to absorb nutrients and requires time to adapt (Magnuson, Parry, &

Chwals, 2011). The inability to establish some degree of enteral intake further complicates the risk of bowel atrophy, putting the infant at greatest risk for cholestasis related to TPN and central-line infection, further prolonging the ability to achieve bowel health (Perks & Abad-Jorge, 2008).

For a description of what portion of the small bowel is responsible for secretion and absorption of various nutrients, see Table 13.6. It is important to mention here that although there is some overlap regarding what is absorbed in the jejunum and the ileum, the jejunum does not compensate for the loss of the ileum. In other words, the ileum does a good job of compensating for the loss of the jejunum but the reverse is not true.

The symptoms of SBS, as mentioned in Box 13.7, are related to a lack of absorptive surface area. This leads to fluid and nutrient losses because of poor absorption when the volume of intake exceeds the ability to absorb it. The rapidly moving small bowel contents is hyperosmolar, as it enters the bowel this creates an osmotic draw that leads to diarrhea. This is further complicated by the fermentation of dietary sugars into acids by colonic flora (Georgeson, 1998). Lack of bile salt reabsorption decreases fat and fat-soluble vitamin absorption with ileal loss and further complicates symptoms related to secretory diarrhea. Malabsorption then leads to electrolyte disturbances, dehydration, and failure to thrive (Perks & Abad-Jorge, 2008).

The small bowel has a remarkable ability to adapt; however, different segments of the small bowel adapt better than others, as previously mentioned and as presented in Table 13.6. In Case 13.4, the infant has lost all of the ileum. The remaining proximal small bowel does not adapt to the loss of ileal function well. The ileum is responsible for absorption of macronutrients, vitamin B_{12}, zinc, reabsorption of bile salts, and the secretion of hormones that adjust motility. In addition, in this case, the ileocecal valve, which helps slow the passage of intestinal contents and guard against the reflux of colonic bacteria, has been removed. This puts the infant at risk of rapid transfer of food and nutrients and exposes the colon to a high osmotic load, increasing diarrhea and nutrient losses. In Case 13.4, two thirds of the jejunum remain as does the duodenum. This will allow for absorption of macronutrients, water- and fat-soluble vitamins, minerals, intestinal hormones, pancreatic enzymes, and bile salts. However, these losses will continue if there is rapid transit interfering with adequate absorption time. Therefore, every effort has to be made to slow the transit time.

For this infant, the transit time is the key to absorption, while establishing some enteral intake is key to decreasing liver disease and limiting exposure to hyperalimentation. According to Wessel and Kocoshis (2007), infants are more sensitive to volume than concentration. Therefore, enteral feedings need to be advanced very slowly at 5 to no more than 10 mL/kg/d so as to not exceed the bowels' ability for absorption. Furthermore, the degree of threshold is different for each infant and, as mentioned before, is very dependent on damage to the epithelial cell lining and condition of the brush boarder necessary for absorption (Adamkin, 2009; Magnuson et al., 2011). The bowel can adapt by increasing crypt depth and villus height by way of mucosal hyperplasia with exposure to enteral substrate. Eventually, the bowel will lengthen and hypertrophy will increase the surface area available for absorption; however, how long that will take depends on the ability to establish enteral intake (Georgeson, 1998).

TESTING

Monitoring stool output is essential; the volume should remain less than 30 mL/kg/d. A sign of increased organic acids from the breakdown of carbohydrate (CHO) can be measured by stool pH and is positive with a pH less than 5.5. If diarrhea should occur, measuring stool for reducing substances can be useful to evaluate for CHO malabsorption (Adamkin, 2009). Fats

Table 13.6 Function of the Small Bowel

Section of Bowel	Stomach	Duodenum	Jejunum	Ileum
Secretion	Hydrochloric acid to digest proteins and add a protective barrier; diverse amines support growth and differentiation, digestion, and regulation (Magnuson et al., 2011)	Pancreatic enzymes/bile acid and intestinal hormone regulation (Magnuson et al., 2011)		Intestinal hormones control gut motility and transit time; ileocecal valve slows transit and prevents reflux of bacteria from colon (deSilva et al., 2006; Magnus et al., 2011)
Absorption	Vitamin B_{12}	Fat-soluble vitamins and digestion of fats	Carbohydrate, protein, and fat Vitamin B_{12}, zinc, and the reabsorption of bile salts (Zeigler, 1986); fat-soluble vitamins/minerals, including Fe, Ca, and Mg	Carbohydrate, protein, and fat Greatest absorption of vitamin B_{12}, zinc, and reabsorption of bile salts

Box 13.7 Symptoms of SBS

- Diarrhea
- Steatorrhea
- Electrolyte disturbances
- Metabolic acidosis
- Failure to thrive
- Dehydration

SBS, short bowel syndrome.

are better tolerated than CHO, because the fermentation of CHO can cause bloating and increase osmotic draw, which leads to diarrhea. A reducing substances test is positive if greater than 1/2% and is a concern for SBS. Close monitoring and correction of fluid, electrolyte, and metabolic abnormalities are imperative. It is equally important to recognize that enteral calories for growth need to be at least 10% higher than parenteral calories to account for lack of nutrient absorption and the calorie expenditure of digestion. In addition, keep in mind that after NEC or bowel resection caloric demands can be 10% to 50% higher than in other infants of the same gestation (Perks & Abad-Jorge, 2008). Monitoring of fat-soluble vitamins as well as zinc and copper levels is also important (Adamkin, 2009). Infants with SBS are also at risk of metabolic bone disease and require monitoring of calcium and phosphorous levels. Liver and bone disease necessitate the need to monitor for coagulation abnormalities. It is recommended to get baseline coagulation studies and to continue this testing periodically thereafter until the infant is off TPN and labs are normal. Determining baseline liver functions and continuing to test every other week is recommended to assess TPN tolerance (Perks & Abad-Jorge, 2008; Price, 2000).

TREATMENT

It is always best to start by treating the underlying cause of SBS if this is known (Gomella, 2013). Often the cause is related to exceeding the threshold of the enteral intake. Identifying this threshold volume is difficult and can take some trial and error. This is further complicated by the need to establish enteral intake to encourage bowel healing and improve motility as well as enzyme and hormone production. The establishment of beneficial bacterial growth and bowel length is also dependent on enteral feeding. Although maternal breast milk is the gold standard for infant nutrition, the severity of the diarrhea and metabolic derangements may require changing feedings to an elemental formula to maintain some degree of enteral intake, at least temporarily. Some infants will tolerate bolus feedings, but most with significant bowel loss will require continuous feeding, which allows for saturation of the bowel lining and increases exposure to available surface area for absorption (Adamkin, 2009; Perks & Abad-Jorge, 2008).

It is paramount to first provide nutritional support to establish a normal growth pattern and support healing. This will require the use of hyperalimentation and central-line access. The next step is to establish enteral intake beginning at a rate of 5 to 10 mL/kg/d. This may require maintaining only elemental feedings for long periods while monitoring electrolytes and stooling pattern to avoid diarrhea. Daily weights and strict intake and output are also essential. After there has been some establishment of enteral intake, the addition of soluble fiber in the form of pectin, green beans, or guar gum can help decrease transit time. In the colon, fiber ferments to short chain fatty acids, which provide multiple benefits for the colon, including the stimulation of sodium transport, which reduces colonic water and decreases diarrhea (Adamkin, 2009).

Carbohydrate malabsorption can lead to gastric acid hypersecretion secondary to loss of the negative feedback. Acid hypersecretion in the stomach is secondary to markedly elevated gastrin levels, which contribute to the increased osmotic load presented to the distal bowel. Therefore, an H_2 blocker can be considered when the stool pH is less than 5.5 (Vanderhoof, Zach, & Adrian, 2005).

Cholestyramine is another possible treatment for infants who have severe diarrhea. This is an ion exchange resin used to control diarrhea because it binds bile salts that contribute to diarrhea. Caution is required with this therapy as there can be an increase in fat malabsorption, risk of metabolic bone disease, and the potential for constipation (Adamkin, 2009; Perks & Abad-Jorge, 2008). Steatorrhea, indicating poor fat absorption, raises concern for a low bile salt pool and the need to assess adequate absorption of fat-soluble vitamins and zinc (Adamkin, 2009). With SBS and long-term hyperalimentation (TPN), infants are also at risk of deficiency of vitamins A, E, K, B_{12}, and zinc. It is important to recognize that the preterm infant with SBS has increased susceptibility to calcium, phosphorus, sodium, and zinc losses and even depletion. This indicates the need for close monitoring (Wessel & Kocoshis, 2007).

Infants who develop cholestatic liver disease from TPN and only tolerate low enteral intake may benefit from the use of phenobarbital and ursodeoxycholic acid to enhance liver function and bile secretion (Magnuson et al., 2011). Cycling of TPN is potentially another way of decreasing liver damage if the infant can maintain adequate glucose levels (Adamkin, 2009; Perks & Abad-Jorge, 2008).

Last options for those infants who are unable to establish adequate enteral nutrition and lack of bowel growth are surgical procedures to lengthen the small bowel to increase surface area. A procedure known as *longitudinal intestinal lengthening and tapering* (LILT) increases bowel surface area and carries a variable improved survival of 30% to 100%. The serial transverse enteroplasty procedure (STEP) involves using staples to narrow an area of dilated bowel, improving absorption and surface area. The treatment of last resort is bowel transplant (Magnuson et al., 2011).

RELATED COMPLICATIONS

Mortality is approximately 20% in infants who experience SBS because of related risks of infection from central-line access complicated by overall poor nutrition. Lack of intravenous access presents another very difficult complication. Liver disease and cholestasis secondary to long-term TPN, if severe, lead to death within the first year of life (Adamkin, 2009). As mentioned previously, the bowels' ability to compensate for the loss of small intestine depends on the functional portion of small bowel that remains and whether or not the infant has retained the ileocecal valve. In addition, without terminal ileum, the patient is susceptible to gall stone formation as well as oxalate renal stones resulting from increased oxalate absorption in the colon. Children colonized with lactobacilli convert excess CHO to D-lactate dehydrogenase, which is poorly metabolized, resulting in significant D-lactic acidosis, which can lead to coma and death (Vanderhoof et al., 2005).

Some infants, especially those who have 40 cm of small bowel or less, are more likely to require TPN upon discharge and for some time thereafter. These infants require multiple follow-up appointments coordinated by their pediatrician, including pediatric surgery, nutrition, and gastroenterology. Visiting and block nursing are often put in place. The family will need education, support, and counseling by the APN related to central-line and TPN management, risks and signs of infection, as well as feeding intolerance and dehydration. Equally important will be initiating consult with a social worker and establishing social support prior to discharge.

MECONIUM ILEUS

Case 13.5

A former 37 4/7-gestation male Caucasian infant was born to a 32-year-old gravida 1, now para 1 mother by way of normal spontaneous vaginal delivery after an uncomplicated pregnancy. The infant presents in the newborn nursery at 48 hours of life with bilious vomiting, gross distention, and persistent poor feeding. The pediatrician on call orders a two-view abdominal x-ray and consults with both radiology for an upper gastrointestinal (UGI) series and the neonatal intensive care unit (NICU) for further recommendations and potential transfer. The abdominal film is significant for calcifications noted over the right upper quadrant and gross small bowel distention. The distended bowel loops have a soap bubble appearance.

The infant's birth weight was 3.2 kg and the Apgar scores were 9 and 9 at 1 and 5 minutes, respectively. The infant had been eating fairly well at the breast over the past 24 hours. He has not passed stool and has been voiding adequately.

1. **What x-ray finding is concerning for meconium peritonitis?**

   ANSWER: Calcifications over the right upper quadrant. *This finding can be a sign of complicated meconium ileus with perforation in utero. The calcification is the by-product of healing process.*

2. **What interventions would you consider to help stabilize this patient while waiting for further radiographic and possibly surgical intervention?**

   ANSWER: Make the infant nothing by mouth (NPO), place an oral gastric tube to suction for decompression and intravenous fluids. *These interventions should be initiated immediately prior to transfer where additional radiographic studies and lab testing will be performed.*

DIFFERENTIAL

Given the findings on the abdominal x-ray ordered for the infant in Case 13.5, the radiologist recommends starting with a BE, given the appearance of distal small bowel obstruction, to be followed by a UGI if necessary. Listing the presenting symptoms, history, and available study results with corresponding potential diagnoses for each helps the clinician develop a list of tests that will guide further testing in an attempt to determine the cause of the infant's symptoms. An immediate study for this case presentation is a two-view abdominal x-ray in addition to other tests performed concurrently, as listed in Table 13.7.

Table 13.7 **Concerning Symptoms, Differential Diagnoses, and Corresponding Testing for Case 13.5**

Symptom/History	Differential	Testing
Bilious vomiting/ abdominal distention/ bowel calcifications with a soap bubble appearance on x-ray/ failure to pass meconium	In utero meconium peritonitis, malrotation with or without volvulus, until proven otherwise Small bowel obstruction distal to the ampulla of Vater Ileus (second to infection) Meconium plug Meconium ileus Reflux Hirschsprung's disease Idiopathic	Full examination, UGI is the gold standard, two-view KUB required if UGI is not immediately available Barium enema is preferred to start with this case, given the bowel gas noted in the distal small intestine (deSilva et al., 2006) Full electrolyte panel to assess dehydration, acidosis (Barksdale et al., 2011) Hirschsprung's unlikely given the infant has stooled, but very possible
Abdominal distention/ poor feeding, bilious vomiting	Sepsis with possible ileus	CBC with differential (American Academy of Pediatrics, 2015), test results will determine further studies and treatment Abdominal (two-view) x-ray
Bowel obstruction, concern for meconium ileus, Caucasian male	Cystic fibrosis	Chromosomal analysis, newborn screening, parental screening, sweat test

CBC, complete blood count; KUB, kidney, ureters, and bladder; UGI, upper gastrointestinal.

DIFFERENTIAL DIAGNOSES

To evaluate the potential causes for the abdominal distention and bilious vomiting seen in the infant in Case 13.5, a differential diagnostic list is compiled using the diagnoses identified in Table 13.7. Potential diagnoses are ordered from most to least likely to help the practitioner prioritize testing. A list of diagnoses can be found in Box 13.8.

PATHOPHYSIOLOGY

This ileus is caused by thick tenacious meconium creating hard sticky pellets that adhere to the bowel wall lining, usually in the distal ileum, that cause obstruction. These pellets are also referred to as *inspissated meconium*. Conditions that would cause the meconium to be dry, such as a pancreatic enzyme deficiency, result in a tenacious sticky meconium that leads to blockage (deSilva et al., 2006; van der Doef, Kokke, van der Ent, & Houwen, 2011).

With simple meconium ileus, the infant has inspissated meconium that blocks the distal small intestine. This can be seen in infants who are small for gestational age, premature, or who have CF. The meconium blocks the passage of intestinal contents, which leads to

| **Box 13.8 *Differential Diagnoses for Case 13.5*** |

- Meconium ileus
- Cystic fibrosis
- Meconium plug
- Small bowel atresia
- Proximal colonic atresia
- Total colonic Hirschsprung's disease
- Congenital hypothyroidism

Source: Barksdale et al. (2011).

abdominal distention, vomiting with or without bile, and often results in failure to pass stool. In complicated meconium ileus, there is obstruction in utero significant enough to cause distention and ischemia, which leads to perforation and/or volvulus. When perforation occurs, the bowel contents enter the peritoneum, causing inflammation and a chemical reaction. This reaction leads to the appearance of echogenic bowel seen on prenatal ultrasound, which is calcification that occurs with healing. The calcifications can then be seen on an abdominal x-ray. This finding is concerning for perforation, but can be seen for other reasons as well, such as with infection. The calcifications can be located in one isolated area or scattered throughout the abdomen. Perforation in utero can also lead to a meconium pseudocyst. This occurs when the meconium that spills into the peritoneum forms what appears as a cyst at the site of perforation and may be palpated on examination as a mass. Perforation can also lead to bowel adhesions that create further obstruction (deSilva et al., 2006; Parry, 2015). If volvulus should occur early enough in gestation, the affected portion of the bowel can be absorbed, presenting with an atresia at birth. Both uncomplicated and complicated meconium ileus present with microcolon, which results from a colon of disuse (deSilva et al., 2006; Puder, 2009). An x ray presenting this finding can be found in deSilva et al. (2006). These infants will typically present with bilious vomiting, failure to pass stool, and abdominal distention. The maternal history may also include polyhydramnios and often a family history of CF (Puder, 2009). Other associated diseases, CF, and meconium plug warrant mention here to identify the relationship and distinct differences of each.

CF Causing Meconium Ileus

Infants who present with meconium ileus are at high risk for CF. Patients with CF have a very high content of sodium in their sweat, which is normally hypotonic. The gene mutation leads to poor permeability of chloride, therefore, salt cannot be reabsorbed (Cuthbert, 1992). The high salt content leads to very dry viscous secretions in the glands affected. This occurs at the level of epithelial cells within mucus-secreting glands and exocrine cells of the pancreas. This disease also affects the epithelia of the respiratory tract, intestinal tract, male genital tract, and hepatobiliary system. CF is an autosomal recessive inherited disease that requires two gene mutations. In Whites, one in 20 individuals is a carrier, making it most common in Caucasians living in the northern hemisphere (Larson-Nath, Gurram, & Chelimsky, 2015). Seventy percent of patients with CF will have the gene mutation at position 508, known as *ΔF508*. However, there are over 1,600 mutations that account for the additional 30%, making universal screening impossible (Larson-Nath et al., 2015).

Meconium Plug Syndrome

Infants with meconium plug syndrome may present with delayed stooling and abdominal distention. This is a disease of the distal colon and rectum, most often associated with prematurity, which results in immature motility of the intestine. This is also seen in the infants of diabetics and is considered small left colon syndrome. On abdominal x-ray, there may be small and large bowel obstruction without air fluid levels (Gomella, 2013). A meconium plug is distinctly different from meconium ileus in that the plug, which appears white like a mucus bullet, when evacuated relieves the symptoms. A BE can again be effective in evacuating the plug and relieving the obstruction. The BE is also helpful in demonstrating the small left colon. If after evacuation normal bowel function expected for the infant's maturity level does not occur, testing for CF or a biopsy for Hirschsprung's disease should be considered (Parry, 2015).

TESTING

The classic "soap bubble" appearance on x-ray, which represents air or fluid mixed with the meconium, and the distal small bowel location will lead the radiologist to suggest a BE before a UGI, even in those infants who present with bilious vomiting (deSilva et al., 2006; Parry, 2015; Puder, 2009). The BE works both to diagnose and to treat. First, a colon of disuse is discovered, followed by the inspissated meconium, which is relieved by the contrast solution. Although 20% to 30% of infants with CF will have a meconium ileus (deSilva et al., 2006), 90% of infants with meconium ileus have CF (Puder, 2009; van der Doef et al., 2011). Therefore, it is imperative that all infants with a meconium ileus have a genetics consult and genetic testing. However, testing for the CF gene can be inconclusive given the multiple mutations, therefore all infants will need to have a "sweat test," which is the gold standard for detecting CF (Puder, 2009).

TREATMENT

Initial treatment should include bowel decompression with a gastric tube to continuous suction. The examination of electrolytes for dehydration and metabolic acidosis is necessary given poor feeding, vomiting, and concerns for bowel necrosis. Rehydration with intravenous fluids should be initiated immediately. A sepsis workup should be initiated and antibiotics started, if indicated. If the infant demonstrates free air on the x-ray, immediate surgical intervention is required to relieve the obstruction and remove any necrotic bowel (Parry, 2015).

The contrast solution used for a BE can be very effective in mobilizing the inspissated meconium as it draws water into the bowel, and therefore is effective in clearing the obstruction and outlining the microcolon in uncomplicated meconium ileus. Depending on the degree of evacuation, the infant may need additional enemas with N-acetylcysteine (Mucomyst) to further evacuate inspissated meconium. With complicated meconium ileus, the infant will almost always require surgery to examine the bowel for obstruction, to evacuate the meconium, resect any atretic or necrotic bowel, and correct volvulus if one is present. This may or may not result in the need for an ostomy (deSilva et al., 2006; Puder, 2009).

Hyperalimentation will be necessary if the infant is expected to be NPO for any extended period of time. Enteral feedings with human milk or an elemental formula may be initiated once bowel function has been restored. Pancreatic enzymes should be considered when feeding is established, unless there is a good reason to not consider CF (Parry, 2015).

Related Complications

Infants who have complicated meconium ileus will almost always require surgical intervention as a result of adhesions, atresia, and/or volvulus. Therefore, additional risks associated with surgery, recovery, and healing are a concern. Some will require an ostomy, putting them at risk of SBS (see Case 13.4 on SBS). This is dependent on the degree of injury and how much bowel is removed. Problems associated with poor wound healing, long-term TPN, the risk of associated cholestasis, further obstruction secondary to adhesions, as well as line infection warrant close monitoring. All infants with meconium ileus will require a genetic consult and genetic testing for CF.

Following surgery, the infant may have an ileus, which prolongs the ability to start enteral intake. Slow transit times and dyskinetic bowel are always a concern and are dependent on recovery of any proximally dilated bowel, which can make the establishment of full enteral feedings difficult (Parry, 2015). Prolonged hospital stay can be significant for infants with meconium ileus if it is associated with CF as it can be difficult to establish positive weight gain in these babies. Infants with CF will require pancreatic enzymes and fat-soluble vitamin replacement. However, it does not end there; van der Doef et al. (2011) describe the lifelong problems associated with constipation that CF patients experience as a result of slow intestinal transit coupled with poor digestion, which leads to impaction. Therefore, stooling patterns require close monitoring in support of adequate bowel health. Long-term nursing services and additional surgery to reverse the ostomy may be required. There will be a need for family education, support, and counseling by the APN, as well as follow-up with genetics, pulmonary, and CF clinics to coordinate a full range of care services.

HIRSCHSPRUNG'S DISEASE (GI OBSTRUCTION)

Case 13.6

Baby L is a former 38-week-gestation female infant born by normal spontaneous vaginal delivery to a 32-year-old gravida 1, now para 1. Maternal history was significant for known trisomy 21 with a moderately sized membranous ventricular septal defect (VSD). Her birth weight was 3.005 kg. The infant was cared for in the well-baby nursery and was nursing well at the breast prior to discharge home on day of life (DOL) 2. Baby L had adequate urine output and stooled two times prior to discharge.

Now on DOL 9, Baby L has only had two stools since discharge. She has had some vomiting, occasionally yellow/green in color. The pediatrician instructed the parents to give Baby L a glycerin suppository daily and changed the feedings to 24 cal/oz of elemental formula, as the infant's weight is now 2.855 kg, down 5% from birth. Now at 2 weeks of life, Baby L continues to vomit, and is feeding and stooling poorly. The stools are very small in volume and watery. At 3 weeks of life, the parents bring Baby L to the emergency room given concerns for poor feeding, abdominal distention, persistent vomiting (yellow-green), and lethargy. At this time, her weight is now 2.556 kg, down 15% from her birth weight.

In the emergency room, she was given intravenous fluids (IVF) because of concerns for dehydration. She presented with gross abdominal distention, which prompted an

(continued)

Case 13.6 (*continued*)

abdominal x-ray and upper gastrointestinal (UGI) series, which showed no sign of obstruction, malrotation, or volvulus, but there was gross bowel distention with air fluid levels. The infant was admitted to the NICU. Upon admission, Baby L was put on nothing by mouth (NPO) status and a nasogastric tube with low continuous suction was started in addition to the IVF. Serial abdominal x-rays were followed that became concerning for a transition zone. Surgery and pediatric gastroenterology were both consulted on this case.

1. **Within how many hours of life do 98.5% of term infants have their first stool?**

   ANSWER: 24 hours.

2. **What does a "transition zone" on an abdominal x-ray represent?**

   ANSWER: An area from where there is gross distention to normal caliber bowel. *This area of transition indicates the grossly distended normal bowel that then transitions to the normal caliber abnormal bowel that does not contain ganglion cells.*

DIFFERENTIAL

Given the findings on the abdominal x-ray of Baby L in Case 13.6, both the surgeon and the radiologist recommended performing a BE to further evaluate the rectal/sigmoid region given the concern for a transition zone on the abdominal x-ray. Listing the presenting symptoms, history, and available study results with corresponding potential diagnoses for each helps the clinician develop a list of tests to help guide further testing in an attempt to determine the cause of the infant's symptoms. Immediate study for this presentation is a two-view abdominal x-ray in addition to other studies performed concurrently, as listed in Table 13.8.

DIFFERENTIAL DIAGNOSES

To evaluate the potential causes for abdominal distention and bilious vomiting of the infant in Case 13.6, a differential diagnostic list is compiled using the diagnoses identified in Table 13.7. Potential diagnoses are placed in order of most to least likely, helping the practitioner to prioritize testing. A list of diagnoses can be found in Box 13.9

PATHOPHYSIOLOGY

Examination of the history for the stooling pattern when an infant presents with distention and/or vomiting can be most revealing. In the full-term infant, 98.5% of all infants will stool in the first 24 hours of life, whereas 100% of full term and 98.8% of preterm (> 32 weeks gestation) infants will stool by 48 hours. Typically, a newborn will stool four times per day for the first week of life (Gomella, 2013). Therefore, this symptom can help guide testing and narrow the differential diagnostic list. The most common cause of intestinal obstruction of the neonate is Hirschsprung's disease, also known as *megacolon*, which occurs in one in 5,000 live births. This disease is an abnormality of development, with an arrest of the

Table 13.8 Concerning Symptoms, Differential Diagnoses, and Corresponding Testing for Case 13.6

Symptom/History	Differential	Testing
Constipation/gross abdominal distention	Imperforate anus; maternal medications that decrease motility (e.g., magnesium sulfate, morphine), Hirschsprung's disease, large bowel obstruction, hypothyroidism, dehydration, electrolyte abnormalities (hyponatremia, hypokalemia, hypoglycemia; Gomella, 2013)	Physical examination, examination of infant and maternal history, electrolytes, abdominal x-ray
Initial lack of weight gain, weight down 5% from BW at 9 days, then down 15% from BW at 3 weeks of life	Poor feeding and low tone second to trisomy 21 Poor feeding and vomiting second to obstruction, or sepsis	Full neuro examine with attention to root/suck/Moro reflexes; monitor weight twice weekly; with persistent weight loss needs more detailed testing given other symptoms
Yellow/green emesis and spitty with feeding; trisomy 21 with moderate membranous VSD	Bilious vomiting risk of malrotation and volvulus until proven otherwise, high risk for duodenal atresia or Hirschsprung's disease given prenatal diagnosis of trisomy 21; also need to consider: Hypoganglionosis Neuronal intestinal dysplasia type A (Gomella, 2013) Small bowel obstruction distal to the ampulla of Vater Ileus Meconium plug Reflux Idiopathic disease	UGI gold standard, two-view KUB required if UGI is not immediately available Barium enema may be necessary if symptoms persist and previous studies are not diagnostic or if other findings indicate distal obstruction Hirschsprung's disease less likely given the infant has stooled
Lack of stool requiring glycerin suppositories	Hirschsprung's, anorectal malformation with fistula (Gomella, 2013)	Two-view KUB followed by barium enema

(continued)

Table 13.8 Concerning Symptoms, Differential Diagnoses, and Corresponding Testing for Case 13.6 (*continued*)

Symptom/History	Differential	Testing
Persistent bilious vomiting, weight loss, dehydration, lack of stool, lethargy, gross abdominal distention	Sepsis with ileus Bowel obstruction, given lack of stool consider Hirschsprung's disease Hypoganglionosis Neuronal intestinal dysplasia type A (Gomella, 2013) Meconium plug syndrome Severe reflux Hypothyroidism Maternal magnesium administration	CBC with differential (American Academy of Pediatrics, 2015), test results will determine further studies and treatment; abdominal (two view) x-ray followed by barium enema; magnesium crosses the placenta decreasing bowel motility

BW, birth weight; CBC, complete blood count; KUB, kidney, ureters, and bladder; UGI, upper gastrointestinal; VSD, ventricular septal defect.

Box 13.9 *Differential Diagnoses for Case 13.6*

- Hirschsprung's disease
- Hypoganglionosis
- Dehydration
- Small left colon
- Neuronal intestinal dysplasia
- Small and large bowel stenosis/atresias
- Anal rectal malformation with fistula
- Sepsis with ileus
- Megacystis—microcolon with hypoperistalsis (Berdon's syndrome)
- Hypothyroidism
- Meconium ileus
- Meconium plug syndrome
- Idiopathic

Sources: Barksdale et al. (2011), Gomella (2013).

---

myenteric nervous system as the neural crest cells fail to migrate between the fifth and 12th weeks of gestation, which results in aganglionosis. Ganglion cells are necessary for peristalsis, the propulsion of the bolus of food through the GI track. Typically, the anal sphincter is triggered to relax and allow for stool evacuation once the rectum fills with stool. However, with Hirschsprung's disease the absence of parasympathetic ganglion cells removes the trigger for the sphincter to relax, the muscle becomes hypertrophied, and stool is unable to move forward. This causes a backup and distention of the proximal bowel and the affected area remains small from lack of stool and disuse (deSilva et al., 2006; McAlhany & Popovich, 2007). This area of the bowel is seen as the transition zone on a radiograph and can be found in deSilva et al. (2006).

The distal colon is the most commonly affected portion of the bowel and can account for up to 15% of infants who fail to pass stool within 48 hours of birth (Gomella, 2013). However, more proximal segments can be affected beginning distally at the rectum and moving more proximally, including the entire colon and rarely a portion of the small bowel (deSilva et al., 2006; McAlhany & Popovich, 2007). Therefore, the disease is described as either short- or long-segment Hirschsprung's depending on the amount of bowel involved. Short segment usually only involves the rectosigmoid region. The most common associated genetic disease is trisomy 21 occurring in 8% to 16% of infants with this congenital anomaly (McAlhany & Popovich, 2007; Parry, 2015). The disease is more common in males than females (4:1) and most common among White males (Gomella, 2013; McAlhany & Popovich, 2007). Genetics consult is very important for families of these infants, because there is an increased risk of 4% to 8% for Hirschsprung's disease in siblings (deSilva et al., 2006; Parry, 2015).

TESTING

As previously mentioned, a two-view abdominal x-ray will provide the clinician with information about bowel gas pattern, distention, or possible perforation. An infant with Hirschsprung's disease will have a dilated bowel with air fluid levels and lack of air in the rectum. Up to 91% of infants with Hirschsprung's disease will have abdominal distention and as many as 37% will have bilious vomiting. Most infants will have failed to pass meconium within 48 hours of life. With bilious vomiting, a UGI to rule out malrotation and volvulus is imperative. If the UGI is reassuring, the next step is to perform a BE to evaluate the lower GI tract and, in Case 13.6, is important given the degree of distention. Although in some cases the KUB (kidney, ureters, and bladder) can be very helpful if a transition zone is noted, thereby redirecting the choice to perform a BE first, as in this case presentation. Infants with Hirschsprung's disease who do not present at birth present later in infancy with a history of constipation and foul-smelling ribbon-like stools and failure to thrive, as in Case 13.6 (McAlhany & Popovich, 2007). The BE can be not only diagnostic, but also therapeutic as it helps evacuate the obstruction should the infant have a meconium plug or meconium ileus (Parry, 2015).

If the initial studies are inconclusive, following the infant with serial abdominal x-rays to monitor evacuation of the contrast is helpful. If the infant has Hirschsprung's disease, an area known as the *transition zone* will appear with marked proximal dilatation followed by significant distal narrowing, described as funneling, which occurs where the bowel becomes aganglionic (deSilva et al., 2006). In the infant who presents beyond the immediate newborn period, the bowel can take on a ragged appearance noted on the BE, which is consistent with enterocolitis (deSilva et al., 2006). If the radiographic testing is suspicious for Hirschsprung's disease or if the infant continues to have dilation without improvement with conservative therapy, a suction biopsy, which has high sensitivity and specificity, is performed. This procedure collects two to three samples of the mucosal lining of the bowel for examination. If negative and still highly suspicious, a full-thickness rectal biopsy is necessary to make the diagnosis. The samples are then examined for the presence of ganglion cells. If ganglion cells are absent and acetyl cholinesterase–positive hypertrophic nerve fibers are present (on staining), the diagnosis is positive for Hirschsprung's disease (Gomella, 2013; McAlhany & Popovich, 2007).

TREATMENT

Initially the infant will require fluid resuscitation. Close monitoring of electrolytes is necessary as well as measurement of intake and output. Consideration should be given to the administration of hyperalimentation dependent on the degree of growth failure as with Case 13.6, with a plan for surgery. Bowel decompression with nasogastric suction should begin immediately as bowel perforation secondary to gross overdistention can occur in 3% to 4% of these infants (Gomella, 2013). The treatment for Hirschsprung's disease requires the removal of the aganglionic segment. Therefore, all of these infants will require surgery, as the ultimate goal is to remove the obstruction, return normal bowel function, and preserve continence. The type of surgical repair is dependent on how proximal ganglion cells are found within the bowel and on surgeon preference.

There are two types of repair. When the colon is absent of ganglion cells up to or beyond the splenic flexure, a diversion colostomy is typically performed known as the transabdominal approach (TAA). This procedure will require repeat staged surgery as the infant grows until the colostomy is reversed. The more common procedure is the transanal endorectal pull through (TERP), which has been shown to decrease length of stay and decrease cost. There are two types of TERP. The first takes place close to the time of diagnosis. The second is used when the patient is stable; there is a preference for the delayed approach. When delayed, the goal is to get the infant to grow to double the birth weight with the use of some enteral feeding, with TPN support when needed. This is achieved with the use of rectal irrigations to keep the bowel decompressed (Kim et al., 2010).

RELATED COMPLICATIONS

Enterocolitis is a potential and serious complication of Hirschsprung's disease that occurs when the bowel is unable to be adequately decompressed. This complication can occur before or after repair and is a major cause of morbidity and mortality in these patients. Although surgery is not an emergency, adequate decompression and bowel evacuation are a must to preserve bowel integrity. As with any surgery, poor wound healing, infection, abdominal distention, obstruction and anal stenosis, anastomotic stricture or leak, and hernia are concerns and more or less likely depending on the type of procedure performed. The infant who requires a diverting colostomy will require reversal and a pull-through procedure at some point, usually within the first year of life (McAlhany & Popovich, 2007).

If the infant should have the pull-through procedure, the patient may still experience long-term problems with constipation, fecal incontinence, and enterocolitis (Kim et al., 2010; Levitt, Dickie, & Pena, 2010). Parents need to be educated on what to watch for and when to notify the pediatrician. Infants who experience any of these complications require further evaluation of the anatomy and, in some situations, need additional surgery to correct the dysfunction. Stricture at the anastomosis may require regular dilatation. Discharge instructions will need to include educating the family on how to perform the rectal dilatation (McAlhany & Popovich, 2007). Abdominal distention and enterocolitis can lead to failure to thrive further, thereby complicating an infant's recovery. Some patients with incontinence go on to require diet modification to encourage constipation and daily enemas in an attempt to regulate bowel function. Kim et al. (2010) examined 281 infants who underwent either a TAA or TERP procedure for Hirschsprung's disease and found the risk of incontinence to be the same regardless of the approach. Therefore, stretching of the anal sphincter during the TERP procedure does not seem to be a risk for later incontinence. Children who go on to have difficulty with incontinence may have social difficulty and experience emotional distress, requiring further support (Levitt et al., 2010). These infants require ongoing examination and evaluation of their growth and bowel continence. Education, medical management, emotional support, and follow-up can be managed and supported by the APN.

CONCLUSIONS

Anomalies occurring along the intestine interrupt the body's ability to consume, digest, and absorb nutrients necessary for our very survival. Abnormalities that cause obstruction, such as duodenal atresia, malrotation with volvulus, meconium ileus, and Hirschsprung's disease, can be corrected surgically, whereas acquired diseases, such as NEC and SBS, can cause injury, leading to long-term disability and even death. Malformations or diseases discussed in the chapter have the potential for complications that result in long-term disability requiring ongoing medical and nursing care. The APN care many of these patients will need, as they strive to regain maximum bowel function.

ACKNOWLEDGMENTS

To my husband, James, and children, Heidi, Jessica, and Daniel, who have encouraged and supported me throughout my professional career. To my grandchildren, may they grow to know and understand the importance of sharing knowledge.

REFERENCES

Adamkin, D. H. (2009). *Nutritional strategies for the very low birth weight infant*. New York, NY: Cambridge University Press.

American Academy of Pediatrics. (2015). *Red book report of the committee on infectious diseases* (30th ed., p. 683). Elk Grove Village, IL: Author.

Barksdale, E. M., Chwals, W. J., Magnuson, D. K., & Parry, R. L. (2011). The gastrointestinal tract: Part 3 Selected gastrointestinal anomalies. In R. J. Martin, A. A. Fanaroff, & M. C. Walsh (Eds.), *Fanaroff and Martin's neonatal-perinatal medicine: Diseases of the fetus and infant* (9th ed., pp. 1400–1430). St. Louis, MO: Mosby.

Bell, M. J., Ternberg, J. L., Feigin, R. D., Keating, J. P., Marshall, R., Barton, L., & Brotherton, T. (1978). Necrotizing enterocolitis: Therapeutic decisions based upon clinical staging. *Annals of Surgery, 187*(1), 1–7.

Bingham, E. M. (2012). Optimizing nutrition in the neonatal intensive care unit: A look at enteral nutrition and the prevention of necrotizing enterocolitis. *Topics in Clinical Nutrition, 27*(3), 250–259.

Caplan, M. S. (2015). Neonatal necrotizing enterocolitis. In R. J. Martin, A. A. Fanaroff, & M. C. Walsh (Eds.), *Fanaroff and Martin's neonatal-perinatal medicine: Diseases of the fetus and infant* (10th ed., pp. 1423–1432). Philadelphia, PA: Saunders.

Committee on Infectious Diseases and Committee on Fetus and Newborn (CIDCFN). (2011). Policy statement for the prevention of perinatal group B streptococcal (GBS) disease. *Pediatrics, 128*(3), 611–616.

Cooney, D. R. (1998). Defects of the abdominal wall. In J. A. O'Neill, M. I. Rowe, J. L. Grosfeld, E. W. Fonkalsrud, & A. G. Coran (Eds.), *Pediatric surgery* (5th ed., pp. 1045–1069). St. Louis, MO: Mosby.

Cuthbert, A. W. (1992). The biochemical defect in cystic fibrosis. *European Respiratory Journal, 85*(19), 2–5.

deSilva, N. T., Young, J. A., & Wales, P. W. (2006). Understanding neonatal bowel obstruction: Building knowledge to advance practice. *Neonatal Network, 25*(5), 303–318.

Donahue, L. (2007). Spontaneous intestinal perforation. *Neonatal Network, 26*(5), 335–351.

Filston, H. C., & Kirks, D. R. (1981). Malrotation the ubiquitous anomaly. *Journal of Pediatric Surgery, 16*(4, Suppl. 1), S614–S620.

Georgeson, K. E. (1998). Short-bowel syndrome. In J. A. O'Neill, M. I. Rowe, J. L. Grosfeld, E. W. Fonkalsrud, & A. G. Coran (Eds.), *Pediatric surgery* (5th ed., pp. 1223–1232). St. Louis, MO: Mosby.

Gephart, S. M., & Hanson, C. K. (2013). Preventing necrotizing enterocolitis with standardized feeding protocols, not only possible but imperative. *Advances in Neonatal Care, 13*(1), 48–54.

Gephart, S. M., McGrath, J. M., Effken, J. A., & Halpern, M. D. (2012). Necrotizing enterocolitis risk: State of the science. *Advances in Neonatal Care, 12*(2), 77–87.

Gephart, S. M., Poole, S. H., & Crain, D. R. (2014). Qualitative description of neonatal expert perspectives about necrotizing enterocolitis risk. *Newborn & Infant Nursing Reviews, 14*, 124–130.

Gomella, T. L. (2013). *Neonatology, management, procedures, on-call, problems, diseases, and drugs* (7th ed.). New York, NY: McGraw-Hill.

Good, M., Sodhi, C. P., Hackam, D. J. (2014). Evidenced feeding strategies before and after the development of necrotizing enterocolitis. *Expert Review of Clinical Immunology, 10*(7), 875–884. doi:10.1586/1744666X.2014.913481

Gordon, P. V., Swanson, J. R., Attridge, J. T., & Clark, R. (2007). Emerging trends in acquired intestinal disease: Is it time to abandon Bell's criteria? *Journal of Perinatology, 27*, 661–671.

Henry, M. C. W., & Moss, R. L. (2009). Necrotizing enterocolitis. *Annual Review of Medicine, 60*, 111–124.

Horton, K. K. (2005). Pathophysiology and current management of necrotizing entercolitis. *Neonatal Network, 24*(1), 37–46.

Kim, A. C., Langer, J. C., Pastor, A. C., Zhang, L., Sloots, C. E. J., Hamilton, N. A., . . . Teitelbaum, D. H. (2010). Endorectal pull-through for Hirschsprung's disease—A multicenter long term comparison of results: Transanal vs transabdominal approach. *Journal of Pediatric Surgery, 45*, 1213–1220.

Kimberlin, D. W., Brady, M. T., Jackson, M. A., & Long, S. S. (2015). *Red book: 2015 report of the Committee on Infectious Diseases* (30th ed., p. 683). Elk Grove Village, IL: American Academy of Pediatrics.

Larson-Nath, C., Gurram, B., & Chelimsky, G. (2015). Disorders of digestion in the neonate. In R. J. Martin, A. A. Fanaroff, & M. C. Walsh (Eds.), *Fanaroff and Martin's neonatal-perinatal medicine: Diseases of the fetus and infant* (10th ed., pp. 1379–1394). Philadelphia, PA: Saunders.

Levitt, M. A., Dickie, B., & Pena, A. (2010). Evaluation of the patient with Hirschsprung's disease who is not doing well after a pull-through procedure. *Seminars in Pediatric Surgery, 19*(2), 146–153.

Lucas, A., & Cole, T. J. (1990). Breast milk and neonatal necrotizing enterocolitis. *Lancet, 336*(8730), 1519–1523.

Magnuson, D. K, Parry, R. L., & Chwals, W. J. (2011). The gastrointestinal tract. In R. J. Martin, A. A. Fanaroff, & M. C. Walsh (Eds.), *Fanaroff and Martin's neonatal-perinatal medicine: Diseases of the fetus and infant* (9th ed., pp. 1375–1400). St. Louis, MO: Mosby.

McAlhany, A., & Popovich, D. (2007). Hirschsprung disease. *Newborn & Infant Nursing Reviews, 7*(3), 151–154.

Moore, K. L., Persaud, T. V. N., & Torchia, M. G. (2016). *The developing human: Clinically oriented embryology* (10th ed.). Philadelphia, PA: Elsevier.

Moore, T. A., & Wilson, M. E. (2011). Feeding intolerance a concept analysis. *Advances in Neonatal Care, 11*(3), 149–154.

Morgan, J., Bombell, S., & McGuire, W. (2013). Early trophic feeding versus enteral fasting for very low birth weight infants (Review). *Cochrane Collaboration, 13*, 1–24.

Moss, R. L., Kalish, L. A., Duggan, C., Johnston, P., Brandt, M. L., Dunn, J. C. Y., . . . Sylvester, K. G. (2008). Clinical parameters do not adequately predict outcome in necrotizing enterocolitis: A multi-institutional study. *Journal of Perinatology, 28*, 665–674.

Neu, J. (2014). Necrotizing enterocolitis. In B. Koletzko, B. Poindexter, & R. Uauy (Eds.), *Nutritional care of preterm infants: Scientific basis and practical guidelines (World review of nutrition and dietetics)* (Vol. 110, pp. 264–277). Basel, Switzerland: S. Karger. doi:10.1159/ 000358475

Parry, R. L. (2015). Selected gastrointestinal anomalies in the neonate. In R. J. Martin, A. A. Fanaroff, & M. C. Walsh (Eds.), *Fanaroff and Martin's neonatal-perinatal medicine: Diseases of the fetus and infant* (10th ed., pp. 1395–1422). Philadelphia, PA: Saunders.

Patole, S. K., & de Klerk, N. (2005). Impact of standardized feeding regimens on incidence of neonatal necrotizing enterocolitis: A systematic review and meta-analysis of observational studies. *Archives of Disease in Childhood—Fetal and Neonatal Edition, 90,* 147–151.

Perks, P., & Abad-Jorge, A. (2008). Nutritional management of the infant with necrotizing enterocolitis. *Practical Gastroenterology,* 46–60. Retrieved from https://med.virginia.edu/ginutrition/wp-content/uploads/sites/199/2015/11/PerksArticle-Feb-08.pdf

Price, P. (2000). Parenteral nutrition: Administration and monitoring. In S. Groh-Wargo & J. H. Cox (Eds.), *Nutritional care of high risk newborns* (pp. 96–101). Chicago, IL: Precept Press.

Puder, M. (2009). General consideration: Part 2: Surgical considerations. In A. Hansen, & M. Puder (Eds.), *Manual of neonatal surgical intensive care* (2nd ed., pp. 13–23). Shelton, CT: Peoples Medical Publishing House.

Ross A. J. (2004). Organogenesis of the gastrointestinal tract. In R. A. Polin, W. W. Fox, & S. H. Abman (Eds.), *Fetal and neonatal physiology* (3rd ed., pp. 1101–1110). Philadelphia, PA: Saunders.

Shaw, A. M. (2008). Bicarbonate and chloride equilibrium and acid–base balance in the neonate. *Neonatal Network, 27*(4), 261–266.

Trotter, C. (2011). Abnormalities of the gastrointestinal tract. Congenital anomalies of the gastrointestinal tract, Part II: The small bowel. In C. Trotter (Ed.), *Neonatal radiology basics* (2nd ed., pp. 4-6–4-28). Petaluma, CA: NICU Ink.

van der Doef, H. P. J., Kokke, F. T. M., van der Ent, C. K., & Houwen, R. H. J. (2011). Intestinal obstruction syndromes in cystic fibrosis: Meconium ileus, distal intestinal obstruction syndrome, and constipation. *Current Gastroenterology Report, 13,* 265–270. doi:10.1007/s11894-011-0185-9

Vanderhoof, J. A., Zach T. L., & Adrian, T. E. (2005). Gastrointestinal disease. In M. G. MacDonald, M. M. K. Seshia, & M. D. Mullet (Eds.), *Avery's neonatology, pathopysiology & management of the newborn* (6th ed., pp. 940–964). Philadelphia, PA: Lippincott Williams & Wilkins.

Walsh, M. C., & Kliegman, R. M. (1986). Necrotizing enterocolitis: Treatment based on staging criteria. *Pediatric Clinics of North America, 33*(1), 179–201.

Wessel, J. J., & Kocoshis, S. (2007). Nutritional management of infants with short bowel syndrome. *Seminars in Perinatology, 31,* 104–111.

Zeigler, M. M. (1986). Short bowel syndrome in infancy: Etiology and management. *Clinics in Perinatology, 13*(1), 163–173.

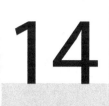

14

Infectious Diseases Cases

Karen Wright

Chapter Objectives

1. Identify the prevalent epidemiologic factors contributing to neonatal sepsis
2. Differentiate between early-onset sepsis (EOS) and late-onset sepsis
3. Discuss appropriate diagnostic modalities for the detection of sepsis
4. Discuss preventative and empiric therapy used to treat infants with suspected sepsis
5. Appraise case study evidence and prescribe appropriate management for sepsis
6. Apply evidence-based practice criteria to analyze case study questions

SEPSIS

EPIDEMIOLOGY

Although rare, neonatal sepsis is considered in multiple differential diagnoses in the neonatal intensive care unit (NICU). Neonates are empirically treated for sepsis as a part of the management consideration and exclusionary diagnosis. Despite the low incidence of sepsis, it is a significant cause of morbidity and mortality of newborns, resulting in frequent treatment of the presumption of sepsis.

The incidence of neonatal sepsis is estimated to range from one to five cases per 1,000 live births (Phares et al., 2008). The range in incidence is explained by the varied incidence by gestational age, and the differing incidence between EOS and late-onset sepsis. Based on the data from the National Institute of Child Health and Human Development Neonatal Research Network, the incidence of primary (early-onset) sepsis is approximately 2% per 1,000 live births but in late-onset sepsis the incidence is 36% (Pammi & Haque, 2015).

Based on these data, the overall mortality rate of neonatal sepsis is 13% to 25% and is higher in premature infants. Because of high mortality rate associated with sepsis, neonatal nurse practitioners (NNPs) practice with a low threshold for evaluation, and treatment is universal in all infants (presumptive sepsis) (Adair et al., 2003).

PATHOPHYSIOLOGY/ONSET OF SEPSIS

The classification of neonatal sepsis is done primarily by age. *EOS* is defined by the Centers for Disease Control and Prevention (CDC) as an infection that occurs during the first week of life. The incidence of EOS has fallen with the refinement of the intrapartum antibiotic prophylaxis guidelines that were initially identified in 1996 and updated most recently in 2010. Late-onset sepsis presents at greater than 3 days of life and is transmitted by environmental horizontal transmission.

EOS is acquired vertically, by transmission in utero whereby the organism is acquired during the antepartum or intrapartum period, transplacentally, hematogenously, or during birth. In addition, with ruptured membranes, organisms may ascend to colonize the fetus and amniotic fluid, resulting in chorioamnionitis (Verani, McGee, Schrag, & Division of Bacterial Diseases, National Center for Immunization and Respiratory Diseases, CDC, 2010).

The primary organism associated with EOS is group B *Streptococcus* (GBS), which is the primary cause of neonatal death by infection in the United States (Verani et al., 2010). GBS is a gram-positive bacteria with 10 serotypes (1a–IX), designated by the type of polysaccharide capsule or surface proteins of the specific strains. The pathogenic strains identified in the United States are Ia, Ib, II, III, and V (Fluegge, Supper, Siedler, & Berner, 2005).

In the very low-birth-weight population, however, the enteric bacteria *Escherichia coli* are more prevalent (Bizzarro et al., 2005). Other pathogens responsible for EOS include *Klebsiella*, *Hemophilus*, and *Enterobacter*.

Table 14.1 **A Comparison of Gram-Positive and Gram-Negative Organisms, Including Commonly Identified Shapes**

Gram-Positive Organisms	Gram-Negative Organisms
Cocci (sphere shaped) in clusters— *Staphylococcus*	Bacilli (rod shaped)—*Escherichia coli, Klebsiella, Proteus, Salmonella, Shigella, Acinetobacter, Campylobacter* (rods), *Enterobacter* (rod), *Pseudomonas, Hemophilus, Proteus*
Cocci in chains—*Streptococcus, Enterococcus*	Intracellular—*Chlamydia*
Tetrad—*Micrococcus*	Diplococcus—*Neisseria*
Rods—*Corynebacterium, Clostridium, Listeria*	Spirochete—*Treponema pallidum*

MICROBIOLOGY/ETIOLOGIC AGENTS

The identification of bacterial pathogens is based on the difference in bacterial wall structure. Bacteria with cell walls thickened with peptidoglycan can be stained with violet and are therefore gram-positive organisms. In contrast, gram-negative organisms have a more impenetrable wall, making these bacteria more resistant to antibodies. Other differences include a thick outer wall membrane and relatively high lipoprotein content in gram-negative organisms (endotoxins) as opposed to gram positives, which produce exotoxins. Overall, this indicates that gram-negative organisms are likely to be pathogenic and more resistant to antibiotics than gram-positive organisms. Gram-positive organisms are sometimes nonpathogenic and are primarily cocci or sphere shaped, and gram-negative pathogens are primarily bacillus or rods. The organisms are classified in Table 14.1.

Case 14.1

As the neonatal nurse practitioner, you are called to see a 40-hour-old newborn who was rushed to the neonatal intensive care unit by the mother–baby nurse as a result of a report from mother that her baby was bleeding from his mouth and nose. Your quick assessment finds the newborn pale and asystolic. You intubate the newborn immediately after estimating his weight to be 3 kg and insert the endotracheal tube (ETT) to 9 cm, and initiate positive pressure ventilation. Upon insertion of the ETT, you note bright-red blood in the ETT. After 1 minute, the heart rate rises to greater than 100 beats per minute (bpm) but the baby remains poorly perfused, ashen, and flaccid. The chest is hyperexpanded with audible rales throughout. Further information reveals that the mother is a 28-year-old gravida 3, now para 3, O+, rubella immune, HIV negative, HBsAg (hepatitis B surface antigen) negative, rapid plasma regain nonreactive (RPR NR), group B *Streptococcus* negative. Mother presented in labor with spontaneous rupture of membranes 4 hours prior to delivery and was afebrile. Pregnancy was complicated by pregnancy-induced hypertension.

1. *How should this baby be managed?*

   A. Provide oxygenation and ventilation and supportive measures such as blood pressure and thermal support
   B. Obtain a full diagnostic evaluation: chest x-ray, complete blood count, blood culture, and coagulation panel
   C. Begin empiric antibiotic coverage
   D. All of the above

   ANSWER: D. *The comprehensive management of this neonate progresses rapidly from establishing support of oxygenation and ventilation, beginning IV fluids, providing a fluid bolus, and maintaining a neutral thermal environment. Rapid diagnostics allow for stat treatment with empiric antibiotics.*

(continued)

Case 14.1 *(continued)*

2. *Based on the gestational age, timing and presentation, what is the differential diagnosis for this infant?*

A. Fulminant early onset sepsis with disseminated intravascular coagulopathy
B. Spontaneous pulmonary hemorrhage
C. Late-onset septicemia
D. Congenital cytomegalovirus (CMV)

ANSWER: A. *Based on this severe presentation of a term infant, this baby likely has fulminant septicemia with disseminated intravascular coagulopathy (DIC). Early-onset sepsis is defined as septicemia presenting within the first 7 days of life, which excludes late-onset septicemia as a diagnosis for this 40-hour-old infant. DIC is a secondary process resulting in hemorrhage due to damage to the endothelium and activation of the clotting cascade. Bleeding from the gums and mouth indicates a systemic problem and based on the presentation of this baby disseminated intravascular coagulopathy would most likely be suspected as a complication of fulminant sepsis. A further consideration would be to consider a coinciding inborn error of metabolism and other metabolic factors that contribute to septicemia such as hypoxia and acidosis. Spontaneous pulmonary hemorrhage is normally seen as a complication of preterm infants who have received surfactant.*

RISK FACTORS

Information surrounding the maternal course of labor and delivery is paramount to the detection of the neonatal risk of sepsis. Table 14.2 describes the risk factors for neonatal sepsis and indications for antimicrobial therapy (Schuchat, Zywicki, Dinsmoor et al., 2000). The CDC describes maternal colonization with GBS as the primary risk factor for sepsis. In addition, prolonged rupture of membranes is associated with a higher incidence of sepsis (Herbst & Källén, 2007).

GBS Disease Screening

In 2010, the CDC updated the protocol for GBS screening and maternal intrapartum antibiotic prophylaxis. Following this update, the incidence of GBS has steadily decreased (Ohlsson & Shah, 2014) to 0.27 per 1,000 intrapartum women in 2013. Stoll and colleagues found that despite the decrease in GBS-related sepsis, the organism remains the most prevalent bacteria in neonatal sepsis of term infants, followed by *E. coli* in preterm infants; and despite antibiotic prophylaxis, one half of the babies developed EOS (Stoll et al., 2011).

VIRAL ETIOLOGIES

Similar to neonatal sepsis, neonatal viral infections may be congenital or acquired by nosocomial transmission. Because viral studies are not routinely obtained, the incidence of neonatal viral infections may be higher than reported (Verbon, 2006).

Table 14.2 **Risk Factors for Neonatal Sepsis**

Maternal	*Maternal colonization with GBS (vagino/rectal, urine) (primary risk factor) *Previous delivery of newborn with GBS sepsis *PROM > 18 hours *Intrapartum maternal fever > 100.4°F *Preterm delivery prior to 37 weeks ROM prior to labor Silent or leaking membranes Chorioamnionitis Inadequate antibiotic treatment prior to delivery History of UTI
Newborn	Intrauterine fetal monitoring Fetal distress (tachycardia, MAS, traumatic delivery, resuscitation) Gestational age <37 weeks Low birth weight Multiple gestation Invasive procedures Metabolic disorders

*Indications for inadequate antibiotic prophylaxis.

GBS, group B *Streptococcus*; MAS, meconium aspiration syndrome; PROM, premature rupture of membranes; ROM, rupture of membranes; UTI, urinary tract infection.

Case 14.2

An infant is delivered at term to a 27-year-old gravida 1, para 0. Serology is negative with the exception of a positive group B *Streptococcus* (GBS) screen. Rupture of membranes occurred at home 30 hours prior to spontaneous vaginal delivery with a maternal fever noted to 101.4°F on admission. The mother was given one dose of ampicillin, which was completed 1 hour prior to delivery. The baby is asymptomatic.

1. *Which of the following is true about this case scenario?*
    A. The mother has chorioamnionitis
    B. There was adequate treatment for GBS prior to delivery
    C. A complete blood count (CBC) with differential and blood culture should be drawn
    D. Antibiotics are not indicated at this time

    A. A
    B. A and C
    C. All of the above

(continued)

Case 14.2 *(continued)*

ANSWER: B. *Maternal fever is an important maternal clinical indication of chorioamnionitis and is present in 95% to 100% of clinical cases. Most clinicians consider a maternal fever of more than 100.4°F to be an abnormal clinical finding during pregnancy, but considering that sometimes a low-grade fever may be present during labor. Other contributing factors in this scenario include fetal tachycardia and unknown length of ruptured membranes. There is no indication that mother was treated for GBS prior to delivery. Based on the most recent Centers for Disease Control guidelines for the prevention of perinatal GBS disease, a CBC with blood culture should be drawn, and antibiotics are indicated for this newborn at this time.*

2. *Should a C-reactive protein (CRP) be sent?*

   A. YES, an elevated CRP would be diagnostic of sepsis
   B. A CRP should be sent at 12 to 24 hours of life
   C. A CRP is not indicated at this time

   ANSWER: B. *A CRP is a non-specific inflammatory marker that is increased in inflammatory conditions. Although there are a variety of noninfectious causes for an elevated CRP level, obtaining a CRP level may be helpful as information, which contributes to the diagnosis of sepsis. CRP levels may also help the clinician to determine the length of treatment of antibiotics. If the CRP level is persistently low, then the diagnosis of sepsis is not likely. In order to obtain the most valid findings, CRP levels are generally not drawn until 12 hours of life.*

TORCH VIRUSES

TORCH is an acronym designating possible neonatal viral infections, including toxoplasmosis, other (syphilis, varicella-zoster, parvovirus), rubella, cytomegalovirus (CMV), and herpes. These infections are considered together because they present similarly at birth. Because other perinatal viral infections exist (enterovirus, varicella), approaching the individual etiology of the virus may be a more common and cost-effective practice approach (de Jong, Vossen, Walther, & Lopriore, 2013).

Toxoplasmosis

Toxoplasmosis is a protozoan parasite that is derived from a feline host. Perinatal infections from toxoplasmosis are only mildly symptomatic and generally affect immunocompromised women. Babies may be asymptomatic until the first few months of life or into childhood, or present with hydrocephalus chorioretinitis and intracranial calcifications. Most infants with toxoplasmosis are asymptomatic at birth; however, more severe infection at birth yields intrauterine growth restriction, jaundice, hepatosplenomegaly, and cutaneous lesions. The less common presentation is considered the classic presentation of chorioretinitis, hydrocephalus, and cerebral calcifications. Clinical evaluation of neonates with toxoplasmosis includes ophthalmic examination, neurologic evaluation, and hearing screening (Tamma, 2007).

Toxoplasmosis is a common neonatal infection and a member of the herpes virus family. As with toxoplasmosis, the neonatal presentation of CMV may be asymptomatic.

Other Agents

The category of "other" refers primarily to the vertical transmission of syphilis, which is caused by the spirochete *Treponema pallidum*. Syphilis carries a high morbidity and thus is routinely screened for in pregnancy by use of the RPR/VDRL (rapid plasma reagin/Venereal Disease Research Laboratory) tests, and in high-risk cases, again during the second trimester and at delivery (Workowski, Bolan, & CDC, 2015). Treating the expectant mother with penicillin 30 days prior to delivery is of paramount importance to influence neonatal infection. Common to other TORCH infections, infants with syphilis may be asymptomatic at birth. Those who have symptoms may present with hepatosplenomegaly, snuffles (syphilitic rhinitis), and skin lesions. Treatment of syphilis at any age is with penicillin G (American Academy of Pediatrics [AAP], 2015).

Other manifestations considered within the consideration of "other" include varicella (chickenpox) and lymphocytic choriomeningitis (LCM) virus (from house mice). Like the aforementioned viruses, both present with similar symptoms such as chorioretinitis. However, newborns with varicella present with cicatricial (scarred) skin lesions and/or a generalized pruritic, vesicular rash, whereas infants with LCM present with manifestations similar to other TORCH infections such as hydrocephalus, chorioretinitis, intracranial calcifications, and microcephaly (AAP, 2015). Infants exposed to varicella-zoster are treated with varicella-zoster immune globulin, and then with acyclovir for 10 days (CDC, 2006). In contrast, treatment for LCM is supportive care.

Rubella

The rubella virus is a highly contagious ribonucleic acid (RNA) virus sometimes called *German measles*. Maternal infection with the rubella virus generally occurs following a maternal primary infection during the first trimester and may affect every fetal organ. The manifestation of the rubella virus is based on gestational timing. Perinatal infection with the rubella virus may vary from congenital rubella syndrome with its multiple neonatal problems. The clinical features of congenital rubella infection are widely varied and include intrauterine growth restriction, cloudy cornea, blueberry muffin spots (dermal extramedullary hematopoiesis), deafness, and central nervous system (CNS) damage. Diagnosis is by isolation of the rubella antibody or by detection of higher levels of rubella immunoglobulin G (IgG) or IgG antibodies. The CDC mandates reporting of the rubella virus whenever it is isolated (AAP, 2015). Congenital rubella syndrome is a consideration in the differential diagnosis of any infant with symmetric intrauterine growth restriction without clear cause.

Cytomegalovirus

Like Epstein–Barr virus, CMV is a member of the herpes virus family and is more commonly asymptomatic and latent, whereas 10% of babies delivered with CMV are born with clinical manifestations such as intrauterine growth restriction, jaundice, thrombocytopenia, microcephaly, and cerebral calcifications (Boppana, 2013). Possible routes of neonatal transmission include vertical transmission (transplacentally, from the vaginal mucosa, or via breast milk), or by transfusion of infected blood products. Transmission early in pregnancy is more highly associated with long-term consequences such as sensory neural hearing loss and poor developmental outcomes. To date, CMV remains the leading cause of nonhereditary sensorineural hearing loss (Goderis et al., 2014). In asymptomatic infants, a failed newborn hearing screen may be the first signal of CMV infection. Diagnosis may be by isolation of the CMV in the urine or saliva. Neonatal treatment of CMV with oral valganciclovir for 6 months has demonstrated improved neurodevelopmental outcome at 2 years of life (AAP, 2015).

Herpes Simplex Virus

Acquired herpes simplex virus (HSV) is primarily transmitted perinatally by vertical transmission. Other less common methods of transmission include intrauterine (presenting as symmetric growth restriction, neurologic damage, and chorioretinitis) and postnatal (nosocomial) transmission. Neonatal HSV transmission is, to a large extent, preventable by cesarean delivery in the presence of active lesions. However, disruptions in skin, such as by the use of fetal scalp electrodes, may reduce the natural barrier to HSV. Neonatal HSV can be classified clinically as either localized (skin, eyes, mouth); neurologic, which presents as encephalitis; or disseminated, which has significant mortality (Kimberlin, 2007). For the most optimal neurodevelopmental outcome, treatment of HSV includes parenteral acyclovir for 21 days followed by 6 months of oral acyclovir. Following ophthalmologic consult to screen for retinitis, infants should be treated with a topical ophthalmic drug such as 1% trifluridine, 0.1% idodeoxyuridine, or 0.15% ganciclovir (AAP, 2015).

CLINICAL MANIFESTATIONS OF SEPSIS

Signs and symptoms of neonatal EOS generally present unevenly, ranging from indistinct signs of sepsis to septic shock. In the delivery room, fetal tachycardia is associated with chorioamnionitis. The presentation of sepsis is generally nonspecific and includes respiratory distress, irritability, lethargy, temperature instability, poor perfusion, hypotension, and shock. Fever is not generally a finding within the first 24 hours of life. The presence of pneumonia is a less common finding with intrapartum antibiotic prophylaxis (IAP) (Phares et al., 2008).

PREVENTION AND APPROACH

The key concept of the CDC 2010 guidelines involves identification of mothers at risk and administration of parenteral antibiotic prophylaxis more than 4 hours prior to delivery. Identification of mothers carrying GBS may be by two methods: (a) rectovaginal cultures or (b) by risk factors. Screening of mothers by culture is recommended between 35 to 37 weeks of pregnancy unless a GBS urinary tract infection has been diagnosed in the mother during the current pregnancy or the mother has a history of a previous delivery with GBS disease (Boyer, Gadzala, Kelly, Burd, & Gotoff, 1983). The screening is completed near delivery so that results are available prior to the onset of labor (Verani et al., 2010). Screening by risk factors is less desirable as half of women delivering infants infected with GBS have no risk factors (Stone et al., 2003).

Case 14.3

As a health care provider, you are called to see a term baby following delivery in the emergency department. The mother had regular prenatal care, but following a brief labor, delivered precipitously just after arrival. Mother is a 30-year-old gravida 2, para 1, O+, rubella immune, rapid plasma reagin nonreactive (RPR NR), HBsAg negative, group B *Streptococcus* (GBS) positive. Assigned Apgar scores are 8 and 8 at 1 and 5 minutes, respectively. The

(continued)

Case 14.3 *(continued)*

baby is meconium stained and noted to be awake and alert, pink, and with mild tachypnea and retractions. The emergency room nurse reports that mother's temperature is 101.4°F. Mother reports that her water broke en route to the hospital.

1. *How should this baby be managed?*

   A. Obtain a chest x-ray (CXR), complete blood count (CBC) and blood culture, begin ampicillin and gentamicin, admit for observation
   B. Admit baby for 24-hour observation. Complete a septic workup if symptomatic
   C. Obtain a CBC and blood culture and observe for 24 hours
   D. Routine newborn care.

ANSWER: A. *This rationale is based on the current CDC guidelines for the prevention of perinatal GBS disease. In the scenario, the baby is tachypneic with retractions. This baby is at risk for septicemia due to GBS-positive status with inadequate treatment and maternal fever. The baby was also meconium stained and at risk for coinciding meconium aspiration syndrome (MAS). Based on this rationale, the newborn should be admitted and treated empirically. If the baby were asymptomatic, the next step would be considered based on the likelihood or chorioamnionitis, which is presumed due to maternal fever. Based on the guidelines antibiotic therapy would still be indicated. If the baby were asymptomatic and the mother afebrile without prolonged rupture of membranes, but is GBS positive without treatment, the baby requires 48-hour observation but antibiotics are not required at this time. Routine newborn care is not indicated due to the symptomatic nature of the infant.*

2. *What is the differential diagnosis for this baby?*

   A. Transient tachypnea of the newborn
   B. Meconium aspiration syndrome
   C. Hypoxic ischemic encephalopathy
   D. A and B only
   E. All of these

ANSWER: D. *This baby is presenting with tachypnea and mild retractions at birth. Although transient tachypnea is a retrospective diagnosis, it is a diagnosis worth consideration in this scenario. The baby was also noted to have meconium-stained fluid following precipitous delivery necessitating the inclusion of meconium aspiration prior to delivery as a consideration. Hypoxic ischemic encephalopathy is associated with birth asphyxia but this baby had Apgar scores of 8 and 8, indicating that the baby was not in need of resuscitation at birth.*

DIAGNOSIS AND EVALUATION

Diagnosis of neonatal sepsis is problematic considering the length of time needed to reach a diagnosis, sensitivity of the test, and the consideration of false-negative evidence.

BLOOD CULTURE

Blood is considered a sterile body fluid and blood culture is the gold standard of neonatal sepsis. A positive blood culture yields identification of the culprit and establishes a definitive diagnosis of sepsis. Blood cultures may be drawn by venous or arterial puncture, or from a newly inserted vascular line such as an umbilical artery catheter. The general consensus is that only one aerobic culture is needed prior to the beginning of empirical antibiotic therapy.

For all infants, the volume of blood needed to optimize blood culture results is based on the weight of the infant. The minimum sample amount is 1 mL, but to increase the accuracy, consider that the volume of distribution is greater in larger infants, indicating that a larger sample for larger babies will improve the accuracy of the test by preventing a false-negative report because of a low colony count, and decrease the false-positive ratio to 1% (Schelonka et al., 1996). Blood cultures are monitored by automated systems and become positive within 24 to 36 hours (Garcia-Prats, Cooper, Schneider, Stager, & Hansen, 2000). Other confounding variables of blood culture results include intrapartum antibiotic administration of antibiotic that crosses to neonates prior to delivery (Schelonka et al., 1996).

COMPLETE BLOOD COUNT

The white blood cell (WBC) count and differential of neutrophils are also standard measurements for neonatal sepsis, The most useful index of WBC analyses is the immature-to-total neutrophil (I/T) ratio, but this has a wide range of abnormal values. A higher I/T ratio is indicative of depleted bone marrow reserves, indicating a septic process. The absolute neutrophil count may be elevated or diminished in the presence of neonatal sepsis. These values have been associated with neonatal sepsis when both are abnormal. Despite the value of these findings, the test is fairly nonspecific for neonatal sepsis and has poor predictive value, indicating that CBC has more value in the exclusion of sepsis (Hornik et al., 2012).

CEREBROSPINAL FLUID

Cerebrospinal fluid (CSF) is another sterile body fluid that, based on unit practices, may or may not be analyzed to diagnose for neonatal sepsis. CSF is obtained by lumbar puncture, a stressful procedure that may be withheld if the newborn is unstable. The study of CSF includes Gram's stain, culture, white and red blood cell counts with differential, and protein and glucose levels. These values vary with gestational age and day of life. The utility of C-reactive protein (CRP) measurement in spinal fluid is controversial (Corrall, Pepple, Moxon, & Hughes, 1981; Philip & Baker, 1983; Pourcyrous et al., 1993) and is poorly correlated with serum (Polin & the Committee on Fetus and Newborn, 2012).

BIOMARKERS OF SEPSIS

Adding to the challenge of diagnosing neonatal sepsis, it is estimated that blood cultures are positive in less than 40% of cases (Schelonka et al., 1996). Given this fact, combined with the poor predictive value of the CBC, the identification of a biomarker for the expeditious diagnosis of sepsis and the ability to discern infected from noninfected neonates would be beneficial. Acute-phase reactants, also known as *cytokines*, are components of the complement systems currently studied as biomarkers for neonatal sepsis (Bhatti, Chu, Hagerman, Schreiber, & Alexander, 2012). These cytokines are actually proteins released from various physiologic modalities in response to cellular responses to sepsis and inflammation. Currently, under review are the most encouraging CRPs, interleukin 6 and 8 (IL-6 and 8) and procalcitonin (PCT). To identify a cytokine or a combination of cytokines that are highly sensitive with an early response to sepsis would be very beneficial. Although highly sensitive, these markers are nonspecific, which limits their predictive value (Edgar et al., 1994).

CRP is a pentraxin protein and a nonspecific acute-phase reactant that is synthesized from the fetus but derived from the humoral immune system. A common value considered to be a positive CRP is 10 mg/L or higher. CRP levels are measured in the blood and are highest 6 to 18 hours with peak values that range from 8 to 60 hours. Because of this range, CRP levels are considered to have a lower level of sensitivity during the beginning of sepsis. For this reason, a single measurement of CRP is less useful than sequential assessment. Although highly sensitive, CRP, however nonspecific, may be elevated in circumstances other than sepsis (Pourcyrous et al., 1993).

IL-6 and IL-8 are cytokines that provide a proinflammatory response to inflammation and are produced by mononuclear phagocytes, endothelial cells, and fibroblasts. IL-6 is a precursor of CRP and peaks at 2 to 3 hours after provocation and is measurable using umbilical cord blood (Messer et al., 1996). When tested, IL-6 is 100% predictive of blood culture positive sepsis if measured prior to 1 hour after birth. The drawback is that it is also predictive of but not distinctive for other inflammatory processes such as respiratory distress syndrome (Kallman, Ekholm, Eriksson, Malmstrom, & Scholin, 1999). Tumor necrosis factor (TNF-alpha) is a precursor to IL-6 but is only partially accurate in the diagnosis of EOS and late-onset sepsis (Edgar et al., 1994).

Conversely, IL-8 is produced by monocytes, macrophages, and endothelial cells and also in response to inflammation. As with IL-6, IL-8 is sensitive but lacks specificity for neonatal sepsis, but, unlike IL-6 and CRP, IL-8 is less sensitive at birth and more sensitive at 24 or 48 hours of age (Laborada et al., 2003).

Like CRP, PCT is an acute-phase reactant and is formed by monocytes and hepatocytes with a delayed response of 4 to 6 hours after introduction to bacteria. PCT is more sensitive to late-onset sepsis than EOS (81%, 90%; Vouloumanou, Plessa, Karageorgopoulos, Mantadakis, & Falagas, 2011).

MOLECULAR DIAGNOSIS

The PCR (polymerase chain reaction) is the molecular microarray that is used most often to support the diagnosis of neonatal sepsis. The advantage of this study is that the test is rapid (9 hours), requires a smaller amount of blood (200 mcL), and, most important, is not impacted by maternal antibiotics given prior to delivery. However, the downside of using PCR is the cost and availability of the test (Jordan & Durso, 2005).

SCREENINGS THAT ARE NOT RECOMMENDED

Gastric Aspirates and Body Surface Cultures

Many screens for sepsis are less useful, particularly in EOS. Gastric aspirates may contain white blood cells, but this may be a result of ingestion of maternal white blood cells present in the amniotic fluid that are not related to neonatal sepsis (Mims, Medawar, Perkins, & Grubb, 1972). Body surface cultures have been found to have poor predictive value for sepsis (Evans et al., 1988).

The exception is found in the case of suspected HSV. In this circumstance, surface cultures using one swab beginning with the eye (conjunctivae), mouth, nasopharynx, then rectum may be useful if obtained between 12 to 24 hours of life. Positive cultures suggest viral replication (Kimberlin, 2004).

DIFFERENTIAL DIAGNOSIS

Because of the nonspecific presentation of neonatal sepsis, there are multiple systemic differential diagnoses related to the hallmark presentations of cardiorespiratory distress, temperature instability, and neurologic symptoms. Less common diagnoses that need to be considered are nonbacterial infections such as herpes simplex, enteroviruses, CMV, influenza viruses, respiratory syncytial virus, syphilis, and candidiasis (Nizet & Klein, 2010).

Considering that EOS presents as respiratory distress, differential or possibly simultaneous diagnoses that are noninfectious include transient tachypnea, respiratory distress syndrome, meconium aspiration, pneumothorax, congenital anomalies such as transient temperature instability, as well as asphyxia, dehydration, and cardiac etiologies (Nizet & Klein, 2010).

Temperature instability may also be associated with environmental adaptation, dehydration, neonatal abstinence syndrome, asphyxia, hypothyroidism, or congenital adrenal hypoplasia. Finally, neurologic impersonators of sepsis include hypoglycemia, hypocalcemia, hypermagnesemia, seizures, and inborn errors of metabolism (Nizet & Klein, 2010).

ANTIBIOTIC THERAPY

Because neonatal sepsis has a high mortality rate but lower incidence, the decision to start antibiotic therapy is multifactorial. Considerations include clinical evaluation, risk factors, and diagnostic studies. Of these considerations, ill-appearing infants are treated during the process of exclusion of other possible etiologies such as congenital heart disease or neurologic conditions (Polin & the Committee on Fetus and Newborn, 2012).

Antibiotic coverage for early-onset neonatal sepsis is systemic with provision of broad coverage of the most anticipated gram-positive (i.e., GBS) and gram-negative (i.e., *E. coli*) pathogens. The suggested dosage of ampicillin is 100 mg/kg intravenously every 12 hours. Gentamicin is nephrotoxic and ototoxic and is therefore dosed by gestational age and days of life. The recommended dosage of gentamicin is a 4- to 5-mg/kg/dose every 24 to 36 hours based on gestational age (Young & Magnum, 2011).

Late-onset sepsis of infants who have been continuously hospitalized since birth requires antibiotic coverage for more organisms that may be antibiotic resistant. Vancomycin is given in place of ampicillin with the dosage based on age, weight, and possibly serum creatinine (Young & Magnum, 2011). Further, addition of a third antibiotic may be warranted.

ADJUNCTIVE THERAPIES

Although multiple adjunctive immunotherapeutic therapies are available, there is no evidence supporting the use of these therapies. Adjunctive therapies for neonates include intravenous immunoglobulin (IVIG), granulocyte-colony stimulating factor (G-CSF), and pentoxifylline.

IVIG has multiple actions, including stimulating the complement system and improving neutrophil function. G-CSF is a naturally occurring cytokine given to stimulate the production of neutrophils and monocytes (Carr, Brocklehurst, Dore, & Modi, 2009). Pentoxifylline is a xanthine derivative related to inhibition of the release of protein integral to systemic gram-negative infection. The clinical use of this therapy is in the initial stages so data are limited; however, existing data suggest an improvement in neonatal mortality (Pammi & Haque, 2015).

Supportive Therapy

Supportive care is centered around providing adequate oxygenation and organ perfusion. Oxygenation may be by via supplemental oxygen or supportive ventilation. In some cases, critically ill infants may require surfactant replacement to improve oxygenation (Finer, 2004).

Infants with poor perfusion indicative of septic shock may need inotropic therapy with a crystalloid solution (normal saline, 10 mls/kg × 2 doses), progressing to a colloid infusion (albumin, fresh frozen plasma) following the initiation of a dopamine infusion if perfusion is not recovered. The inotropic action of dopamine is dose directed. Starting with an intermediate neonatal continuous IV dose (5–10 mcg/kg/min), dopamine increases cardiac contractility and mildly increases systemic vascular resistance by promoting norepinephrine release as the dose is increased (Young & Magnum, 2011).

Dobutamine is a synthetic catecholamine and a potent inotrope that may be added to dopamine therapy to increase myocardial oxygen consumption. Dobutamine is commonly given by continuous IV infusion at 2 to 5 mcg/kg/min (Young & Magnum, 2011).

Critically ill newborns who become resistant to the use of vasopressors may have adrenal insufficiency. The use of corticosteroids is a further yet judicious step to the management of hypotension (Fanaroff & Fanaroff, 2006). Hydrocortisone is an adrenal corticoid, which increases the articulation adrenergic receptors in the vascular wall. The dosage is calculated by body surface area dosing (23–30 mg/m^2) or 1 mg/kg/dose every 8 hours (Young & Magnum, 2011). The duration of action of hydrocortisone is approximately 2 hours (Young & Magnum, 2011). Although not without complications, corticosteroids address adrenal insufficiency by raising cortisol levels (Fanaroff & Fanaroff, 2006).

CORE CONCEPTS

The effective management of neonatal sepsis requires an understanding of the underlying core concepts:

1. Neonatal sepsis is managed with antibiotics and supportive therapies.

2. Adjunctive therapies are available but lack evidence for definitive use.

3. A positive blood culture is diagnostic of sepsis.

4. The use of CRP and cytokine levels is currently under study.

5. Broad spectrum antibiotics remain the best strategy to cover organisms that are most likely the cause of neonatal sepsis

6. When screening infants for TORCH, test for the most likely organism as opposed to testing for all.

7. Chorioretinitis is a treatable inflammatory process related to perinatally acquired infections, and treatment should be considered in the presence of eye drainage with intrauterine growth restriction or suspicion of a perinatally acquired viral infection.

8. Sepsis is a retrospective diagnosis of exclusion so therefore it is a consideration in the diagnosis of most early onset and later onset neonatal illnesses.

Case 14.4

A 24-year-old gravida 1 presents in labor at 40 weeks gestational age. Her prenatal record states that she is O+, rubella immune, HBsAg negative, rapid plasma reagin nonreactive (RPR NR), HIV negative, group B *Streptococcus* (GBS) positive. She presents with rupture of membranes (ROM) of undetermined length with delivery imminent. Mother has a temperature of 102.2°F and fetal tachycardia is noted. In 1 hour, she spontaneously delivers a late preterm infant; Apgar scores were 8 and 8 at 1 and 5 minutes, respectively. The baby breathes spontaneously and is pink in room air. On examination, you find that the baby has a birth weight of 2,475 g, length of 46 cm, and head circumference of 31 cm. Upon closer inspection you note that this baby has vesicles clustered randomly on the scalp and purulent eye drainage.

1. *Each of the following is associated with congenital viral infection except:*

   A. Symmetric intrauterine growth restriction
   B. Premature rupture of membranes (PROM)
   C. Vesicular lesions
   D. Eye drainage

   ANSWER: B. *A classic finding of congenital viral infections is small for gestational age (< 10%) including toxoplasmosis, congenital rubella, and congenital cytomegalovirus (CMV). Vesicular lesions are more specific to herpes simplex virus (HSV). PROM is nonspecific and not directly associated with congenital viral infection.*

2. *Treatment with acyclovir warrants laboratory surveillance of:*

   A. Platelet count
   B. Creatinine and white blood cell count
   C. Sodium and potassium
   D. Calcium and magnesium

   ANSWER: B. *Acyclovir is an antiviral agent that is the most recommended for treatment of neonatal HSV infections, and decreases neonatal mortality from congenital HSV infection. Neonates are treated with acyclovir beginning whenever congenital HSV is suspected. The dose is 60 mg/kg/d and the duration of treatment is based on clinical response and manifestation of HSV. Monitoring the neonate receiving acyclovir includes renal function to prevent toxicity and assess hydration. Neutrophils should also be monitored for neutropenia, which may result, while on acyclovir. In addition, a peripheral IV infusion site is at risk for ulceration if acyclovir infiltrates. Platelets, sodium, potassium, calcium, and magnesium are not directly impacted by acyclovir.*

REFERENCES

Adair, C. E., Kowalsky, L., Quon, H., Ma, D., Stoffman, J., McGeer, A., . . . Davies, H. (2003). Risk factors for early-onset group B streptococcal disease in neonates: A population-based case-control study. *Canadian Medical Association Journal, 169,* 198.

American Academy of Pediatrics. (2015). Rubella. In D. W. Kimberlin, M. T. Brady, M. A. Jackson, & S. S. Long (Eds.), *Red book: 2015 Report of the committee on infectious diseases* (30th ed.). Elk Grove Village, IL: Author.

Bhatti, M., Chu, A., Hagerman, J., Schreiber, M., & Alexander, K. (2012). Future directions in the evaluation and management of neonatal sepsis. *NeoReviews, 13*(2), e103–e110.

Bizzarro, M., Raskind, C., Baltimore, R., & Gallagher, P. G. (2005). Seventy-five years of neonatal sepsis at Yale: 1928–2003. *Pediatrics, 116*, 595–602.

Boppana, S. B., Ross, S. A., & Fowler, K. B. (2013). Congenital cytomegalovirus infection: Clinical outcome. *Clinical Infectious Diseases, 57*(Suppl. 4), S178–S181.

Boyer, K. M., Gadzala, C. A., Kelly, P. D., Burd, L. I., & Gotoff, S. P. (1983). Selective intrapartum chemoprophylaxis of neonatal group B streptococcal early-onset disease. I. Epidemiologic rationale. *Journal of Infectious Diseases, 148*, 795.

Carr, R., Brocklehurst, P., Dore, D., & Modi, N. (2009). Granulocyte macrophage colony stimulating factor administered as prophylaxis for reduction of sepsis in extremely preterm, small for gestational age neonates: A single-blind, multicenter, randomized controlled trial. *Lancet, 373*, 1–23.

Centers for Disease Control and Prevention (CDC). (2006). A new product (VariZIG) for postexposure prophylaxis of varicella available under an investigational new drug application expanded access protocol. *Morbidity and Mortality Weekly Report, 55*, 209.

Centers for Disease Control and Prevention (CDC), Active Bacterial Core Surveillance. (2013). ABCs report: Group B *Streptococcus*. Retrieved from http://www.cdc.gov.ezproxy.rush.edu/abcs/reports-findings/survreports/gbs13.html

Corrall, C., Pepple, J., Moxon, E., & Hughes, W. (1981). C-reactive protein in spinal fluid of children with meningitis. *Journal of Pediatrics, 99*, 365–369.

de Jong, E. P., Vossen, A. C., Walther, F. J., & Lopriore, E. (2013). How to use . . . neonatal TORCH testing. *Archives of Disease in Childhood—Fetal and Neonatal Edition, 98*, 93.

Edgar, J., Wilson, D., McMillan, S., Crockard, A., Halliday, M., Gardner, K., . . . McNeil, T. (1994). Predictive value of soluble immunological mediators in neonatal infection. *Clinical Science, 87*(2), 165–171.

Evans, M. E., Schaffner, W., Federspiel, C. F., Cotton, R. B., McKee, K. T., Jr., & Stratton, C. W. (1988). Sensitivity, specificity, and predictive value of body surface cultures in a neonatal intensive care unit. *Journal of the American Medical Association, 259*(2), 248–252.

Fanaroff, J., & Fanaroff, A. (2006). Blood pressure disorders in the neonate: Hypotension and hypertension. *Seminars in Fetal & Neonatal Medicine, 11*, 65.

Finer, N. (2004). Surfactant use for neonatal lung injury: Beyond respiratory distress syndrome. *Paediatric Respiratory Review, 5*(Suppl. A), S289.

Fluegge, K., Supper, S., Siedler, A., & Berner, R. (2005). Serotype distribution of invasive group B streptococcal isolates in infants: Results from a nationwide active laboratory surveillance study over 2 years in Germany. *Clinical Infectious Diseases, 40*, 760.

Garcia-Prats, J., Cooper, T., Schneider, V., Stager, C., & Hansen, T. (2000). Rapid detection of microorganisms in blood cultures of newborn infants utilizing an automated blood culture system. *Pediatrics, 105* (3, Pt. 1), 523.

Goderis, J., DeLeenheer, E., Smets, K., Van Hoecke, H., Keymeulen, A., & Dhooge, I. (2014). Hearing loss and congenital CMV infection: A systematic review. *Pediatrics, 134*, 972.

Herbst, A., & Källén, K. (2007). Time between membrane rupture and delivery and septicemia in term neonates. *Obstetrics & Gynecology, 110*, 612.

Hornik, C., Benjamin, D., Becker, K., Li, J., Clark, R., Cohen-Wolkowiez, M., & Smith, P. (2012). Use of the complete blood cell count in early-onset neonatal sepsis. *Pediatric Infectious Disease Journal, 31*(8), 803–807.

Jordan, J., & Durso, M. (2005). Real-time polymerase chain reaction for detecting bacterial DNA directly from blood of neonates being evaluation for sepsis. *Journal of Molecular diagnostics, 7*, 525.

Kallman, J., Ekholm, I., Eriksson, M., Malmstrom, B., & Scholin, J. (1999). Contribution of interleukin-6 in distinguishing between mild respiratory disease and neonatal sepsis in the newborn infant. *Acta Pediatrics, 88*(8), 880–884.

Kimberlin, D. W. (2004). Neonatal herpes simplex infection. *Clinical Microbiology, 17*, 1.

Kimberlin, D. W. (2007). Herpes simplex virus infections of the newborn. *Seminars in Perinatology, 31*, 19.

Laborada, G., Rego, M., Jain, A. Guliano, M., Stavola, J., Balladbh, P., . . . Nesin, M. (2003). Diagnostic value of cytokines and C-reactive protein in the first 24 hours of neonatal sepsis. *American Journal of Perinatology, 20*(8), 491–501.

Messer, J., Eyer, D., Donato, L., Gallati, H., Matis, J., & Simeon, U. (1996). Evaluation of interleukin-6 and soluble receptors of tumor necrosis factor for early diagnosis of neonatal infection. *Journal of Pediatrics, 129*(4), 574–580.

Mims, C., Medawar, S., Perkins, J., & Grubb, W. (1972). Predicting neonatal infections by evaluation of the gastric aspirate: a study in two hundred and seven patients. *American Journal of Obstetrics & Gynecology, 114*(2), 232–238.

Nizet, V., & Klein, J. (2010). *Bacterial sepsis and meningitis. Infectious diseases of the fetus and newborn infant* (7th ed.). Philadelphia, PA: Elsevier Saunders.

Ohlsson, A., & Shah, V. S. (2014). Intrapartum antibiotics for known maternal group B streptococcal colonization. *Cochrane Database of Systematic Reviews, 2014*(6), CD007467.

Pammi, M., & Haque, K. (2015). Pentoxifylline for treatment of sepsis and necrotizing enterocolitis in neonates. *Cochrane Database of Systematic Reviews, 3,* CD004204.

Phares, C. R., Lynfield, R., Farley, M. M., Mohle-Boetani, J., Harrison, L., Petit, S., . . . Schrag, S. (2008). Epidemiology of invasive group B streptococcal disease in the United States, 1999–2005. *Journal of the American Medical Association, 299,* 2056.

Philip, A., & Baker, C. (1983). Cerebrospinal fluid C-reactive protein in neonatal meningitis. *Journal of Pediatrics, 102,* 715–717.

Polin, R., & the Committee on Fetus and Newborn. (2012). Management of neonates with suspected or proven early-onset bacterial sepsis. *Pediatrics, 129*(5), 1006–1015.

Pourcyrous, M., Bada, H., Korones, S., Baselski, V., & Wong, S. (1993). Significance of serial C-reactive protein: A systematic review of modern diagnostic tests for neonatal sepsis. *Archives of Pediatrics and Adolescent Medicine, 92,* 431.

Schelonka, R., Chai, M., Yoder, B., Hensley, D., Brockett, R., & Ascher, D. (1996). Volume of blood required to detect common neonatal pathogens. *Journal of Pediatrics, 129*(2), 275.

Schuchat, S., Zywick, S., Dinsmoor, M., Mercer, B., Romaquera, J., O'Sullivan, M., . . . Levine, O. (2000). Risk factors and opportunities for prevention of early-onset neonatal sepsis: A multicenter case-control study. *Pediatrics, 105,* 21.

Stoll, B. J., Hansen, N. I., Sánchez, P. J., Faix, R. G., Poindexter, B. B., Van Meurs, K. P., . . . Eunice Kennedy Shriver National Institute of Child Health and Human Development Neonatal Research Network. (2011). Early onset neonatal sepsis: The burden of group B Streptococcal and E. coli disease continues. *Pediatrics, 127*(5), 817.

Stone, P., Gupta, A., Loughrey, M., Della-Latta, P., Cimiotti, J., Larson, E., . . . Saiman, L. (2003). Attributable costs and length of stay of an extended-spectrum beta-lactamase-producing Klebsiella pneumonia outbreak in a neonatal intensive care unit. *Infectious Control & Hospital Epidemiology, 24,* 601.

Tamma, P. (2007). Toxoplasmosis. *Pediatrics in Review, 28,* 470.

Verani, J. R., McGee, L., Schrag, S., & Division of Bacterial Diseases, National Center for Immunization and Respiratory Diseases, Centers for Disease Control and Prevention (CDC). (2010). Prevention of perinatal group B streptococcal disease—Revised guidelines from CDC. *MMWR Recommendations and Reports, 59,* 1–34.

Verboon-Maciolek, M., Krediet, T., Gerards, L., Fleer, A., & van Loon, T. (2005). Clinical and epidemiologic characteristics of viral infections in a neonatal intensive care unit during a 12-year period. *Pediatric Infectious Disease Journal, 24,* 901–904.

Vouloumanou, E., Plessa, E., Karageorgopoulos, D., Mantadakis, E., & Falagas, M. (2011). Serum procalcitonin as a diagnostic marker for neonatal sepsis: A systematic review and meta-analysis. *Intensive Care Medicine, 37*(5), 747–762.

Workowski, K., Bolan, G., & Centers for Disease Control and Prevention (CDC). (2015). Sexually transmitted diseases treatment guidelines, 2015. *MMWR Recommendations and Reports, 64,* 1.

Young, T., & Magnum, B. (2011). *NeoFax 2011.* Montvale, NJ: Thomson Reuters.

15

Musculoskeletal System Case Studies

Kathryn R. McLean and Maureen F. McCourt

Chapter Objectives

1. Review embryology and pathophysiology of the musculoskeletal system
2. Apply knowledge of common defects of the musculoskeletal system to effectively communicate and relay information to parents
3. Analyze case studies to determine differential diagnoses and develop a plan of care
4. Review American Academy of Pediatrics (AAP) guidelines on developmental dysplasia of the hip (DDH) to formulate a plan of care

This chapter reviews the development of the musculoskeletal system and pathophysiology of the most common disorders and defects. The disorders and defects presented in this chapter include inherited disorders, malformations or deformities, and birth injuries. Inherited disorders include osteogenesis imperfecta (OI), achondroplasia, and thanatophoric dwarfism. Malformations or deformities caused by physical constraints include clubfeet, arthrogryposis, and DDH. Birth injuries include fractures and Erb's palsy. Case studies are presented to allow integration of the information provided on these disorders into diagnoses and plans of care for each case.

EMBRYOLOGY

The development of the musculoskeletal system is influenced by many factors. Structural defects are classified as malformations, deformations, or disruptions. Malformations involve abnormal tissue formation. Genetics, teratogens, and the fetal environment can all contribute to malformations. Examples of malformations include the skeletal dysplasias such as achondroplasia and thanatophoric dysplasia. Deformations occur when altered mechanical forces interfere with formation of parts of the body. Examples of malformation include arthrogryposis secondary to oligohydramnios, clubfeet, and plagiocephaly. Disruptions involve breakdown or destruction of normal tissues. Loss of a limb caused by an amniotic band is an example of a disruption. Normal morphogenesis requires proper cell division and migration, appropriate interaction between adjacent tissues, aggregation of similar cell types, normal hormonal influence, and appropriate mechanical factors. Malformations occur early in gestation (first 8 to 12 weeks), but deformations or disruptions often occur as the pregnancy progresses (Moore, Persaud, & Torchia, 2015).

The skeletal system arises from the embryonic mesoderm and neural crest cells (Butler & Mullins, 2014; Moore et al., 2015). The mesoderm gives rise to the mesenchyme, which differentiates into fibroblasts, chondroblasts, and osteoblasts. Various genes affect condensation of mesenchymal cells into the cartilage bone models (Table 15.1). Cartilage first appears during the fifth week of gestation. Homeobox-containing genes (HOX) regulate the patterning of limbs. Digits are formed by 8 weeks of life. Ossification centers appear in bone

Table 15.1 **Genes and Molecules Involved in Cartilage Bone Model Formation**

Genes	Growth Factors, Enzymes, and Hormones
Homeobox-containing genes: CHox-1, Hoxd-3, Hoxa-2, MHox, CHox-4, Hoxd-13	BMP-2, BMP-4, BMP-5
Msx-1, Msx-2	TGF-β
Barx-1	Activan
	Syndecan-1, Syndecan-2, Syndecan-3
Ck-erg	Versican
	Tenascin
Cart-1	GDF-5
	Fibronectin, hyaluronan, hyaladherin
	Cell adhesion molecules: N-CAM, N-Cadherin

BMP, bone morphogenetic protein; GDF, growth differentiation factor; N-CAM, neural cell adhesion molecule; TGF, transforming growth factor.

Adapted from Moore et al. (2015).

models by 8 weeks. Calcium and phosphorus stores from the mother affect this process. Ossification continues throughout life until approximately age 25. The length of the bones, and subsequently the height of the person, is complete by approximately age 20. Diet, vitamin D levels, and human growth hormone levels influence this growth (Moore et al., 2015). The skeleton is reshaped and remodeled throughout life through the interaction of osteoblasts (bone-forming cells) and osteoclasts (bone-degrading cells; Swarr & Sutton, 2010).

The synovial joints, necessary for movement, begin to develop by 6 weeks. The interzonal mesenchyme between the bones differentiates into the capsule and ligaments surrounding a cavity that contains lubricating fluid. Any abnormal intrauterine environment that restricts movement may cause joint fixation and deformity (Moore et al., 2015). This is the typical mechanism that occurs with arthrogryposis and clubfeet.

The development of the skeletal muscles involves differentiation of the mesoderm into myoblasts. Various genes and the MyoD family of muscle-specific basic helix–loop–helix (bHLH) transcription factors are activated to influence this differentiation. Myoblasts organize into myotubes. Myotubes enlarge and develop myofilaments. Growth of the myofilaments leads to muscle fibers. The number and size of muscle fibers continues to grow postnatally (Butler & Mullins, 2014). The continued development of the skeletal muscles requires proper innervation in order to prevent muscle wasting.

EVALUATION OF THE SKELETAL SYSTEM USING RADIOLOGIC IMAGING

A typical skeletal survey involves the following views: anteroposterior (AP) and lateral skull, AP and lateral thoracolumbar spine, AP of chest, AP of pelvis, upper and lower limbs, hands, and feet. One must look at the shape of the rib cage, number and shape of the ribs, presence of any vertebral anomalies, presence of any abnormal shape or length of long bones, presence of any fractures, and any abnormalities of the hands or feet. Shortening of part of the body is referred to as rhizomelia (proximal), mesomelia (middle), or acromelia (distal; Swarr & Sutton, 2010).

SKELETAL DYSPLASIAS: ACHONDROPLASIA AND THANATOPHORIC DYSPLASIA

Both achondroplasia and thanatophoric dysplasia are examples of primary dysplasias that result from mutations in genes. Once the mutations occur, inheritance is autosomal dominant with a risk of 50:50 inheritance in offspring of the affected patient. Both disorders involve the fibroblast growth factor-3 (FGFR3) gene (Swarr & Sutton, 2010).

Thanatophoric dysplasia is a potentially lethal skeletal dysplasia that presents with a very narrow thorax with consequent pulmonary hypoplasia, short limbs, normal trunk length, prominent forehead, and depressed nasal bridge. Cupped long bones on x-ray are a classic finding and differentiate this type of dwarfism from other nonlethal types. Craniosyntosis may be present. Death may occur related to respiratory failure secondary to the pulmonary hypoplasia. Surviving infants may have mental retardation or seizures related to megalencephaly or other cerebral anomalies (Swarr & Sutton, 2010).

Achondroplasia is the most common form of dwarfism (Butler & Mullins, 2014). Clinical findings include disproportionately short limbs compared with the rest of the body, normal trunk size, disproportionately large head, and "trident hands" (phalanges are short, wide, and cone-shaped). In infancy, the patient can have hypotonia and may have respiratory difficulties. In some patients, stenosis of the foramen magnum may place them at risk for brain stem compression with subsequent cardiorespiratory arrest. Hearing loss, recurrent otitis media, and speech delay may occur. Intellectual development is normal (Swarr & Sutton, 2010).

OSTEOGENESIS IMPERFECTA

Collagen, the major protein of connective tissue, provides a matrix for bone formation and is involved in healing fractures. OI is a genetic disorder in which the type I collagen is defective, creating easily fractured bones and other connective tissue problems (Glorieux et al., 2007). The major types of OI, clinical findings, and inheritance are described in Table 15.2.

OI often occurs as a spontaneous mutation. It is autosomal dominant in the majority of cases. With survival the patient's chance of having an offspring with the same disorder is 50:50. The majority of OI cases involve the genes that code for type I collagen (COL1A1 and COL1A2; Glorieux et al., 2007). Other forms of OI, many are of which recessive inheritance, are caused by mutations in CRTAP, LEPRE1, SERPINF1, FKBP10, and WNT1 genes (Amor et al., 2011; Baldridge et al., 2008; Barnes et al., 2012; Bodian et al., 2009; Cabral et al., 2012; Homan et al., 2011; Keupp et al., 2013). There are nine identified types the first four (I–IV) of which are most common (Table 15.2; Glorieux et al., 2007). The number of types will expand as new mutations are identified.

Diagnosis begins with identification of clinical findings. Future testing may include skin biopsy or genetic testing for the specific chromosomes implicated in OI (Glorieux et al., 2007). Both tests are time-consuming, and the practitioner should not wait until diagnosis is confirmed before initiating gentle care.

Table 15.2 **Types of Osteogenesis Imperfecta**

Type	Major Clinical Findings	Inheritance	Severity
I	Blue sclera; mild bone fragility; fractures often not seen until child begins to walk, bruises easily, slightly shorter-than-average stature; loose joints and low muscle tone; hearing loss in the 20s and 30s	Autosomal dominant	Mild
II	High perinatal mortality; fractures occur in utero; respiratory distress caused by underdeveloped lungs; severe bone deformities and numerous fractures; blue sclera	Autosomal dominant	Severe to lethal
III	Severe bone fragility with fractures, often in utero; progressive bone deformities; extremely short stature (< 5th percentile); respiratory distress sometimes occurs with chest deformities; white or blue sclera; dentinogenesis imperfecta (defective dental enamel) may be present	Autosomal dominant	Severe

(continued)

Table 15.2 **Types of Osteogenesis Imperfecta (***continued***)**

Type	Major Clinical Findings	Inheritance	Severity
IV	Moderate bone fragility; fractures may occur before ambulation but rare in utero; short stature (< 5th percentile); white to light-blue sclera; dentinogenesis imperfecta (defective dental enamel) may be present	Autosomal dominant	Moderate
V	Fracture occurrence and frequency similar to type IV; hypertrophic callus formation with fractures or spontaneously; calcification of the interosseous membrane between the radius and ulna restricting forearm rotation and potential dislocation of the radial head	Autosomal dominant	Moderate
VI	Similar findings as type IV; characteristic mineralization defect seen on bone biopsy	Autosomal recessive	Moderate; very rare
VII	Varied expression: Some cases are similar to type II, whereas others are more like type IV but with white sclera, small heads, and round faces; short stature; short humeri and femora	Autosomal recessive, mutation in the CRTAP gene	Moderate to severe to lethal
VIII	Similar to type II or III, but sclera are white; severe growth deficiency; extreme undermineralization of the skeleton	Autosomal recessive, mutation in the LEPRE1 gene	Severe
IX	Similar to type III and IV	Autosomal recessive, mutation in the peptidyl-prolyl isomerase B (PPIB) gene	Moderate, very rare

Adapted from Barnes et al. (2012) and Glorieux et al. (2007, pp. 4–10).

Fractures, pain management, and prevention of additional fractures will be an issue throughout the child's life. Circulation of affected extremities needs monitoring if splints or casting required. Casts may create additional fractures because of their weight so are often not utilized in the neonatal period (Glorieux et al., 2007). Narcotics may be required during acute episodes of fracture for pain management. Pamidronate, a bisphosphonate, reduces the number of new fractures, increases bone density, and improves mobility and ambulation (Allgrove, 2002; Astrom & Sonderhall, 2002; Giraud & Meunier, 2002; Glorieux, 2001). Administration of human growth hormone shows mixed results (Glorieux et al., 2007). Stem cell therapy may provide treatment in the future (Jones et al., 2014; Ramachandra et al., 2014).

Careful handling is an essential component of care to minimize pain and prevent or minimize risk of additional fractures. Avoid lifting the infant by holding beneath the armpits or by the arms or legs. Lift by placing one hand under the buttocks and the other behind the head. Spread the fingers of your hands to minimize pressure points and increase support. Support the legs against your forearms. When changing diapers, avoid holding by ankles—lift from the buttocks instead. Avoid vigorous burping—use a rocking motion while in a semiupright position or gently rub the abdomen to help expel gas. The manipulation required to dress an infant may cause fractures. Parents can alter clothing to provide additional seams, sealed by Velcro or snaps, to reduce this manipulation. Gel mattresses reduce pressure (Hartman, 2003).

Future issues include potential hearing loss as the child nears young adulthood. Dentition is often affected because of poor enamel formation (Glorieux et al., 2007).

Parents will require substantial education to care for their infants. They need to learn careful handling techniques, signs and symptoms of fractures, and administration of any analgesics. The Osteogenesis Imperfecta Foundation website (www.oif.org) is one source of parental teaching material.

Death is a possible outcome in several types of OI. Mortality is usually related to respiratory failure secondary to deformity of the thoracic cavity. Palliative care programs may be beneficial. After discharge, parents will need emotional support from all care providers and be made aware of available resources.

DEVELOPMENTAL DYSPLASIA OF THE HIPS

The proper formation of the hip joint depends on mechanical forces, genetic predisposition, and hormonal influences. The head of the femur must lie in a specific area and position on the hip in order for the acetabulum to shape correctly. A cleft between the acetabulum and head of the femur appears by 8 weeks gestation. Though the hip joint is formed by 11 weeks, the shape of the acetabulum continues to evolve after birth (Moore et al., 2015). Normal development of the hip requires a deep concentric position of the femoral head in the acetabulum. Breech position of the hip and other in utero mechanical forces place the femoral head lower on the hip, stretching the capsule and creating a shallow acetabulum. The hormone relaxin affects the tightness of the capsule. Female infants have increased receptors to relaxin, making them more at risk for hip instability (Wilkinson & Wilkinson, 2010).

The Ortolani and Barlow tests are the two maneuvers used in the newborn period to evaluate for DDH. Examination of the hip is done one hip at a time. Place the infant on his or her back with the legs in a frog-like position with hips bent 90°. The examiner's middle fingers are kept over the trochanter. The hip is abducted with gentle inward and upward pressure (Ortolani). Next, the hip is adducted using the thumb to apply outward and backward pressure over the inner thigh (Barlow). A clunk may be heard during reduction or dislocation (positive sign; Wilkinson & Wilkinson, 2010).

Other physical finding may indicate the presence of congenital hip dysplasia. When the legs are held together, determine whether creases line up. Asymmetry of skin folds may occur with DDH. The Barlow and Ortolani signs may not be present if the hips are completely dislocated and not able to reduce. A difference in leg length may also occur with dislocated hips. Determine whether the range of motion of the hips is normal—a reduction in range of motion may occur if the hip is dislocated (Wilkinson & Wilkinson, 2010). Re-examination of the hips should occur with each future examination.

Detection of suspected hip dysplasia involves identification of risk factors. Investigate family history to determine whether there is any DDH. A female infant in breech position born by cesarean section is at higher risk for DDHs. Per American Academy of Pediatric (AAP) guidelines, asymptomatic breech female infants should have a hip ultrasound at 6 weeks of life (Committee on Quality Improvement, Subcommittee on Developmental Dysplasia of the Hip, 2000). Soft clicks are equivocal findings and just warrant monitoring. Positive Ortolani or Barlow tests warrant an orthopedic referral. Should the infant show evidence of developmental dysplasia at any point, the treatment involves use of a Pavlik harness (Gulati et al., 2013; Wilkinson & Wilkinson, 2010). A Pavlik harness maintains the hips in flexion and abduction while allowing some motion. It also reduces the risk of dislocation. The length of treatment is usually 3 to 9 months (Gulati et al., 2013). Triple diapers are not recommended (Committee on Quality Improvement, Subcommittee on Developmental Dysplasia of the Hip, 2000). Failure to detect DDH places the infant at risk for hip dislocation, premature osteoarthritis of the hip in early adulthood, and avascular necrosis of the head of the femur (Wilkinson & Wilkinson, 2010).

TALIPES EQUINOVARUS (CLUBFOOT)

Talipes equinovarus is commonly called "clubfoot." Clubfoot has four main components: equinovarus deformity of the foot and ankle; variable rigidity of the deformity; mild calf atrophy; and mild hypoplasia of the tibia, fibula, and bones of the foot. Clubfoot is more common in boys (2:1) and half of the cases are bilateral, with increased risk among family members. The etiology of clubfoot is unknown although genetic and environmental factors appear to play a multifactorial role (Dobbs & Gurnett, 2009; Hart, Grottkau, Rebello, & Albright, 2005; Son-Hing & Thompson, 2015).

The classifications for clubfoot are positional, congenital, and teratogenic. The most common is positional clubfoot caused by intrauterine positioning late in pregnancy, which resolves quickly. Congenital clubfoot with multifactorial etiology is the most common and has intermediate severity. Teratologic clubfoot, associated with other conditions, is the most severe form. Although clubfoot is typically an isolated birth defect, it can be associated with neuromuscular disorders such as myelodysplasia or arthrogryposis. It may also be part of multiple congenital abnormalities. These are usually associated with teratologic clubfoot (Dobbs & Gurnett, 2009; Hart et al., 2005; Son-Hing & Thompson, 2015).

The typical diagnostic process for clubfoot is determining the classic four components noted above on physical exam. It is also often diagnosed on prenatal ultrasound around 16 to 20 weeks, which helps with management planning and eases parental anxiety. Clubfoot is a deformity of the foot and entire lower leg that presents in mild to severe forms. X-rays are used in the assessment of clubfoot. AP and lateral standing or simulated weight bearing help determine line measurements to ascertain the position of the unossified navicular bone (primary site of deformity) and overall alignment of the foot (Dobbs & Gurnett, 2009; Hart et al., 2005; Son-Hing & Thompson, 2015).

All newborns with clubfoot should be referred for orthopedic consultation. Nonoperative treatment options include taping, malleable splints, and serial plaster casts. Serial casting is the most common treatment with foot manipulation toward the correct position and cast changes every 1 to 2 weeks. This allows for progressive correction, confirmed by x-ray, with the process complete by 3 months of age. Holding casts are used for an additional 3 to 6 months with orthotics or corrective shoes used until the child is walking. Operative treatment is indicated if nonoperative options are unsuccessful. The Ponsetti Method is now the most common treatment option, which uses early manipulation and plaster-of-paris casting weekly for 4 to 6 weeks. When required, this method is combined with percutaneous tendo Achilles tenotomy. For the most optimal outcome, this is followed by prolonged bracing for 2 to 4 years. The overall outcome for newborns with positional and congenital clubfoot is good. Outcomes with the teratologic form are more difficult with cases and outcome dependent on the associated conditions (Hart et al., 2005; Son-Hing & Thompson, 2015).

TORTICOLLIS

Torticollis is a painless condition associated with shortening of the sternocleidomastoid muscle which results in the head tilting to the tightened side and the tilting chin toward the opposite side. There can be an associated palpable mass within the affected muscle during the first few weeks of life and flattening of the head, slight facial asymmetry, as well as plagiocephaly. The exact etiology of torticollis is unknown, but intrauterine malposition, birth trauma, muscle fibrosis, and venous abnormalities are implicated. DDH and metatarsus adductus can be associated with torticollis. Torticollis may also result from congenital cervicovertebral anomalies, including Klippel–Feil syndrome and congenital scoliosis (Liu & Thompson, 2015).

Torticollis is diagnosed by physical exam. Cervical spine x-rays and sometimes computed tomography are indicated to rule out congenital cervicovertebral anomalies as the etiology of torticollis because the treatment plan will be different in these cases.

The treatment plan for torticollis when underlying skeletal abnormalities have been ruled out includes a stretching exercise program to lengthen the contracted muscle. The head should be tilted toward the opposite shoulder and the chin rotated toward the affected side and maintained for 5 to 10 seconds. Usually, this is repeated 10 to 15 times in a gentle fashion as quickly after diagnosis as possible, four times a day. Torticollis usually resolves within 6 months with an exercise program begun within 3 months. Programs begun after 18 months are typically unsuccessful. If an exercise program is unsuccessful, a surgical release of the sternocleidomastoid contracture is indicated. Torticollis associated with congenital cervical anomalies is more complex and may need further surgical intervention, such as a surgical fusion, with less optimal outcomes. Facial asymmetry related to head tilting is unlikely to resolve (Liu & Thompson, 2015).

CONGENITAL SCOLIOSIS

Congenital scoliosis is curvature of the spine related to deformities in the coronal plane secondary to failure of vertebrae formation (hemivertebrae), failure of segmentation (unsegmented bars), or a combination of these. Scoliosis in children younger than 3 years of age is rare, but vertebral segmentation is relatively common and can lead to scoliosis development later in life. Scoliosis occurs more commonly in families, in boys, and with curvatures to the left side. Risk factors for congenital scoliosis include anoxia and environmental toxins, cancer or spinal tumors, connective tissue disorders, diaphragmatic hernia, hypotonia, maternal diabetes, maternal medications, rickets or malnutrition, and spinal cord malformations (Brand, 2008; Son-Hing & Thompson, 2015).

The conditions associated with abnormal vertebral segmentation, which can lead to congenital scoliosis, include achondroplasia, Alagille syndrome, camptomelic dysplasia, diaphanospondylostosis, OI type II, Robinow syndrome, spondylocostal dysostosis/spondylothoracic dysostosis, trisomy 9, 8, 18, and 21, and VATER/VACTERL syndrome (Brand, 2008). Congenital genitourinary malformations, congenital heart disease, and spinal dysraphism occur more frequently in newborns with congenital scoliosis (Son-Hing & Thompson, 2015).

The diagnostic process starts with a physical exam; newborns with congenital scoliosis may or may not have curvature of the spine depending on the severity of the curve. The spine should also be examined for any associated spinal dysraphism. These newborns should be assessed for chest asymmetry and resultant respiratory distress that can occur with severe scoliosis associated with pneumothorax or diaphragmatic hernia. Careful assessment for presence of a murmur to rule out associated congenital heart disease and palpation of the kidneys with good urine output to rule out congenital genitourinary malformations are important (Brand, 2008; Son-Hing & Thompson, 2015).

Diagnostic imaging for infants with suspected congenital scoliosis includes plain films of the thoracic and lumbar spine, which can diagnose spinal deformities. Magnetic resonance imaging is often done to evaluate the spinal canal and spinal cord for lesions. Echocardiogram may be useful to check for congenital heart disease and renal ultrasound to detect any associated congenital genitourinary anomalies. A renal ultrasound following urine output and laboratory tests will assist in ruling out congenital genitourinary anomalies (Brand, 2008; Son-Hing & Thompson, 2015).

Newborns with congenital scoliosis must be referred for orthopedic consultation. Sequential weight-bearing radiographs are necessary to monitor scoliosis progression, often using the "Cobb Angle." Cobb angles of 10° diagnose scoliosis and angles up to 25° are unlikely to progress. Often Cobb angles greater than 45° in young children require surgery. Conservative management includes use of orthotics and casting; surgery is required when these interventions are no longer successful. Congenital scoliosis tends to be the most progressive, is resistant to correction, and results in larger deformities than other types of scoliosis. Orthopedic follow-up is critical to optimize patient outcomes (Brand, 2008; Son-Hing & Thompson, 2015).

BIRTH INJURIES

Macrosomic infants are more at risk for all types of birth injuries. Soft tissue injuries, such as cephalhematomas and bruising, are most common. The clavicle fracture followed by fracture of the humerus are the most common long-bone fractures. Brachial plexus injuries involve damage to the nerves in the neck and shoulders. In Erb–Duchenne paralysis, the affected arm is limp, elbow is extended, and arm is internally rotated. With Klumpke's paralysis, the hand and wrist are paralyzed (Butler & Mullins, 2014). If a brachial plexus injury is suspected, the infant should be referred to a neurologist and for occupational therapy.

OSTEOMYELITIS

Osteomyelitis is an infection of the bone that can occur as a result of bacteremia, direct inoculation from a puncture wound, or spread from adjacent areas of infection. In neonates, the most common route for transmission is from infected blood traveling to the metaphysic, where there is an area of sluggish blood flow providing a perfect setup for bacteria to get trapped and proliferate. In addition, sinusoidal vessels can transmit infection to the growth plate, which can impact long-term bone growth. Infection and inflammation can cause abscess formation and, with rupture of the abscess, it can lead to a joint space infection known as *septic arthritis.* The most common bones involved in neonatal osteomyelitis are the femur and tibia; the most common organism is *Staphylococcus aureus.* Other organisms associated with neonatal osteomyelitis include methicillin-resistant *S. aureus* (MRSA), streptococci and enteric aerobic bacilli, and *Candida albicans* (Fisher, 2011; Gilmore & Thompson, 2015).

Risk factors for osteomyelitis include birth weight less than 2,500 g or gestational age less than 37 weeks, delivery via emergency cesarean delivery, respiratory distress syndrome (RDS), hyperbilirubinemia, umbilical lines, asphyxia, scalp laceration after vacuum extraction, and renal vein thrombosis (Fisher, 2011; Gilmore & Thompson, 2015).

When infection is suspected, the diagnostic process involves a complete sepsis evaluation, including a complete blood count with differential, blood culture, a urine test, and cerebral spinal fluid test. A thorough physical exam is indicated when osteomyelitis is suspected. Typically, there is decreased movement of the limb and swelling or possible redness at the site, general signs of sepsis, ranging from mild to severe, are seen. Radiography (shows signs of bone destruction), ultrasound, MRI, CT scan, and bone scans can be useful in the diagnosis of osteomyelitis. Bone-needle aspiration of purulent material will lead to confirmation of the diagnosis and provide material for culture and susceptibility testing (Fisher, 2011; Gilmore & Thompson, 2015).

Broad-spectrum antibiotic therapy (oxacillin or nafcillin and an aminoglycoside such as gentamicin or tobramycin) should be started with suspected osteomyelitis, and treatment should be altered according to culture results and antibiotic sensitivities. Antibiotics should be adjusted to the organism and sensitivities found in the bone-needle aspiration material. Treatment should be of 4 to 6 weeks duration (Fisher, 2011; Gilmore & Thompson, 2015).

Many neonates with osteomyelitis go on to have permanent sequelae regardless of prompt diagnosis and treatment. The growth plate can be damaged causing disparities in the both the affected and nonaffected limbs. Certain outcomes may not be apparent until age 9 or 10 (Fisher, 2011; Gilmore & Thompson, 2015).

CONCLUSIONS

This chapter outlines some of the disorders and defects that can occur with the neonatal musculoskeletal system. Early identification by the neonatal team and follow-up by an orthopedic subspecialist are essential in establishing a collaborative treatment plan to optimize patient outcomes. It is critical to communicate the plan of care with the family and to include them in the care of their infant. Communication and participation in care will decrease parental anxiety and ensure appropriate care of the infant after discharge.

Case 15.1

The neonatal team was called to a spontaneous vaginal delivery at 34 weeks gestation. The labor and delivery nurses reported a prenatal ultrasound showing "shortened and thickened femurs." The vaginal delivery was uneventful. At delivery, the infant was limp with no spontaneous respirations. The infant received positive pressure ventilation by Ambu bag, and was subsequently intubated with a 3.5-mm endotracheal tube at 4 minutes of life. The heart rate remained more than 100 beats per minute throughout resuscitation. Apgar scores were 2 at 1 minute, 6 at 5 minutes, and 6 at 10 minutes of age. The

(continued)

Case 15.1 *(continued)*

physical exam was notable for the following findings: right foot laterally rotated and immobile at the ankle, swelling at multiple sites along the extremities, shortened lower limbs. On arrival to the neonatal intensive care unit (NICU), the infant was placed on mechanical ventilation. The infant demonstrated spontaneous respirations in addition to mechanical breaths. Spontaneous movement of extremities was present, but limited, especially in the limbs that exhibited localized swelling. The female infant weighed 2,300 g.

The diagnostic images obtained are seen in Figures 15.1, 15.2, 15.3, and 15.4. This infant's malformations include a bowing deformity of the right femur and contracture of the right ankle. Generalized osteopenia is present. Wormian bones (small irregular bones located in the cranial sutures) are seen. Fractures in various states of healing are evident on multiple ribs, the clavicles, both humeri, and left ulna.

1. *What is the most likely musculoskeletal disorder in this case?*

   A. Thanatophoric dwarfism
   B. Osteogenesis imperfecta (OI)
   C. Birth trauma

   ANSWER: B. *The multiple fractures present from birth are most consistent with OI (Butler & Mullins, 2014).*

2. *What diagnostic tests would you obtain?*

   A. Chest x-ray, MRI of the head, muscle biopsy
   B. No additional tests required—defects are obvious with inspection
   C. Full skeletal series: chest x-ray, skull, all limbs

   ANSWER: C. *A full skeletal series will document all fractures present at birth, the presence of wormian bones in the skull, and any deformities of rib cage and limbs (Butler & Mullins, 2014).*

3. *What initial laboratory tests would you order?*

   A. Arterial blood gas, blood culture, complete blood count, serum glucose
   B. Clotting studies, blood gas, electrolytes
   C. Blood culture and complete blood count only

   ANSWER: A. *As the infant has respiratory distress, laboratory tests to evaluate gas exchange, sepsis, and possible hypoglycemia are required.*

4. *What are the implications/problems associated with this diagnosis?*

   A. Increased risk of infection resulting from immunodeficiency
   B. Respiratory distress, increased risk of future fractures, pain management
   C. Respiratory distress related to surfactant deficiency, increased calorie/nutrient requirement, hypocalcemia

   ANSWER: B. *Deformities of the rib cage can limit lung expansion. The fragility of bones continues beyond the newborn period and especially can occur when child begins to ambulate, and pain occurs with fractures (Glorieux et al., 2007).*

(continued)

Case 15.1 (continued)

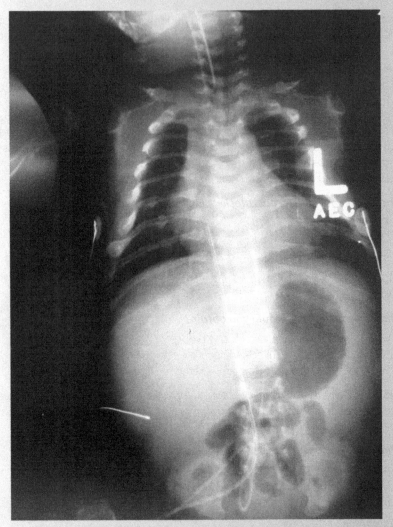

Figure 15.1 Chest and Abdominal Film

5. *What specialists could assist in the management of this infant?*

A. Genetics, occupational therapy, pediatric orthopedics, social servicesInfectious disease, pulmonology

B. Orthopedics only

C. Neonatologists are familiar with this common disorder and can manage the infant without consultation with specialists

ANSWER: A. *This condition requires a multidisciplinary approach (Glorieux et al., 2007).*

(continued)

Case 15.1 (continued)

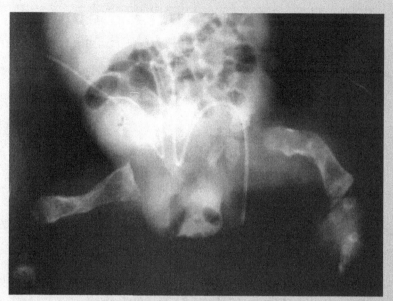

Figure 15.2 Lower Extremities Film

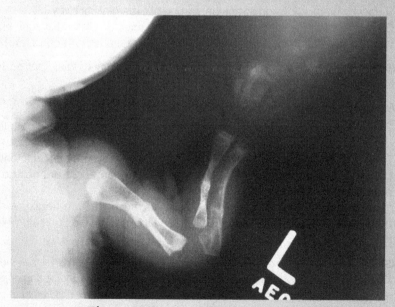

Figure 15.3 Left Upper Extremity Film

(continued)

Case 15.1 *(continued)*

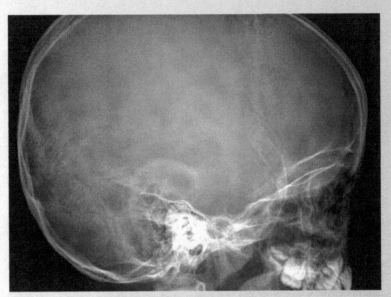

***Figure* 15.4** Skull Film of Infant

6. *What would the clinical management of this infant include?*

  A. Withdrawal of support as disorder is not compatible with life
  B. Surfactant preparation administration, casting of extremity fractures
  C. Careful handling to minimize pain and future fractures, ventilator management and weaning, antibiotics until blood culture is negative or sepsis/pneumonia resolves

ANSWER: C. *Refer to recommendations contained in the body of this chapter (Glorieux et al., 2007).*

7. *This baby's mother asks you "How did this happen?" You respond:*

  A. "This is a genetic disorder that causes brittle bones. Most cases are spontaneous mutations. There is nothing you did during pregnancy to cause this."
  B. "Your baby is premature. The respiratory distress is caused by a surfactant deficiency. Premature infants are fragile, so fractures can occur during the birth process."
  C. "Your diet didn't include enough calcium, so the bones are fragile. With the proper diet for your baby the fractures will heal and there won't be a problem in the future."

ANSWER: A. *The cases are autosomal dominant in types I-V, autosomal recessive in types VI-IX. The majority are spontaneous mutations. Genetic counseling and testing of parents will be beneficial to aid parents in their decision on whether to have children in the future (Glorieux et al., 2007).*

(continued)

Case 15.1 (continued)

8. Based on the clinical findings described and the information in Table 15.2, what is the most likely type of this particular disorder?

A. Type I
B. Type II or III
C. Type IV

ANSWER: B. *The severity of fractures and respiratory distress present from birth supports clinical findings of Type II or III (Glorieux et al., 2007).*

Case 15.2

The neonatal team is called to a shoulder dystocia delivery. You arrive after the delivery and find a crying infant actively moving but the right arm is extended and limp. Examination of both clavicles demonstrated crepitus and a "step-off" (difference in elevation of two parts of the clavicle) upon palpation of the right clavicle. The infant weighed 4,825 g.

1. What diagnosis do you suspect?

A. Muscle strain that will resolve with time
B. Fractured right clavicle with possible brachial plexis injury
C. Fractured right humerus

ANSWER: B. *Limitation of arm movement is present in both temporary and permanent nerve injury. Crepitus and "step-off" are often palpable with clavicle fractures (Butler & Mullins, 2014).*

2. What diagnostic test would you order?

A. Chest and right arm x-rays
B. MRI of upper body
C. Electromyography of the right arm

ANSWER: A. *X-rays are confirmatory. The entire limb should be included to rule out additional fractures (Butler & Mullins, 2014).*

3. What is the recommended management of the skeletal condition?

A. Casting
B. No special care required
C. Limitation of movement by keeping the right arm of the t-shirt pinned across the chest

ANSWER: C. *Limitation of movement reduces pain. The fracture heals on its own without casting (Butler & Mullins, 2014).*

Case 15.3

Baby girl J is a 40 2/7-week-gestation 3,285-g infant in the newborn nursery. She was delivered by cesarean section for breech presentation. Her mother is a 22-year-old gravida 1, para 0 to 1 with normal serology and a benign medical history. Baby girl J has a normal physical exam and is pink in room air with no distress. She has no clicks or clunks on hip examination.

1. *Name the procedures you used to determine the presence of hip clicks or clunks.*

   A. Govanni and Hayes
   B. Auscultation of the hip joint
   C. Ortolani and Barlow

   ANSWER: C. *A description of how to perform these maneuvers is contained within this chapter (Wilkinson & Wilkinson, 2010).*

2. *What other details would you look for while performing the exam?*

   A. Symmetry of leg creases and leg length, degree of movement of hip joint
   B. Legs kept extended and positioned toward head
   C. Hyperextension of the knee

   ANSWER: A. *Dislocated hips result in uneven leg creases and decreased hip movement (Wilkinson & Wilkinson, 2010).*

3. *What would your management plan include?*

   A. Placement of a Pavlik harness
   B. Triple diapers
   C. Examination of hips with each visit and hip ultrasound at 6 weeks

   ANSWER: C. *As the infant shows no evidence of developmental dysplasia of the hip (DDH) at present, there is no need for a Pavlik harness. Triple diapers are never recommended. DDH may become evident over time and a breech female is at highest risk; therefore, frequent hip examination and future hip ultrasound are recommended (Committee on Quality Improvement, Subcommittee on Developmental Dysplasia of the Hip, 2000).*

4. *What complications can occur if a provider fails to identify the condition?*

   A. None—this condition is self-resolving
   B. Hip dislocation, premature osteoarthritis of the hip, and avascular necrosis of the head of the femur
   C. Locked hip, Erb's palsy

   ANSWER: B. *Rationale for this answer is contained in the body of this chapter (Wilkinson & Wilkinson, 2010).*

Case 15.4

Baby boy J was born at 40 weeks weighing 3,500 g via a normal vaginal delivery after an uncomplicated pregnancy; Apgar scores are 9 at 1 minute and 9 at 5 minutes of life. He was transferred to the newborn nursery and on physical exam was noted to have equinovarus deformity of the foot and ankle; variable rigidity of the deformity; mild calf atrophy; and mild hypoplasia of the tibia, fibula, and bones of the foot. Baby J's stiffness and movement appear intermediate in nature without any other abnormalities.

1. **What is Baby J's diagnosis?**

    A. Metatarsus adductus
    B. Calcaneovalgus foot
    C. Talipes equinovarus (clubfoot)

    ANSWER: C. *Talipes equinovarus is commonly called* clubfoot. *Clubfoot has four main components: equinovarus deformity of the foot and ankle, variable rigidity of the deformity, mild calf atrophy, and mild hypoplasia of the tibia, fibula, and bones of the foot (Son-Hing & Thompson, 2015).*

2. **What is the typical diagnostic process for Baby J's orthopedic diagnosis and what should you see on physical exam?**

    A. Diagnosis is typically made by physical exam findings that include equinovarus deformity of the foot and ankle; variable rigidity of the deformity; mild calf atrophy; and mild hypoplasia of the tibia, fibula, and bones of the foot
    B. Diagnosis made by x-rays of lower extremities
    C. Diagnosis made by MRI

    ANSWER: A. *The typical diagnostic process for clubfoot is determining the classic four findings on physical exam, which include equinovarus deformity of the foot and ankle, variable rigidity of the deformity, mild calf atrophy, and mild hypoplasia of the tibia, fibula, and bones of the foot. It is also often diagnosed on prenatal ultrasound around 16 to 20 weeks, which helps with management planning and eases parental anxiety (Son-Hing & Thompson, 2015).*

3. **What are the associated anomalies of Baby J's orthopedic diagnosis?**

    A. It is typically an isolated birth defect but can be associated with neuromuscular disorders such as myelodysplasia or arthrogryposis
    B. It has no associated anomalies
    C. It is often associated with cardiac anomalies

    ANSWER: A. *Although clubfoot is typically an isolated birth defect, it can be associated with neuromuscular disorders, such as myelodysplasia or arthrogryposis. It may also be part of multiple congenital abnormalities (Dobbs & Gurnett, 2009).*

(continued)

Case 15.4 (continued)

4. What imaging studies are required for Baby J's orthopedic diagnosis?

A. MRI aids in the diagnosis process

B. X-rays are used in the assessment process

C. Ultrasound is required for diagnosis

ANSWER: B. *X-rays are used in the assessment of clubfoot. AP and lateral standing or simulated weight bearing help determine line measurements to ascertain the position of the unossified navicular bone (primary site of deformity) and overall alignment of the foot (Son-Hing & Thompson, 2015).*

5. What is the most common treatment option for clubfoot?

A. Surgical repair

B. Ponsetti Method

C. Usually resolves spontaneously, no treatment required

ANSWER: B. *The Ponsetti Method is now the most common treatment option, which uses early manipulation and plaster-of-paris casting weekly for 4 to 6 weeks. This is combined with percutaneous tendo Achilles tenotomy when required, and is followed by prolonged bracing for 2 to 4 years for the most optimal outcome (Son-Hing & Thompson, 2015).*

6. What is Baby J's prognosis?

A. Outcome is poor with Baby J's physical exam findings of bilateral inversion and adduction of the forefoot, inversion of the heel and hindfoot, equinus (limited extension) of the ankles and joints, and internal or medial rotation of the legs

B. Prognosis is guarded as surgery will be the first approach needed and used

C. Overall outcome is good as Baby J's stiffness and movement appear intermediate in nature without any other abnormalities

ANSWER: C. *The overall outcome for newborns with positional and congenital clubfoot is good. Outcomes with the teratologic form are more difficult cases and outcome dependent on the associated conditions (Son-Hing & Thompson, 2015).*

Case 15.5

Baby girl A was born at 30 weeks weighing 1,270 g to a 39-year-old gravida 2, para 1 now 2, blood type B positive, antibody screen negative, rapid plasma reagin (RPR) nonreactive, rubella immune, hepatitis B surface antigen negative, HIV negative, group B *Streptococcus* unknown, chlamydia negative, gonorrhea negative mother. Pregnancy was uncomplicated, and mother received routine prenatal care with no past medical history. Preterm labor occurred with premature rupture of membranes. There was a maternal tempera-

(continued)

Case 15.5 (*continued*)

ture of 103°F. Antibiotics and bethamethasone were given. Fetal bradycardia was noted and an emergency cesarean section was performed. Baby emerged depressed and required intubation in the delivery room. She was transferred to the neonatal intensive care unit (NICU). Baby A's NICU course was complicated by respiratory distress syndrome (RDS) for which surfactant replacement was given. She required umbilical arterial and venous lines. Baby A received 7 days of antibiotic therapy, although blood cultures were negative. Baby A was extubated to continuous positive airway pressure (CPAP) and placed on nasogastric feedings. She required phototherapy for 3 days. On day of life 20, Baby A began having apnea requiring reintubation along with temperature instability. A sepsis evaluation was initiated and she was placed on oxacillin and gentamicin. Baby A had a positive blood culture, *Staphylococcus aureus*. She was also noted to have swelling of the right leg and limited movement of the extremity.

1. **Baby A's current diagnoses list includes prematurity, RDS, apnea of prematurity, and blood sepsis. What new diagnosis would you add to this list?**

    A. Rule out joint injury from birth trauma

    B. Rule out osteomyelitis

    C. Rule out osteoporosis

    ANSWER: B. *Osteomyelitis is an infection of the bone that can occur as a result of bacteremia, direct inoculation from a puncture wound, or spread from adjacent areas of infection. In neonates, the most common route for transmission is from infected blood traveling to the metaphysic, where there is an area of sluggish blood flow providing a perfect setup for bacteria to get trapped and proliferate (Gilmore & Thompson, 2015).*

2. **What factors place Baby girl A at risk for this new diagnosis?**

    A. History of a difficult delivery causing injury

    B. Poor nutrition related to prematurity and blood sepsis

    C. Prematurity, birth weight of 1,270 g, delivery via emergency cesarean section, RDS, hyperbilirubinemia, umbilical arterial catheter (UAC) and umbilical venous catheter (UVC) lines, and blood infection

    ANSWER: C. *Risk factors for osteomyelitis include birth weight less than 2,500 g or gestational age less than 37 weeks, delivery via emergency cesarean delivery, respiratory distress syndrome (RDS), hyperbilirubinemia, umbilical lines, asphyxia, scalp laceration after vacuum extraction, and renal vein thrombosis (Gilmore & Thompson, 2015).*

3. **What is the diagnostic process for Baby A's new diagnosis?**

    A. Radiography, ultrasound, MRI, computerized tomography (CT) scan, and bone scans can aid in diagnosis with bone needle aspiration of purulent material confirming diagnosis

    B. Nutrition labs

    C. No further testing required since current treatment will resolve new diagnosis

(*continued*)

Case 15.5 (continued)

ANSWER: A. *When infection is suspected, the diagnostic process involves a complete sepsis evaluation, including a complete blood count with differential, blood culture, a urine test, and cerebral spinal fluid test. A thorough physical exam is indicated when osteomyelitis is suspected. Typically, there is decreased movement of the limb and swelling or possible redness at the site, general signs of sepsis, ranging from mild to severe, are seen. Radiography (shows signs of bone destruction), ultrasound, MRI, CT scan, and bone scans can be useful in the diagnosis of osteomyelitis. Bone-needle aspiration of purulent material will lead to confirmation of the diagnosis and provide material for culture and susceptibility testing (Fisher, 2011).*

4. What is the treatment for Baby girl A?

   A. Immobility of the extremity
   B. Nutritional supplements depending on lab test results
   C. Antibiotics adjusted to organism and sensitivities found in the bone need aspiration material, 4 to 6 weeks duration

ANSWER: C. *Broad-spectrum antibiotic therapy (oxacillin or nafcillin and an aminoglycoside such as gentamicin or tobramycin) should be started with suspected osteomyelitis, and treatment should be altered according to culture results and antibiotic sensitivities. Antibiotics should be adjusted to the organism and sensitivities found in the bone-needle aspiration material. Treatment should be of 4 to 6 weeks duration (Gilmore & Thompson, 2015).*

5. What is the long-term outcome for Baby girl A?

   A. Poor prognosis with ongoing continued issues
   B. Certain outcome may not be apparent until age 9 or 10 since growth plate can be damaged
   C. Good prognosis when injury recovers

ANSWER: B. *Many neonates with osteomyelitis go on to have permanent sequelae regardless of prompt diagnosis and treatment. The growth plate can be damaged causing disparities in both the affected and nonaffected limbs. Certain outcomes may not be apparent until age 9 or 10 (Gilmore & Thompson, 2015).*

Case 15.6

Baby girl N was born at 32 weeks weighing 1,500 g to a 20-year-old gravida 1, para 0 now 1, blood type AB positive, antibody screen negative, RPR nonreactive, rubella immune, hepatitis B surface antigen negative, HIV negative, group B *Streptococcus* unknown, chlamydia

(continued)

Case 15.6 (*continued*)

negative, gonorrhea negative mother. The maternal history was significant for maternal diabetes, no drug use or alcohol use but cigarette smoking (one package per day). Pregnancy was uncomplicated until preterm labor at 32 weeks, labor progressed and Baby N emerged depressed after delivery with a nuchal cord. Apgar scores were 1 at 5 minutes and 8 at 10 minutes of life. Baby N was transferred to the neonatal intensive care unit in 40% oxygen via face mask for prematurity and respiratory distress. Upon admission, a chest x-ray was performed showing eight-rib expansion, a ground-glass appearance of lungs, air bronchograms, normal heart size, and segmented vertebrae with slight curvature of the spine. Baby N's physical exam is noted to be within normal limits for gestational age.

1. *Baby N's differential diagnoses include prematurity, respiratory distress syndrome, and what orthopedic diagnosis?*

   A. Congenital kyphosis
   B. Congenital scoliosis
   C. Sacral agenesis

   ANSWER: B. *The diagnosis of congenital scoliosis starts with a physical exam; newborns with congenital scoliosis may or may not have curvature of the spine depending on the severity of the curve. Diagnostic imaging for infants with suspected congenital scoliosis includes plain films of the thoracic and lumbar spine, which can diagnose spinal deformities which include hemivertebrae, unsegmented bars, or a combination of the two (Brand, 2008).*

2. *What are the current risk factors for Baby N's orthopedic diagnosis?*

   A. Maternal diabetes and cigarette smoking
   B. Prematurity
   C. None of the above

   ANSWER: A. *Risk factors for congenital scoliosis include anoxia and environmental toxins, cancer or spinal tumors, connective tissue disorders, diaphragmatic hernia, hypotonia, maternal diabetes, maternal medications, rickets or malnutrition, and spinal cord malformations (Brand, 2008).*

3. *What conditions are associated with abnormal vertebral segmentation, which can lead to Baby's N's orthopedic diagnosis?*

   A. Achondroplasia, Alagilles syndrome, camptomelic dysplasia, dysostosis/spondylothoracic dysostosis, VACTER/VACTERL syndrome
   B. Trisomy 9, 8, 18, 21
   C. All of the above

   ANSWER: C. *The conditions associated with abnormal vertebral segmentation, which can lead to congenital scoliosis, include achondroplasia, Alagille syndrome, camptomelic dysplasia, diaphnaospondylostosis, OI type II, Robinow syndrome, spondylocostal dysostosis/spondylothoracic dysostosis, trisomy 9, 8, 18, and 21, and VATER/VACTERL syndrome (Brand, 2008).*

(continued)

Case 15.6 (continued)

4. **What diagnostic imaging is needed for Baby N?**
   A. X-rays of the thoracic and lumbar spine and MRI
   B. Ultrasound and CT scan of the thoracic and lumbar spine
   C. No diagnostic imaging needed

   ANSWER: A. *Diagnostic imaging for infants with suspected congenital scoliosis includes plain films of the thoracic and lumbar spine, which can diagnose spinal deformities which include hemivertebrae, unsegmented bars, or a combination of the two (Brand, 2008).*

5. **What are Baby N's follow-up needs?**
   A. Orthopedic follow-up, sequential weight-bearing, radiographs showing "Cobb angle"
   B. Pediatric follow-up sufficient with physical exam monitoring curvature of spine
   C. No follow-up needed

   ANSWER: A. *Newborns with congenital scoliosis must be referred for orthopedic consultation. Sequential weight-bearing radiographs are necessary to monitor scoliosis progression, often using the "Cobb Angle." Cobb angles of 10° diagnose scoliosis and angles up to 25° are unlikely to progress. Often Cobb angles greater than 45° in young children require surgery. Conservative management includes use of orthotics and casting; surgery is required when these interventions are no longer successful (Brand, 2008).*

Case 15.7

Baby girl M was born at 38 weeks weighing 3,300 g after an uncomplicated pregnancy via a normal vaginal delivery with Apgar scores of 8 at 1 minute and 9 at 5 minutes. She was transferred to the newborn nursery and on physical exam was noted to have a head tilted to the right with a tight sternocleidomastoid muscle and chin toward the left. Slight flattening of the head and slight facial asymmetry were noted. No other anomalies were seen.

1. **What is Baby M's diagnosis?**
   A. Congenital kyphosis
   B. Sacral agenesis
   C. Congenital muscular torticollis

   ANSWER: C. *Torticollis is a painless condition associated with shortening of the sternocleidomastoid muscle which results in the head tilting to the tightened side and the tilting chin toward the opposite side (Liu & Thompson, 2015).*

(continued)

Case 15.7 (continued)

2. What imaging studies are required for Baby M?

A. None indicated

B. Cervical spine x-rays to rule out congenital cervicovertebral anomalies

C. MRI

ANSWER: B. *Cervical spine x-rays and sometimes computed tomography are indicated to rule out congenital cervicovertebral anomalies as the etiology of torticollis because the treatment plan will be different in these cases (Liu & Thompson, 2015).*

3. What is the treatment plan and prognosis for Baby M?

A. When underlying skeletal abnormalities are ruled out, a stretching exercise program is needed. The prognosis is good, with resolution typically in 6 months.

B. Surgery is usually required with good prognosis.

C. No treatment is necessary—this condition will resolve on its own, and there will be a good prognosis.

ANSWER: A. *The treatment plan for torticollis when underlying skeletal abnormalities have been ruled out includes a stretching exercise program to lengthen the contracted muscle. The head should be tilted toward the opposite shoulder and the chin rotated toward the affected side and maintained for 5 to 10 seconds. Usually, this is repeated 10 to 15 times in a gentle fashion as quickly after diagnosis as possible, four times a day. Torticollis usually resolves within 6 months with an exercise program begun within 3 months (Liu & Thompson, 2015).*

REFERENCES

Allgrove, J. (2002). Use of bisphosphonates in children and adolescents. *Journal of Pediatric Endocrinology and Metabolism, 15*(Suppl. 3), 921–928.

Amor, I. M. B., Rauch, F., Gruenwald, K., Weis, M., Eyre, D. R., Roughley, P., . . . Morello, R. (2011). Severe osteogenesis imperfecta caused by a small in-frame deletion in CRTAP. *American Journal of Medical Genetics, 155A*(11), 2865–2870.

Astrom, E., & Soderhall, S. (2002). Beneficial effect of long term intravenous bisphosphonate treatment of osteogenesis imperfecta. *Archives of Disease in Childhood, 86*(5), 356–364.

Baldridge, D., Schwarze, U., Morello, R., Lennington, J., Bertin, T. K., Pace, J. M., . . . Lee, B. (2008). CRTAP and LEPRE1 mutations in recessive osteogenesis imperfecta. *Human Mutation, 29*(12), 1435–1442. Retrieved from http://www.ncbi.nlm.nih.gov/pmc/articles/PMC2671575

Barnes, A. M., Cabral, W. A., Weis, M., Makareeva, E., Mertz, E. L., Leikin, S., . . . Marini, C. (2012). Absence of FKBP10 in recessive type XI osteogenesis imperfecta leads to diminished collagen cross-linking and reduced collagen deposition in extracellular matrix. *Human Mutation, 33*(11), 1589–1598. Retrieved from http://www.ncbi.nlm.nih.gov/pmc/articles/PMC3470738

Bodian D. L., Chan, T-F., Poon, A., Schwarze, U., Yang, K., Byers, P. H., . . . Klein, T. E. (2009). Mutation and polymorphism spectrum in osteogenesis imperfecta type II: Implications for genotype-phenotype relationships. *Human Molecular Genetics, 18*(3), 463–471. Retrieved from http://www.ncbi.nlm.nih.gov/pmc/articles/PMC2638801

Brand, M. C. (2008). Examination of the newborn with congenital scoliosis. *Advances in Neonatal Care, 8*(5), 265–273.

Butler, J. M., & Mullins, B. (2014). Musculoskeletal system. In C. Kenner & J. Lott (Eds.), *Comprehensive neonatal nursing care* (5th ed., pp. 376–391). New York, NY: Springer Publishing.

Cabral, W. A., Barnes, A. M., Adeyemo, A., Cushing, K., Chitayat, D., Porter, F. D., Marini, J. C. (2012). A founder mutation in LEPRE1 carried by 1.5% of West Africans and 0.4% of African Americans causes lethal recessive osteogenesis imperfecta. *Genetics in Medicine, 14*(5), 543–551. Retrieved from http://www.ncbi.nlm.nih.gov/pmc/articles/PMC3393768

Committee on Quality Improvement, Subcommittee on Developmental Dysplasia of the Hip. (2000). Clinical practice guideline: Early detection of developmental dysplasia of the hip. *Pediatrics, 105*(4), 896–905.

Dobbs, M. B., & Gurnett, C. (2009). Update on clubfoot: Etiology and treatment. *Clinics in Orthopedic Related Research, 467*(5), 1146–1153.

Fisher, R. G. (2011). Neonatal osteomyelitis. *NeoReviews, 12*(7), e374–e380. Retrieved from http://neoreviews.aappublications.org

Gilmore, A., & Thompson, G. H. (2015). Bone and joint infections in neonates. In R. J. Martin, A. A. Fanaroff, & M. C. Walsh (Eds.), *Fanaroff and Martin's neonatal-perinatal medicine: Diseases of the fetus and infant* (10th ed., pp. 1784–1788). Philadelphia, PA: Saunders.

Giraud, F., & Meunier, P. (2002). Effect of cyclical intravenous pamidronate therapy in children with osteogenesis imperfecta: Open-label study in seven patients. *Joint Bone Spine, 69*(5), 486–490.

Glorieux, F. (2001). The use of bisphosphonates in children with osteogenesis imperfecta. *Journal of Pediatric Endocrinology and Metabolism, 14*(Suppl. 6), 1491–1495.

Glorieux, F. (Ed.). (2007). Guide to osteogenesis imperfecta for pediatricians and family practice physicians. Retrieved from http://www.oif.org

Gulati, V., Eseonu, K., Sayani, J., Ismail, N., Uzoigwe, C., Choudhury, M. Z., . . . Tibrewal, S. (2013). Developmental dysplasia of the hip in the newborn: A systematic review. *World Journal of Orthopedics, 4*(2), 32–41.

Hart, E. S., Grottkau, B. E., Rebello, G. N., & Albright, M. B. (2005). The newborn foot: Diagnosis and management of common conditions. *Orthopaedic Nursing, 24*(5), 313–321.

Hartman, J. (Ed.). (2003). Osteogenesis imperfecta: A guide for nurses. Retrieved from http://www.oif.org/site/Docserver/Web_Version.pdf?docID=181

Homan, E. P., Rauch, F., Grafe, I., Doll, J. A., Dawson, B., Bertin, T., . . . Lee, B. (2011). Mutations in SERPINF1 cause osteogenesis imperfecta type VI. *Journal of Bone and Mineral, 26*, 2798–2803. Retrieved from http://www.ncbi.nlm.nih.gov/pmc/articles/PMC3214246

Jones, G. N., Moschidou, D., Abdulrazzak, H., Kalirai, B. S., Vanleene, M., Osatis, S., . . . Guillot, P. V. (2014). Potential of human fetal chorionic stem cells for the treatment of osteogenesis imperfecta. *Stem Cells and Development, 23*(3), 262–276. Retrieved from http://www.ncbi.nlm.nih.gov/pmc/articles/PMC3904514

Keupp, K., Beleggia, F., Kayserili, H., Barnes, A. M., Steiner, M., Semler, O., . . . Wollnik, B. (2013). Mutations in WNT1 cause different forms of bone fragility. *American Journal of Human Genetics, 92*(4), 565–574.

Liu, R. W., & Thompson, G. H. (2015). Musculoskeletal disorders in neonates. In R. J. Martin, A. A. Fanaroff, & M. C. Walsh (Eds.), *Fanaroff and Martin's neonatal-perinatal medicine: Diseases of the fetus and infant* (10th ed., pp. 1776–1783). Philadelphia, PA: Saunders.

Moore, K. L., Persaud, T. V. N., & Torchia, M. G. (2015). *The developing human: Clinically oriented embryology* (10th ed., pp. 337–378, 457–486). Philadelphia, PA: Elsevier.

Ramachandra, D. L., Shaw, S. S. W., Shangaris, P., Loukogeorgakis, S., Guillot, P. V., De Coppi, P., & David, A. L. (2014). In utero therapy for congenital disorders using amniotic fluid stem cells. *Frontiers in Pharmacology, 5*, 270. Retrieved from http://www.ncbi.nlm.nih.gov/pmc/articles/PMC4271591

Son-Hing, J. P., & Thompson, G. H. (2015). Congenital abnormalities of the upper and lower extremities and spine. In R. J. Martin, A. A. Fanaroff, & M. C. Walsh (Eds.), *Fanaroff and Martin's neonatal-perinatal medicine: Diseases of the fetus and infant* (10th ed., pp. 1789–1808). Philadelphia, PA: Saunders.

Swarr, D. T., & Sutton, V. R. (2010). Skeletal dysplasias in the newborn: Diagnostic evaluation and developmental genetics. *NeoReviews, 11*(6), e290–e305. Retrieved from http://neoreviews.aappub lications.org/content/11/6/e290

Wilkinson, A. G., & Wilkinson, S. (2010). Neonatal hip dysplasia: A new perspective. *NeoReviews, 11*(7), 349–362.

16

Inherited Metabolic Disorders and Endocrine Disease

Elena Bosque

Chapter Objectives

1. Provide a basic definition of inherited metabolic disorder (IMD), or in layperson's terms, endocrine disease
2. Suggest at least one reason why the diagnosis of these cases is so challenging for clinicians
3. Explain why some of these disorders appear early, and why some appear later
4. Suggest at least three possible symptoms of IMD before a diagnosis is made
5. Offer at least one important question that can be posed to the mother, or parent, about maternal or family history
6. Based on the cases that are presented, suggest at least two tests that can be performed on a neonate if IMD or endocrine disease is suspected, before a subspecialist, such as a pediatric endocrinologist, is contacted
7. Apply what was learned from the cases to suggest how a neonatal nurse practitioner (NNP) would approach parents during a conversation when their baby is symptomatic, tests are pending, and no diagnosis is yet available

Inherited metabolic disorders (IMDs) are also known as *inborn errors of metabolism* and encompass both metabolic and biochemical genetic diseases. Some of the expressions of IMD overlap with endocrine disorders, such as hypothyroidism and congenital adrenal hyperplasia, so they are often grouped together (Champion, 2010; Wilcken, 2011). Most of these conditions involve a mutation of a gene, cause an absent or defective enzyme, and lead to abnormal physiology and biochemical function (Ramachandran, 2009).

Many of these disorders present during the neonatal period, as the protective effect of the maternal placenta ceases. Many of the disorders can be difficult to diagnose and have profound negative consequences for the individual. Because some of these disorders can be corrected with diet or medication if diagnosed early, blood screening at birth, the newborn screen, has become the standard practice in many countries (Kaye et al., 2006; Lee & Cook, 2006). Because some of the metabolic and endocrine diseases present early, before the results of the newborn screen are known, or are not identified by the screen, it is important for health care providers to be able to identify clinical manifestations of these disorders and to provide initial care before subspecialists are involved (Champion, 2010).

It is beyond the scope or goals of this chapter to a provide comprehensive description of all metabolic or endocrine disorders. There exist many reputable references for that purpose. Rather, the goal is to provide an overview of the problem in conceptual terms and a general approach to care that can be applicable to cases that the NNP care provider may encounter. It is not expected or feasible for the NNP to be able to remember and respond to specific information for all metabolic or endocrine disorders. The expectation is that the student, and practicing NNP, will be able to identify typical clinical expressions of these disorders, describe appropriate first-line interventions in collaboration with a neonatologist, refer to a subspecialist, and talk to parents about these problems.

In this chapter an overview of IMDs or endocrine disorders is presented, including definition, incidence, principles of consideration of the problem, and basic concepts of pathophysiology. Reasons for the challenging nature of diagnosing IMDs or endocrine disorders are suggested. A strategy for evaluation and treatment of these disorders is presented, including first-line investigations, second-line investigations, short- and long-term management options, referrals, discharge planning, and follow-up. Throughout, the focus is on the priority issues that should be considered by the NNP to support the infant and family with IMD, which are emphasized by the cases presented.

DEFINITION

IMDs, also called *inborn errors of metabolism*, involve problems with the mechanisms by which specific major foodstuffs are converted to energy or cellular building blocks and degraded for excretion (Ramachandran, 2009). A gene mutation leads to an absent or defective gene product or enzyme and results in the accumulation of the precursor of the enzyme or by-product, a shortage of the product of the enzymatic reaction, or both (Cederbaum, 2012). The metabolic mechanisms involved in these processes are depicted in Figure 16.1. The site of the disorder or multiple disorders can occur at any location along this process.

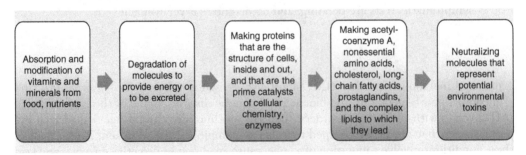

Figure 16.1 Inherited Metabolic Disorders Possible Sites: Conversion Mechanisms Required for Food→Energy→Excretion

INCIDENCE

Collectively, the incidence of IMD is less than one per 2,000 live births. Approximately 12,500 infants are identified each year with IMD. Most common disorders, such as phenylketonuria, occur approximately one per 10,000 live births. Conversely, some disorders occur rarely, such as homocystinuria, which is diagnosed in approximately one per 200,000 live births. It is possible that the incidence of IMD is underestimated if conditions are undetected (Adamkin, 2015; Ramachandran, 2009).

ALTERNATIVE PRINCIPLES OF CONSIDERATION OF IMD

Various structured approaches to the consideration and evaluation of IMD have been developed. In Table 16.1, examples of the effects and disorders that arise from single- gene or enzyme defects are presented. These include problems that arise because of defects of production or function of enzymes, receptor or transport proteins, or structural proteins. These defects will result in accumulation of substrate or lack of a necessary product or gene that disrupts structure and function. But many abnormalities are complex and involve multiple functional proteins and enzymes (Champion, 2010; Suadubray, Sedel, & Walter, 2006).

Some researchers and clinicians consider IMD with the view that many acquired diseases have one or several genetic bases or predispositions. Others believe that metabolic disorders develop only after two or three things go wrong. Ramachandran (2009, p. 1) stated, "Diseases are intellectual constructs, not reality. . . . The reality of medicine is the sick patient."

Table 16.1 **Example of Single Gene Disorders and Enzyme Defects**

Defect	*Pathophysiology*	*Disorder*
Enzyme defect	• Accumulation of substrate • Lack of product • Failure to inactivate protein, which causes damage	Most IMDs, e.g., PKU
Receptor/transport protein defect	Absent genes in lipoprotein pathway cause disrupted clearance of low-density lipoprotein	For example, familial hypercholesterolemia
Structural protein defect	Affects protein • Structure • Function • Quantity	For example, Marfan's, Ehlers–Danlos
Enzyme defect with variable expression, with food or drug susceptibility	Absent catalyst enzyme in red blood cell oxidative pathway causes hemolysis in response to certain illnesses, foods, medications	For example, G6PD

G6PD, glucose-6-phosphate deficiency; IMDs, inherited metabolic disorders; PKU, phenylketonuria.

This approach fits nicely with the "family-centered" perspective that is valued by advanced practice neonatal nurses. The NNP is taught to treat and support the family that has a sick or premature infant. When an infant presents with symptoms of IMD, in many cases, it will be weeks, if ever, before a diagnosis is reached. Often, the goals of the collaborative team are functional. These goals include cardiopulmonary and metabolic stability, then oral or gastric feeding, with the hope of discharge to home and subspecialist follow-up later.

IMD PATHOPHYSIOLOGY

Normally, enzyme proteins catalyze metabolic processes. Thousands of enzymes are required to perform critical biochemical reactions for processing or transport of amino acids, carbohydrates, or fatty acids. The substance upon which the enzyme acts is the substrate.

With absence or deficiency of these enzymes, the substrate molecules accumulate and may be converted to products that are not usually present. Also, alternative end products interfere with normal metabolic processes. Finally, there is an inability to degrade end products. Symptoms result from increased levels of normal substrate that become toxic or lack normal end products necessary for cellular function.

The toxic levels of metabolites or deficient cellular function can lead to mental retardation, decreased muscle tone, seizures, organ failure, blindness, deafness, and death. Specific pathophysiology of various disorders, organized within groups, is presented.

Although various strategies for evaluation and treatment have been suggested, IMDs or endocrine disorders are classified by group as suggested by Saudubray et al. (2006; Table 16.2). The classification groups include disorders that give rise to intoxication, those involving energy metabolism, and those involving complex molecules.

The inborn errors of intermediary metabolism that lead to acute or progressive intoxication usually manifest early. They result from the accumulation of toxic compounds before the block in the metabolic pathway or process. These include disorders such as aminoacidopathies, organic acidurias, urea cycle defects, galactosemia, and hereditary fructose intolerance. The infant may be symptom free initially. Later, the infant presents with increased drowsiness and poor feeding after the metabolite accumulates, with stress, or when feeds are introduced. Without intervention full decompensation will occur with acidosis, seizure, obtundation, coma, and death.

Energy deficiencies may manifest early or later. These include disorders such as fatty acid oxidation defects, disorders of ketogenesis, glycogen storage disease type I, and disorders of gluconeogenesis. Mitochondrial disorders and long-chain fatty acid oxidation defects can present with many symptoms, especially neurological or cardiac ones, but may also include disruptions of energy metabolism. Infants may present at birth or later with hypoglycemia, lactic acidosis, or cardiac decompensation.

Disorders of disturbed metabolism of complex molecules usually manifest later and may be associated with normal laboratory data. These disorders include lysosomal storage disease, peroxisomal disorders, or disorders of glycosylation. These complex molecules are key to embryogenesis, so infants with these disorders present with dysmorphic features, which may be subtle at birth but become more pronounced as storage material accumulates (Ramachandran, 2009; Saudubray et al., 2006).

WHAT MAKES DIAGNOSIS CHALLENGING?

Diagnosis of IMD is challenging for most nonsubspecialist clinicians. Many are intimidated because of the fear of making an incorrect diagnosis. Nonspecific presentations and individual rarity of diseases means limited exposure for clinicians. IMDs or endocrine disorders

Table 16.2 Example of Classification System for Inherited Metabolic Disorders

Group	Metabolic Problem	Disorder	Timing of Presentation	Treatment
1: Disorders that give rise to intoxication	• Inborn error of intermediary metabolism • Acute or chronic intoxication • Most are treatable	Include aminoacidopathies, organic acidurias, urea cycle disorders, sugar intolerances, metal disorders, and porphyrias	• Neonatal or later through late adulthood • Can present intermittently	• Diet • Extracorporeal procedures • Drugs • Vitamins
2: Energy deficiency disorders: those that involve energy metabolism	Inborn errors of intermediary metabolism that affect the cytoplasmic and mitochondrial energetic processes	Include: • Cytoplasmic defects encompass those affecting glycolysis, glycogenosis, gluconeogenesis, hyperinsulinisms (most treatable) • Creatine (partly treatable) and pentose phosphate pathways (untreatable) • Mitochondrial defects include respiratory chain disorders, and Krebs cycle and pyruvate oxidation defects (mostly untreatable) • Disorders of fatty acid oxidation and ketone bodies (treatable)	• Most at birth • A few present later with stress • Some of these affect embryological development	• For some, dextrose, diet, supplements • For others, no treatment
3: Disorders involving complex molecules	Involves cellular organelles	Include lysosomal, peroxisomal, glycosylation, and cholesterol synthesis defects, e.g., Gaucher's, Niemann–Pick type A or type B, Pompe's, Krabbe's, Fabry's diseases, or mucopolysaccharidosis I; or X-linked adrenoleukodystrophy or Zellweger spectrum syndrome	• Many present at birth but are permanent and progressive	• Mostly untreatable • Some new or experimental enzyme, organ transplant, or gene therapy

357

will not be diagnosed unless specific investigations for that disorder are undertaken. It becomes important to understand the basic pathophysiology of IMDs and, upon presentation of symptoms, to develop an approach to the investigation (Champion, 2010; Leonard, 2006).

CLINICAL PRESENTATION

TIMING WHEN IMD PRESENTATION IS LIKELY

IMDs, depending on the defect, can present at any time in life (Table 16.2). Fifty percent of individuals present after the first year of life (Saudubray et al., 2006). Infants may present during the neonatal period, when first introduced to substrate or following stress of birth. Some infants may present during weaning of breastfeeding because of increased oral intake and increased protein load. Metabolic pathways are stressed with growth spurts and illness, and these conditions may lead to the presentation of some disorders. The end of the first year is a possible presentation time. At this time there is slowing of growth rate, which means more protein is catabolized for the same intake, so there is a greater load on metabolic pathways.

Infection may trigger IMD at any time in life, but especially during early childhood, when the infant and young child are vulnerable because of decreased natural immunity. Illness causes increased metabolic stress and is often associated with decreased intake and vomiting or diarrhea.

Hormonal changes can trigger presentation of IMD. Puberty causes alterations in growth rate and changes in hormonal milieu. During the postnatal period women may present with disorders. One example is the urea cycle defect, which may have been previously asymptomatic, but the disorder is triggered after delivery because involution of placenta causes a significant protein load (Champion, 2010; Valayannopoulos & Poll-The, 2013).

COMMON PRESENTING SYMPTOMS

The most common presenting symptoms include dysmorphic features, hypoglycemia, poor feeding, vomiting, poor growth, jaundice, acidosis, cardiomyopathy, respiratory distress, lethargy, hypotonia, seizures, encephalopathy, obtundation, coma, and sudden death (Adamkin, 2015; Saudubray et al., 2006; Valayannopoulos & Poll-The, 2013). Since some of these symptoms, if displayed early, or subtly, may be caused by some common neonatal problem such as breastfeeding difficulty, jaundice, benign cardiac murmur, or infection, it becomes clear why a consistent, thorough, differential, and systematic approach is necessary for the assessment of all infants. The clinician may not be able to identify the specific disorder, but he or she should be able to describe and document a complete physical and first-line laboratory and radiographic evaluation. Any infant who presents with hypoglycemia, acidosis, lethargy, or seizures should be considered to, possibly, have an IMD.

PHYSICAL EXAM BY SYSTEMS

PHYSICAL EXAM

The physical exam should be performed with a consistent, thorough approach. Various systematic approaches are taught, and most include some variation of general evaluation, and then a "head-to-toe" exam.

General Assessment

It is important to start with a general assessment of the infant for evaluation of phenotype and activity. There may or may not be phenotype abnormalities with specific IMDs, but a thorough evaluation may reveal physical dysmorphology that is present with some disorders.

Also, it is important to initiate a neurological evaluation of the infant at rest in terms of position, tone, and activity before the infant is disturbed.

A complete physical exam, of all organs or systems, should be performed to identify all abnormalities to assist in the evaluation and care of the infant. It is possible to have confounding problems as in the case, for example, of an infant with a metabolic disorder, who, also, has respiratory distress because of meconium aspiration syndrome. In this chapter, only the organs or systems most commonly affected by IMD, which may be identified during a physical exam, are presented. A more complete description is presented in Table 16.3 (Champion, 2010; Valayannopoulos & Poll-The, 2013).

Eye

An eye exam may reveal or suggest galactosemia, sphingolipidoses, mitochondrial cytopathies, Kearns–Sayre syndrome, and other IMDs. Infants with these conditions may present with cataracts, cherry spots, retinopathies, or abnormal gaze. Without dilation of the pupils, it is possible to miss some of these anomalies during the initial eye exam, so if an IMD is suspected, a referral to a pediatric ophthalmologist is appropriate.

Table 16.3 Presenting Signs of IMD in Infants Less Than 3 Months of Age

Organ System Mainly Involved	Presenting Sign	Metabolic Disease
Eye	Cataracts	• Galactosemia
	Cherry spots	• Sphingolipidoses
	Retinopathies	• Mitochondrial cytopathies, fat oxidation defects, and peroxisomal disorders
	Abnormal movements or gaze	• Mitochondrial cytopathies or Gaucher's syndrome
Cardiac	Cardiac failure	• Long-chain FAO defects
	Cardiomyopathy Arrhythmias	• Carnitine palmitoyltransferase type II • Very long-chain acyl-CoA dehydrogenase deficiency • Long-chain 3-hydroxy-acyl-CoA dehydrogenase deficiency • Trifunctional protein deficiency • Carnitine acyl translocase deficiency • Kearns–Sayre syndrome

(continued)

Table 16.3 Presenting Signs of IMD in Infants Less Than 3 Months of Age (*continued*)

Organ System Mainly Involved	Presenting Sign	Metabolic Disease
Hepatic	Liver failure	• Galactosemia • Hereditary fructose intolerance • Tyrosinemia type I • Phosphomannoisomerase
	Jaundice, cholestasis	• Galactosemia • Long-chain 3-hydroxy-acyl-CoA Dehydrogenase deficiency • Bile acid synthesis defects • Cerebrotendinous xanthomatosis
	Hepatosplenomegaly	• Congenital erythropoietic porphyria
Endocrine	Hepatosplenomegaly • Metabolic acidosis • Hypoglycemia	• Glycogenosis type I/III • Fructose bisphosphatase deficiency
	Severe hypoglycemia • Ambiguous genitalia	• Congenital hyperinsulinism • Congenital adrenal hyperplasia
	Cardiac involvement	• Fatty acid oxidation defects • Carnitine uptake defect

Neurologic	Encephalopathy
	• Coma
	• Abnormal movements
		• Branched-chain amino acid disorders
		  ■ Maple syrup urine disease
		  ■ Methylmalonic acidemia
		  ■ Propionic acidemia
		  ■ Isovaleric acidemia
		  ■ Multiple carboxylase deficiency
		• Glutaric aciduria type II
		• Urea cycle disorders
		• Hyperornithinemia–hyperammonemia–homocitrullinuria syndrome (triple H)

	Seizures	• Vitamin B_6-responsive seizures • Pyridoxamine-5-phosphate oxidase • Multiple carboxylase deficiency • Folinic acid–responsive seizures • Congenital magnesium malabsorption
	Seizures + microcephaly	• 3-phosphoglycerate dehydrogenase • Glucose transporter type 1 deficiency

CoA, coenzyme A; FAO, fatty acid oxidation; IMD, inherited metabolic disorder.

Cardiac

A cardiac exam should be performed in any infant with suspected metabolic disorder. However, for some IMDs, the cardiac problem, when accompanied by hemodynamic instability, is the presenting symptom. There may be significant cardiac problems and symptoms with mitochondrial disorders, for example, mitochondrial respiratory chain disorders, or glycogen storage disease, for example, Pompe's disease. The symptoms of IMD with cardiac involvement may include cardiac murmur, arrhythmia, cardiomyopathy with signs of failure, or hemodynamic decompensation.

Gastrointestinal/Liver

Abdominal distension, associated with vomiting or diarrhea, may be assessed for many of the intoxication disorders. Liver or spleen involvement is common in many IMDs. Signs of liver failure may be seen with disorders such as galactosemia and tyrosinemia. Hepatosplenomegaly may be seen with congenital erythropoietic porphyria or lysosomal storage diseases, for example, Gaucher's disease.

Genitourinary

Genitalia should be assessed for appropriateness for gestational age and for any abnormalities. Abnormalities, such as ambiguous genitalia in a female, may be associated with endocrine disorders such as congenital adrenal hyperplasia. Other abnormalities may be related to other sex development disorders.

Neurologic

Many infants with IMDs present with abnormal neurological signs. Sometimes these signs are as subtle and ubiquitous as "poor feeding." However, infants may present with progressive or significant neurological symptoms. With maple syrup urine disease and many of the acidemia disorders, the infant will present with hypotonia, seizures, obtundation, and may progress to coma.

Those with IMDs may also have accompanying abnormal, distinctive odors of urine, breath, saliva, or sweat. Abnormal odor may be an important diagnostic feature of some disorders, such as phenylketonuria, which presents with a stale, barn-like smell, or tyrosinemia, which presents with a rancid smell (Champion, 2010; Valayannopoulos & Poll-The, 2013).

FURTHER EVALUATION AND CARE

OBTAIN HISTORY

Both family and pregnancy history should be obtained. Both parents and family members, if present, should be asked about neonatal death or sudden, unexplained death of any infant or child. The family members should be asked, specifically, whether any family member had mental retardation, developmental delay, or heart problems. It is helpful to remember that X-linked conditions have male predominance but females may have milder forms, so it may be important to listen, carefully, to how mild abnormalities are described, especially of female relatives. Parents should be asked whether they are related at all. Autosomal recessive disorders are more likely to occur with parental consanguinity.

Although pregnancy history may be available in the medical record, parents should still be questioned as information may be lacking or prenatal care may have been received elsewhere without transfer of records. Infants with IMD are often born to mothers with normal pregnancies. However, in some cases, the pregnancies may have had associated severe hyperemesis, liver dysfunction, fatty liver of pregnancy, or HELLP (hemolysis, elevated liver enzymes, and low platelet count) syndrome. Fetal ultrasound results may have revealed congenital malformations associated with genetic metabolic disorders (Champion, 2010).

FIRST-LINE INVESTIGATIONS

Initially, other disorders, which may be concomitant, should be investigated. These include common problems, such as poor maternal feeding, physiologic jaundice, and benign cardiac murmurs, as well as less common and more serious problems such as persistent pulmonary hypertension, cardiac lesions, sepsis, gastrointestinal tract obstruction, liver problems, or central nervous system problems, for example, hypoxic ischemic encephalopathy (HIE), nonaccidental trauma, or brief resolved unexplained events (BRUEs).

At this stage, if IMD is suspected, the goal is to promote cardiopulmonary and metabolic stability and to obtain some basic measures that are routinely available, before proceeding with more specialized investigation. First, investigations of blood often include complete blood glucose levels, pH, arterial carbon dioxide, bicarbonate, base deficit, complete blood count, lactate, ammonia, serum amino acids, liver function studies, and clotting screen. First-line investigations of urine include ketones, organics acids (including orotic acid), reducing substances (if suspecting galactosemia), and amino acids. Even if the NNP is uncertain about ordering some of these first-line studies before discussion with a neonatologist, much may be revealed by, at least, blood sugar levels and arterial blood gas tests, as well as some other commonly ordered metabolic tests (Table 16.4; Champion, 2010; Valayannopoulos & Poll-The, 2013).

If any of the physical exam findings or laboratory test results are abnormal, or if the clinician is concerned despite normal results, then this may be the appropriate time to ask for a consult from a pediatric subspecialist. Depending on the case and stability of the infant, it may be appropriate to request a consult from a pediatric endocrinologist, geneticist, neurologist, cardiologist, gastroenterologist, infectious disease specialist, dermatologist, and so on (Leonard & Morris, 2006; Saudubray et al., 2006; Valayannopoulos & Poll-The, 2013).

SECOND-LINE INVESTIGATIONS

Second-line investigations are usually performed as a result of the consultants' recommendations. Depending on the resources at the facility where the infant was born or evaluated, sometimes the infant must be transported to a regional pediatric medical center for some of these tests. Second-line investigations may include urine, cerebral spinal fluid, or serum samples for metabolites or markers, such as urine succinylacetone, cerebral spinal fluid glycine, serum acylcarnitines, and other markers or metabolites. Chromosomes and other specific genetic studies may be requested. Specific imaging may include tandem mass spectrometry as well as other radiographic or ultrasound studies. Organ- or organelle-specific investigations may include studies such as long-chain fatty acids, transferrin isoelectric focusing, peroxisomal function tests, and so forth. Skin, muscle, and liver biopsies may be performed at this time, if possible, or during postmortem studies.

For the second-line investigations, it is important to determine with the collaborative team an appropriate medical order to prevent excessive exsanguination and handling. It is also important to contact the laboratory personnel in the facility to determine whether the

Table 16.4 **Basic Metabolic Screening Tests of IMDs or Endocrine Disorders That Should Be Considered by the NNP Before Further Investigations**

Test	Reason	Clinical Importance: Abnormalities May Be Associated With Disorders
Glucose—IMD or endocrine disorders should be suspected in any infant with prolonged, persistent hypoglycemia	Normal, low, or high	• Intoxication disorders: ↓ glucose with poor feeding; obtundation • Energy deficiency disorders: ↓, normal, or ↑ • Complex molecules disorders: may be normal • Endocrine: hypoglycemia
Arterial blood gas	To determine metabolic acidosis	• Intoxication disorders: ↓ pH, ↑ CO_2 with coma and respiratory failure, or ↓ CO_2 with hyperventilation • Energy deficiency disorders: ↓ pH with lactic acidosis, ↑ base deficit, ↓ carbon dioxide with alkalosis • Complex molecules disorders: may be normal
Electrolytes	Especially serum bicarbonate to determine metabolic acidosis To determine anion gap with acidosis	• Intoxication disorders: abnormal electrolytes with vomiting and acidosis • Energy deficiency disorders: ↓ bicarbonate, abnormal with acidosis • Complex molecules disorders: may be normal • Endocrine: hyponatremia, hyperkalemia
Liver function studies with bilirubin, coagulopathy studies	To determine liver involvement and jaundice	• Intoxication disorders: ↑ liver function tests • Energy deficiency disorders: ↑ liver function tests • Complex molecules disorders: ↑ bilirubin or normal
Ammonia	May be elevated	• Intoxication disorders: ↑ • Energy deficiency disorders: ↑ • Complex molecules disorders: ↑ or normal
Lactate	May be elevated	• Intoxication disorders: ↑ lactate • Energy deficiency disorders: ↑ lactate • Complex molecules disorders: may be normal
Urinary ketones	To determine if present, which is abnormal	• Intoxication disorders: ↑ ketones • Energy deficiency disorders: normal or ↑ ketones • Complex molecules disorders: may be normal

CO_2, carbon dioxide; IMDs, inherited metabolic disorders; NNP, neonatal nurse practitioner.

tests are analyzed at that facility, or must be sent out, to be able to plan for optimum collection and processing of the samples. To accomplish this goal, one must establish proper timing (e.g., not before a long weekend if the sample needs to be sent to another lab), confirm proper tubes, proper handling (e.g., does sample need to be placed on ice?), and notify the lab technologists when these tests are to be sent so that they are processed immediately (Champion, 2010).

Acute Management

The goals of acute management are to stop further decompensation and buildup of toxic metabolites. Any food or drug that cannot be metabolized properly should be reduced or eliminated from the diet. Missing or inactive enzymes or other chemicals should be replaced, if possible. Toxic products of metabolism that accumulate as a result of the metabolic disorder should be removed.

If the infant's oral feedings are stopped at the time of evaluation, 10% dextrose with electrolytes should be administered. This strategy would be excepted if congenital lactic acidosis or mitochondrial disorders were suspected, as higher carbohydrates exacerbate acidosis. In that situation, 5% dextrose with electrolytes should be administered. If fat oxidation defects are excluded from the evaluation, then provide lipids. If the infant is hyperglycemic, insulin should be considered rather than decreasing the dextrose infusion rate (mg/kg/min).

Electrolytes should be monitored because of intravenous fluid therapy and underlying conditions. If acidotic, potassium levels should be monitored because potassium falls as acidosis is corrected. Both sodium and potassium should be ordered if certain endocrine disorders that alter electrolyte balance are suspected.

With certain disorders, it may be necessary to remove or divert toxic metabolites. For organic acidemias, carnitine is administered to conjugate with organic acids and improve renal clearance. With isovaleric acidemia, glycine is provided for the same effect. With urea cycle defects, sodium benzoate administration is alternated with sodium phenylbutyrate for the same effect. For many intoxication disorders with neurological symptoms, filtration and dialysis will be considered. All of these interventions can be determined in collaboration with the neonatologist and appropriate subspecialist consultants (Champion, 2010; Kaye et al., 2006; Leonard, 2006; Raghuveer, Garg, & Graf, 2006; Saudubray et al., 2006; Valayannopoulos & Poll-The, 2013).

Long-Term Management

Lifelong treatment may include diet management, provision of a deficient substance, or vitamin therapy. Vitamin supplements include vitamin B_{12}, biotin, riboflavin, thiamine, pyridoxine, or folate. Psychological support for family, genetic counseling, and continued follow-up with the pediatrician and appropriate pediatric subspecialists, depending on the case. Some of the treatments for IMD and endocrine disorders are listed in Table 16.5 (Champion, 2010; Kaye et al., 2006; Leonard, 2006; Raghuveer et al., 2006; Saudubray et al., 2006; Valayannopoulos & Poll-The, 2013).

Importance and Issues of Newborn Screening

Newborn screening is a successful public health program that began in 1963 with drops of blood on filter paper and a process of bacterial inhibition assay to detect phenylketonuria,

Table 16.5 Supplemental Treatments for IMDs or Endocrine Disorders

Medication, Metabolite, or Vitamin	Disorder
Agalsidase alfa and beta	Fabry's disease
Allopurinol	Hyperuricemia synthetase superactivity and deficiency
Betaine	Homocystinuria
Biotin	Biotinidase deficiency
Chenodeoxycholic acid	3βDD; 3-ORD; CTX
Cholesterol	Smith–Lemli–Opitz syndrome
Cholestyramine	Familial hypercholesterolemia
Cholic acid	3-ORD
Copper histidine	Menkes disease
Creatine monohydrate	Guanidinoacetate methyltransferase, arginine:glycine amidinotransferase deficiencies
Cysteamine/ phosphocysteamine	Cystinosis
Dextromethorphan	Nonketotic hyperglycinemia
Diazoxide	Persistent hyperinsulinism
Dichloroacetate	Primary lactic acidosis
Entacapone: BH_4	Disorders of BH_4 synthesis, PAH deficiency

(continued)

Table 16.5 **Supplemental Treatments for IMDs or Endocrine Disorders (*continued*)**

Medication, Metabolite, or Vitamin	Disorder
Ezetimibe	Familial hypercholesterolemia
Folinic acid	Hereditary orotic aciduria, methylene synthase deficiency, methionine synthase deficiency, folate malabsorption, cobalamin disorders, cerebral folate transporter disorders
Galsulfase	Mucopolysaccharidosis type VI
Granulocyte cell stim factor	Glycogen storage disease
Glycine	Isovaleric academia
Haem arginate	Acute porphyrias
Vitamin B_{12}	Cobalamin metabolism disorders
5-Hydroxytryptophan	Disorders of neurotransmitter synthesis
Imiglucerase	Gaucher's disease
Ketamine	Nonketotic hyperglycinemia
L-Arginine	Urea cycle disorders
Laronidase	Mucopolysaccharidosis type I
L-Carnitine	Carnitine disorders
L-Citrulline	Carbamoyl phospate synthase deficiency and ornithine carbamyl transferase deficiency

(*continued*)

Table 16.5 **Supplemental Treatments for IMDs or Endocrine Disorders** **(*continued*)**

Medication, Metabolite, or Vitamin	Disorder
L-Dopa	Disorders of L-dopa synthesis
L-Lysine-hydrochloric acid	Lysinuric protein intolerance
L-Serine	3-phosphoglycerate dehydrogenase deficiency
L-Tryptophan	Nonketotic hyperglycinemia
Magnesium	Primary hypomagnesemia with secondary hypocalcemia
Mannose	Congenital disorder of glycosylation
Mercaptopropionylglycine	Cystinuria
Metronidazole	Propionic and methylmalonic acidemia
Miglustat	Gaucher
N Carbamoylglutamate	*N*-acetylglutamate synthase deficiency
Nicotinamide	Hartnup's disease
Nicotinic acid	Hyperlipidemia
Nitisinone (NTBC)	Tyrosinemia
Octreotide	Persistent hyperinsulinemia
Pantothenic acid	Type II 3 methylglutaconic aciduria
Penicillamine	Wilson's disease: cystinuria

(continued)

Table 16.5 **Supplemental Treatments for IMDs or Endocrine Disorders** *(continued)*

Medication, Metabolite, or Vitamin	Disorder
Pyridoxine	Gamma-cystathionase deficiency, cystathionine beta synthase deficiency, pyridoxine dependency with seizures, OAT deficiency, X-linked sideroblastic anemia, primary hyperoxaluria type I
Pyridoxal phosphate	Pyridox(am)ine 5′-phosphate oxidase deficiency
Riboflavin	Glutaric aciduria I, electron-transferring-flavoprotein dehydrogenase deficiencies, SCAD deficiency, congenital lactic acidosis
Selegiline	Used with 5-hydroxytryptamine and L-dopa in tetrahydrobiopterin defects
Statins	Hyperlipidemias; some used experimentally in Smith–Lemli–Opitz syndrome
Sodium benzoate; sodium phenylbutyrate	Hyperammonemia
Thiamin	Maple syrup urine disease, pyruvate dehydrogenase deficiency, complex I deficiency
Triethylenetetramine	Wilson's disease
Triheptanoin	VLCAD, pyruvate carboxylase deficiencies

3βDD, 3-beta-dehydrogenase deficiency; 3-ORD, Δ⁴–ooxosteroid 5-beta-reductase deficiency; BH_4, tetrahydrobiopterin deficiency; CTX, cerebrotendinous xanthomatosis; IMDs, inherited metabolic disorders; OAT, ornithine aminotransferase deficiency; PAH, phenylalanine hydroxylase deficiency; SCAD, short-chain acyl-CoA dehydrogenase; VLCAD, very long-chain acyl-CoA dehydrogenase.

a preventable cause of mental retardation. Screening tests were developed to detect a few more conditions in the following years. Treatment and follow-up recommendations were established (Adamkin, 2015; Kaye et al., 2006; Marsden, Larson, & Levy, 2006; Wilcken, 2011).

In the 1990s, with the application of tandem mass spectrometry, many metabolic and hematological disorders could be detected, and the list of conditions in the newborn screen was broadened. Examples of some of the disorders that can be detected include endocrine disorders, hemoglobinopathies, immunodeficiencies, cystic fibrosis, as well as phenylketonuria and other inborn errors of metabolism.

Newborn screening is widely accepted in most developed and in many developing countries. Validity and follow-up recommendations have been established. However, unequivocal long-term benefit has not been confirmed for some rare disorders. Some experts question whether there exists clear scientific evidence of long-term benefit of screening and treatment. Controversies exist among experts in different countries about the benefits and risks of certain therapies, especially with disparate availability of resources, and about which disorders should be included in the screen (Adamkin, 2015; Scala, Parenti, & Andria, 2012; Wilcken, 2011).

Presently, in the United States, newborn screening programs are mandated in most states, and more than 50 conditions are included. The goal is to screen all infants and provide the necessary follow-up evaluation and intervention to prevent death or disability. The concept of "newborn screening" has been broadened to include other technologies, such as hearing screening with automated auditory brainstem response to screen for hearing loss, and critical congenital heart disease screening with pulse oximetry (Glidewell et al., 2015; Kaye et al., 2006).

In the future, it may be possible to perform a genetic and mutational scan across the whole genome of the fetus, in a noninvasive manner, by analyzing cell-free fetal DNA in maternal blood as early as the fifth week of gestational age. This technology and approach remain controversial because of methodological, ethical, and political issues.

COMMUNICATION WITH PARENTS

It has been demonstrated that parents of infants in the neonatal intensive care unit (NICU) have high informational needs (De Rouck & Leys, 2009). Parents of infants in the NICU with suspected IMD or endocrine problems may be distressed because of the uncertainty of diagnosis, uncertainty of outcome, lengthy time for receipt of laboratory results, prolonged hospitalization, and, sometimes, complex supportive care skill-acquisition needs. Communication with parents should be honest and should include open-ended questions and detailed explanations in understandable language. A reassuring, empathetic, and caring style of communication has been considered to be most effective (De Rouck & Leys, 2009).

NNP CARE PROVIDER APPROACH TO CARE OF INFANTS WITH IMD

Because the care of the infant with suspected IMDs and endocrine disorders can feel overwhelming, it is helpful to emphasize the priorities and interventions of the NNP within the scope of practice granted by state licensure (Table 16.6). These priorities include identification of abnormal symptoms, evaluation, stabilization, communication with parents, notification of colleagues and consultants, consideration of need for transport, and discharge planning. All of these efforts will involve collaboration with the neonatologist.

Table 16.6 Zellweger Spectrum Peroxisomal Biogenesis Disorder

Overview	
Other name	Also known as infantile Refsum's disease
Incidence	One case per every 50,000 to 100,000 births
Cause and pathophysiology	Peroxisomal biogenesis disorder resulting from deficiencies in the catabolism of very long-chain fatty acids and branched chain fatty acids and phospholipid plasmalogen biosynthesis; symptoms caused by degeneration of myelin
Symptoms	Hypotonia, feeding problems, hearing loss, vision loss, and seizures; radiological finding: characteristic bone spots known as *chondrodysplasia punctata*
Physical exam	Includes large fontanel; distinctive facial features, including a flattened face; broad nasal bridge; and high forehead
Onset	Onset is most commonly in childhood and adolescence with a progressive course, although periods of stagnation and remission occur
Treatment	General supportive care; diet modification

Case 16.1

History

The infant is a 38-week-gestational-age male born via cesarean section for fetal decelerations and uterine rupture. The infant's birth weight is 3.55 kg. He is born to a 25-year-old with the following history: gravida 6, para 6, blood type O+, antibody negative, hepatitis B surface antigen negative, rubella immune, rapid plasma reagin negative (RPR), HIV negative, chlamydia negative, gonococcal negative, group B *Streptococcus* (GBS) unknown. The mother is admitted for induction because of preeclampsia. Apgar scores are 0, 4, 5, 5, 7 (at 1, 5, 10, 15, and 20 minutes of age, respectively).

(continued)

Case 16.1 (continued)

He is intubated and received chest compressions for 1 to 2 minutes. The umbilical cord arterial blood gas result is: pH 6.55, carbon dioxide 194, bicarbonate 17, base deficit −26. Umbilical arterial and venous catheters are placed. The initial blood sugar level is 30 mg/dL. He receives normal saline and sodium acetate boluses. The infant is placed on a high-frequency oscillator ventilator. He has bloody tracheal aspirates. The chest x-ray reveals expansion to the eighth rib, mild reticular granular, streaky densities.

The mean arterial blood pressure is 41. There is a low resting heart rate of 80 to 100 beats per minute. The creatine phosphokinase (CPK) level is 339 (normal is 10–120 mcg/L), creatine phosphokinase–myocardial band (CPK-MB) isoenzyme, particular for myocardium, is 11.2 (normal is 0–3 mcg/L). The initial hematocrit is 53%. The complete blood count results are within normal limits and platelet count is 347,000. Blood culture is pending.

The infant presents with tonic–clonic seizure activity within the first hours of life associated with hypoglycemia, which is confirmed by electroencephalogram. He receives a loading dose of phenobarbital and hypothermia treatment is started. Parents are Spanish speaking and have five small children at home.

Initial Assessment and Plan

1. **If you are nervous about how to proceed on admission of this infant, what two tests are the most important ones to reveal the possibility of inherited metabolic disorders (IMDs) or metabolic disorders?**

   A. Arterial blood gas and blood sugar

   B. Cerebral spinal fluid glycine and blood culture

   C. Plasma long-chain fatty acids and triglyceride level

   ANSWER: A. *Severe acidosis or severe hypoglycemia, especially associated with seizure activity, should signal the possibility of IMD or metabolic disorder. However, these conditions can be explained by other causes (Champion, 2010).*

2. **What is your initial assessment and plan of care, by systems?**

   ANSWER: Possible responses should be ordered by systems and may include:

   Fluid/electrolyte/nutrition:
   Assessment: hypoglycemia related to stress and hypoxic ischemic encephalopathy (HIE) versus IMD or metabolic disorder; (2) risk of intestinal hypoxic damage and electrolyte imbalance caused by acidosis.
   Plan: (1) nothing by mouth (NPO) status; (2) order fluids of 10% dextrose at 80 mL/kg/d; (3) follow chemistries and check urine output; (4) consider placing a Foley urinary catheter because of decreased tone and probable need for sedation; (5) for hypoglycemia give D10 bolus 2 mL/kg and intravenous dextrose infusate (later the blood sugar level was 62 mg/dL, normal).

   Respiratory:
   Assessment: (1) respiratory depression and pulmonary hemorrhage related to stress and HIE versus; (2) IMD with coagulopathy.

(continued)

Case 16.1 (*continued*)

Plan: (1) order blood gases, x-rays, and adjust ventilator setting accordingly; (2) consider increased mean airway pressure to tapenade pulmonary blood vessels to treat pulmonary hemorrhage.

Cardiovascular:

Assessment: This infant is hemodynamically stable, with elevated cardiac enzymes from HIE versus metabolic disorder.

Plan: (1) he needs to be monitored; (2) consider lactate and blood gases to follow acidosis; (3) consider pressors, if hypotensive.

Gastrointestinal/hematological:

Assessment: Stable hematocrit and platelet count despite pulmonary hemorrhage, which may be acute and transient, because of HIE versus IMD with coagulopathy.

Plan: (1) order coagulopathy panel; (2) consider transfusion if results are abnormal or there is further bleeding; (3) consider ranitidine later, in total parenteral nutrition, if he remains NPO.

Infectious disease:

Assessment: Blood culture pending. Some may consider this a case of possible sepsis.

Plan: (1) order antibiotics because of unknown GBS status although some might consider this case as a low risk for infection because of known uterine rupture as a cause of fetal distress and perinatal depression; (2) follow blood culture and continue antibiotics; (3) consider lumbar puncture.

Metabolic:

Assessment: Possible IMD because of symptoms of hypoglycemia, acidosis, neurological depression, abnormal enzyme levels, and seizure activity.

Plan: (1) follow blood gases and acid–base balance; (2) consider correction of acidosis per sodium acetate bolus or correction via total parental nutrition; (3) obtain newborn screen.

Neurological:

Assessment: Obtundation with seizure activity related to HIE versus IMD or endocrine disorder.

Plan: (1) continue phenobarbital and monitor for further seizure activity; (2) proceed with hypothermia; (3) obtain electroencephalogram (EEG) later and consult with neurologist; (4) consider more head imaging.

Health care maintenance:

Assessment: Normal screening is needed before discharge.

Plan: (1) obtain newborn screen; (2) confirm that aquamephyton and eye prophylaxis were given; (3) offer hepatitis B vaccine before discharge.

Psychosocial:

Assessment: Need to address parental need of information and support.

Plan: (1) consider use of a language interpreter; (2) provide parents with an explanation of events, possible diagnoses, and plan of care; (3) involve them as much as possible in care and promote lactation; (4) consider breast milk oral care; (5) refer to the social worker for support; (6) consider a family conference, when appropriate.

(continued)

Case 16.1 (continued)

Diagnoses

3. **Select an appropriate diagnosis for this infant.**

   A. Meningitis
   B. Hyperglycemia
   C. Significant initial respiratory and metabolic acidosis, resolving

   ANSWER: C. *Possible responses may include: (a) 38-week appropriate-for-gestational-age (AGA) male with neonatal encephalopathy in the setting of uterine rupture; (b) hypoglycemia that has been resolved; (c) significant initial respiratory and metabolic acidosis, resolving; (d) possible sepsis; (e) pulmonary hemorrhage; (f) possible IMD; (g) seizure activity; (h) need for psychosocial support of family (Champion, 2010).*

Hospital Course

By the second week of life, the infant tolerated initial feedings supported with total parenteral nutrition. The Foley catheter had been removed. There was a history of hypoalbuminemia treated with nutrition and hypermagnesemia, which resolved. He had received furosemide for mild anasarca, which was resolving. The last electrolytes were normal. Hypothermia was discontinued after 72 hours and he had been extubated by the sixth day. He had been weaned to room air by the seventh day. Blood pressure remained normal after discontinuation of dopamine on the fourth day of life. His blood culture was negative. He had received antibiotics for 72 hours. Although his coagulopathy panel was normal during the second week of life, he had required two packed red blood cell and three fresh frozen plasma transfusions for mild coagulopathy and anemia. His last hematocrit was 43%, last fibrinogen level was 210 mg/dL, and last platelet count was 165 x 10³/microliter.

His metabolic and neurological status was still of concern. He had decreased tone, poor suck, prolonged obtundation. The newborn screen was normal. He had further seizure activity and electroencephalogram was markedly abnormal. He continued to receive phenobarbital and Keppra. The head ultrasound showed edema. The nuclear magnetic resonance imaging showed few areas of ischemia and edema.

Further Assessment and Plan

4. **What is your assessment and plan in terms of metabolic, neurological, health care maintenance, and psychosocial systems?**

   ANSWER: Possible responses should be ordered by selected systems and may include:

   Metabolic: *Continued symptoms that may be consistent with IMDs and history of abnormal cardiac enzymes.* Obtain endocrine consult, based on recommendations consider lactate, ammonia, serum amino acids, urine organic acids.

   Neurological: *Continued abnormal neurological status related to resolving HIE versus IMD.* Continue support of breast and nipple feeding. Follow up with neurologists.

(continued)

Case 16.1 (*continued*)

Continue phenobarbital and levetiracetam. Obtain phenobarbital levels. Levetirace-tam levels are not usually monitored.

Health care maintenance: *Need for health care maintenance no matter what the eventual diagnosis is.* Obtain further newborn screens, as indicated, for postblood transfusions. Obtain hearing screen. Offer hepatitis B vaccine.

Psychosocial: *Address short- and long-term supportive needs.* Arrange for the interpreter to be present at care conference regarding the infant's condition, plan of care, and long-term care needs. Consider and discuss the possibility of need for nasogastric or gastric tube. Plan for follow-up appointments with neurology, genetics, or endocrine (possibly) specialists, a developmental clinic, and pediatrician.

Hospital Course

Results of metabolic workup: newborn screen: normal; lactic acid: 1.3 (normal <2 mmol/L); ammonia level: 36 (norm <50 g); serum amino acids: normal (normal values are 10s–100s, not 1000s); urine organic acids: normal.

5. What are other explanations for prolonged obtundation?

ANSWER: Possible responses may include elevated phenobarbital level or resolving HIE.

Key Concepts

The key concepts in the case of the infant with hypoglycemia, seizures, and obtundation are that there may be other causes of symptoms that may also be attributed to IMDs or endocrine disease. The care provider may not have all of the test results, but if one approaches each case using a systems approach to problems, and investigates abnormal symptoms or laboratory results with different possible diagnoses in mind, then problems will not be overlooked. In this case, the symptoms were attributed to the HIE. However, confounding and coexisting problems are possible, so it was important that metabolic causes of hypoglycemia, elevated cardiac enzymes, and neurological symptoms were investigated and ruled out.

Case 16.2

This infant was born at 41 1/7 weeks gestation, appropriate for gestational age (AGA). The infant's birth weight was 3.32 kg. He was born to a 31-year-old woman with the following history: gravida 1, para 1, blood type O+, antibody negative, hepatitis B surface antigen neg-ative, rubella immune, RPR negative, HIV negative, chlamydia negative, gonococcal negative, group B *Streptococcus* (GBS) negative. The pregnancy was complicated by abnormal triple

(continued)

Case 16.2 (*continued*)

screen, risk for trisomy 21, negative polyhydramnios. The parents refused further testing. The fetal ultrasound had no markers for trisomy 21. The mother received prenatal vitamins.

There was spontaneous rupture of membranes for 6 hours prior to delivery with clear fluid and spontaneous vaginal delivery. The baby had spontaneous respirations and normal activity. The Apgar scores were 8 and 9 (at 1 and 5 minutes, respectively).

The infant was admitted to the neonatal intensive care unit (NICU) at 48 hours for feeding difficulties. After admission he was observed to have stridor, airway instability, feeding dyscoordination, and required gavage support. The physical exam was notable for split sutures, mildly flattened face, broad nasal bridge, high forehead, bilateral single palmar creases, and mild hypotonia.

Hospital Course at 3 Weeks of Age Is Presented by Systems

Fluid/electrolyte/nutrition: The infant was supported by gavage feedings. A barium swallow study on day 8 was normal. At 2 weeks of age, his weight was 3.172 kg. He was still taking only one third of feeding volumes by nipple.

Respiratory: The stridor had worsened and was associated with occasional oxygen desaturation and increased work of breathing. The blood gas was normal. A chest x-ray was relatively normal except for a slightly increased density of the right lung and mild eventration of the right lung. Nasal cannula oxygen was required from days 7 to 9.

Cardiovascular: An echocardiogram on day of life 7 was normal and the infant remained hemodynamically stable.

Gastrointestinal/hematological: The total and direct bilirubin on day 4 was 4.9 and 0.7 mg/dL, respectively. The total and direct bilirubin on day 18 was 1.8 and 1.2 mg/dL, respectively. The abdominal x-ray revealed a normal gas pattern. There were no signs of clinical bleeding.

Infectious disease: A complete blood count on day 4 was normal.

Metabolic/genetics: Newborn screens were sent and pending. The blood sugars and blood gases were normal.

Neurological: There was continued moderate hypotonia. The anterior fontanel was mildly wide. The cranial sutures were mildly wide.

Psychosocial: Parents were actively involved in infant's care.

Assessment and Plan

1. *What is your assessment and plan of care, by systems?*

   ANSWER: Possible responses should be ordered by systems and may include:

   Fluid/electrolyte/nutrition: *Feeding difficulties and failure to thrive* as it is abnormal to be less than birth weight at 3 weeks of age. Fortify feedings. Continue to support nippling, per cues, and support with gavage feedings. Order a feeding specialist evaluation.

   Respiratory: *Stridor, resolving.* Provide oxygen per nasal cannula to keep oxygen saturation 93% to 98% as needed.

(*continued*)

Case 16.2 *(continued)*

Cardiovascular: *Congenital heart disease ruled out:* monitor.

Gastrointestinal: *Cholestatic jaundice* in the infant who had not received total parenteral nutrition. Obtain liver function studies and follow bilirubin. Consider ursodiol if direct bilirubin is greater than 2.0 mg/dL. Obtain coagulation studies. Consider liver ultrasound.

Metabolic/genetics: *Inborn error of metabolism is suspected.* Obtain better family history. When asked, mother said she has a cousin with infantile Refsum's disorder who is a 19-year-old graduating from a special education program. Send blood for karyotype (46XY). Follow newborn screen result (found to be normal). Send blood for thyroid function studies, serum organic acids, urine organic acids, lactate, pyruvate, ammonia, creatine kinase analyses. Based on endocrine consult recommendations, send blood for methylation studies for Prader–Willi, ferritin levels, very long-chain fatty acid profile to rule out peroxisomal biogenesis disorder.

Neurological: *Continued hypotonia observed.* Obtain consultation with a neurologist. Based on the neurology consult recommendations, order magnetic resonance imaging, electroencephalogram, long-bone x-rays, liver ultrasound, renal ultrasound, and eye exam.

Psychosocial: *Address short- and long-term supportive needs.* Support parents and arrange for family conference with long-term care, referral, and follow-up plans.

Diagnoses

2. *Select an appropriate diagnosis for this infant.*

   A. Respiratory alkalosis

   B. Indirect hyperbilirubinia of unknown origin

   C. Mild hypotonia

   ANSWER: C. *Possible responses may include (a) 1-month-old former 41 and 1/7-week AGA male with feeding difficulty, failure to thrive; (b) mild respiratory distress with stridor and mild oxygen desaturation events; (c) cholestasis of unknown origin; (d) mild hypotonia; (e) mild dysmorphology, including a flattened face, broad nasal bridge, and high forehead (Champion, 2010; Raghuveer, Garg, & Graf, 2006).*

3. *What would you say to the parents at this point when they ask what is wrong with the baby?*

   ANSWER: Possible responses may include something like: "I realize that you are very concerned about your baby and the fact that he is not eating or growing well. We are also concerned because, since he was born at full term and did not have problems at birth, it is unusual for him to still have these difficulties. Because of what we learned about your cousin with Refsum's disorder, it is possible that your baby may have something similar. We are going to order some tests and ask a specialist to evaluate your baby. We don't have answers right now but we will tell you of any results as soon as we have them. For now we are going to support feeding and growth with your breast milk, and

(continued)

Case 16.2 (continued)

support the respiratory difficulty. Sometimes we do not have the diagnoses before a baby is ready to go home, but our goal is to get him home with you, when he is stable, and to refer you and him to all of the experts who can help him after he goes home. What are your concerns or questions? What are you most worried about?"

Hospital Course at 1 Month of Age

Fluid/electrolyte/nutrition: The feeding difficulties and failure to thrive were both resolving. The infant did not tolerate fortified feedings so was changed back to breast-milk feedings. He tolerated ad lib demand feedings by 1 month of life with adequate volumes and slow weight gain, but was not yet at the ideal growth trajectory.

Respiratory: The stridor was still present by improving. The infant was in room air with the last mild oxygen desaturation event at day of life 24.

Cardiovascular: Congenital heart disease was ruled out, but cardiac function will need to be monitored.

Gastrointestinal: Mild cholestatic jaundice did not require pharmacologic treatment but did require further monitoring. Liver function studies included elevated values for aspartate aminotransferase (633 units per liter), alanine aminotransferase (303 units per liter), and gamma-glutamyl transferase (32 units per liter). The peak direct bilirubin was 1.2 mg/dL and ferritin level was 2,997 ng/mL. The liver ultrasound and coagulations studies were normal.

Metabolic/genetics: Confirmed inherited metabolic disorder (IMD). Confirmed Refsum's disease peroxisomal biogenesis disorder (spectrum of Zellweger's disorder; see Table 16.7): Very long-chain fatty acids were abnormal: high C26 2.59 (normal 0.05–0.91), high C26/C22 0.3 (normal < 0.02), high C24/C22 1.9 (normal 0.6–1.1). All of the following studies

Table 16.7 NNP Priorities and Interventions for Infant With Suspected IMD

Priority	Intervention
Proper *identification* of abnormal symptoms	• Complete physical assessment and documentation of abnormalities • Obtain family, maternal, pregnancy, and labor and delivery histories.
Initial *evaluation*	• Obtain first-line investigatory lab tests; at least, obtain arterial blood gas sample and blood sugar level. • Obtain other tests as indicated (radiological, pulse oximetry, echocardiogram, etc.).

(continued)

Case 16.2 (*continued*)

Priority	Intervention
Initial *stabilization*	• Provide basic stabilization per neonatal resuscitation program guidelines and systems approach to problems; treat acid/base imbalances. • If IMD is suspected, consider nothing per mouth and intravenous dextrose infusion. • Do not transfuse without consultation with at minimum, the neonatologist, as genetic studies may be required before transfusion.
Communicate with parents initially	• Provide honest description of what is observed as abnormal findings • Do not offer a diagnosis unless it is confirmed. • Reassure parents that further tests will be performed; infant will be supported; and specialists are available, if needed. • *Remember, you are not expected to be a subspecialist, but are expected to support the infant and obtain resources to benefit the infant.*
Proper *notification* of colleagues	• Notify the neonatologist per institutional and practice expectations.
Consider *need for transport*	• Based on the stability of the infant and resources in this institution, consider need for transport to regional children's hospital with subspecialist support at this time.
Further *evaluation*	• Consider the remainder of first-line investigation studies, if not already obtained.
Consideration of *need for subspecialist* consult	• If symptoms persist, or worsen, and diagnosis is unclear, consider subspecialist consultation request. The type of consultation depends on the case presentation and systems involved.
Support recommendations of consultant	• Based on discussion with team, as recommended by consultants, order further diagnostic tests. • Provide supportive interventions per recommendations.

(*continued*)

Case 16.2 (continued)

Priority	Intervention
Family conference	• Once a diagnosis is made, or plan for diagnostic tests is made, conduct an interdisciplinary family conference to answer all questions, provide information regarding possible differential diagnoses, and identify goals of hospitalization, for example, cardiorespiratory stability, feeding (oral, nasogastric, etc.), and discharge to home or eventual transport. • If necessary, discuss the need for transport to regional children's hospital.
Plan for *functional goals*	• Identify appropriate plan for functional goals for this infant. • Communicate plan to entire team (neonatology, nursing, support staff). • Refer to the social worker for support.
Discharge planning	• Identify a pediatrician who is comfortable following an infant with this disorder. • Plan for support, if appropriate, for example, home oxygen, home support for tube feedings. • Support nurses in writing a specific discharge teaching plan. • Plan for discharge medications, metabolites, vitamins, diet, etc., and allow time to obtain necessary supplements before discharge. • Avoid discharge on weekend or holiday unless all necessary items are obtained.
Make appropriate *referrals and follow-up* appointments	*If able to be discharged from your institution without transport to regional children's hospital, then:* • Make pediatrician follow-up appointment. • Complete referral documentation for subspecialist outpatient clinic referrals. • If appropriate, complete paperwork to obtain special formulas through government-funded programs. • If necessary, make first appointments at subspecialist clinics. • If diagnosis is known, refer parents to appropriate support groups.

IMD, inherited metabolic disorder; NNP, neonatal nurse practitioner.

(continued)

Case 16.2 (*continued*)

were normal: thyroid function studies, serum ammonia, lactate, pyruvate, creatine phosphokinase (CPK), acylcarnitine profile, serum amino acids and urine organic acids, methylation studies for Prader–Willi and Angelman's syndromes, cortisol, and red blood cell plasminogen studies. Long-bone x-rays were negative for patellar stippling, and there were no cystic lucencies of bilateral talus. Antioxidant therapy was not recommended yet.

Neurological: Hypotonia was improving. The MRI showed a subarachnoid hemorrhage. The following tests were normal: electroencephalogram, long-bone x-rays, liver ultrasound, renal ultrasound (no cortical cysts), eye exam (no cysts). He passed his hearing screen.

Psychosocial: The parents accepted the diagnosis and were relieved that there was an explanation for the problems that had required a prolonged hospitalization. They were prepared to support the discharge and follow-up plan that would require continued visits to the pediatric geneticist/metabolic specialist, pediatric gastroenterologist, pediatric neurologist, nutritionist, and pediatrician.

Key Concepts

The key concepts in the case of the infant with poor feeding are that, prospectively, his feeding difficulty symptoms were subtle and common to many newborns, so it is important to remember that IMD and endocrine disorders may present with subtle signs. Despite the fact that there was dysmorphology, the features were mild and, prospectively, could have been attributed to familial likeness. What stood out in this case, and what should reassure care providers that it is unlikely to miss such a diagnosis, is that there was no explanation for the prolonged feeding difficulties and hypotonia as this was a normal delivery of a term infant. When one cannot discharge a term infant because of feeding problems, other causes must be investigated.

In this case, the thorough family history and evaluation by system revealed other information that provided support for subspecialist consultation and for a specific diagnosis. Finally, even if the care provider does not have a diagnosis, it is important to be honest with parents, share whatever information is available, provide a plan of care that may include subspecialists, and focus on functional goals.

Case 16.3

This male infant was born at 38 2/7 weeks gestation and he was large for gestational age (LGA). The infant's birth weight was 4.025 kg (91–96th percentile). He was born to a 17-year-old woman with the following history: gravida 1, para 1, blood type O+, antibody negative, hepatitis B surface antigen negative, rubella immune, RPR negative, HIV negative, chlamydia negative, gonococcal negative, group B *Streptococcus* (GBS) positive. The pregnancy was

(*continued*)

Case 16.3 (continued)

complicated by type 1 diabetes and suboptimal glycemic control with hemoglobin A1C of 6.8% to 8.1%. Maternal medication included metformin, insulin, prenatal vitamins, cefazolin, and penicillin.

There was spontaneous rupture of membranes for 7 hours prior to delivery with clear fluid. Labor was complicated by fetal intolerance to labor. The infant was delivered via cesarean section under general anesthesia. The infant was nonvigorous at birth but responded quickly to positive pressure ventilation for 1 minute. The infant's activity improved but was admitted to the neonatal intensive care unit (NICU) because of respiratory distress. The Apgar scores were 4 and 9 (at 1 and 5 minutes, respectively). The infant required continuous positive airway pressure and minimal inspired oxygen for only 4 minutes then was stable, off respiratory support, in room air, by 4 minutes of age. The blood sugar was 61 mg/dL at 1 hour of age and the infant tolerated a small amount of formula, so was transferred to the mother/baby unit.

The infant was transferred back to the NICU at 11 hours of age because of persistent hypoglycemia despite breastfeeding and adequate provision of formula supplementation, with blood glucose levels of 31 to 35 mg/dL.

Hospital Course by Systems

Fluid/electrolyte/nutrition: The infant was supported by oral feedings but required high dextrose infusion up to 15 mg/kg/min (normal dextrose infusion index in newborns is 5 to 8 mg/kg/min) via an umbilical venous catheter for recalcitrant hypoglycemia during the first week of life. He developed dilutional hyponatremia, treated with normal saline infusion, and transient hypocalcemia, both corrected. At the end of the first week, the intravenous dextrose was slowly weaned and the infant remained euglycemic with breastfeeding and bottle-feeding. He was ready for discharge on day of life 9.

Respiratory: There was no further respiratory distress.

Cardiovascular: There was an audible murmur at 11 hours of age with normal blood pressure and perfusion. The murmur was only heard intermittently and not appreciated at discharge.

Infectious disease: A sepsis evaluation was performed because of the infant's presentation of persistent hypoglycemia. The only identifiable risk factor was maternal positive GBS carrier status, for which she had received adequate intrapartum prophylaxis with penicillin and delivered by caesarian section. The complete blood count was unremarkable, serial C-reactive proteins were normal, and blood culture was negative. The sepsis evaluation was considered negative and final.

Endocrine: Evaluation for adrenal dysfunction and pan-hypopituitarism were initiated because of the persistent hypoglycemia despite substantial intravenous dextrose support. Serum cortisol, insulin, and growth hormone levels were drawn when the infant's blood glucose level dropped to less than 50 mg/dL despite ongoing dextrose infusion rate of 12 mg/kg/min. The cortisol level was low, so an adrenocorticotropic (ACTH) hormone level was measured to evaluate for adrenal insufficiency and pan-hypopituitarism. The ACTH stimulation test was normal and the hypoglycemia was considered to be likely the result of hyperinsulinism from maternal diabetes.

(continued)

Case 16.3 (*continued*)

Metabolic/genetic: Newborn screens were sent and pending. The infant was feeding well, euglycemic, and without intravenous dextrose for more than 48 hours before discharge. The infant was eumorphic per physical exam.

Psychosocial: The mother was a 17-year-old adolescent and the father was 19 years of age. Both maternal and paternal grandmothers were involved and supportive. Social services followed this family and offered support and resources.

Discharge Diagnoses

1. What are your discharge diagnoses?

ANSWER: Possible responses may include (a) 8-day-old former 38 2/7-week LGA male; (b) recalcitrant hypoglycemia treated with intravenous dextrose up to 15 mg/kg/min, now resolved and stable; (c) cardiac murmur, transient; (d) sepsis evaluation negative and final; (e) probable hyperinsulinism associated with infant of diabetic mother, resolved; (f) adolescent parents with support systems in place.

2. How could this infant's cortisol level be low with a normal ACTH?

ANSWER: Possible responses may include: There is controversy about what constitutes a "normal" cortisol level in a newborn and may be affected by the time of day, degree of stress, and other factors. The cortisol level, insulin, and growth hormones are often obtained in cases of hypoglycemia, but are thought to be most useful when the serum is collected at a time of very low blood sugar, such as less than 30 mg/dL. In this case, the normal ACTH was reassuring, especially with resolution of the hypoglycemia.

Hint: The approach may vary per institution or practice style, but one may consider obtaining a serum sample to measure cortisol level, insulin, and growth hormone any time the blood sugar is less than 30 mg/dL. Often the provider will order interventions to treat the hypoglycemia appropriately, with the hope that the problem will be resolved completely. However, in the rare cases in which the hypoglycemia is recalcitrant, yet treated, the infant may not experience blood sugars less than 30 mg/dL again collected when the tests yield the most revealing results. So, when in doubt, one should ask one's colleagues whether it is appropriate to order these tests.

Key Concepts

The key concepts in the case of the infant who presents with hypoglycemia are that the same systems approach should be considered for every infant evaluated, along with proper identification of risk factors. In this case, the infant was stabilized in the NICU after birth, but despite the maternal history of insulin-dependent type 1 diabetes, he was not automatically admitted because his physical assessment and blood sugar level were normal. The support of the stable mother–baby dyad and breastfeeding is a priority and often infants of diabetic mothers remain euglycemic with their mothers.

On the other hand, the neonatal provider must always review the maternal history and identify the risk factors for possible problems. In this case, it was not surprising that

(continued)

Case 16.3 (continued)

this infant had significant hypoglycemia because the mother was a type 1 diabetic, as opposed to a gestational diabetic, and because there was not optimal glycemic control, as reflected by the elevated hemoglobin A1C levels. Depending on the system of care in individual hospitals, it might be common for the neonatal care provider to check in with the infant's nurse or pediatrician in the first 24 hours, in anticipation of a possible need for NICU care.

As in the other endocrine/metabolic cases, one must not presume the cause of the presenting symptom. In this case, the presenting symptom for NICU admission was hypoglycemia. Because infection can present with hypoglycemia, and especially because this infant also presented with transient respiratory distress, a sepsis evaluation was appropriate. Because the respiratory distress resolved so quickly, and because there were other possible causes of the hypoglycemia, many providers would not necessarily start antibiotics as in this case (although some might have).

Finally, the neonatal nurse practitioner (NNP) does not need to remember which test to order to evaluate for adrenal insufficiency or pan-hypopituitarism. The NNP is expected to know such information as initial interventions for hypoglycemia, normal dextrose infusion levels for a term infant, when to consider insertion of a central intravenous catheter, or when to collaborate with a neonatologist or pediatric endocrinologist to care for an infant such as the one described in this case.

CONCLUSIONS

The evaluation and treatment of IMDs and endocrine disorders can be daunting for the care provider because of nonspecific, rare presentations and the complexities of these disorders. An overview of IMDs or endocrine disorders has been presented, including a strategy for evaluation and treatment, to guide the NNP. This approach includes a thorough assessment, first-line investigations, second-line investigations, short- and long-term management options, referrals, discharge planning, and follow-up. The key concepts presented in exemplar cases are that an infant may have subtle symptoms of IMDs or endocrine problems that may be in common or coexist with other problems. If a thorough systems approach is applied, and referrals to consultants are made at appropriate times, then one does not need to feel intimidated by these problems. As with all other neonatal problems, the aim is to support the infant and family with the goal of discharge to home with the necessary support, follow-up care, and referrals.

REFERENCES

Adamkin, D. H. (2015). Metabolic screening and postnatal glucose homeostasis in the newborn. *Pediatric Clinics of North America, 62,* 385–409.

Cederbaum, S. (2012). Metabolic and endocrine disorders of the newborn. In C. A. Gleason & S. U. Devaskar (Eds.), *Avery's disease of the newborn* (pp. 209–214). Philadelphia, PA: Elsevier Saunders.

Champion, M. (2010). An approach to the diagnosis of inherited metabolic disease. *Archives of Disease in Childhood, 95,* 40–46.

De Rouck, S., & Leys, M. (2009). Information needs of parents of children admitted to a neonatal intensive care unit: A review of literature (1990–2008). *Patient Education and Counseling, 76*(2), 159–173.

Glidewell, J., Olney, R. S., Hinton, C., Pawelski, J., Sontag, M., Wood, T., . . . Hudson, J. (2015). State legislation, regulations, and hospital guidelines for newborn screening for critical congenital heart disease—United States 2011–2014. *Morbidity and Mortality Weekly Report, 64*(23), 625–656.

Kaye, C. I., Committee on Genetics, Accurso, F., La Franchi, S., Lane, P.A., Hope, N., . . . Michele, A. (2006). Newborn screening fact sheets. *Pediatrics, 118*(3), 934–963.

Lee, P. J., & Cook, P. (2006). Frequency of metabolic disorders: More than one needle in the haystack. *Archives of Disease in Childhood, 91*, 879–880.

Leonard, J. V. (2006). Komrower lecture: Treatment of inborn errors of metabolism: A review. *Journal of Inherited Metabolic Disease, 29*, 275–278.

Leonard, J. V., & Morris, A.A. (2006). Diagnosis and early management of inborn errors of metabolism presenting around the time of birth. *Acta Paediatrica, 95*(1), 6–14.

Marsden, D., Larson, C., & Levy, H. L. (2006). Newborn screening for metabolic disorders. *Journal of Pediatrics, 148*, 577–584.

Raghuveer, T. S., Garg, U., & Graf, W. D. (2006). Inborn errors of metabolism in infancy and early childhood: An update. *American Family Physician, 73*(8), 1981–1990.

Ramachandran, T. S. (2009). Inherited metabolic disorders overview. Retrieved from emedicine.medscape.com/article/1183253-overview

Scala, I., Parenti, G., & Andria, G. (2012). Universal screening for inherited metabolic diseases in the neonate (and the fetus). *Journal of Maternal–Fetal & Neonatal Medicine, 25*(Suppl. 5), 4–6.

Suadubray, J. M., Sedel, F., & Walter, J. H. (2006). Clinical approach to treatable inborn metabolic diseases: An introduction. *Journal of Inherited Metabolic Disease, 29*, 261–274.

Valayannopoulos, V., & Poll-The, B. T. (2013). Diagnostic work-up in acute conditions of inborn errors of metabolism and storage diseases. *Handbook of Clinical Neurology, 113*, 1553–1562.

Wilcken, B. (2011). Newborn screening: How are we travelling, and where should we be going? *Journal of Inherited Metabolic Disease, 34*, 569–574.

Health Care Maintenance and Role Preparation Through Case-Based Learning

17

Health Promotion: Newborn Through the First Year of Life

Bobby Bellflower

Chapter Objectives

1. Discuss the importance of optimal nutrition through the first year of life
2. Explain the necessity of vaccinations for this patient population
3. Apply the knowledge gained into practice to provide families with information to promote safety for the infant after discharge home. This will include car seat safety, safe sleep practices, smoke and drug exposure, as well as infection control

The birth of an infant is an exciting time for families. Discharge home from the safety of the hospital can be overwhelming. As health care providers, it is our responsibility to provide accurate, up-to-date information to promote the healthy growth and development of the infant and family unit. The information available to families is voluminous but it is not always easy to separate truth from fallacy. To ensure a safe passage from newborn to toddler, there are many aspects of infant care that need to be addressed throughout the first year of life.

    I. Safety
        A. Car seat safety
        B. Safe sleep practices and environments
        C. Smoke exposure
        D. Bathing practices

II. Infection control
    A. Prevention at home
    B. Vaccine schedule (Centers for Disease Control and Prevention [CDC] recommendations)
    C. "Catch up" recommendations

III. Nutritional support
    A. Nutritional goals for optimal growth
    B. Feeding issues
    C. Oral care for infants

SAFETY ISSUES

CAR SEAT SAFETY

The American Academy of Pediatrics (AAP) recommends the use of child safety seats for all newborns, infants, and children (AAP, 2011a). Although there has been a long, sustained national campaign to encourage parents to use car safety seats (CSSs) for all children, motor vehicle accidents continue to be the leading cause of death for children 4 years of age and older (AAP, 2011a). Studies indicate that child safety seats reduce the risk of injury by 71% to 82% and reduce the risk of death by 28% when compared with children of similar ages in seat belts (Elliott, Kallan, Durbin, & Winston, 2006; Zaloshnja, Miller, & Hendrie, 2007). Booster seats reduce the risk of injury among 4- to 8-year-old children by 45% compared with seat belts (Arbogast, Jermakian, Kallan, & Durbin, 2009).

Five evidence-based recommendations for best practice in the use of child safety seats are listed by the AAP and are as follows.

- All infants and toddlers should ride in a rear-facing CSS until they are 2 years of age or until they reach the highest weight or height allowed by the manufacturer of their CSS. The car seats should be infant-only or convertible car seats (AAP, 2011a).

- All children 2 years or older, or those younger than 2 years old who have outgrown the rear-facing weight or height limit for their CSS, should use a forward-facing CSS with a harness for as long as possible, up to the highest weight or height allowed by the manufacturer of their CSS. Many of the current car seats can accommodate children who weigh up to 65 to 80 lb. (AAP, 2011a).

- All children whose weight or height is above the forward-facing limit for their CSS should use a belt-positioning booster seat until the vehicle lap-and-shoulder seat belt fits properly, typically when they have reached 4 ft., 9 in. in height and are between 8 and 12 years of age (AAP, 2011a).

- When children are old enough and large enough to use the vehicle seat belt alone, they should always use lap-and-shoulder seat belts for optimal protection (AAP, 2011a).

- All children younger than 13 years old should be restrained in the rear seats of vehicles for optimal protection (AAP, 2011a).

Parents often find it difficult to properly install CSSs into their vehicle; therefore, it is important for the practitioner to either know how to instruct parents to place the seat in the vehicle or to provide information on how to find experts to help insert the CSS in the vehicle. In many communities, certified child passenger safety technicians (CPSTs) are available to provide help and instructions to properly install child safety seats (AAP, 2015a). Other resources are found on www.healthychildren.org and include:

- NHTSA (National Highway Traffic Safety Administration) or call NHTSA Vehicle Safety Hotline at 888/327-4236
- SeatCheck (or call 866/SEATCHECK [866/732-8243])
- National Child Passenger Safety Certified Technicians (or call 877-366-8154)—This site provides information in Spanish and also provides a list of CPSTs with enhanced training in protection of children with special needs.

These resources are readily available and are dedicated to the safety of our children. In today's society, most parents are computer savvy and appreciate sites using and sources to gather information.

SAFE SLEEP PRACTICES AND ENVIRONMENTS

In 1992, the AAP issued guidelines for safe sleep practices and environments because of a relatively high rate of sudden infant death syndrome (SIDS), defined as an infant death that cannot be explained after a thorough case investigation, including a scene investigation, autopsy, and review of the clinical history (AAP, 2011b). Almost 4,000 infants die from unexplained deaths in the United States and, after an extensive investigation, close to half of these deaths are diagnosed as SIDS (Goldstein, Trachtenberg, Sens, Harty, & Kinney, 2016). In the United States, SIDS is the leading cause of postneonatal mortality (between 1 month and 1 year of age) and the fourth leading cause of infant mortality (Matthews, MacDorman, & Thomas, 2015). Most SIDS deaths occur between 1 month and 4 months of age and about 90% of SIDS deaths occur by 6 months of age, although SIDS can occur up to 1 year of age (National Institute of Child Health and Human Development [NICHD], 2015). African American and American Indian/Alaska Native infants have a higher incidence of SIDS compared to Hispanic, Asian, or White babies (NICHD, 2015).

After the guidelines were issued in 1992, the AAP and NICHD promoted a Safe-to-Sleep initiative aimed at promoting nonprone sleeping practices. In the United States between 1992 and 1996, nonprone sleeping decreased from 70% to 24% and the SIDS rate decreased by 38% in those 4 years (Goldstein et al., 2016). According to the study by Goldstein and colleagues (2016), the SIDS postneonatal (after 28 days of life) infant mortality rate from 1982 to 2012 decreased 71.3% from 1.357 per 1,000 live births (4,902 deaths) to 0.390 per 1,000 live births (1,534 deaths). Over the past decade, SIDS rates in the United States have essentially held steady, thus the AAP has expanded the recommendations from safe sleeping practices to encompass multiple factors in the sleep environment that may affect SIDS and other sudden infant unexpected deaths such as suffocation and strangulation (AAP, 2011b).

The pathophysiology of SIDS is unclear, but many scientists and researchers subscribe to the hypothesis of the triple-risk model (Filiano & Kinney, 1994). According to the triple-risk model (NICHD, 2015), SIDS may occur through an interaction or convergence of three factors:

- A vulnerable infant—Intrinsic factors, such as unknown brain anomaly or homeostatic abnormalities, especially in the brain stem area that controls temperature, heart rate, and respiratory rate, may inhibit the infant's ability to respond to external stressors that all infants experience. Examples include an increase in hypercarbia (rebreathing CO_2) as a result of prone sleeping or soft bedding, overheating, or bed-sharing. Infants with neurologic abnormalities may not be able to move their heads or increase their respiratory rate in response to hypercarbia resulting from sleeping prone on a soft surface.

- Critical developmental period—During the initial 6 months of life, infants are in a rapid growth phase and their homeostatic systems change rapidly and may be compromised in the ability to respond to hazardous situations, thus some infants may not be able to respond to common stressors.

- External stressors—Environmental stressors, such as a prone sleeping position, second- and third-hand tobacco exposure, overheating, bed-sharing, soft sleep surfaces, or an upper respiratory infection may be overwhelming for a vulnerable infant during the critical development phase (NICHD, 2015). One study from Norway found that almost 50% of infants who died from SIDS had an upper airway infection (Arnestad, Anderson, Vege, & Rognum, 2001).

The AAP has updated and expanded their recommendations for safe sleep practices and environments (AAP, 2011b). The AAP committee responsible for updating the recommendations reviewed all of the present literature and found no data to support changes from the 2011 recommendations. Twelve of the 18 recommendations are based on Level A evidence, meaning they are the result of consistent scientific evidence and are unlikely to change based on future research (U.S. Preventive Services Task Force, 2013). Three of the recommendations are based on Level B evidence, implying the recommendations are based on inconsistent scientific evidence, but the current evidence has an impact on health outcomes. Some of the studies may be insufficient because of size or quality, therefore further research might change the recommendations (U.S. Preventive Services Task Force, 2013). The last three recommendations are Level C recommendations, indicating they are based primarily on expert opinion and consensus (U.S. Preventive Services Task Force, 2013).

LEVEL A RECOMMENDATIONS

I. *Back to sleep for every sleep*—To reduce the risk of SIDS, infants should be placed for sleep in a supine position (wholly on the back) for every sleep by every caregiver until 1 year of life. Side sleeping is not safe and is not advised (AAP, 2011b).
   A. Parents may worry about the baby choking while sleeping on his or her back, but infants have airway protective mechanisms, including infants with gastroesophageal reflux (Tablizo et al., 2007). Only infants with severe anatomic airway difficulties, such as type 3 or 4 laryngeal clefts, might benefit from prone positioning (AAP, 2011b). Increasing the head of the bed has not been shown to be effective for gastroesophageal reflux and may result in the baby sliding to the bottom of the bed in a prone position.
   B. Preterm and low-birth-weight babies are at an increased risk for SIDS and should be placed supine as soon as they are medically stable and certainly by 32 weeks postmenstrual age. Caregivers in the hospital should model the correct sleeping position as soon as possible, because parents copy the behavior of the hospital caregivers (AAP, 2011b). Babies will become acclimated to sleeping on their backs and parents will model the behavior. These concepts are well documented and are best practice with high levels of evidence backing

them, but many health care providers continue to place well babies and growing preterm babies in a prone position (Grazel, Phalen, & Polomano 2010). Knowing the recommendations and encouraging health care providers to follow the recommendations may help increase compliance with supine sleeping positions, and thus reduce deaths from SIDS.

C. Newborn babies in the well-baby nursery or rooming-in with mother should be placed on their backs immediately. There is no evidence that placing newborn babies on the side helps to clear amniotic fluid (AAP, 2011b).

D. Infants should be placed supine to sleep until they are 1 year old, but when they roll over they can be left in that sleeping position (AAP, 2011b).

II. *Use a firm sleep surface*—A firm crib mattress, covered by a fitted sheet, is the recommended sleeping surface to reduce the risk of SIDS and suffocation (AAP, 2011b).

A. Only cribs, bassinettes, or play yards approved by the Consumer Product Safety Commission are recommended (Consumer Product Safety Commission, n.d.).

B. Broken cribs or cribs with missing parts should not be used as these present a choking and strangulation hazard (AAP, 2011b).

C. Only a firm mattress specifically designed for a particular crib should be used and the mattress should be covered with a tight fitted sheet to prevent strangulation and suffocation (AAP, 2011b). No soft surfaces, such as pillows, quilts, comforters, stuffed toys, or blankets, should be in the bed with the baby (AAP, 2011b).

D. Infants should not be placed on a bed or sofa to sleep because of the risk for suffocation and entrapment. No bedrails to keep the infant from rolling off the bed should be used because of the risk of entrapment (AAP, 2011b).

E. The infant's crib should be in an area without cords, wires, or window coverings because of the risk of entanglement and strangulation (AAP, 2011b).

F. Infants should not sleep in sitting devices, including CSSs, swings, and bouncy seats. Infants less than 4 months of age are at an extreme risk if they fall asleep in a sitting device because they may fall asleep in positions that might increase risk for suffocation and airway constriction. Parents must be careful when carrying a baby in a sling to prevent the material from covering the nose and causing suffocation (AAP, 2011b).

III. *Room-sharing without bed-sharing* is important in the quest to prevent SIDS. Studies indicate that room-sharing without bed-sharing may help decrease SIDS by 50% (Tappin, Ecob, & Brooke, 2005). Placing the infant's crib in the room with parents and close to the parent's bed may help in monitoring, feeding, and parental fatigue while safeguarding the baby from suffocation, strangulation, and entrapment in the soft bed (AAP, 2011b).

A. Devices that claim to make bed-sharing safe are not recommended (AAP, 2011b)

B. Mothers may feed the baby in bed, but the baby should be placed back in the crib once feeding is complete. The risk of SIDS is extremely high on sofas and armchairs, therefore infants should not be fed on the sofa or armchair if the parent is at risk of falling asleep (AAP, 2011b).

C. Although there is no evidence to support bed-sharing to prevent SIDS, there is evidence to support *no bed-sharing* in specific situations. These situations may increase the risk of SIDS dramatically and include the following:

1. Bed-sharing with infants less than 3 months of age
2. Bed-sharing with a smoker or if mother smoked during the pregnancy
3. Bed-sharing with anyone who is very tired and at risk of rolling over on the baby
4. Bed-sharing with anyone using many types of medications such as antidepressants, pain medicine, alcohol, or illicit drugs
5. Bed-sharing with more than one person, including other children
6. Bed-sharing on a soft surface such as a waterbed or old mattress
7. Bed-sharing on a bed with pillows, quilts, or other soft surfaces that may increase risk of entrapment, suffocation, or SIDS (AAP, 2011b).

IV. *Soft objects and loose bedding should not be in the infant's crib.* These include soft stuffed animals, pillows, blankets, and quilts that may increase the risk of SIDS, suffocation, and strangulation (AAP, 2011b).
   A. Loose blankets and sheets should not be used as these present a strangulation and suffocation hazard.
   B. Clothing that keeps the baby warm without covering the face is recommended instead of sheets and blankets.
   C. It is recommended that no bumper pads around the crib be used. There is no evidence that bumper pads prevent harm and bruising of the baby and they are a strangulation and suffocation hazard (AAP, 2011b).

V. *There is evidence to indicate that regular prenatal care reduces the risk of SIDS* (AAP, 2011b).

VI. *Smoke exposures during pregnancy and in the infant's sleep environment are major risk factors for SIDS.* Health care providers should encourage the family to maintain a smoke-free home and car and should counsel parents on the hazards of smoking for the family and the baby.
   A. Smoking during pregnancy increases risk for SIDS.
   B. Second- and third-hand smoke increases the risk for SIDS.
   C. Bed-sharing with an adult smoker poses a particularly high risk of SIDS for any infant (AAP, 2011b).

VII. *Exposure to alcohol and illicit drug use during and after pregnancy increases the risk of SIDS.* Encourage mothers to seek help in abstaining from alcohol during pregnancy to consider drug withdrawal programs (AAP, 2011b).
   A. Bed-sharing and alcohol or illicit drug use pose a high risk of SIDS.
   B. Now that marijuana is legal in some areas, there are questions about the use of marijuana during pregnancy. A review of known literature revealed that there are some consequences of marijuana use throughout pregnancy including growth restriction, learning disabilities, and memory impairment (Wu, Jew, & Lu, 2011). There are ongoing studies in the states where marijuana is now legal and the practitioner will need to access the latest data because this will be a question many pregnant mothers and families will ask.

VIII. *Breastfeeding is recommended* because the evidence shows that breastfeeding reduces the risk of SIDS (AAP, 2011b).
   A. Exclusive breastfeeding without formula or any other food until the baby is 6 months old is best.
   B. Any breastfeeding will decrease the risk of SIDS (AAP, 2011b).

IX. *Consider offering a pacifier.* Although the mechanism of action is unclear, the evidence indicates that sucking on a pacifier when going to sleep may decrease the risk of SIDS (AAP, 2011b).

   A. If the pacifier falls out, there is no need to reinsert it.

   B. Do not use pacifier holders as they may present a risk for strangulation.

   C. For breastfeeding infants, wait to introduce a pacifier until breastfeeding is firmly establish, usually around 3 to 4 weeks (AAP, 2011b).

X. *Avoid overheating infants.* Infants should not require more than one layer of clothing beyond what an adult requires to be comfortable.

   A. There is evidence that overheating increases the risk of SIDS, but because the studies all used different temperatures, there is not a recommended room temperature to follow.

   B. Not enough evidence is available to recommend using a fan to decrease the risk of SIDS (AAP, 2011b).

XI. *Do not use home cardiopulmonary monitors to reduce the risk of SIDS.* There is no evidence that monitoring babies in the hospital can identify babies at risk for SIDS and that home monitors prevent SIDS. For specific situations, there are infants who may benefit from home monitoring, but home monitoring to prevent SIDS is not recommended (AAP, 2011b).

XII. *The national campaign to reduce the incidence of SIDs should be embraced and discussed by all health care providers.* The Safe-to-Sleep (formerly Back-to-Sleep) program has been very effective and is easy for parents and families to understand (NICHD, 2015). All heath care providers should participate in the program and know enough about it to promote the program in public and policy arenas (AAP, 2011b).

Level B Recommendations

I. *All infants should be immunized according to the AAP and Centers for Disease Control and Protection (CDC) guidelines.*

   A. There is no evidence that immunization contributes to SIDS and there is some evidence that immunization may decrease the risk of SIDS (AAP, 2011b).

II. *Do not use commercial devices that claim to reduce the risk of SIDS.* There is no evidence that any device decreases the incidence of SIDS (AAP, 2011b).

III. *Infants should have supervised, awake tummy time* to facilitate physical development and decrease postural plagiocephaly (AAP, 2011b).

Level C Recommendations

I. *Media sites and manufacturers should follow the Safe-to-Sleep guidelines in their messaging and products* (AAP, 2011b).

   A. Because many families and parents are exposed to hours of TV, movies, websites, and other media daily, it is important that all media present current guidelines. Many families are influenced greatly by what they hear and see in the media (AAP, 2011b).

II. *Expand the Safe-to-Sleep campaign* (AAP, 2011b).

   A. All caregivers, including parents, grandparents, day-care workers, and anyone who provides care for babies should be included in Safe-to-Sleep education.

B. The campaign should focus on African American and American Indian/Alaska Native populations because these groups have the highest incidence of SIDS.

C. The national campaign should concentrate on increasing breastfeeding while decreasing bed-sharing and exposure to tobacco smoke.

D. The campaign should be started before pregnancy and ideally should be part of high school education for both boys and girls (AAP, 2011b).

III. *Continue research and surveillance on the risk factors, causes, and pathophysiology of SIDS* and other causes of sudden infant death (AAP, 2011b).

Although the Safe-to-Sleep campaign has been effective from the introduction, SIDS rates have been static over the past decade. It is important to make the recommendations part of daily practice and that all family members are educated about the crucial aspects of Safe-to-Sleep.

SMOKE EXPOSURE

Exposure to tobacco smoke during pregnancy, at delivery, and after delivery may have life-long effects on infants. Smoking during pregnancy may cause low birth weight, preterm delivery, orofacial clefts (cleft lip/cleft palate), and stillbirth (AAP, 2015b). Exposure to tobacco during pregnancy may cause placenta previa, placenta abruptio, and death at delivery (AAP, 2015b). After delivery, babies exposed to tobacco smoke during pregnancy have an increased risk of SIDS, respiratory disorders, asthma, and other breathing problems (AAP, 2015b). Infants born to smoking mothers are at increased risk of obesity and diabetes (Anblagan et al., 2013). The pathophysiology of fetal and neonatal harm as a result of smoking during pregnancy involves at least two of the major components of tobacco smoke: nicotine and carbon monoxide. Research indicates that carbon monoxide and nicotine cross the placenta and are present in fetal circulation, amniotic fluid, and the breast milk of smoking mothers (Anblagan et al., 2013). There is evidence that the amount of nicotine in fetal circulation can be up to 15% higher than in maternal circulation and the amount of nicotine in the amniotic fluid can be up to 88% higher than in maternal circulation (Anblagan et al., 2013). Nicotine causes (a) vasoconstriction of the uteroplacental vasculature resulting in diminished oxygen and nutrient supply via the placenta to the fetus; (b) suppression of maternal appetite, thus decreasing maternal and fetal nutrient and energy intake; and (c) alterations in growth of peripheral and central nervous systems (Anblagan et al., 2013). Carbon monoxide binds with hemoglobin to form carboxyhemaglobin resulting in diminished oxygen to the fetus (Anblagan et al., 2013). Diminished oxygen to the fetus results in possible placental insufficiency, low birth weight, and prematurity, among other problems. About 20% of women smoke during pregnancy (Anblagan et al., 2013). According to Anblagan et al. (2013), maternal smoking during pregnancy may result in lower volume of some neonatal organs, including the brain, lungs, and kidneys, compared to same gestational age infants born to nonsmoking mothers. Studies summarized by the 2014 Surgeon General's report (CDC, 2014) indicate that smoking during pregnancy and exposure to second- and third-hand smoke may delay or prevent maturation of brain cells and impair the infant's response to hypoxia, thus explaining one reason for SIDS. Current General Surgeon's reports are important sources of information for health care providers and the general public. The reports synthesize and analyze current literature to make recommendations for care and management.

Second-hand smoke and third-hand smoke are detrimental to most people, especially newborns and infants. *Second-hand smoke* is defined as smoke from burning tobacco products, such as cigarettes or cigars, and exhaled smoke from active smokers (CDC, 2015e). Third-hand smoke is the residue left from second-hand smoke such as found on the clothes and hair of smokers, wall, carpets, furniture, and drapes (AAP, 2015b). Exposure to second- and third-hand smoke may expose infants to more than 4,000 chemicals and lead to problems such as an increased incidence of SIDS, respiratory disorders, asthma and other breathing problems, tooth decay, pneumonia, ear aches, sleep problems, and developmental delays (AAP, 2015b, 2015e).

Unfortunately, many children in the United States are exposed to second- and third-hand smoke (CDC, 2015f). The only way to prevent the hazards of prenatal smoking and second-hand smoke is to stop smoking, but that is not always easy for parents or grandparents. Discuss the hazards of smoking with the family and the significant health consequences of smoking for both the parent and the baby. Offer suggestions for smoking cessation and give parents information about smoking-cessation programs. Many families have situations in which they have little control of second-hand smoke exposure for their infant. In these situations, give suggestions on the best way to limit exposure to second-hand smoke. Make sure parents have appropriate referrals to smoking-cessation programs and websites that discuss the hazards of smoking and ways to limit exposure to second-hand smoke. The CDC and AAP are great sources for health care professionals and families to use to learn about the consequences of smoking and how to stop smoking.

BATHING PRACTICES

Many parents are excited yet concerned about giving their baby a bath at home. Although bathing is not considered a major issue, there are a few concepts that are important to remember. Most babies will only need to bathe three times a week to prevent dry skin ("Bathing and Skin," 2015). Remind parents to sponge bathe babies until the umbilical stump dries and falls off, usually within the first week or 2 of life. During a sponge bath, babies need to be covered with a towel or blanket and one section bathed and dried at a time to prevent heat loss and cold stress ("Bathing and Skin," 2015). After the umbilical stump dries, the baby may be placed in a tub bath with 2 in. of warm water in the basin ("Bathing and Skin," 2015). Parents need to turn on the cold water first when starting the bath and turn off the cold water last when turning off the water. The temperature of the water coming out at the faucet level should be no more than 120°F to prevent burns ("Bathing and Skin," 2015). As the baby grows, parents may consider buying and using a bathtub ring. The bathtub ring is designed to help the baby sit in an adult tub and is not a safety device. Parents may develop a false sense of security and leave the baby in the bathtub for a few minutes. If the ring tips over, it may trap the baby causing the baby to drown. The AAP does not recommend the use of bathtub rings ("Bathing and Skin," 2015). Bath time can be fun for parents and the baby, but safety in the bathtub is paramount.

INFECTION CONTROL

PREVENTION AT HOME

The most important way to prevent infection is to practice good hand hygiene by washing hands with soap and running water, or if soap and water are not available, using a 60% alcohol-based hand sanitizer (CDC, 2015a). Because most organisms are spread via hands, effective hand hygiene may prevent many respiratory and diarrheal illnesses in babies (CDC, 2015a). There is no evidence that antibacterial soap is more effective than regular soap (National Resource Center for Health and Safety in Childcare and Early Education, 2015). Effective handwashing is the most important infection-prevention concept to get across to parents and families. Parents are the best advocates for their baby; therefore, they can insist that everyone wash his or her hands prior to touching the baby. According to the CDC

(2015a), hands should be washed before and after preparing food, after going to the bathroom, after changing diapers, after touching garbage, and after handling tissues. Paper towels should be used to turn faucet handles off and to open bathroom doors after washing hands (National Resource Center for Health and Safety in Childcare and Early Education, 2015). Other factors, such as cleaning surfaces and toys that the baby comes in contact with, are important, but handwashing is the most effective way to prevent infection in the home or childcare center.

VACCINE SCHEDULES

Vaccines for babies, families, and health care workers are an important aspect of infection prevention at home, in health care arenas, and in public areas. Every year the Advisory Committee on Immunization Practices (ACIP) publishes recommendations for vaccines for children from birth through 18 years of age (CDC, 2015e). The vaccine recommendations are approved by the AAP, ACIP, American College of Obstetricians and Gynecologists, and the American Academy of Family Physicians each year. It is important that all health care providers check the CDC website for vaccine recommendations in January or February of each year (CDC, 2015e). Vaccine schedules are published with specific guidance on the age to start each vaccine and a catch-up vaccine schedule for missed vaccines. The CDC has vaccine schedules to download on smartphones and has specific calendars for parents to download to maintain vaccination schedules (CDC, 2015e). The following vaccine information is taken directly from the 2015 CDC vaccine website and is subject to change when new information is available:

    I. Hepatitis B vaccine is the only vaccine recommended at birth. For routine vaccination of hepatitis B, see the following from CDC (2015e):

    At birth:

    A. Administer monovalent HepB vaccine to all newborns before hospital discharge.

    B. For infants born to hepatitis B surface antigen (HBsAg)-positive mothers, administer HepB vaccine and 0.5 mL of hepatitis B immune globulin (HBIG) within 12 hours of birth. These infants should be tested for HBsAg and antibody to HBsAg (anti-HBs) 1 to 2 months after completion of the HepB series at age 9 through 18 months (preferably at the next well-child visit).

    C. If mother's HBsAg status is unknown, within 12 hours of birth administer HepB vaccine regardless of birth weight. For infants weighing less than 2,000 g, administer HBIG in addition to HepB vaccine within 12 hours of birth. Determine mother's HBsAg status as soon as possible and, if mother is HBsAg-positive, also administer HBIG for infants weighing 2,000 g or more as soon as possible, but no later than age 7 days.

    Doses following the birth dose:

    A. The second dose should be administered at age 1 or 2 months. Monovalent HepB vaccine should be used for doses administered before age 6 weeks.

    B. Infants who did not receive a birth dose should receive three doses of a HepB-containing vaccine on a schedule of 0, 1 to 2 months, and 6 months starting as soon as feasible. See CDC Catch-up Schedule (www.cdc.gov/vaccines/schedules/hcp/imz/catchup.html).

    C. Administer the second dose 1 to 2 months after the first dose (minimum interval of 4 weeks), administer the third dose at least 8 weeks after the second dose *and* at least 16 weeks after the *first* dose. The final (third or fourth) dose in the HepB vaccine series should be administered *no earlier than age 24 weeks*.

D. Administration of a total of four doses of HepB vaccine is permitted when a combination vaccine containing HepB is administered after the birth dose.

Catch-up hepatitis B vaccination:
A. Unvaccinated persons should complete a three-dose series.
B. A two-dose series (doses separated by at least 4 months) of adult formulation Recombivax HB is licensed for use in children aged 11 through 15 years (CDC, 2015e).

II. For rotavirus (RV) vaccines, the minimum age to start is 6 weeks for both RV1 (Rotarix) and RV5 (RotaTeq). RV vaccine is a live virus and should not be administered in the neonatal intensive care unit (NICU) because the risk of shedding the virus via stool outweighs the benefits (Committee on Infectious Diseases, AAP, 2009). Recommendations for RV vaccinations are as follows:

Routine vaccination:
Administer a series of RV vaccine to all infants as follows:
A. If Rotarix is used, administer a two-dose series at 2 and 4 months of age.
B. If RotaTeq is used, administer a three-dose series at ages 2, 4, and 6 months.
C. If any dose in the series was RotaTeq or vaccine product is unknown for any dose in the series, a total of three doses of RV vaccine should be administered.

Catch-up RV vaccination:
A. The maximum age for the first dose in the series is 14 weeks, 6 days; vaccination should not be initiated for infants aged 15 weeks, 0 days or older.
B. The maximum age for the final dose in the series is 8 months, 0 days (CDC, 2015e).

III. For diphtheria, tetanus toxoids, and acellular pertussis (DTaP) vaccine, the minimum age to administer is 6 weeks.

Routine vaccination:
A. Administer a five-dose series of DTaP vaccine at ages 2, 4, 6, 15 through 18 months, and 4 through 6 years. The fourth dose may be administered as early as age 12 months, provided at least 6 months have elapsed since the third dose. However, the fourth dose of DTaP need not be repeated if it was administered at least 4 months after the third dose of DTaP.

Catch-up vaccination:
A. The fifth dose of DTaP vaccine is not necessary if the fourth dose was administered at age 4 years or older (CDC, 2015e).
B. For tetanus and diphtheria toxoids and acellular pertussis (Tdap) vaccine, the minimum age is 10 years for both Boostrix and Adacel (CDC, 2015e).

IV. For *Haemophilus influenzae* type b (Hib) conjugate vaccine, the minimum age is 6 weeks for PRP-T (ACTHIB, DTaP-IPV/Hib [Pentacel] and Hib-MenCY [Men-Hibrix]) and PRP-OMP (PedvaxHIB or COMVAX) and 12 months for PRP-T (Hiberix).

Routine vaccination:
A. Administer a two- or three-dose Hib vaccine primary series and a booster dose (dose 3 or 4 depending on vaccine used in primary series) at age 12 through 15 months to complete a full Hib vaccine series.
B. The primary series with ActHIB, MenHibrix, or Pentacel consists of three doses and should be administered at 2, 4, and 6 months of age. The primary series with PedvaxHib or COMVAX consists of two doses and should be

administered at 2 and 4 months of age; a dose at age 6 months is not indicated.

C. One booster dose (dose 3 or 4 depending on vaccine used in primary series) of any Hib vaccine should be administered at age 12 through 15 months. An exception is Hiberix vaccine. Hiberix should only be used for the booster (final) dose in children aged 12 months through 4 years who have received at least one prior dose of Hib-containing vaccine.

D. For recommendations on the use of MenHibrix in patients at increased risk for meningococcal disease, please refer to the meningococcal vaccine footnotes (CDC, 2015e).

Catch-up vaccination:

A. If dose 1 was administered at ages 12 through 14 months, administer a second (final) dose at least 8 weeks after dose 1, regardless of Hib vaccine used in the primary series.

B. If both doses were PRP-OMP (PedvaxHIB or COMVAX), and were administered before the first birthday, the third (and final) dose should be administered at age 12 through 59 months and at least 8 weeks after the second dose.

C. If the first dose was administered at age 7 through 11 months, administer the second dose at least 4 weeks later and a third (and final) dose at age 12 through 15 months or 8 weeks after second dose, whichever is later.

D. If first dose is administered before the first birthday and second dose administered at younger than 15 months, a third (and final) dose should be given 8 weeks later.

E. For unvaccinated children aged 15 months or older, administer only one dose.

Vaccination of persons with high-risk conditions:

A. Children aged 12 through 59 months who are at increased risk for Hib disease, including chemotherapy recipients and those with anatomic or functional asplenia (including sickle cell disease), HIV infection, immunoglobulin deficiency, or early component complement deficiency, who have received either no doses or only one dose of Hib vaccine before 12 months of age, should receive two additional doses of Hib vaccine 8 weeks apart; children who received two or more doses of Hib vaccine before 12 months of age should receive one additional dose.

B. For patients younger than 5 years of age undergoing chemotherapy or radiation treatment who received a Hib vaccine dose(s) within 14 days of starting therapy or during therapy, repeat the dose(s) at least 3 months following therapy completion.

C. Recipients of hematopoietic stem cell transplant (HSCT) should be revaccinated with a three-dose regimen of Hib vaccine starting 6 to 12 months after successful transplant, regardless of vaccination history; doses should be administered at least 4 weeks apart.

D. A single dose of any Hib-containing vaccine should be administered to unimmunized* children and adolescents 15 months of age and older undergoing an elective splenectomy; if possible, vaccine should be administered at least 14 days before procedure.

---

* *Patients who have not received a primary series and booster dose or at least one dose of Hib vaccine after 14 months of age are considered unimmunized* (CDC, 2015e).

E. Hib vaccine is not routinely recommended for patients 5 years or older. However, one dose of Hib vaccine should be administered to unimmunized persons aged 5 years or older who have anatomic or functional asplenia (including sickle cell disease) and unvaccinated persons 5 through 18 years of age with HIV infection.

V. For pneumococcal vaccines (PCV), the minimum age is 6 weeks for PCV13 and 2 years for PPSV23.

Routine vaccination with PCV13:

A. Administer a four-dose series of PCV13 vaccine at ages 2, 4, and 6 months and at age 12 through 15 months.

B. For children ages 14 through 59 months who have received an age-appropriate series of seven-valent PCV (PCV7), administer a single supplemental dose of 13-valent PCV (PCV13).

Catch-up vaccination with PCV13:

A. Administer one dose of PCV13 to all healthy children aged 24 through 59 months who are not completely vaccinated for their age.

   i. The minimum interval between doses of PCV (PCV7 or PCV13) is 8 weeks.

   ii. For children with no history of PPSV23 vaccination, administer PPSV23 at least 8 weeks after the most recent dose of PCV13 (CDC, 2015e).

VI. Inactivated poliovirus vaccine (IPV) is important because live virus vaccine cannot be administered in the NICU and the minimum age to receive IPV is 6 weeks.

Routine vaccination:

A. Administer a four-dose series of IPV at ages 2, 4, 6 through 18 months, and 4 through 6 years. The final dose in the series should be administered on or after the fourth birthday and at least 6 months after the previous dose.

Catch-up vaccination:

A. In the first 6 months of life, minimum age and minimum intervals are only recommended if the person is at risk for imminent exposure to circulating poliovirus (i.e., travel to a polio-endemic region or during an outbreak).

B. If four or more doses are administered before age 4 years, an additional dose should be administered at age 4 through 6 years and at least 6 months after the previous dose.

C. A fourth dose is not necessary if the third dose was administered at age 4 years or older and at least 6 months after the previous dose.

D. If both oral polio vaccine (OPV) and IPV were administered as part of a series, a total of four doses should be administered, regardless of the child's current age. IPV is not routinely recommended for U.S. residents aged 18 years or older (CDC, 2015e).

VII. For influenza vaccines, the minimum age is 6 months for inactivated influenza vaccine (IIV) and 2 years for live, attenuated influenza vaccine (LAIV).

Routine vaccination:

A. Administer influenza vaccine annually to all children beginning at age 6 months. For most healthy, nonpregnant persons aged 2 through 49 years, either LAIV or IIV may be used. However, LAIV should *not* be administered to some persons, including (a) persons who have experienced severe allergic reactions to LAIV, any of its components, or to a previous dose of any other influenza vaccine; (b) children 2 through 17 years receiving aspirin or aspirin-containing products; (c) persons who are allergic to eggs; (d) pregnant women; (e) immunosuppressed persons; (f) children 2 through 4 years of age with asthma or who had wheezing in the past 12 months; or (g) persons who have taken influenza antiviral medications in the previous 48 hours. For all other contraindications and precautions to use of LAIV, see Grohskopf et al. (2014).

For children aged 6 months through 8 years:
A. For the 2015 to 2016 season, administer two doses (separated by at least 4 weeks) to children who are receiving influenza vaccine for the first time. Some children in this age group who have been vaccinated previously will also need two doses. For additional guidance, follow dosing guidelines in the 2014 to 2015 ACIP influenza vaccine recommendations and see Grohskopf et al. (2014).

VIII. The minimum age for measles, mumps, and rubella (MMR) vaccine is 12 months for routine vaccination.

Routine vaccination:
A. Administer a two-dose series of MMR vaccine at ages 12 through 15 months and 4 through 6 years. The second dose may be administered before age 4 years, provided at least 4 weeks have elapsed since the first dose.
B. Administer one dose of MMR vaccine to infants aged 6 through 11 months before departure from the United States for international travel. These children should be revaccinated with two doses of MMR vaccine, the first at age 12 through 15 months (12 months if the child remains in an area where disease risk is high), and the second dose at least 4 weeks later.
C. Administer two doses of MMR vaccine to children aged 12 months and older before departure from the United States for international travel. The first dose should be administered on or after age 12 months and the second dose at least 4 weeks later.

Catch-up vaccination:
A. Ensure that all school-aged children and adolescents have had two doses of MMR vaccine; the minimum interval between the two doses is 4 weeks (CDC, 2015e).

IX. For varicella (VAR) vaccine, the minimum age is 12 months.

Routine vaccination:
A. Administer a two-dose series of VAR vaccine at ages 12 through 15 months and 4 through 6 years. The second dose may be administered before age 4 years, provided at least 3 months have elapsed since the first dose. If the second dose was administered at least 4 weeks after the first dose, it can be accepted as valid.

Catch-up vaccination:
A. Ensure that all persons aged 7 through 18 years without evidence of immunity (see CDC, 2007), have two doses of varicella vaccine. For children aged 7 through 12 years, the recommended minimum interval between doses is 3 months (if the second dose was administered at least 4 weeks after the first dose, it can be accepted as valid); for persons aged 13 years and older, the minimum interval between doses is 4 weeks (CDC, 2015e).

X. For hepatitis A (HepA) vaccine, the minimum age is 12 months.

Routine vaccination:

A. Initiate the two-dose Hep A vaccine series at 12 through 23 months; separate the two doses by 6 to 18 months.

B. Children who have received one dose of Hep A vaccine before age 24 months should receive a second dose 6 to 18 months after the first dose.

C. For any person aged 2 years and older who has not already received the HepA vaccine series, two doses of HepA vaccine separated by 6 to 18 months may be administered if immunity against hepatitis A virus infection is desired.

Catch-up vaccination:

A. The minimum interval between the two doses is 6 months (CDC, 2015e).

For all vaccinations, please go to the CDC website to read the latest recommendations for vaccination. The ACIP is an ongoing committee that synthesizes scientific information and studies to update recommendations for current immunizations with appropriate vaccines. *The presented information on vaccines is meant to provide the neonatal nurse practitioner (NNP) student with an understanding of the importance and complexity of vaccinations and is not meant to be a source for providing vaccines to babies. Only the ACIP via the CDC website should be used as a current source of vaccine administration.*

Pain and fever are major concerns for parents and babies during vaccine administration. Although some providers and clinics routinely administer acetaminophen as an antipyretic and pain control medication, there is some research indicating that the administration of acetaminophen prior to vaccine administration may diminish the antibody response in babies and children (Prymula et al., 2009). Discuss the hazards of routine administration of acetaminophen before casually telling parents to give it before administering vaccines. There are myriad ways to prevent or decrease pain during administration of vaccines, including breastfeeding immediately before, during, and after administration; using appropriate-size needles; holding and talking to the baby; and kangaroo care for preterm babies (Taddio et al., 2015).

MATERNAL VACCINATIONS

In recent years, pertussis outbreaks have been seen in different part of the United States and there has been an increase in the number of cases, almost 33,000 cases in 2014 alone (CDC, 2015c). The highest incidence of pertussis is in babies and most deaths occur in babies less than 3 months old (CDC, 2015c). Because there is no pertussis vaccine for newborns, research has focused on ways to prevent pertussis in babies younger than 6 months of age. There are two main focus areas to prevent pertussis in young babies: cocoon the baby by vaccinating people around the baby and giving pregnant women a pertussis vaccine between 27 and 36 weeks gestation (CDC, 2015d). Because it is difficult to make sure people around the baby get vaccinated, the CDC recommends giving mothers the pertussis vaccine during every pregnancy. Efficacy and safety of the vaccine has been tested and immunizing mothers during pregnancy is expected to decrease hospitalization and death cased by pertussis (Amirthalingam et al., 2014; Munoz et al., 2014). Antibodies form after maternal administration and pass through the placenta to the baby affording effective protection until the baby can receive the vaccination series by 6 months of age. This is a relatively new recommendation (2012) and not all mothers are receiving the vaccination yet, but it is important to know. Good practice includes encouraging all family members, health care workers, and childcare worker to get vaccinated, but vaccinating the mother during pregnancy may be the most effective way to save babies from death as a result of pertussis (CDC, 2015d).

NUTRITIONAL SUPPORT

OPTIMAL GOALS FOR GROWTH

Rapid growth occurs during the first year of life and the first 6 months is the most rapid phase of growth in life ("Nutrition Supervision," 2014). Most babies will double their birth weight by 6 months of life and triple their birth weight by 12 months of age ("Nutrition Supervision," 2014). During the first 6 months, babies gain around 4 to 7 ounces per week and grow in length around 1 inch per month ("Nutrition Supervision," 2014). From 6 to 18 months, babies gain around 3 to 5 ounces per week and grow about 1/2 inch per month ("Nutrition Supervision," 2014). Breastfed babies tend to grow faster than formula-fed babies during the first 6 months, but grow slower from 6 to 12 months ("Nutrition Supervision," 2014). Around 40% to 50% of the calories in breast milk and formula come from fats, thus providing essential fatty acids, calories, and fat-soluble vitamins ("Nutrition Supervision," 2014). Infant growth depends on many factors, including nutrition, genetic factors, and prenatal factors ("Nutrition Supervision," 2014).

All mothers should be encouraged to breastfeed, at least for the first 6 months of life. If there are reasons that the mother cannot breastfeed, formula should be given to the baby. In the United States, about 73% of mothers initiate breastfeeding, but only about 40% breastfeed at 6 months of age ("Nutrition Issues and Concerns," 2014). Breastfeeding may decrease the number and severity of bacterial and viral illnesses in babies and it may provide a protective effect against some chronic diseases such as Crohn's disease, type 1 diabetes mellitus, lymphoma and leukemia, and celiac disease ("Nutrition Issues and Concerns," 2014). There is mounting evidence that breastfeeding decreases the incidence of otitis media and asthma, thus indicating that the immunologic effects last long past the newborn period ("Nutrition Issues and Concerns," 2014). Breastfeeding may help prevent obesity and many studies have shown that breastfed babies have increased cognitive functions, including higher IQs and better academic performance in school ("Nutrition Issues and Concerns," 2014). Long-term benefits of breastfeeding for the mother include decreased incidence of ovarian cancer, premenopausal breast cancer, hip fractures, and osteoporosis ("Nutrition Issues and Concerns," 2014).

Although there are few contraindications for breastfeeding, the contraindications should be discussed with the mother and she should be strongly counseled not to breastfeed. The strongest contraindication is an inherited metabolic disorder such as galactasemia ("Nutrition Issues and Concerns," 2014). Other contraindications include HIV, active untreated tuberculosis, certain medications such as specific antibiotics, chemotherapeutic drugs, and certain antipsychotic drugs ("Nutrition Issues and Concerns," 2014). Hepatitis A, B, and C are not transmitted via breast milk, therefore babies born to mothers with hepatitis B should be allowed to breastfeed (CDC, 2015b).

VITAMIN AND MINERAL ADMINISTRATION

All breastfed babies should have vitamin D started within a few days of life ("Vitamin D," 2015). Many mothers are vitamin D deficient and cannot provide enough for their babies via breast milk. Vitamin D deficiency may lead to rickets in babies, thus it is imperative that all babies, including formula-fed babies, receive vitamin D, 400 international units (IU) per day ("Starting Solid Food," 2015b). Over the past several years, studies indicate that almost all children are vitamin D deficient, therefore the AAP has recommended that all children receive vitamin D 400 IU daily ("Vitamin D," 2015). Breastfed babies are at risk for iron deficiency and should have an iron supplement of 1 mg/kg/d started around 4 months of age ("Nutrition Supervision," 2014).

FEEDING ISSUES

All babies should exclusively breastfeed or receive formula until 6 months of age (AAP, 2015c). Solid food can be introduced around 6 months of age or after the baby shows signs or cues that he or she is ready to start solid-food feedings ("Starting Solid Food," 2012). Indications to start solid-food introduction include: can the baby hold his or her head up and sit in a high chair? Does he or she open mouth when food is present? Can he or she move food from the spoon to the throat? and Has he or she doubled in birth weight ("Starting Solid Food," 2012). Single-grain cereal should be started first—oatmeal, rice, or barley—fruits and vegetables can be added one at a time after cereal ("Starting Solid Food," 2012). After tolerating cereal, some pediatricians advocate starting vegetables instead of fruit in order to diminish a preference for sweet foods, but there is no evidence to support the validity of that practice, therefore it does not matter in what order they are introduced ("Starting Solid Food," 2012). Parents should offer a single food and observe for 3 to 5 days for allergic reactions before offering another food ("Nutrition Supervision," 2014). Introducing solid food too early may lead to obesity, allergies, and eczema (AAP, 2015c). Pureed fruits, vegetables, and meats can be added to the diet one by one (AAP, 2015d). Caution parents to be careful about offering bite-size food that can cause choking such as hard candy, grapes, popcorn, and hotdogs ("Nutrition Supervision," 2014). Babies do not need fruit juice or extra water while exclusively bottle or formula feeding ("Nutrition Supervision," 2014). After 6 months of age, if parents choose to give fruit juice, it should be in a sippy cup and not in a bottle so as to prevent dental caries ("Nutrition Supervision," 2014).

Bright Futures is an AAP program with specifics about newborn and infant nutrition and is an excellent source for best practices for nutrition in infants. Not only does it give evidence-based nutrition recommendations, the program provides tools for the provider to use when discussing all aspects of nutrition with mothers and other family members (AAP-Bright Futures, 2016).

ORAL HEALTH

Oral health should begin early in life because dental caries is the most common chronic disease in childhood (AAP, 2014). By 2 years of age more than 24% of children have dental caries (AAP, 2014). Dental caries is a multifactorial disease process that involves demineralization and remineralization of the tooth enamel (AAP, 2014). Multiple factors, including sugar, bacteria, saliva, and fluoride, are involved in maintaining a healthy balance between demineralization and remineralization of the tooth enamel (AAP, 2014). *Streptococcus mutans* is the organism most closely associated with dental carries and this organism has the ability to ferment sugar, thereby creating an acidotic environment that predisposes the tooth to other organisms (AAP, 2014). The acidotic environment leads to demineralization, but saliva and fluoride can help mediate the effect of organisms and an acidotic environment (AAP, 2014). Saliva essentially washes food particles out of the mouth and removes the sugar that ferments and creates an environment conducive to bacteria and demineralization (AAP, 2014). Fluoride inhibits demineralization at the tooth surface, enhances remineralization, which results in a more acid-resistant tooth surface, and inhibits the formation of bacterial enzymes (AAP, 2014).

In order to prevent dental caries, parents should start brushing teeth twice a day with a smear or rice-sized portion of fluoridated toothpaste as soon as the first tooth erupts (AAP, 2014). Other recommendations are to exclusively breastfeed for 6 months, not to put a child to bed with a bottle, limit sugary drinks and food to mealtime, wean bottle by 1 year of age, limit fruit juice to 4 to 6 oz. per day at mealtime, and discourage the intake of carbonated beverages (AAP, 2014). The use of a pacifier or sucking on fingers is not associated with dental issues unless the practice continues past 3 years of age. Pacifiers should be offered at naptime and sleep time to decrease SIDS (AAP, 2014). If parents have dental caries, they should not give the baby anything that they have had in their mouths. Parents need to be vigilant in providing oral health for their baby in order to prevent dental caries.

CONCLUSIONS

From birth to 1 year of life is a time of rapid growth and change. Parents have multiple sources of information, including the Internet, family, and friends to obtain answers to their questions. Many sources do not give current or correct information. It is important that as health care providers, NNPs provide current, evidence-based, responsive, and accurate information to parents and caregivers. Almost all parents and caregivers will go to the Internet for information; therefore, it is imperative that NNPs provide websites that provide current and evidence-based information. Answering the questions for the case studies and accessing the references and websites provided will enable you to assure parents they have current, evidence-based, and best-practice information to care for their baby.

Case 17.1

You get a call from the nurse in the well-baby nursery and she asks you to go talk to a mother who does not want her baby to get any shots because the baby is only a few hours old. Baby G is a 1-hour-old, 39 4/7-weeks term, female baby born to gravida 1, now para 1 mother with no prenatal care. Lab work, including hepatitis B, was drawn from the mother on admission. The lab work is back and reveals that the mother has a positive HbsAg.

1. *What do you order for the baby to limit transmission of hepatitis B to the baby?*

   A. Hepatitis B vaccine
   B. Hepatitis B vaccine and hepatitis B immune globulin (HBIG)
   C. HBIG

   ANSWER: B. *In order to prevent or mitigate the transmission of hepatitis B to the baby from mother, the baby must receive hepatitis B vaccine within 12 hours of delivery. HBIG can be given at the same time (in a different site). If the mother's hepatitis B status is unknown, check her hepatitis B status via lab draw and give hepatitis B vaccine within 12 hours of delivery. Although HBIG is more effective if given within 12 to 24 hours after delivery, it is effective if given up to 7 days post-delivery (CDC, 2015e).*

(continued)

Case 17.1 (continued)

2. The mother would like to breastfeed her baby. The nurses are confused about allowing her to breastfeed and call you to clarify. What do you advise the nurses to tell the mother?

A. Yes, she may breastfeed immediately (CDC, 2015b)
B. No
C. Only after the baby has received hepatitis B vaccine and HBIG

ANSWER: A. *Yes, mothers can breastfeed with hepatitis B. There have been no reports of transmission of hepatitis B to the baby via breast milk. Hepatitis B is transmitted through contact with the mother's blood (CDC, 2015b).*

At 4 weeks of age, the mother planned to take Baby G for her well-baby check-up. The mother called the nursery and asked to speak to the NNP who talked to her about the hepatitis B vaccine while she and the baby were hospitalized. The mother wants to know what she can do to prevent pain when her baby gets her immunizations.

3. *What is the best answer to decrease or prevent the pain associated with injections and immunizations?*

A. Tylenol—35 mg orally (baby weighs 3.5 kg)
B. Bottle of fruit juice because the sweet taste will diminish the pain of the injection
C. Start breastfeeding about 5 minutes before and during administration of the vaccine per injection

ANSWER: C. *Preventing or attenuating pain in newborns is a very important topic that is not addressed often. There are several nonpharmacological pain-management techniques that are available for parents and caregivers to use. Breastfeeding before, during, and after administration of vaccines has been shown to be very effective in preventing and relieving pain in term babies. Tylenol should not be given prior to vaccine administration as it has been shown to decrease the amount of antibody formation from the vaccine, thus it decreases the effectiveness of the vaccination (Prymula et al., 2009; Taddio et al., 2015).*

Case 17.2

Baby B is a 6-week-old African American female infant born to a 25-year-old, gravida 3, now para 3, mother at 30 weeks gestational age. The baby required oxygen at 0.5 L/min/bi-nasal cannula for 12 days and has been in room air for over a month. Her weight is 2.2 kg and she is bottle feeding well. Mother does not want to breastfeed. Mild gastroesophageal

(continued)

Case 17.2 (*continued*)

reflux with no evidence of aspiration is her only issue and the remainder of her hospital course has been uneventful. Baby B is ready for discharge within the next few days. You are the neonatal nurse practitioner (NNP) and you talk to the mother about putting her baby on her back to sleep. The mother tells you that her other two children (both premature) slept on their stomach and she does not see a reason why this baby cannot sleep on her stomach. In fact, she tells you that because the baby spits up a lot, sleeping on her stomach might keep her from choking.

1. *What is the best sleep position for preterm babies without medical problems?*
   A. The baby can sleep on her side instead of her back
   B. Studies show that preterm babies sleeping on their backs have a lower rate of sudden infant death syndrome (SIDS) and will not aspirate formula into their lungs
   C. The baby can sleep on her stomach with the head of her bed increased at a 30° angle

   ANSWER: B. *The American Academy of Pediatrics (AAP) recommends that all babies sleep supine, including term and preterm babies. Preterm babies in the neonatal intensive care unit should be on their backs from 32 weeks to discharge to model the back-to-sleep position for parents and caregivers. Side sleeping is considered unsafe because many of the babies end up prone on the abdomen. The head of the bed should not be raised as preterm babies may slide or scoot to the end of the bed and end up in a precarious position. The AAP recommendations were changed and updated in 2011 and reaffirmed without change in 2015. All recommendations are well referenced, evidence based, updated, and available for health care professionals and parents on the AAP website. It is important for NNPs and health care providers to stay updated on current recommendations (AAP, 2011b).*

After you talk to the mother a little longer, she tells you that the grandmother is going to keep all three of the children during the day when mother goes to work. You ask if anyone in the home smokes and the mother tells you that the grandfather smokes, but the grandmother does not. During the summer, the grandfather always goes outside, but during the winter he will often smoke in the house.

2. *How can second- and third-hand smoke affect infants?*
   A. Second-hand and third-hand smoking do not pose a risk to babies
   B. Causes increased incidence of SIDS, respiratory disorders, asthma and other breathing problems, tooth decay, pneumonia, ear aches, sleep problems, and developmental delays
   C. May cause SIDS, constipation, asthma, reflux, and colic

   ANSWER: B. *Multiple studies have documented the hazards of second- and third-hand smoke. Caregivers may try to smoke outdoors, but there are always instances when they will smoke in the house. Cigarette smoke has been associated with the development of multiple problems in newborns, both preterm and term. Because preterm babies are more vulnerable, it is important to be aware of the hazards of cigarette smoke and alert parents to those*

(continued)

Case 17.2 (continued)

effects (AAP, 2015b, 2015e). Second- and third-hand cigarette smoke always pose a risk to everyone, including term and preterm babies, but so far it has not been associated with constipation or colic (AAP, 2015b, 2015e).

Case 17.3

Bianchi, the baby in Case 17.2, is now 3.5 months old. Bianchi wakes up every 3 hours to feed and Ms. Gray is working daily, thus she is desperate for some sleep! After talking to her mother about what to do, Ms. Gray calls you. Bianchi's grandmother told Ms. Gray to mix "some cereal and baby food in her bottle" before Bianchi goes to bed so she would be full and sleep longer. The mother read in some of the literature from the hospital that babies should not get baby food before 4 months of age. You are in the developmental follow-up clinic and receive the call from Ms. Gray. She wants to know what she should do.

1. **What are the recommendations for feeding solid foods to infants?**
   A. Cereal at 3 months, but no baby food until 4 months of age
   B. Cereal and applesauce at 4 months of age, vegetables at 5 months, and meat at 6 months
   C. No solid food until 6 months old

   ANSWER: C. *The American Academy of Pediatrics (AAP) recommends that babies receive only breast milk or formula until 6 months of age, delaying introduction of cereal and baby food. Anything other than breast milk or formula is considered solid food. Juice, soft drinks, and tea are not appropriate for babies less than 6 months of age. The AAP changed the recommendation for no solid food to 6 months from 4 months in 2015. The recommendations were based on solid studies and are available on the AAP website. It is important to stay updated on current recommendations based on the evidence and best practice (AAP, 2015d).*

Ms. Gray asks you why she cannot give her baby cereal. She fed her other children cereal at 3 months of age and they are okay. Ms. Gray tells you that formula in expensive and inconvenient and the sooner Bianchi takes solid food, the better it is for her family. You explain to her why it is important not to start solid food (including cereal) too early.

2. **What harm can come from early feeding of solid food to a baby?**
   A. Obesity, allergies, and eczema
   B. Obesity, ear infections, and bronchiolitis
   C. Obesity, rhinitis, and bronchiolitis

   ANSWER: A. *Obesity, allergies, and eczema have been associated with early feeding and the AAP recommends no solid food (including cereal) until 6 months of age (AAP, 2015b). Bronchiolitis has not been associated with early feedings (AAP, 2015c).*

Case 17.4

James is a 6-month-old baby and is the youngest of three boys in a busy working family. Although James is a healthy, growing baby, his mother has some questions. Because James was an unexpected addition to their family, his siblings are 10 and 12 years older than him. James is growing rapidly and at his check-up at 6 months of age his height is at the 75th percentile on the growth chart. His mother said he is still in a rear-facing car seat in the back seat, but she is ready to turn him around so she can see him. She asks you for advice on when she can change the car seat to front facing.

1. *How long should a child stay in a rear-facing car seat in the back seat of a vehicle?*

   A. One year of age
   B. Eighteen months of age
   C. Two years or until the child outgrows the height and weight of the specific car seat

   ANSWER: C. *The American Academy of Pediatrics (AAP) recommends that children stay in a rear-facing seat until 2 years of age or until they outgrow the parameters of the car seat. Each brand of car safety seat (CSS) has height and weight parameters specific for that seat, thus you may need to caution parents to read the guidelines that come with the CSS. Health care providers need to stay updated on current recommendations for care safety seat recommendations. Parents report that they get different recommendations from different providers, thus it is important that all providers give parents current, evidence-based, best-practice recommendations from the AAP. The recommendations on the website are well referenced and updated based on the most current evidence available. Although the reference is cited as 2011, it was reaffirmed in 2015 with discussion of the latest evidence (AAP, 2011a).*

As his mother continued to ask questions during the well-child visit, she wondered when James could ride in the front seat. She seemed surprised at your answer because her other boys were riding in the front seat at 4 and 5 years of age.

2. *When can children sit in the front seat of a vehicle assuming they are properly restrained?*

   A. At 6 years of age
   B. At 8 years of age
   C. At 13 years of age

   ANSWER: C. *Although neonatal nurse practitioners care for and manage children up to 2 years of age, many families have older children. It is important to know the recommendations for babies and older children, because families will ask. Never put a baby in a CSS in the front seat of a vehicle. No child under the age of 13 should ride in the front seat according to the AAP guidelines (reaffirmed in 2015). Some parents are not aware that the seat belts do not fit younger children well and the deployment of air bags may cause great harm to a younger child in the 6- to 8-year-old range (AAP, 2011b). AAP has developed specific guidelines for parents, but many do not know how to access the information. Therefore, it is important to provide information on how to access the most current guidelines (AAP, 2011a).*

ACKNOWLEDGMENTS

I would like to thank the co-editors of this book for the opportunity to participate in writing case studies and pioneering a technique to enhance learning and critical-thinking skills for NNPs. Dr. Sheldon Korones was my mentor, professor, and friend for many years and he is the reason I am an NNP now. He knew that NICUs were only as good as the nurses and NNPs who provided care and management for babies. I will always be grateful for his belief in nurses. NNPs have been a vital part of care and management of neonates for more than 40 years. They deserve acknowledgment and much appreciation for paving the way for today's NNP. On a personal note, I am grateful for the support and understanding of my parents, Bobby and Wilodene Burrell, and my husband and son, Dale and Will Bellflower. Life with them has been an adventure!

REFERENCES

American Academy of Pediatrics (AAP). (2011a). Policy statement: Child passenger safety. *Pediatrics, 127*(4), 788–793. Reaffirmed in *Pediatrics,* Feb 2015, *135*(2) e558. doi:10.1542/peds.2014-3717

American Academy of Pediatrics. (2011b). SIDS and other sleep-related infant deaths: Expansion of recommendations for a safe infant sleeping environment. *Pediatrics, 129*(5), 1030–1039. Reaffirmed in *Pediatrics,* April 2015, *135*(4). doi:10.1542/peds.2011-2285

American Academy of Pediatrics (AAP). (2014). Maintaining and improving the oral health of young children. *Pediatrics, 134,* 124–1229. doi:10.1542/peds.2014-2984

American Academy of Pediatrics (AAP). (2015a). Car seats: Information for families for 2015. Retrieved from https://www.healthychildren.org/English/safety-prevention/on-the-go/Pages/Car-Safety -Seats-Information-for-Families.aspx

American Academy of Pediatrics (AAP). (2015b). Effects of tobacco on children. Retrieved from http://www2.aap.org/richmondcenter/EffectsOfTobaccoOnChildren.html

American Academy of Pediatrics (AAP). (2015c). Infant allergies and food sensitivities. Retrieved from https://www.healthychildren.org/English/ages-stages/baby/breastfeeding/Pages/Infant-Aller gies-and-Food-Sensitivities.aspx

American Academy of Pediatrics (AAP). (2015d). Infant food and feeding. Retrieved from https://www.aap.org/en-us/advocacy-and-policy/aap-health-initiatives/HALF-implementation-Guide/Age-Specific-Content/Pages/Infant-Food-and-Feeding.aspx#none

American Academy of Pediatrics. (2015e). Second hand smoke and children. Retrieved from http://www2.aap.org/richmondcenter/pdfs/SecondhandHandout.pdf

American Academy of Pediatrics-Bright Futures. (2016). Bright Futures guidelines and pocket guide. Retrieved from https://brightfutures.aap.org/materials-and-tools/guidelines-and-pocket-guide/Pages/default.aspx

Amirthalingam, G., Andrews, N., Campbell, H., Ribeiro, S., Kara, E., Donegan, K., . . . Ramsay, M. (2014). Effectiveness of maternal pertussis vaccination in England: An observational study. *Lancet, 384*(9953), 1521–1528. doi:10.1016/S0140-6736(14)60686-3

Anblagan, D., Jones, N. W., Costigan, C., Parker, A. J. J., Allcock, K., Aleong, R., . . . Coyne, L. H. (2013). Maternal smoking during pregnancy and fetal organ growth: A magnetic resonance imaging study. *PLOS ONE, 8*(6), e67223. doi:10.1371/journal.pone.0067223

Arbogast, K. B., Jermakian, J. S., Kallan, M. J., & Durbin, D. R. (2009). Effectiveness of belt positioning booster seats: An updated assessment. *Pediatrics, 124*(5), 1281–1286.

Arnestad, M., Anderson, M., Vege, A., & Rognum, T. O. (2001). Changes in the epidemiological pattern of sudden infant death syndrome in southeast Norway, 1984–1998: Implications for future prevention and research. *Archives of Disease in Childhood, 85,* 108–115.

Bathing and skin care. (2015). Retrieved from https://www.healthychildren.org/English/ages-stages/baby/bathing-skin-care/Pages/default.aspx

Centers for Disease Control and Prevention. (2007). Prevention of varicella. *Morbidity and Mortality Weekly Report.* Retrieved from http://www.cdc.gov/mmwr/pdf/rr/rr5604.pdf

Centers for Disease Control and Prevention (CDC). (2014). Chapter nine: Reproductive outcomes. In *2014 Surgeon General's report: The health consequences of smoking—50 years of progress* (pp. 459–498). Retrieved from http://www.cdc.gov/tobacco/data_statistics/sgr/50th-anniversary/index.htm

Centers for Disease Control and Prevention (CDC). (2015a). Handwashing: Clean hands save lives. Retrieved from http://www.cdc.gov/handwashing/when-how-handwashing.html

Centers for Disease Control and Prevention (CDC). (2015b). Hepatitis B virus infection. Retrieved from http://www.cdc.gov/breastfeeding/disease/hepatitis.htm

Centers for Disease Control and Prevention (CDC). (2015c). Pertussis outbreak trends. Retrieved from http://www.cdc.gov/pertussis/outbreaks/trends.html

Centers for Disease Control and Prevention (CDC). (2015d). Provide the best prenatal care to prevent pertussis. Retrieved from http://www.cdc.gov/pertussis/downloads/fs-hcp-provide-prenatal-care.pdf

Centers for Disease Control and Prevention (CDC). (2015e). Recommended immunization schedules for persons aged 0 through 18 years, United States, 2015. Retrieved from http://www.cdc.gov/vaccines/schedules/downloads/child/0-18yrs-child-combined-schedule.pdf

Centers for Disease Control and Prevention (CDC). (2015f). Secondhand smoke facts. Retrieved from http://www.cdc.gov/tobacco/data_statistics/fact_sheets/secondhand_smoke/general_facts

Center for Disease Control and Prevention-Morbidity and Mortality Weekly Report. (2007). Prevention of Varicella. Retrieved from http://www.cdc.gov/mmwr/pdf/rr/rr5604.pdf

Committee on Infectious Diseases, American Academy of Pediatrics (AAP). (2009). Prevention of rotavirus disease: Updated guidelines for use of rotavirus vaccine. *Pediatrics, 123*(5), 1412–1420.

Consumer Product Safety Commission. (n.d.). Safe-to-Sleep: Crib information center. Retrieved from http://www.cpsc.gov/en/Safety-Education/Safety-Education-Centers/cribs

Elliott, M. R., Kallan, M. J., Durbin, D. R., & Winston F. K. (2006). Effectiveness of child safety seats vs seat belts in reducing risk for death in children in passenger vehicle crashes. *Archives of Pediatric and Adolescence Medicine, 160*(6), 617–621. [Published correction appears in *Archives of Pediatric and Adolescence Medicine* 2006, *160*(9), 952]

Filiano, J. J., & Kinney, H. C. (1994). A perspective on neuropathologic findings in victims of the sudden infant death syndrome: The triple-risk model. *Biology of the Neonate, 65*(3–4), 194–197.

Goldstein, R. D., Trachtenberg, F. L., Sens, M. A., Harty, B. J., & Kinney, H. C. (2016). Overall postnatal mortality and rates of SIDS. *Pediatrics, 1*(137), e20152298. doi:10.1542/peds.2015-2298

Grazel, R., Phalen, A. G., & Polomano, R. C. (2010). Implementation of the American Academy of Pediatrics recommendations to reduce sudden infant death syndrome risk in neonatal intensive care units: An evaluation of nursing knowledge and practice. *Advances in Neonatal Care, 10*(6), 332–342. doi:10.1097/ANC.0b013e3181f36ea0

Grohskopf, L. A., Olsen, S. J., Sakolow, L. Z., Bresee, J. S., Cox, N. J., Broder, K. R, . . . Walter, E. B. (2014). Prevention and control of seasonal influenza with vaccines: Recommendations of the Advisory Committee on Immunization Practices (ACIP)—United States, 2014–2015 influenza season. *Morbidity and Mortality Weekly Report, 63*(32), 691–697. Retrieved from http://www.cdc.gov/mmwr/pdf/wk/mm6332.pdf#page=11

Matthews, T. J., MacDorman, M. F., & Thomas, M. E. (2015). Infant mortality statistics from the 2013 period linked birth/infant death data set. *National Vital Statistics Report, 64*(9), 1–30.

Munoz, F. M., Bond, N. H., Maccato, M., Pinell, P., Hammill, H. A., Swamy, G. K., . . . Baker C. J. (2014). Safety and immunogenicity of tetanus diphtheria and acellular pertussis (Tdap) immunization during pregnancy in mothers and infants: A randomized clinical trial. *Journal of the American Medical Association, 311*(17), 1760–1769. doi:10.1001/jama.2014.3633

National Institute of Child Health and Human Development. (2015). Safe-to–Sleep: Research on possible causes of SIDS. Retrieved from https://www.nichd.nih.gov/sts/campaign/science/Pages/causes.aspx

National Resource Center for Health and Safety in Childcare and Early Education. (2015). Caring for our children: National health and safety performance standards and guidelines for early care and education programs, Standard 3.2.2.2. Retrieved from http://cfoc.nrckids.org/StandardView/3.2.2.2

Nutrition issues and concerns. (2014). Retrieved from https://brightfutures.aap.org/Bright%20 Futures%20Documents/BFNutrition3rdEdition_issuesConcerns.pdf

Nutrition supervision. (2014). Retrieved from https://brightfutures.aap.org/Bright%20Futures%20 Documents/BFNutrition3rdEditionSupervision.pdf

Prymula, R., Siegrist, C. A., Chlibek, R., Zemlickova, H., Vackova, M., Smetana, J., . . . Schuerman L. (2009). Effect of prophylactic paracetamol administration at time of vaccination on febrile reactions and antibody responses in children: Two open-label, randomised controlled trials. *Lancet*, *374*(9698), 1339–50. doi:10.1016/S0140-6736(09)61208-3

Starting solid food. (2012). Retrieved from https://www.healthychildren.org/English/ages-stages/ baby/feeding-nutrition/Pages/Switching-To-Solid-Foods.aspx

Tablizo, M. A., Jacinto, P., Parsley, D., Chen, M. L., Ramanathan, R., & Keens, T. G. (2007). Supine sleeping position does not cause clinical aspiration in neonates in hospital newborn nurseries. *Archives of Pediatric and Adolescence Medicine*, *161*(5), 507–510.

Taddio, A., McMurtry, M., Shah, V., Riddell, R. P., Chamber, C. T., Noel, M., . . . Bleeker, E. V. (2015). Reducing pain during vaccine injections: Clinical practice guideline. *Canadian Medical Association Journal*, *187*(13), 975–982. doi:10.1503/cmaj.150391

Tappin, D., Ecob, R., & Brooke, H. (2005). Bedsharing, roomsharing, and sudden infant death syndrome in Scotland: A case control study. *Journal of Pediatrics*, *147*(1), 32–37.

U.S. Preventive Services Task Force. (2013). Grade definitions. Retrieved from http://www.uspre ventiveservicestaskforce.org/Page/Name/grade-definitions

Vitamin D: On the double. (2015). Retrieved from https://www.healthychildren.org/English/healthy -living/nutrition/Pages/Vitamin-D-On-the-Double.aspx

Wu, C. S., Jew, C. P., & Lu, H. C. (2011). Lasting impacts of prenatal cannabis exposure and the role of endogenous cannabinoids in the developing brain. *Future Neurology*, *6*(4), 459–480.

Zaloshnja, E., Miller, T. R., & Hendrie, D. (2007). Effectiveness of child safety seats vs safety belts for children aged 2 to 3 years. *Archives of Pediatric and Adolescence Medicine*, *161*(1), 65–68.

18

Developmental Care and Optimizing Neurodevelopmental Outcomes in the Preterm and Critically Ill Infant

Susan M. Quinn and Kimberly Knoerlein

Chapter Objectives

1. Review normal brain development and maturation and discuss how prematurity and/or illness and the interactions between the undeveloped brain and the environment can affect brain growth
2. Identify stressful environmental factors in the neonatal intensive care unit (NICU) environment and describe the effects that can cause adverse neurodevelopment in the premature and high-risk infant
3. Identify and examine the goals of evidence-based care practices that are age-appropriate, nontraumatic, and developmentally supportive for the preterm and high-risk infant and their families in the NICU environment
4. Apply knowledge of appropriate education and teaching of developmentally appropriate care that enhances the neurodevelopment of preterm and high-risk infants through evaluation of case studies

BRAIN DEVELOPMENT

Development and maturation of the central nervous system (CNS; brain and spinal cord) is a complex molecular and cellular process beginning early in gestation and continuing throughout infancy. As the CNS develops and matures, it is continuously affected by its interactions with the surrounding environment. Lack of appropriate stimuli and exposure to adverse factors during the embryonic and fetal period and during infancy can alter brain development causing lifelong neurodevelopmental and behavioral consequences. The embryonic period spans 52 to 60 days from fertilization through completion of major organogenesis, with the fetal period occurring at the end of the embryonic period until birth (MacDonald & Seshia, 1997). During embryological and fetal development, the brain is rapidly growing, leading to proliferation and refinement of neuronal pathways (Gudsnuk & Champagne, 2011). These neuronal pathways, or synapses, are the roadways for communication within the CNS. The CNS develops during a series of events that occur in a specific sequence, with each event dependent on the prior event to enable progress to the next stage of development.

The earliest stage of CNS development begins early in gestation, at approximately 17 days. This is when ectoderm, a primitive layer of cells, begins to rapidly divide forming a thickened mass called the *neural plate* in the dorsal section of the embryo. By day 20, the neural plate folds to form the neural tube, which eventually becomes the brain and spinal cord. With successful closure of the neural tube by the middle of the forth to fifth week of gestation, the anterior, or rostral end, of neural tube gives rise to three primary vesicles: the prosencephalon (forebrain), mesencephalon (midbrain), and the rhombencephalon (hindbrain; Schoenwolf, Bleyl, Brauer, Francis-West, & Philippa, 2015). By the fifth week of gestation, the prosencephalon and rhombencephalon each subdivide into two portions converting the three primary brain vesicles into five secondary brain vesicles (Schoenwolf et al., 2015). The prosencephalon divides into the cranial telencephalon (end-brain) and a caudal diencephalon (between-brain) and the rhombencephalon divides into a cranial metencephalon (behind-brain) and caudal myelencephalon (medulla-brain; Schoenwolf et al., 2015). Cavities within each of the brain vesicles then form into the ventricles of the mature brain. The choroid plexus develops from the blood vessels that invade the ventricles from the diencephalon and the myelencephalon. The rostral neural tube, which is contiguous with the myelencephalon, forms the spinal cord. Formation and maturation of the brain's highly complex sulci and gyri, which define the cerebral hemispheres, is not complete until the 35th week of gestation

After closure of the neural tube, the ectoderm begins to differentiate into more specialized cells with a destined fate within the CNS. Once they begin to differentiate, they continue to divide and eventually begin their migration to their final resting place within the brain or spinal cord, forming the peripheral nerves, roots, and ganglion cells of the peripheral nervous system (Scheibel, 1997). Once migration has occurred and the migrating nerves cells have reached their final destination, they begin to mature and develop extensions from their cells bodies; these extensions are called *dendrites* and *axons*. As the dendrites multiply, they provide an increasing surface area of neuronal pathways to and from other neurons (Scheibel, 1997). The larger the number of neuronal connections or pathways, the higher cognitive functioning will be (Scheibel, 1997). The axon will establish connections with other neurons, some adjacent to the cell body of origin and others to neurons in the lower spinal cord, sometimes a distance of up to 5 ft. (Scheibel, 1997). These neuronal connections or synaptic pathways between the neurons allow for the back-and-forth communication that occurs within the CNS. Another important aspect of brain development is the formation of myelin sheaths around the axons. Myelin is a fatty substance surrounding and insulating the axon that allows for nerve impulses to occur 10 to 100 times more rapidly as would occur along a nonmyelinated axon (Scheibel, 1997). Myelination begins early in gestation and continues throughout adolescence. Myelination that continues throughout infancy allows for the infant to meet developmental milestones such as crawling and walking.

The corpus callosum develops late in gestation and will allow for communication between the two cerebral hemispheres. The two hemispheres have differing, but complementary, roles. The left hemisphere is primarily responsible for semantic and computational aspects of language and the right hemisphere is involved in emotional and prosodic features in speech (Scheibel, 1997). The inability of the hemispheres to interact with each other produces speech that can then sound mechanical and flat, without personal warmth and emotion (Scheibel, 1997).

By approximately 5 to 6 weeks gestation, the first synapses begin forming in a fetus's spinal cord; these early neuronal connections permit the fetus to begin to make spontaneous movements. By approximately 8 to 10 weeks gestation, movements of the toes and fingers begin to appear, as well hiccupping, yawning, sucking, swallowing, grasping, and thumb sucking. During the second semester, critical reflexes vital to sustain life begin to appear such as breathing movements and coordinated sucking and swallowing. The brain stem is also responsible for heart rate (HR) and blood pressure and these are mature by the end of the second semester.

Last of all to develop and mature is the cerebral cortex, which is responsible for human conscious experiences, thinking, memories, and feelings. The cerebral cortex, which arises from the prosencephalon, undergoes rapid growth and maturation between 20 and 37 weeks gestation, particularly in the motor and sensorimotor areas. The cortex consists of numerous folds and fissures that are called *gyri* and *sulci*, which allow for greater surface area and subsequently more neurons in the brain, which is associated with higher functioning. The cerebral cortex is responsible for voluntary actions, thinking, remembering, and feeling and only begins functioning at the end of the third trimester. Premature infants show only basic electrical activity in the sensory and primary motor regions of the cortex. These sensory regions within the cortex are involved in perceiving touch, vision, and hearing and develop as a result of fetal interactions with maternal stimuli within the uterus.

The development of the brain is a complex sequential process affected by a range of intrinsic and extrinsic factors (Figure 18.1). Brain development and maturation can be affected by both the absence of appropriate stimuli and by the presence of adverse factors found in the environment; both can alter optimal brain development before and after birth.

BRAIN DEVELOPMENT OF THE PREMATURE AND CRITICALLY ILL INFANT

> *Recent advances have boosted parents' hopes, but uncertainties remain.*
> —J. Groopman, "A Child in Time"

According to Blencowe et al. (2015), more than one in 10 infants are born prematurely each year, or approximately 15 million infants overall. The majority of these premature infants are born between 32 and 37 weeks of gestation, but 1.6 million are born between 28 and 32 weeks gestation and 780,000 are born extremely premature, before 26 weeks gestation. Neonatology over the past 40 years has made tremendous technological, pharmacologic, and care practice advancements, which has allowed for survival of younger and sicker preterm infants, especially the extremely low-gestational-age neonate (ELGAN) live births less than 28 weeks gestation) and extremely low-birth-weight infants (ELBW, < 1,000 g). Survival of these infants

Embryonic Brain Regions		Brain Structures Present in Adult
Forebrain	Telencephalon	Cerebrum (cerebral hemispheres; includes cerebral cortex, white matter, basal nuclei)
Forebrain	Diencephalon	Diencephalon (thalamus, hypothalamus, epithalamus)
Midbrain	Mesencephalon	Midbrain (part of brainstem)
Hindbrain	Metencephalon	Pons (part of brainstem), cerebellum
Hindbrain	Myelencephalon	Medulla oblongata (part of brainstem)

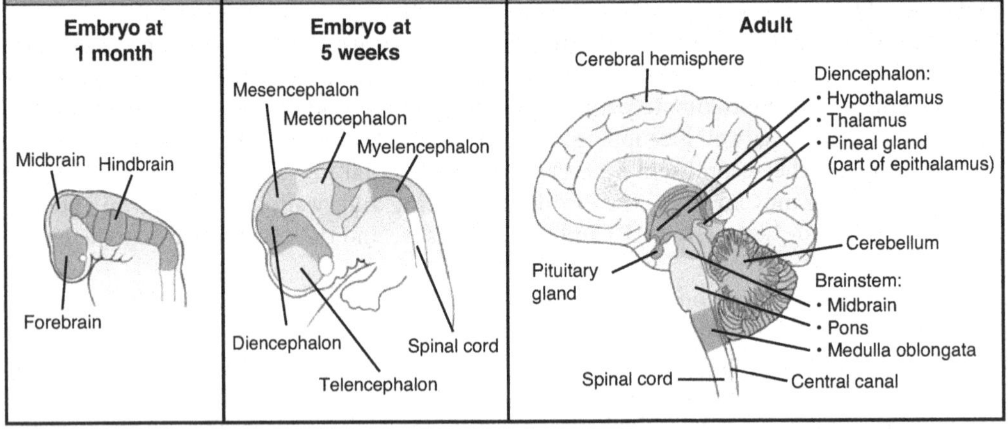

Figure 18.1 Embryonic Brain Development

has increased the uncertainty of the impact of a premature birth on both short- and long-term neurodevelopmental and neurobehavioral outcomes. Prematurity is a known risk factor for neurological impairment (Rosier-van Dunne et al., 2013). According to Spittle and colleagues, it is well known that the period between 20 and 40 weeks gestation is one characterized by rapid vulnerable brain development and growth (Spittle et al., 2014). Infants born prematurely experience an abrupt transition into an environment that is in stark sensory mismatch to their protected in utero environment during a time of extreme vulnerability (McAnulty et al., 2010). Extremely premature and critically ill infants have lengthy stays in the NICU and are developmentally and physiologically unprepared for the many stressful experiences they encounter in this environment (Grunau, Holsti, & Peters, 2006). Infant experiences that both lack appropriate stimuli or cause a stress response could potentially have long-term implications on brain development and growth that have not been fully understood (Jain, 2011).

The environment within the uterus allows for a fetal experience that promotes organized sensory development. The uterine environment allows for stable temperature regulation, optimal nutrition, appropriate neurosensory stimuli, and protection from noxious stimulation. Optimal brain growth and development is largely shaped by early sensory experiences (Webb, Heller, Benson, & Lahav, 2015). A premature birth and hospitalization of an infant in the NICU not only removes the infant from the protection of the uterine environment but also interrupts the important early sensory factors needed for optimal neurodevelopment. Infants hospitalized in the NICU experience continuous exposure to noxious stimuli such as painful procedures, excessive light and noise, and isolation from maternal touch, sound, and smell. Exposure to these adverse and stress-provoking experiences causes physiological instability in the infant. Physiological instability in these premature and high-risk infants can alter optimal brain growth and maturation, which subsequently leads to impaired sensory, cognitive, communicative, and motor sequelae. Obstetrical risk factors can also play a significant role in impairment of brain growth and development during gestation as well. Obstetrical risk factors include chorioamnionitis and premature rupture of membranes (PROM); both have long been associated with brain injury and/or neurodevelopmental impairment (Rosier-van Dunne et al., 2013). Although investigations have been contradictory, impairment in neurodevelopment has also been thought to be associated with intrauterine fetal growth restriction (IUGR) and preeclampsia as well (Rosier-van Dunne et al., 2013).

A preterm birth and hospitalization of an infant constitutes a traumatic life event that has impact on short- and long-term neurobehavioral outcomes (Coughlin, 2014). Research findings suggest a significant proportion of adolescents suffering from traumatic events during infancy have alterations in brain development that have subsequently been found to cause poor long-term cognitive, sensory, communicative, and psychological outcomes (Mahoney et al., 2013). According to Mahoney, Minter, Burch, and Stapel-Wax (2013) cognitive impairment and abnormal brain development are thought to be linked with preterm birth and low birth weight. Infants born prematurely and with low birth weight are at higher risk for disturbances with social interactions, communication, and other psychoaffective disorders in later childhood and adulthood (Mahoney et al., 2013). Early research by Watson (2013) also pointed toward an increased risk of attention deficit hyperactivity disorder (ADHD) in school-aged children who were born prematurely. It is important that the neonatal nurse practitioner understands how the experiences of the fetus and/or infant within its environment affect brain development and growth. This is essential to providing the optimal environment and care practices that will optimize neurodevelopmental outcomes in the preterm and high-risk infant.

Florence Nightingale's publication, *Notes on Nursing*, states, "it may be a strange principle to enunciate as the very first requirement in a hospital is that it should do the sick no harm" (Nightingale, 1863). Unfortunately, hundreds of years later, patients are exposed, sometimes unknowingly, to negligence and harmed more often than not during their hospitalization (Coughlin, 2014). Premature and high-risk infants have very different experiences from their term, healthy infant counterparts. These experiences combined with genetics all play a part in neurodevelopment. Genes are responsible for the overall wiring and formation of the connections among the different brain regions, whereas the environment and repeated experiences are responsible for the fine-tuning and/or pruning of these connections. Noxious stimuli experienced by the fetus and/or the preterm and critically ill infant cause a stress response with disruption development and maturation (fine-tuning and pruning) of the brain architecture and function. By 10 weeks of gestation, the fetus is producing an average of 250,000 neurons per minute with the majority of brain development occurring in the brain stem, cerebellum, and subcortex (Coughlin, 2014). These important structures play critical roles in neurobehavioral and cognitive development throughout an individual's lifetime. Recent studies have indicated that lengthily hospitalizations and stressful experiences during critical stages of brain development can alter gene expression and do this without altering gene sequence. When gene expression is altered without altering the DNA gene sequence of cells, it is called *epigenetic* (Jablonka & Lamb, 2002). Epigenetics is a field of study that examines environmental factors and how they affect gene expression without necessarily causing changes to the DNA sequence of a cell. Epigenetic effects can alter normal brain development and growth.

The survival rate of preterm infants now exceeds 85% with severe neurodevelopmental and neurosensory deficits occurring in 5% to 15% of these survivors (Pickler et al., 2010). Poor neurobehavioral and cognitive outcomes are proportional with gestational age and birth weight, which means the more premature and smaller an infant, the greater chance that he or she will suffer poorer outcomes. A meta-analysis by Watson (2010) revealed 15% of infants with gestational ages between 22 and 27 weeks developed cerebral palsy (CP), whereas only 6% of those born between 32 and 36 weeks, and 0.1% of those born full-term developed CP. According to Pickler and associates (2010), neurodysfunctions, such as learning disorders and behavioral problems, occur in as many as 50% to 70% of children born prematurely. Although the care and technology provided in the NICU is increasing survival of premature and critically ill infants, the environment they experience is not necessarily compatible with optimal brain development and growth. Watson (2010) also found that gestational age and birth weight correlated significantly with poor scores on intelligence tests of cognitive abilities in school-aged children. Adverse events leading to increased morbidity and mortality in this population are a great burden on not only the child and his or her family but on society as well. Preterm birth is one of the most costly and devastating of all health events, with nearly $18 billion spent yearly on initial hospitalization alone with subsequent additional costs added related to later adverse neurobehavioral and cognitive outcomes (Watson, 2010).

The ability of the fetus to experience maternal stimuli, such as her voice and smell, is critical in programming the infant's short- and long-term emotional, psychosocial, and cognitive development. Infants born prematurely miss the necessary exposure to the mother's voice, smell, and tactile stimulation that is so important for normal development and maturation of the neuronal pathways that allow for proper adjustment to the environment after birth. One of the first acoustic sounds a fetus is exposed to is the sound of his or her mother's voice and heartbeat. Webb and colleagues (2015) provide evidence that suggests prenatal exposure to the sounds of the maternal voice and heartbeat paves the way for the development of neuronal pathways in the brain that allow for development of skills for hearing and language. Webb et al. (2015) also suggest that there is evidence that the low-frequency muffled maternal heartbeat in utero provides the fetus with an important rhythmic experience that likely establishes the neuronal pathways for auditory entrainment and synchrony skills necessary for vocal, gestural, and gaze communication. The interruption of these fetal sensory experiences within the uterine environment interferes with optimal neurosensory development and infant–mother attachment and bonding after birth. Webb et al. (2015) theorized that the experience-dependent plasticity of the preterm infant's brain, specifically within the auditory cortex when exposed to maternal sounds, could actually prepare and shape the brain for hearing and learning development after birth. It would therefore be crucial to develop environments within the NICU that allow early maternal involvement in their infant's care so that the infant may experience the mother's heartbeat, voice, and touch, which in turn would continue neurosensory maturation and fine-tuning.

Premature and critically ill infants are vulnerable to forming lower quality attachments to their caregivers; this is a result of disruption of the bonding experience with the mother during prenatal and postnatal development (Sullivan, Perry, Sloan, Kleinhaus, & Burtchen, 2011). After birth, the infant is attracted to the mother's voice and smell, including the scent of amniotic fluid, as a result of their experiences in the uterus. This attachment begins during the last trimester of pregnancy, when olfactory and auditory systems are developing (Sullivan et al., 2011). Preterm and critically ill infants hospitalized in a NICU experience sounds in the environment that deviate from those that healthy term infants experience, possibly interfering with optimal hearing and language development. The maternal voice, sound of her heartbeat, her movement, and smell during gestation allow for a smoother transition to life after birth, which is filled with new sights, sounds, textures, and temperatures for the newborn. The infant exposed in utero to the mother's voice and smell can be soothed by the familiar voice of the mother after birth and breastfeeding is facilitated because of the familiar odor of the mother, which the infant can recognize. The infant's responses to mother's voice and odor also facilitate maternal caregiving allowing for the formation of a trusting relationship between the mother and her infant. Maternal sounds during pregnancy, such as laughing, heartbeat, speech and sounds of breathing, and maternal movement allow the fetus to experience tactile and vestibular stimulation and relate it to the sound and movement from the musculature used to make the sounds after birth. The buffered nature of the uterus allows for the avoidance of overstimulation of sensory input during fetal development. It also allows for the fetus to experience sensory import in an ordered fashion, tactile and vestibular before visual and auditory. Infants born prematurely are not buffered from the noxious environmental stimulus and tactile, vestibular, visual, auditory, and olfactory sensory input occur in an asynchronous manner.

Care practices that promote optimal neurosensory development are challenging within the NICU environment. The premature infant not only misses this period of attachment in utero but also experiences long periods of separation from his or her mother after birth. Noxious stimuli, such as light and noise disrupt maternal–infant bonding, making the formation of a trusting attachment difficult. The exposure to increased sound and light while in the NICU also produces a wide range of physiological instability, which includes increased apnea and bradycardia, changes in blood pressure, and cerebral blood flow (Santos de Carvalho Bonan, da Costa Pimentel Filho, Tristao, Lacerda de Jesus, & Junior, 2014). The visual system is the last system to develop and is not mature and functional until term. Therefore, the visual system of the preterm infant develops and matures while the infant is in the NICU and not prepared for the external visual stimuli, putting him or her at high risk for poor neurosensory and visual development (Graven, 2011). Exposure to artificial lighting not only interferes with visual development but also has been found to increase the incidence of strabismus and can cause changes in circadian rhythm (Graven, 2011). Premature and critically ill infants in the NICU environment are exposed to sounds levels that exceed what they would experience in utero. The fetus is exposed to sound intensity levels of 40 to 60 dB and noise within the NICU can reach 70 to 80 dB (Santos de Carvalho Bonan et al., 2014). These adverse experiences to excessive light and noise put the premature infant at risk for suboptimal visual, hearing, and language development.

The immaturity of the premature infants CNS decreases their autonomic capabilities and subsequently decreases their ability to deal with environmental stimulation such as excessive noise and light. Premature infants inability to autoregulate leaves them unable to limit or select the unpredictable stimuli that they are exposed to, putting these infants at higher risk for abnormal brain development and function. Long-term morbidities resulting from hospitalization in the NICU are not only linked to poor neurodevelopment and psychological outcomes but also to cardiovascular and metabolic complications as well (Coughlin, 2014).

Optimal social and emotional development in infants depends on a nurturing environment and positive attachments to their caregiver. According to Coughlin (2014), the developing brain is a living structure that requires positive stimulation through parental and caregiver interaction, nurturance, and attachment. These positive experiences nurture brain growth and development. The infant's early positive life experiences support and reinforce his or her security, connectedness, attachment, self-regulation, and love later in life (Esch & Stefano, 2011). The first stage of Erik Erikson's stages of psychosocial development is trust versus mistrust. For an infant to develop trust he or she must form an attachment with his or her caregivers, which include bidirectional communication, compassion, consistency, and competence with each infant encounter (Coughlin, 2014).

HISTORY AND ONGOING PROGRESS OF DEVELOPMENTAL CARE FOR PRETERM AND CRITICALLY ILL INFANTS

Caregivers in the 1970s became aware of a possible relationship between neurodevelopment in the premature and critically ill infant and the NICU environment (Als & Brazelton, 1974). In the 1970s, work by Als began to show that the infant was a separate being from his or her environment and could potentially interact with his or her caregivers and physical environment (Als & Brazelton, 1974; Als, Tronick, Lester, & Brazelton, 1977). Developmental care was introduced in the 1980s and 1990s with the aim to minimize the adverse effects experienced in the NICU environment by the premature and ill infant. The work by Als led to the development of the Neonatal Individualized Developmental Care and Assessment Program (NIDCAP; Montirosso et al., 2012). This program was designed by Als to try to minimize the stress premature infants experienced during their time in the NICU. This was done by utilizing observations of the infant before, during, and after caregiving interactions and then providing individualized care that controlled and decreased stressful stimulation for that individual infant. Care practices included clustering of care, positioning and swaddling of the infants.

INFANT SELF-REGULATION

During development and growth of the CNS, neuronal pathways are created between the lower emotional centers of the brain and the higher cognitive centers in the cortex; proper functioning and communication of these pathways is the basis for the infant to self-regulate (Watson, 2010). Self-regulation is the infant's ability to coordinate and organize his or her motor activity, levels of arousal, and attention. Self-regulation is important for learning, planning, decision making, performing complex actions, and resisting temptation later in life (Watson, 2010). The importance of the infant's ability to self-regulate is seen in Als's Synactive Theory of Infant Development, which provides a framework for understanding the behavior of preterm infants. The framework groups the preterm infant's behavior into five subgroups: motor, autonomic, states, attention/interaction, and self-regulatory. The self-regulatory subgroup assesses the infant's ability to successfully achieve and maintain a balance of the other four subsystems. Gibbins, Hoath, Coughlin, Gibbins, and Franck (2008) later reformed Als's theoretical framework with the development of the Universe of Developmental Care Model. Gibbins and colleagues (2008) provide a conceptual model in which the premature infant and the environment are dependent on each other for all caregiving practices (Gibbins et al., 2008). The environment and the experiences of the infant affect the development of the premature brain. These theoretical models are designed to understand and assess each individual infant and his or her specific needs within his or her own environment. Use of these care practices within the NICU environment has been found to lead to better neurodevelopment and neurobehavioral outcomes. Neonatal nurse practitioners implementing theoretical frameworks and conceptual models can then provide evidence-based care for these vulnerable infants in the NICU environment that can best optimize neurodevelopmental outcomes. Implementing evidence-based practices allows for alignment with The Joint Commission, which states that all health care professionals provide age-specific care across the life span. The National Association for Neonatal Nurses published guidelines for age-appropriate care in 2011. The guidelines were developed for practitioners to assist them in providing consistent evidence-based age-appropriate care to the premature and critically ill, hospitalized infant (Coughlin, 2011). The guidelines define and recommend incorporation into practice of the following five core measures: protected sleep, pain and stress assessment and management, attention to age-appropriate activities, family-centered care (FCC), and the healing environment. Understanding and incorporating these core measures into practice will allow practitioners to provide the highest quality of care for infants hospitalized in the NICU (Coughlin, 2011). These five core measures will be described in more detail later in the chapter.

It is critical to look beyond the technical and pharmacological advances that have occurred in the NICU and to focus on the interactions and experiences the infant and parent have within the NICU. Allowing parental involvement in the infant's care, altering care and the environment to suit the infants' needs, and protecting the infant from painful and/or noxious stimuli will lead to better autonomic stability at discharge and improved neurodevelopment outcomes later in life. Care practices should focus on the individual needs of the infant and his or her family and must be developmentally age-appropriate, nontraumatic, and compliant with FCC for this vulnerable population. Studies have shown parental involvement within the NICU, including the ability to room-in, frequency and duration of kangaroo care, and nursing care, can decrease infant energy expenditure and promote autonomic stability. Developmental care includes clustering of care, decreased and appropriately timed sensory stimulation, nonnutritive sucking, kangaroo care, and massage; these care practices attempt to allow the infant to achieve calm alert states (Watson, 2010). Kangaroo care has been shown to be beneficial to both the premature infant and his or her mother by decreasing the infant's physiologic responses to painful and noxious stimuli and increasing maternal milk production. The ability of the infant to achieve a calm alert state optimizes the infant's ability to self-regulate his or her HR rhythms and sleep/wake cycles, leading to overall improved physiological stability and nutrition, which improve neurodevelopment and cognitive outcomes (Watson, 2010). Premature and critically ill infants spend more time in states that are not optimal and supportive for learning and development of self-regulation and growing evidence reveals that self-regulation in premature infants is impaired (Clark, Woodward, Horwood, & Moor, 2008). Premature infants spend more time in sleep and agitated states as a result of their experiences with care practices and interactions within their surrounding environment. Their responses to many interactions, such as averting their gaze and thrusting out their hands, do not allow for successful experiences with their caregivers. When infants are able to have successful experiences with their caregivers, learning occurs. These adverse experiences impair the caregiver's ability to read the infant's cues correctly and respond appropriately, quickly, and consistently to needs of the infant (Watson, 2010). When these interactions are unsuccessful and learning does not occur, brain development is impaired and subsequent neurobehavioral and cognitive impairments can occur later in life.

Beginning in the 1970s, developmental care was implemented and practiced, care practices varied and were difficult to identify and measure. Over a decade later, care practices continued to vary and little was known about how developmental care provided related to preterm and critically ill infants' neurodevelopment. Therefore, core measures for developmentally supportive care in NICU were recently developed to provide an evidence-based framework that would allow care practices to be universally defined and allow for comparative analysis of these practices, which would then allow for clinical outcomes to be better measured across health care organizations (Coughlin, Gibbins, & Hoath, 2009). An infant's brain shows great placidity and resilience during brain development, which can have implications for the application of early interventions to ameliorate some of the poorer outcomes that result from these nonoptimal experiences (Mahoney et al., 2013). Care of the infants in the NICU environment needs to focus on recognition of these high-risk infants development of age-appropriate goals and supportive nontraumatic care that will improve short- and long-term neurodevelopmental outcomes in this vulnerable population.

Modification of care practices and the environment should focus on decreasing stressful, traumatic, and nonsupportive experiences and promote developmentally age-appropriate and evidence-based care that will promote optimal neurodevelopment and neurobehavioral outcomes. Incorporating into practice developmentally age-appropriate nontraumatic supportive care will promote optimal brain growth and maturation in the infant. Offering education, support, and guidance to the caregiver will promote self-efficacy in the caregivers and promote the development of a compassionate and trusting attachment. According to Kenner (2012), it is important that the care of these infants and families be synchronized; that medical, nursing, and developmental care in the NICU be blended, consistently implemented, and evidence-based to allow for care that enhances outcomes for these infants. A major goal of developmentally age-appropriate supportive care is to involve parents in their infant's care early. Allowing parents to become an active participant in their infant's care improves their ability to become more sensitive to the unique signals produced by their infant. The mother is a familiar voice, touch, and smell to the infant, which can help negate the negative stimuli that surround the infant in the NICU environment.

Case 18.1

Veronica was delivered at 29 3/7 weeks gestation, with a birth weight of 1.345 kg, to a 26-year-old gravida 1, para 0 now 1 mother whose prenatal labs were remarkable for a vaginal and urine culture positive for group B *Streptococcus* (GBS), for which she received adequate intrapartum antibiotic treatment. The mother presented in preterm labor with evidence of chorioamnionitis with maternal fever and fetal tachycardia. Veronica delivered precipitously via vaginal delivery with Apgar scores of 3 and 9, at 1 minute and 5 minutes, respectively. Veronica was transported and admitted to the neonatal intensive care unit (NICU), where she was intubated for respiratory distress syndrome with hypoxemia and poor ventilation. She received premedication (rapid sequence intubation), which included atropine, fentanyl, and rocuronium prior to placement of her endotracheal tube. She was given a dose of surfactant via her endotracheal tube and placed on a ventilator. She received sucrose and a pacifier for nonnutritive sucking during the placement of a peripheral intravenous catheter. Intravenous fluids were started. As part of an evaluation to rule out a possible infection, blood cultures and a complete blood count (CBC) were drawn via a venous puncture. She was treated with a 48-hour course of ampicillin and gentamicin. Veronica weaned from her respiratory support and was extubated to nasal continuous positive airway pressure with minimal oxygen requirements by 24 hours of age. She was started on enteral trophic feedings of maternal breast milk via nasogastric tube. She was given a prophylactic course of indomethacin because of her risk for intraventricular hemorrhage and patent ductus arteriosus. Caffeine was started prophylactically because of gestational age and the risk for apnea of prematurity. The mother and father visited their newborn in the NICU shortly after birth and mother was able to provide kangaroo care by 12 hours of age. She plans to pump and provide breast milk for Veronica. The parents noted that sometimes Veronica, when being held, responded by thrusting her hands out, covering her face, and averting her gaze. The advanced practice registered nurse explained that these responses are most likely caused by stressful

(continued)

Case 18.1 *(continued)*

stimuli in the environment that the infant cannot control. She encouraged them to minimize the stress the infant was experiencing by clustering her care, and providing proper positioning and swaddling, which would help decrease environmental stimuli that Veronica was exposed to. Veronica's providers and caregivers utilized observations of Veronica before, during, and after care to understand Veronica's cues and needs and together created an individualized care plan for Veronica.

1. *As the nurse practitioner you explain to the bedside nurse that infants exposed repeatedly to which of the following stressful stimuli in the NICU could cause adverse neurodevelopmental outcomes? (Select all that apply)*

   A. Painful procedures
   B. Maternal separation
   C. Loud noises
   D. All of the above

   ANSWER: D. *All the above stimuli, including maternal separation, can cause a stress response in the premature infant, leading to poor neurodevelopmental outcomes.*

2. *As a neonatal nurse practitioner you understand that infants born prematurely experience maternal separation thereby missing important periods of attachment that occur in utero that increase the risk for suboptimal development of which of the following? (Select all that apply)*

   A. Vision
   B. Hearing
   C. Language
   D. Smell

   ANSWER: A, B, and C. *The ability of the fetus to experience maternal stimuli, which includes auditory, vestibular, and olfactory stimulation, is critical in programming the infant's short- and long-term emotional, psychosocial, and cognitive development.*

3. *The Neonatal Individualized Developmental Care and Assessment Program (NIDCAP) was developed by Heidi Als with the goal to: (Select all that apply)*

   A. Create an environment and individualized care plan for the hospitalized infant to decrease the amount of stressful stimuli the infant experiences
   B. Create an environment and individualized care plan for the parents of infants admitted to the NICU
   C. Create an environment and individualized care plan that improves the work-flow of the providers
   D. All of the above

   ANSWER: A. *This program was designed by Als to try to minimize the stress premature infants experienced during their time in the NICU. Infant experiences that both lack appropriate stimuli or cause a stress response could potentially have long-term implications on brain development and growth that have not been fully understood.*

(continued)

Case 18.1 (continued)

4. What types of stimuli are important during gestation for optimal sensory development in utero?

A. Maternal heartbeat, voice, smell, and movement

B. Maternal touch, voice, movement, and sleep cycles

C. Maternal smell, voice, heartbeat, and mood

D. Maternal heartbeat, voice, mood, and sleep cycles

ANSWER: D. *Maternal heartbeat, her voice, mood, and sleep cycles all contribute, in an organized manner, an environment that allows for optimal sensory development in the fetus.*

5. As a neonatal nurse practitioner you understand that which of the following care practices can help decrease energy expenditure and promote autonomic stability, leading to improved neurodevelopment? (Select all that apply)

A. Parental involvement in infant's care

B. Increased frequency and duration of kangaroo care

C. Non-nutritive sucking

D. All of the above

ANSWER: D. *These care practices attempt to allow the infant to achieve calm alert states that allow for decreased energy expenditure and promote autonomic stability.*

6. Which of the following care practices would help to decrease stressful stimuli in the NICU environment and promote optimal neurodevelopmental outcomes in the preterm/high-risk infant? (Select all that apply)

A. Offer nonpharmacological and pharmacological support to the infant during necessary noxious procedures

B. Have parents leave the nursery while painful procedures are being performed

C. Avoid offering nonnutritive sucking and sucrose to prevent the infant from relating sucking to a painful procedure in the future

D. Avoid the use of narcotics to avoid addiction

ANSWER: A. *By offering both nonpharmacological and pharmacological support during painful procedures these will help decrease evoking the stress response and promote optimal neurodevelopmental outcomes.*

7. As a neonatal nurse practitioner you admit a 24-week-gestation infant into the NICU who is in respiratory failure and requires intubation, you ask for premedication (rapid sequence intubation/RSI) prior to intubation and understand that RSI is used for intubation for which of the following reasons? (Select all that apply)

A. To quickly and effectively perform laryngoscopy and tracheal intubation thereby decreasing stressful stimuli such as pain

B. Identifying other stressful procedures that a premature and/or high-risk infant may experience

(continued)

Case 18.1 (continued)

C. To make the parents feel better about their infant undergoing a painful procedure
D. Improve oxygenation

ANSWER: A. *By quickly and effectively preforming intubation, this will decrease stressful stimuli such as pain and hypoxia and avoid the stress response, which has been showed to place infants at high risk for poor neurodevelopmental outcomes.*

8. *As a neonatal nurse practitioner you understand that core measures for developmentally age-appropriate nontraumatic care in the NICU were developed to provide which of the following? (Select all that apply)*

   A. Care practices that can be universally defined
   B. Care practices where comparative analysis can be performed
   C. Clinical outcomes that can be better measured across health care organizations
   D. All of the above

   ANSWER: D. *Understanding and incorporating these core measures into practice will allow practitioners to provide the highest quality of care that is evidence based for infants hospitalized in the NICU.*

9. *As a neonatal nurse practitioner you understand that optimal sleep–wake cycles can improve neurodevelopmental outcomes. Which of the following appropriate care practices would support optimal sleep–wake cycles in the premature infant? (Select all that apply)*

   A. Reduce stresses in the NICU environment such as excessive noise and light
   B. Promote clustering of care
   C. Parental education on how to interpret their infant's cues
   D. All of the above

   ANSWER: D. *These care practices allow the infant to develop an appropriate sleep-wake cycle that can help improve neurodevelopmental outcomes.*

10. *As a neonatal nurse practitioner you are prenatally consulting a mother who is at 24 weeks gestation and refuses to follow medical advice. You are concerned because you know that development that occurs in utero provides the best environment for optimal neurodevelopment because of which of the following? (Select all that apply)*

    A. Stable temperature regulation
    B. Appropriate stimuli that promote organized sensory development
    C. Protection from noxious stimulation such as pain, noise, and light
    D. Appropriate nutrition for growth

    ANSWER: A, B, and D. *In allowing the fetus to develop in utero provides stable temperature regulation, appropriate stimuli to promote organized sensory development, and provides the appropriate nutrients for growth and developments. Development outside the uterus prematurely can cause excessive unorganized sensory stimulation, poor temperature regulation, and inadequate nutrients for growth to occur, putting the infant at risk for poor neurodevelopmental outcomes.*

LATE PRETERM INFANT AND NEURODEVELOPMENT

The American Academy of Pediatrics (AAP), American College of Obstetricians and Gynecologists (ACOG), and National Center for Health Statistics (NCHS) define *late preterm infants* as those who are born between the gestational ages of 34 weeks and 36 weeks and 6 days (Barfield & Lee, 2016; Kugelman & Colin, 2013). Recently, the term *late-term* has replaced *near term* to describe this group of infants, as *near term* incorrectly implies that these infants are "almost term" and only require routine care (Barfield & Lee, 2016). Since 1990, the late preterm birth rate has risen increasing from 10.6% in 1990 to 12.8% of all live births in 2006 (Barfield & Lee, 2016). Late preterm births now consist of approximately 74% of all preterm births within the United States (Barfield & Lee, 2016; Kugelman & Colin, 2013; Woythaler, McCormick, & Smith, 2011). The overall increase in preterm birth rates from 1990 to 2006 was primarily caused by an increase in this subgroup of late preterm births (Barfield & Lee, 2016). These late preterm infants often have been perceived as infants who are at similar risk for morbidity and mortality as term infants. This is concerning given that recent studies have shown late preterm infants are more vulnerable to poor neurodevelopmental outcomes than their term counterparts (Barfield & Lee, 2016; Kugelman & Colin, 2013; Woythaler et al., 2011). The last trimester of pregnancy is a critical period for growth and development of the fetal brain. Studies have shown that the brain weight at 34 weeks is only 65% of that of a term brain and the external surface has fewer sulci (Barfield & Lee, 2016; Kugelman & Colin, 2013). Although thought to have similar risks as term infants, there is growing evidence to suggest that these infants are more vulnerable to brain injury than previously appreciated (Kugelman & Colin, 2013). During in utero growth, the brain of the fetus continues to undergo significant growth and development between 34 and 36 weeks gestation. As with other infants born before 34 weeks gestation, late preterm infants can be exposed to stressful stimuli during times of extreme vulnerability. Factors, such as excessive light and noise, painful stimuli, and alteration in circadian rhythms, can alter development of the late preterm brain. Woythaler and colleagues (2011) concluded that late preterm infants have poorer neurodevelopmental outcomes than term infants and had increased odds to have mental and/or physical developmental delays most likely resulting from brain immaturity and its vulnerability to injury; their study also suggests that late preterm infants have worse academic performance at school age and require special education more frequently than infants born at term (Woythaler et al., 2011). In one study by Morse, Zheng, and Roth (2009), children who were born before 36 weeks and 6 days gestation had an increased risk for developmental delays and school-related problems, such as retention and suspension issues in kindergarten, and were also less likely to finish high school and college (Morse et al., 2009). Studies have shown that a late preterm infant has a threefold higher mortality rate compared with term infants (7.7 vs. 2.5 per 1,000 live births; Morse et al., 2009).

Late preterm infants are at higher risk for postnatal complications such as feeding difficulties, hypoglycemia, temperature instability, apnea, respiratory distress, and hyperbilirubinemia (Barfield & Lee, 2016; Kugelman & Colin, 2013). At the same serum bilirubin concentrations, the late preterm infant is at higher risk for brain injury and kernicterus than term infants because of the immaturity of the blood–brain barrier, lower circulating bilirubin-binding albumin concentrations, and higher risk for concurrent illnesses (Barfield & Lee, 2016). Maternal complications, such as chorioamnionitis, PROM, preeclampsia, diabetes, and maternal tobacco use, are also found to be more common in the late preterm infant (Kugelman & Colin, 2013). These factors put the late preterm infant at higher risk of adverse experiences that could alter both short- and long-term neurodevelopmental and behavioral outcomes. Outcomes include poor attachment to caregivers; increased risk of CP;

intellectual disorders; and disorders of psychological development, behavior, and emotions later in life. These late preterm infants are born during a critical period of brain development and growth and cannot be treated as their term infant counterparts.

One of the key factors in decreasing poor neurodevelopmental outcomes associated with late preterm births is prevention. The ACOG now recommends that induced vaginal and planned cesarean deliveries do not occur before 39 weeks gestation unless medically indicated. Identification of these high-risk infants and implementation of management strategies to provide developmentally age-appropriate and supportive care should be an integral part of the medical management. These infants may be at higher risk for maternal tobacco smoke exposure, nonsupine sleep positioning, and lack of breastfeeding (Barfield & Lee, 2016). Caregivers of these infants need ongoing education regarding their infant's vulnerabilities and the importance of an optimal environment to allow for care practices and interactions that will promote the development of a trusting and compassionate relationship that will promote optimal brain development.

Case 18.2

Sammy is a 1.625-kg, small-for-gestational-age (SGA), 35-week-gestation infant born after induction of labor for premature, prolonged rupture of membranes (PPROM), mild pregnancy-induced hypertension (PIH), and maternal fever. Sammy was delivered via an uncomplicated vaginal delivery to a 32-year-old, gravida 2, para 1 now 2. Prenatal labs were remarkable for GBS positive, O negative/antibody positive (received Rhogam at 28 weeks), all other prenatal labs unremarkable. The mother used tobacco throughout the pregnancy; she denied any alcohol or illicit drug use. History was significant for type 2 diabetes, controlled with oral hypoglycemic and diet. The mother was admitted for premature prolonged rupture of membranes (PPROM). She was noted to have increasing blood pressure and was diagnosed with mild preeclampsia. As a result of PPROM, there were plans for induction and, at the start of the induction, she was noted to be febrile and there was fetal tachycardia. She received adequate group B *Streptococcus* (GBS) prophylactic antibiotic coverage prior to delivery. Labor and delivery were uncomplicated. Sammy was born at 35 weeks gestation with Apgar scores of 8 and 9 (off for tone and color) and 1 and 5 minutes, respectively. Resuscitation included drying, stimulation, and bulb suctioning. Sammy's birth weight was 2.050 kg, he had a head circumference of 29 cm, and length of 41cm. Infant had skin-to-skin contact with his mom and was then admitted to a single-room neonatal intensive care unit (NICU), initially stabilized on an open warmer, and placed in an open crib after 48 hours of life.

Initial blood glucose was 9. A peripheral intravenous (IV) line was placed, dextrose bolus and maintenance fluids were started with repeat blood glucose of 52. A septic workup was done, blood cultures and complete blood count were drawn, and antibiotics were started. His septic workup was negative after 48 hours. Enteral feedings were initiated after birth. The mother pumped and Sammy was started on maternal breast milk (MBM), and was ad lib breastfeeding at time of discharge. At time of discharge, the mother continued to use tobacco daily, refusing any counseling for tobacco-use cessation.

Family involvement in Sammy's care was encouraged. The mother became concerned that Sammy was often sleeping and not waking for feedings. It was noted by the

(continued)

Case 18.2 (*continued*)

nursing staff that when the mother was holding the infant, she would become frustrated because he would not respond and interact with her consistently. She says to the neonatal advanced practice nurse (APN), "Sammy is just not the same as my 2-year-old when he was born." The mother stated she was concerned regarding Sammy's breastfeeding attempts; he seemed especially sleepy after only several minutes of feeding. She was also concerned about his spitting, especially after breastfeeding, and she cannot understand why Sammy cannot lie prone after feeding. She states that she placed her 2-year-old on his stomach when he was an infant and he did fine. Parents were taught the importance of following the APA recommendations for safe sleep and supine positioning for Sammy and the importance of tummy time with parental supervision at home.

There was limited parent visitation during the week because of family obligations at home; on weekends the family, along with the 2-year-old, would visit and stay all weekend. The mother noted that feedings went better on the weekday evening visits than during the weekend.

At 38 weeks adjusted age, Sammy was ready for discharge home. A family practitioner was identified as his primary care provider (PCP). The neonatal APN called and updated the PCP prior to discharge. Visiting nurse services were arranged for the first week of discharge. Hepatitis B was given, and hearing test and congenital heart screening were done. Education and teaching were done with the family.

1. **As the nurse practitioner getting ready to discharge an infant born at 35 weeks gestation, now with a postmenstrual age of 44 weeks, what indications would prompt you to recommend early intervention for this infant? (Select all that apply)**

   A. Born at 35 weeks gestation experiencing a respiratory course complicated by meconium aspiration syndrome and long-term intubation
   B. Bilateral grade III hemorrhages with subsequent posthemorrhagic hydrocephalus
   C. Hyperbilirubinemia requiring 5 days of phototherapy
   D. All of the above

   ANSWER: D. *All the above factors put an infant at high risk for impaired neurodevelopment and these infants would benefit from early intervention.*

2. **The neonatal nurse practitioner can help caregivers develop a trusting attachment with their preterm infant hospitalized in the NICU by encouraging which of the following care practices? (Select all that apply)**

   A. Early family involvement with their infant's care
   B. Kangaroo care
   C. Education on how best to decrease stressful stimulation and allowing for protected sleep times
   D. Education on how to best interpret their infant's cues

   ANSWER: All of the above. *Skin-to-skin contact (kangaroo care) is an intervention that can promote mother–infant attachment and bonding, allowing for the development of a trusting relationship that can enhance neurodevelopment. Stressful events that the infant*

(continued)

Case 18.2 (continued)

experiences can alter neurodevelopment. Educating parents in ways that will improve neurodevelopment outcomes is important and can increase parental confidence in their ability to provide care that is done in the least stressful manner.

3. **Late preterm infants are born between which of the following gestational ages?**

   A. 34–38 6/7 weeks gestation
   B. 23–28 6/7 weeks gestation
   C. 34–36 6/7 weeks gestation
   D. 32–35 6/7 weeks gestation

   ANSWER: C. *The definition of a late preterm infant is 34 to 36 6/7 weeks; these infants are physiologically and metabolically less mature than infants born at term.*

4. **The neonatal nurse practitioner is educating parents regarding the American Academy of Pediatrics (AAP) recommendations for safe sleep practices, what important practices should she include?**

   A. Breastfeeding should be encouraged
   B. Infants should be immunized
   C. Infant should be placed supine for sleep
   D. All of the above

   ANSWER: D. *Educating parents regarding safe sleep practices encourages practices that reduce the risk for sudden infant death syndrome (SIDS). "Tummy time" is playtime and should be practiced when the infant is awake and only when someone is watching him or her.*

5. **The neonatal nurse practitioner caring for a late preterm infant should be aware of which of the following possible outcomes? (Select all that apply)**

   A. Poor neurodevelopmental and behavioral outcomes
   B. Developmental disabilities and school delays
   C. Improved breastfeeding and safe sleeping practices
   D. Increased risk for cerebral palsy

   ANSWER: A, B, and D. *Late preterm infants are physiologically and metabolically less mature than infants born at term, putting them at higher risk for these factors than term infants.*

6. **The neonatal nurse practitioner should be aware that infants born before 36 weeks and 6 days gestation are at greater risk for which of the following complications after birth?**

   A. Hypothermia
   B. Hypoglycemia
   C. Hyperbilirubinemia
   D. All of the above

(continued)

Case 18.2 (continued)

ANSWER: D. *Late preterm infants are physiologically and metabolically less mature than infants born at term, putting them at higher risk for these factors than term infants.*

7. **The change in terminology from near term infant to late preterm infant was done because:**
   A. They are often the same size and weight as term infants
   B. *Near term* incorrectly implies that these infants are almost term and require normal routine care
   C. To prevent confusion in the parents
   D. Only late preterm infants need to follow the AAP recommendations for safe sleeping practices

   ANSWER: B. *Near term implies that infants are physiologically and metabolically mature as a term infant. Instead, these infants are more like a premature infant who is physiologically and metabolically immature and at risk for such factors such as hypothermia, hypoglycemia, and hyperbilirubinemia.*

8. **The neonatal nurse practitioner should understand which care practices decrease stressful stimuli and promote optimal neurodevelopmental outcomes in the late preterm infant include?**
   A. Offering nonpharmacological and pharmacological support during necessary noxious procedures
   B. Have parents leave the nursery during when painful procedures are being performed
   C. Avoid offering nonnutritive sucking and sucrose so that the infant does not relate sucking and sucrose to painful procedures in the future
   D. Avoid narcotics during painful procedures to avoid respiratory depression

   ANSWER: A. *Painful procedures produce the stress response in premature and high-risk infants, putting the infant at risk for impaired neurodevelopmental outcomes.*

9. **What type of stimulation would the neonatal nurse practitioner encourage the parents to provide for their medically stable infant with a gestational age of 35 weeks? (Select all that apply)**
   A. Massage
   B. Skin-to-skin contact
   C. Gentle touch
   D. Vigorous stimulation during a feeding

   ANSWER: A, B, and C. *Vigorous stimulation, especially during a feeding in a preterm and high-risk infant, is considered stressful stimuli and can induce the stress response in these infants putting them at risk for poor neurodevelopmental outcomes.*

10. **What care practices would the neonatal nurse practitioner include in his or her management of a premature or ill infant that will help minimize parental stress? (Select all that apply)**

(continued)

Case 18.2 (continued)

A. Encourage early parental contact and participation in infant's care
B. Provide honest and open communication between the parents and professionals
C. Allow unlimited parent presence
D. Avoid kangaroo care while an infant is on respiratory support

ANSWER: A, B, and C. *These factors, early parental contact and participation in infant's care, open communication among providers and families, and unlimited parental presence, will promote the development of a trusting and compassionate relationship that will promote optimal brain development.*

HYPOXIC ISCHEMIC ENCEPHALOPATHY AND THE TERM INFANT

Hypoxic ischemic encephalopathy (HIE) is a syndrome that entails abnormal neonatal behavior that follows an insult accompanied by decreased oxygen delivery to a fetal or neonatal brain (Finer, Robertson, Richards, Pinnell, & Peters, 1981). An infant with HIE can have alterations in consciousness, muscle tone, and primitive reflexes. HIE occurs in approximately 0.2% of live births of 37 weeks or greater (Finer et al., 1981).

The neuropathology of HIE begins with intrauterine asphyxia that results in decreased fetal PO_2, pH, and blood pressure as well as increased PCO_2. This causes intracellular edema and increased cerebral tissue pressure. In turn, there is a focal decrease in cerebral blood flow and generalized brain swelling. There is an increase in intracranial pressure followed by generalized decreased cerebral blood flow and final brain necrosis. Experts feel that herniation is not seen with the brain swelling because the neonatal brain has more water than myelinated, mature brain (Volpe, 2008)

The Sarnat classification is used to define the clinical stages of encephalopathy. These stages are as follows: Stage 1—characterized by hyperalertness, hyper-reflexia, dilated pupils, tachycardia, and absence of seizures; stage 2—characterized by presence of lethargy, hyperreflexia, bradycardia, seizures, hypotonia, and a weak suck and Moro reflex; stage 3—characterized by stupor, flaccidity, small-to-midposition pupils that react poorly to light, decreased stretch reflexes, hypothermia, and absent Moro and suck responses (Sarnat & Sarnat, 1976). Finer and colleagues found 35% of infants with HIE had moderate to severe handicap or died (Finer et al., 1981). This was less than the 48% reported in a study by Brown et al. The significant factors that predicted poor outcome were Sarnat stages 2 or 3 and neonatal convulsions unresponsive to a single anticonvulsant (Finer et al., 1981). Outcomes for infants with HIE are defined in five categories: 1—Normal—average range of development for age and no evidence of handicap; 2—Mild handicap—variations from normal on neurologic or development exam without specific diagnosis; 3—Moderate handicap—trainable retardation, severe behavioral disorders, seizure disorders, mild or moderate neurosensory deafness, spastic diplegia, hemiplegia, or visual impairment; 4—Severe handicap—spastic quadriplegia, severe psychomotor retardation, or severe neurosensory deafness or blindness; and 5—Death during hospitalization or follow-up period. Follow-up studies have shown that infants with a higher Sarnat stage had moderate or severe handicap (Finer et al., 1981; Robertson & Finer, 1985). The Robertson and Finer study (1985) showed that children with mild HIE in the newborn period did not develop any major handicaps and there were no deaths. Of the children with moderate HIE in the neonatal period, almost 21% developed one or two handicaps by age 3 to 5 years. Children with severe HIE in the neonatal period only 25% survived to age 3 to 5 years and developed one to four handicaps, which included severe convulsive disorder. With the initiation of whole-body hypothermia for neonatal HIE, there has been a decrease in death rates with no increase in severe disability rates among survivors when followed out to 18 to 22 months (Shankaran et al., 2012). Follow-up of infants at 6 to 7 years who received whole-body hypothermia with regard to end point of death or an IQ score of less than 70 was not statistically significant when compared to usual care (Shankaran et al., 2012).

Case 18.3

Evan was born at 40 5/7 weeks gestation to a 27-year-old, gravida 2, para 1 now 2 mother, with an uncomplicated pregnancy and normal prenatal laboratories. Labor included a prolonged second stage. The delivery was complicated by a shoulder dystocia. Evan was born limp, with no respiratory effort and a heart rate (HR) of 60 bpm. Neonatal resuscitation was initiated. Despite effective positive pressure ventilation (PPV) via mask, the HR did not increase. The infant was intubated by 3 minutes of life; the HR remained less than 80 beats per minute with no spontaneous respiratory effort. Chest compressions were started, a low-lying umbilical vein line placed, and the infant received epinephrine × 1 IV. HR was more than 100 but infant still had no spontaneous respiratory effort or spontaneous movement at 10 minutes of life. Apgar scores were 1 (+1 HR) at 1 minute, 2 (+1 HR, +1 color) at 5 minutes, and 3 (+2 HR, +1 color) at 10 minutes.

Evan met criteria for whole-body cooling, which was initiated. Seizure activity was noted at 9 hours of life, anticonvulsants were started, and seizures were controlled on a therapeutic dose. Baseline electroencephalogram showed a burst suppression pattern that improved with time. Evan initially did not have any primitive reflexes but upon re-warming, had a gag and Moro reflex, was hypotonic, and had a poor suck. An MRI was obtained after Evan was re-warmed, which showed some cortical neuronal necrosis.

Evan was successfully extubated, exhibiting normal respiratory effort in room air. He remained seizure free on a therapeutic dose of anticonvulsants. Oral feeding was difficult and after 3 weeks with minimal improvement, a gastrostomy tube was placed to facilitate discharge home. Infant was taking approximately 50% of feeds orally. Feedings were uncoordinated and infant tired easily. Infant had emesis but was able to protect the airway.

1. *As the neonatal nurse practitioner caring for an infant just admitted with hypoxic ischemic encephalopathy (HIE) you understand that the classification system used to define the clinical stages of encephalopathy includes which of the following?*

   A. Apgars
   B. Dubowitz
   C. Sarnet
   D. Brazelton scale

(continued)

Case 18.3 (*continued*)

ANSWER: C. *The Sarnat classification is used to define the clinical stages of encephalopathy. The significant factors that predicted poor outcome were Sarnat stages 2 or 3 and neonatal convulsions unresponsive to a single anticonvulsant (Finer et al., 1981).*

2. **As a neonatal nurse practitioner caring for an infant undergoing whole-body cooling you understand that the term HIE is defined as:**

   A. Posthemorrhagic hydrocephalus resulting from earlier intraventricular hemorrhages
   B. A syndrome that is subsequent to an insult that causes decreased oxygen delivery to a fetal or neonatal brain
   C. A neurometabolic disorder
   D. A rare syndrome that is manifested by poor growth

   ANSWER: B. *HIE is a syndrome that entails abnormal neonatal behavior that follows an insult accompanied by decreased oxygen delivery to a fetal or neonatal brain (Finer, Robertson, Richards, Pinnell, & Peters, 1981).*

3. **As a neonatal nurse practitioner caring for an infant diagnosed with HIE you understand the neuropathology involved begins with intrauterine asphyxia that results in which of the following?**

   A. Decreased fetal pO_2, pH, and blood pressure
   B. Intracellular edema and increased cerebral tissue pressure
   C. Generalized brain swelling
   D. All of the above

   ANSWER: D. *The neuropathology of HIE begins with intrauterine asphyxia that results in decreased fetal PO_2, pH, and blood pressure, as well as increased PCO_2. This causes intracellular edema and increased cerebral tissue pressure. In turn, there is a focal decrease in cerebral blood flow and generalized brain swelling. There is an increase in intracranial pressure followed by generalized decreased cerebral blood flow and final brain necrosis.*

4. **As a neonatal nurse practitioner you understand that studies have shown that by initiating whole-body hypothermia treatment for moderate to severe neonatal encephalopathy has shown to decrease which of the following? (Select all that apply)**

   A. Death rates
   B. Disabilities in survivors
   C. HIE
   D. Hospitalizations of depressed infants at birth

   ANSWER: A and B. *With the initiation of whole-body hypothermia for neonatal HIE, there has been a decrease in death rates with no increase in severe disability rates among survivors when followed out to 18 to 22 months (Shankaran et al., 2012). Initiating whole-body hypothermia does not prevent HIE or hospitalizations of depressed infants at birth.*

(continued)

Case 18.3 (continued)

5. **As a neonatal nurse practitioner it is important that you can identify significant factors that predict poor neurological outcomes in infants with HIE; these factors include which of the following? (Select all that apply)**

   A. Sarnat stage 2 or 3
   B. Neonatal convulsions unresponsive to a single anticonvulsant
   C. Need for intubation
   D. Need for narcotics for comfort during whole-body hypothermia treatment

   ANSWER: A and B. *Infants that are classified as Sarnat stage 2 or 3 and who experience seizures that do not respond to a single anticonvulsant drug are at high risk for poor neurological outcomes. Both are signs of a significant hypoixic event.*

6. **In caring for infants with HIE, it is important that the neonatal nurse practitioner understands that infant can experience alterations in which of the following? (Select all that apply)**

   A. Consciousness
   B. Muscle tone
   C. Primitive reflexes
   D. Temperature control

   ANSWER: A, B, and C. *All of which are important for evaluating criteria for an infant that may require whole-body therapeutic hypothermia (encephalopathy score).*

7. **As a neonatal nurse practitioner you are asked to attend a vaginal delivery of a postterm infant requiring vacuum extraction; you understand that risk factors for HIE include which of the following? (Select all that apply)**

   A. Shoulder dystocia
   B. Meconium aspiration syndrome
   C. Maternal drug use
   D. Poor maternal nutrition

   ANSWER: A and B. *A difficult delivery and/or the presence of meconium at delivery could indicate signs of stress, possibly indicating the infant is hypoxic leading to subsequent HIE.*

8. **The infant's ability to coordinate and organize motor activity and levels of arousal, which are important for learning, decision making, and performing complex actions, is best defined as:**

   A. Self-regulation
   B. State of infant
   C. Successful breastfeeding
   D. Erik Erikson's stages of psychosocial development

   ANSWER: A. *The infant's ability to self-regulate, defined as coordination and organization of motor activities and arousal states, is the cornerstone of the infant's ability to learn, control emotions, make decisions, and perform complex tasks later in life.*

(continued)

Case 18.3 (continued)

9. *As a neonatal nurse practitioner working in the follow-up clinic for your graduates of the neonatal intensive care unit, you understand that cerebral palsy (CP) is a disorder of the body's motor functions that usually results in brain injury and presents as:*

A. Various types of abnormal movements
B. Cognitive impairments
C. Abnormal muscle tone
D. All of the above

ANSWER: D. *CP is a term used for a group of nonprogressive disorders of movement and posture caused by abnormal development of, or damage to, motor control centers of the brain. CP is caused by events occurring prenatally, during labor and delivery, and after birth.*

GOALS OF DEVELOPMENTALLY SUPPORTIVE CARE: CORE MEASURES

Goals of developmentally supportive care in NICUs are to reduce the stressful interactions an infant may have with his environment. Developmentally supportive care for high-risk infants in NICUs has a goal of providing a structured care environment that supports, encourages, and guides the developmental organization of the premature and/or critically ill infants and their families (Coughlin et al., 2009). Coughlin states that developmental care is care that recognizes the physical, psychological, and emotional vulnerabilities and cues of premature and/or critically ill infants and minimizes the potential for short- and long-term complications associated with the NICU experience. Researchers have explored the general hypothesis that the provision of a developmentally appropriate sensory milieu, coupled with minimal disruptions and care based on the infant's cues, improves medical and developmental outcomes (Coughlin et al., 2009)

Coughlin et al. (2009) developed guidelines for age-appropriate care of the premature and critically ill hospitalized patient. These guidelines are the drivers for an exceptional inpatient experience for both infant and family. The five core measure sets for evidence-based developmental care are as follows: (a) protected sleep, (b) pain and stress assessment and management, (c) developmental activities of daily living, (d) FCC, and (e) promoting the healing environment (Coughlin et al., 2009).

PROTECTED SLEEP

Although the NICU environment and its technologies lead to survival of premature and ill newborns, it also leads to constant exposure to light, noise, and painful interventions that can have deleterious effects on sleep in these infants that leads to sleep deprivation. A study by Judge, Chang, and Lammi-Keefe (2015) explored sleep habits during the first 48 hours of life and later developmental milestones throughout infancy and report that assessment of sleep–wake patterns within the first 24 to 48 hours after birth represents the earliest assessment of functional integrity of the developing nervous system. They also concluded poor infant sleep assessed within the first 48 hours of life in term infants was reflective of altered temperament and impaired neurodevelopment throughout the first year of life (Judge et al., 2015). In the neonate sleep has been found to correlate with maturation of the CNS, memory consolidation and learning, maintaining energy, increased protein synthesis, and secretion of growth hormones (Santos de Carvalho Bonan et al., 2014). Sleep and wakefulness states are present before birth as a result of the circadian cycle (CC), which is generated by 18 to 20th weeks of gestation in the anterior hypothalamus and is modulated by exogenous factors such as light (Santos de Carvalho Bonan et al., 2014). According to Santos de Carvalho Bonan et al. (2014), recent studies show that the circadian system is responsive to light by the 24th week of gestation and low-intensity light can regulate the development of the biological clock. In the last trimester of pregnancy, the sleep–wake cycle of the fetus is in line with maternal sleep–wake cycle and the occurrence of a premature birth may alter the development of the circadian rhythm in the child (Santos de Carvalho Bonan et al., 2014). Sleep has been showed to suggest a strong relationship between sleep and brain growth (Santos de Carvalho Bonan et al., 2014). The NICU environment does not support normal sleep–wake patterns in the infant, therefore it does not allow for a normal developmental trajectory for sleep–wake cycles. Infants, in a NICU environment, especially those who are premature, have sleep patterns that are often structured around the stimuli in the environment and the caregiver's schedule and often, early optimal sleep patterns are not promoted. According to Santos de Carvalho Bonan et al., approximately 20% of awakenings in the NICU environment are related to noise and 10% to nursing interventions and these constant interventions create fragmentation of sleep, which can lead to lower total sleep times leading to sleep deprivation. Fetal sleep is divided into three stages, which are active sleep (AS), quiet sleep (QS), and indeterminate sleep (IS). AS sleep is compatible with rapid eye movement (REM) sleep in adults and is the first type of sleep seen during fetal development and characterized by high physiological activity such as irregular breathing and greater supply of oxygen to the brain (Santos de Carralho Bonan et al., 2014). Maturation and differentiation of the CNS and memory consolidation occur and learning patterns of emotional behavior develop during AS sleep (Santos de Carralho Bonan et al., 2014). QS sleep develops in the 36th to 38th week of gestation and is characterized by a rest period, energy maintenance, increased protein synthesis, and release of growth hormones. Clinical behaviors such as sucking movements, smiles, slight blinking are present and breathing rate and HR are regular (Santos de Carvalho Bonan et al., 2014). Premature infants who have reached term have a sleep pattern that is still mostly AS sleep with less QS sleep compared to term infants and severe neurological damage is associated with longer periods of sleep in the AS stage (Santos de Carvalho Bonan et al., 2014). Changes in sleep experiences and poor sleep habits leading to sleep deprivation are suspected of adversely affecting optimal brain growth and development, which alters neurodevelopment outcomes. Developmental care practices that can reduce stressful stimulation and promote organized sleep–wake cycles need to be implemented and consistently practiced by all team members within the NICU environment. Parental support and education in helping parents learn and understand their infant's nonverbal clues are important in supporting optimal neurodevelopment.

PAIN

Pain—An unpleasant sensory and emotional experience associated with actual or potential tissue damage or described in terms of such damage . . .

— Committee on Taxonomy of the International Association for the Study of Pain

Physiologically, pain perception during fetal and neonatal development is much different from pain in the human adult (Lowery et al., 2007). It is unsure whether the fetus, and infants born prematurely, can perceive noxious stimuli at the cortical level, the site where the emotional aspect of the pain is experienced. Activation of the hypothalamic–pituitary–adrenal axis can occur in the absence of cortical development and activation (Lowery et al., 2007). A fetus or premature infant's inability to experience pain or stressful stimuli at the cortical level does not preclude the harmful effects of stressful stimuli during development. The fetus and neonate are not "little adults" and the structures and mechanisms used for pain processing are unique and completely different from those used by older children and adults (Lowery et al., 2007). Today, our understanding of how infants experience pain and the consequences of that experience has grown. Until the 1980s, it was believed by those caring for the vulnerable fetus and newborn that the fetus and newborn did not have the capacity to experience and process pain. These beliefs were challenged by accumulating data on hormonal–metabolic responses (activation of the hypothalamic–pituitary–adrenal [HPA] axis) seen in the fetus and infants undergoing painful surgical procedures with minimal to no anesthesia (Hall, 2014). To experience pain as an older child and adult children requires both nociception and an emotional reaction or ability to interpret pain (Lowery et al., 2007). Nociception requires an intact and functioning sensory system and an emotional reaction requires some form of consciousness (Velde et al., 2006). *Nociception* is the encoding and processing of harmful stimuli in the CNS. Nociceptors, or pain receptors, respond to painful stimuli by sending a signal along the sensory neurons in the spinothalamic and thalamo-cortical pathways to the brain. Nociception triggers a variety of autonomic responses that can be stressful to the fetus and the preterm infant.

Anatomical and functional perception of pain develops throughout the pregnancy (Lowery et al., 2007). Peripheral sensory nerve fibers and receptors develop early and may be evident as early as the seventh week of gestation and are abundant by 20 weeks gestation. During the 10th to 13th week of gestation, the afferent system located in the spinal cord's dorsal horn is developing (Lowery et al., 2007). As early as 8 weeks gestation, the connections between the peripheral receptors and afferent fibers are forming (Lowery et al., 2007). Myelination of these fibers begins after connections are formed and continues during further development. The speed of processing stimuli increases dramatically during infancy and childhood and does not reach full development until around the age of 30. This increase in speed of processing occurs because of the myelination of the nerve cell axons. Myelin is a fatty substance that insulates the axons and this increases the speed of transmission of impulses to and from the brain.

It is known that incomplete myelination of nerve fibers reduces, but does not eliminate, speed of conduction of painful stimuli, but this decrease in speed of conduction is offset by the short length of the nerve fibers (Vitaliti et al., 2012). The spinal reflex arc develops simultaneously with the growth of the peripheral fibers toward the spinal cord and is shown to occur in response to harmful stimuli. This spinal reflex is present by 19 weeks (Lowery et al., 2007). Connections to the thalamus begin at 14 weeks and are completed by 20 weeks, thalamocortical connections are present from 13 weeks and further mature by 26 to 30 weeks. However, it is not possible to measure evoked potentials form the cortex until 29 weeks gestation and many researchers state that it is not until 29 weeks gestation that there is objective evidence that peripheral stimulus can cause cortical activation (Lowery et al., 2007). Neurons in the cerebral cortex migrate from the periventricular area at 8 weeks gestation and by 20 weeks, the cortex has acquired a full complement of neurons with glial perforation that continues throughout childhood (Lowery et al., 2007). Synaptic formation begins at 12 weeks and peaks in the third trimester, with electroencephalographic activity appearing for the first time at 20 weeks gestation. During fetal development it is now known that cutaneous sensory receptors appear between the 7th and 15th week of gestation and that the spinal reflex arc appears by the 8th week of gestation in response to harmful stimulus.

With the advancement of technological and pharmacological practices, more preterm infants are surviving and we now understand that the fetus and young newborn can experience pain. Infants hospitalized in the NICU undergo many painful and stressful procedures. These care practices include suctioning, venipuncture, and heel lances, just to name a few. They also experience separation from their mothers. There is substantial literature demonstrating that newborn infants in the NICU environment undergoing painful procedures without effective nonpharmacological and/or pharmacological practices to relieve pain are at risk for later cognitive, learning, memory, and attention deficits later in life (Grunau, Whitefield, & Petrie, 1998). Anesthesia has been shown to reduce the stress response of pain in both the fetus and the newborn, although proper assessment of pain in the fetus and newborn is challenging. The fetus and newborn cannot tell us whether they are experiencing pain and subsequent stress. In the fetus, activation of the HPA axis (the "stress response") has been used to assess fetal pain (Velde et al., 2006). According to Velde and colleagues, we know that preterm infants have hormonal stress responses following an invasive intervention (Velde et al., 2006). The fetus and newborn undergoing stressful experiences respond by activation of the HPA axis and is expressed by the release of hormones that can be measured. When caring for infants who are in the NICU environment, careful attention needs to be given to decreasing stressful stimuli, including pain, because exposure to painful stimuli has been shown to induce significant adverse short- and long-term neurodevelopmental changes, especially in newborns admitted to the NICU.

Because of possible negative short- and long-term effects of untreated pain, it is important that nurse practitioners who care for these infants be able to assess both acute and chronic pain and attempts should be made to alleviate and minimize adverse effects of pain. The first most effective way to minimize the stressful effects of pain is to eliminate and/or reduce the number of painful experiences. When this is unavoidable, there are many different ways to treat pain in these infants depending on the type of pain being experienced. Nonpharmacologic and pharmacologic methods are used for the treatment of pain in the infant. Nonpharmacologic methods are often underappreciated, underutilized, and understudied (Hall, 2014). Nonpharmacologic methods can be effective in alleviating the pain experienced. Nonpharmacologic methods would include oral sucrose, nonnutritive sucking, breastfeeding, kangaroo care, massage therapy, and facilitated tucking. These nonpharmacologic methods are effective in alleviating pain during short painful procedures, such as skin-breaking procedures, for example, heel sticks. Sucrose, glucose, and breast milk (with or without nonnutritive sucking) have specific analgesic effects for most skin-breaking procedures. Massage therapy decreases pain scores and promotes weight gain in preterm neonates. Studies have shown that these nonpharmacologic methods effectively reduced an infant's crying and fussiness during acute painful procedures. Nonpharmacologic therapies for the treatment of minor pain are effective and are recommended as the first step in management of pain.

Pharmacologic therapies for pain relief include local anesthetics (topical and infiltration), opioids (morphine, fentanyl) and nonopioids (benzodiazepines, midazolam, lorazepam), other sedatives (phenobarbital, propafol, ketamine), acetaminophen, and nonsteroidal anti-inflammatory drugs (NSAIDs). All are used for lessening the painful experience. These pharmacologic methods are often used in conjunction with the nonpharmacologic methods.

DEVELOPMENTAL ACTIVITIES OF DAILY LIVING

Developmental activities of daily living for the preterm infant include positioning, feeding, and skin care. These developmental activities are disrupted as a result of the early removal from the uterine environment—preterm birth (Monterosso, Kristjanson, & Cole, 2002). While in the uterine environment, the infant's movement allows for active and passive muscle power. When exposed to the extrauterine environment of the NICU, active and passive muscle power is disrupted. Prone positioning for prolonged periods of time, gravitational force, neuromuscular immaturity, and global hypotonia are ways in which the active and passive muscle power is disrupted (Monterosso et al., 2002).

Placing a preterm infant in the supine position allows for easy access and observation by the care provider. Several studies showed that the prone position may have beneficial effects on the respiratory status of preterm infants and eventually the prone position became the favored position (Monterosso et al., 2002). Body position has also been shown to affect incidence and type of apnea, sleep–wake cycles, and tolerance to gastric feedings (Monterosso et al., 2002).

The uterine environment of the preterm infant is minimally affected by gravity but once exposed to the extrauterine environment, the preterm infant has inadequate muscle development to counteract the effects of gravity (Monterosso et al., 2002). This inadequate muscle development inhibits the infant from changing position and can lead to muscle imbalances (Monterosso et al., 2002).

Oral feeding is another developmental activity of daily living the preterm infant needs to be able to perform. Preterm infants are fed via a gavage tube until they are able to coordinate sucking–swallowing–breathing. The infant must also be able to maintain cardiovascular stability for a period of time to consume enough of a caloric volume to grow appropriately (McCain, 2003). Once again, the infant's sleep–wake cycle affects how the infant will transition from gavage to oral feeding. At 32 weeks, an infant can express a full range of behavioral states, which include quiet sleep, crying, and maintaining an alert state. Expressing this full range is important for oral feeding because it relates to the infant's ability to sustain an organized, awake behavior (McCain, 2003). Although the suck–swallow–breathe cycle is present at 28 weeks, a fully mature rhythm in a 1:1:1 ratio is not consistently present until after 37 weeks postconceptual age (PCA; McCain, 2003).

Skin is the largest organ of the body and performs many functions for the infant, including thermoregulation, as a barrier against toxins and microorganisms, a reservoir for fat storage and insulation, and is the primary interface for tactile sensation and communication with the mother (Lund & Kuller, 2007). The stratum corneum provides an important barrier function of the skin and contains 10 to 20 layers for a full-term infant, much fewer for a preterm infant based on gestational age (Lund, Brandon, Holden, Kuller, & Hill, 2013). The ability of the infant to receive tactile sensation and communication with the mother is affected by the decreased stratum corneum, especially when it can be compromised so easily. Overhydration, urine, feces, increased skin pH, friction, diet, and age disrupt the stratum corneum. This disruption can lead to epidermal inflammation, significantly in the diaper area but it can affect any part of the body. The stratum corneum formation is rapid with exposure to the dry environment and estimates to complete barrier maturation range from 2 to 9 weeks postnatal age (Visscher et al., 2009). The dermis of the newborn is thinner and not as well developed as that of an adult. Between the epidermis and the dermis are fibrils that connect the two layers and in the premature infant, these fibrils are fewer in number. The decreased cohesion between the epidermis and the dermis places the premature infant at greater risk for skin injury. Caution should be taken when using and removing medical adhesives (Lund et al., 2013). This skin disruption also interferes with tactile sensation and communication with the mother.

FAMILY-CENTERED CARE

Pregnancy, delivery, and postpartum are sensitive periods in a woman's life. There is a physiological and psychological aspect associated with this period as well as the physical changes that occur, all of which can provoke emotional instability. When a woman delivers a normal and healthy infant she adapts her idealized image of the baby to the real baby. This adaptation is more difficult when an infant is born prematurely (Correia, 2007). Giving birth to a preterm infant is considered to be a stressful event not only for the mother, but also the father. Several studies have shown increased levels of stress in mothers of preterm infants when compared to mothers who delivered full-term infants. Another study showed increased depressive symptoms among fathers of preterm infants (Kaaresen, Ronning, Ulvund, & Dahl, 2006).

Knowledge and concern are increasing about the long-term outcomes of infants born prematurely. Cognitive delay and behavioral and emotional problems are being reported in a large percentage of preterm infants. A risk factor for later behavioral problems has been the increased parental stress during the first year of life (Kaaresen et al., 2006). The stresses experienced by parents include sense of loss of anticipated delivery of a healthy infant, uncertainty of infant's outcome, foreign environment of the NICU, parental role alteration, and the infant's appearance and behavior. These stresses occur while in the NICU but many stresses continue and more occur once the infant is discharged to home (Doucette et al., 2004).

To minimize the stress of parents of a preterm infant, neonatal care practices have begun to change. Parents are encouraged to have early contact and be active participants in the care of the infant (Correia, 2007). FCC is an approach to medical care rooted in the belief that optimal outcomes are achieved when patients' and family members play an active role in providing emotional, social, and developmental support (AAP Committee on Hospital Care and Institute for Family-Centered Care, 2003). The principles for family-centered neonatal care include (a) open and honest communication between parents and professionals; (b) parents need same facts and interpretation of facts as the professionals; (c) in situations involving high mortality and morbidity risk, parents have the right to make decisions regarding aggressive treatment; and (d) antepartum parents should be given information about adverse outcome risk and given the right to state treatment preferences in advance (Harrison, 1993). Some ways to provide FCC are kangaroo care, unlimited parental presence, breastfeeding support, sibling support, transition to home, and parents' accompaniment on rounds.

HEALING ENVIRONMENT

The healing environment is the entire environment that surrounds the infant and the family. This includes but is not limited to the physical surroundings, the people who come in contact with the infant and family, and the organizational system that provides quality and consistent care.

As noted in previous core measures, protected sleep plays a critical role in development. Having a quiet, properly lit environment promotes protected sleep, which, in turn, promotes improved developmental outcomes. Noise levels in the NICU have always been of concern, increasing infant risk for hearing loss and disruption of sleep as well as affecting staff's attention, communication, and risk for errors (Laudert et al., 2007). Direct ambient light also has a negative effect on the infant's visual and neural development as well as possible adverse effects on other neurosensory systems (Laudert et al., 2007). More recently, attention to single-patient rooms to enhance the healing environment has been the focus for the developmental care of the infant. The single-patient room can be tailored to the infant and the family. There are many studies showing both the benefits and possible downsides of the single-patient room. Studies by Harris, Shepley, White, Kolberg, and Harrell (2006) and Walsh, McCullough, and White (2006) both showed increased parent privacy and presence as well as staff satisfaction with use of single-patient rooms. With regard to developmental outcomes of these infants, there have been conflicting studies. Pineda et al. (2014) showed that neurodevelopmental outcomes at age 2 years for infants in single-patient rooms were not improved, whereas Lester et al. (2014) found significant improvements in medical and neurobehavioral outcomes at discharge.

The staff of the NICU, those caring for the infant and family, is a big part of the healing environment. Nurses make up the biggest part of this human connection but physicians, advanced care providers, respiratory therapists, as well as so many others are involved with the infant and family care. There needs to be a culture of caring present within the NICU to foster the healing environment, which affects the developmental care of the infant. *Culture* has been defined as the summation and functional expression of the values of an organization, which consists of its decision-making processes, resource allocations, division and alignment of power, authority, and influence (Ohlinger, Brown, Laudert, Swanson, & Fofah, 2003).

THE NICU GRADUATE: OPTIMIZING NEURODEVELOPMENT OUTCOMES

Discharge of the preterm and previously ill infant from the NICU can be both an exciting anticipated event as well as terrifying for families. Becoming a parent is an exciting and joyful experience; however, having a premature infant provokes feelings of anxiety and uncertainty. With the increasing number of premature infants who are born and the improvement in technology, pharmacology, and care practices, more infants survive to discharge. Many times, after discharge home of the premature infant, parents must continue therapies that were initiated in the hospital (Lopez, Hoehn Anderson, & Feutchinger, 2012). These therapies can include oxygen administration, tube feedings, and apnea monitoring (Lopez et al., 2012). The complex care needs of these high-risk infants continue to be challenging, even after discharge, and much of this burden of care is now placed on the family. According to Jeffries and Canadian Paediatric Society, Fetus and Newborn Committee (2014) parents often feel apprehensive and question their ability to care for their infant on their own after discharge from the NICU. All providers involved in an infant's care while in the NICU should be attuned to parental and family interactions with their infant throughout the hospital course to recognize any concerns about the family's ability to provide appropriate supportive and safe care after discharge (Barkemyer, 2015). High-risk social situations should be identified early. A well-planned and comprehensive discharge is imperative to ensure a safe and effective transition to home in which parents can be confident in the care they provide (Jeffries & Canadian Paediatric Society, Fetus and Newborn Committee, 2014). Recommendations from the AAP stress that assessment of the family and home environment prior to discharge needs to identify any high-risk factors that may impact the developmental and behavioral outcomes for these infants. These high-risk factors include poverty, domestic abuse, illicit drug abuse, lack of education, and families with poor social supports. The infants' developmental outcomes ultimately depend on the capacity and ability of the family to support their child in a supportive and safe home environment.

An integrative literature review was conducted by Lopez et al. (2012) that reviewed studies that focused on the transition of premature infants from the NICU to home. The review of the literature found that the need for home visits, child and family assessment methods, methods of keeping in contact with health care providers, educational and support groups, and the primary nurses' role in a transition program were all important aspects of care that allowed for a safe transition to home (Lopez et al., 2012). Home visits by a nurse were found to be a key component in providing education, support, and nursing care (Lopez et al., 2012). The review of the literature identified five components of successful transition programs that allowed for guidance to address the needs of parents and ways to ease the transition from hospital to home for the infant and families. These five components include open and supportive communication between health care providers and the families. The use of technology through videoconferencing, telephone contact, and a pager can allow for parents to stay in the home and still have the support of the health professionals in the NICU (Lopez et al., 2012). Home visits by the primary nurse on the third or fourth day after discharge were found to be effective in preventing re-hospitalizations. Another component in promoting a safe and successful discharge included assessment of the infant and the parenting skills. Included in this assessment were the infant's feeding and development, medication administration, infant's status, maternal health, parenting skills, and home environment factors. Other components included education and educational and support groups and nurse involvement, which was found to be a key element in all of the transitional programs reviewed (Lopez et al., 2012). As the neonatal nurse practitioner, it is important that you have an awareness of the parental NICU experience during their infant's hospitalization. Encouraging parental involvement from the first day of admission to the NICU and providing open honest communication, education, and support can lead to a successful and safe transition to home. A gradual transfer of responsibility from care provider to parent is needed to allow parents to gain confidence in caring for the infant leading to a successful transfer from hospital to home.

DISCHARGE OF THE LATE PRETERM INFANT

The late preterm infant lacks the physiologic maturity of the term infant and is at higher risk of problems such as feeding difficulties, hypoglycemia, hyperbilirubinemia, hypothermia, apnea, and respiratory distress (Barkemyer, 2015). Discharge readiness is determined by the infant's ability to demonstrate functional maturity, which includes the physiological ability to maintain their temperature, control breathing, and the ability to feed well and gain weight (Jeffries & Canadian Paediatric Society, Fetus and Newborn Committee, 2014). Discharge readiness is based on these physiological markers of maturity rather than actual weight or postmenstural age (PMA) criteria. Infants usually reach these milestones between 34 and 36 weeks PMA (Jefferies & Canadian Paediatric Society, Fetus and Newborn Committee, 2014). Problems that the late preterm infant experiences might not be fully resolved at the time of discharge, therefore the need for sooner and more frequent follow-up may be necessary to reduce the possibility of adverse outcomes such as re-hospitalization (Barkemyer, 2015). Ideally, the late preterm infant should be seen within 24 to 48 hours after discharge. Close monitoring of feeding, voiding, and stooling is essential along with serial weight measurements and assessment for any jaundice (Barkemyer, 2015). Jaundice is a common problem in late preterm infants during the first few days of life and can cause adverse neurologic outcomes if not monitored and treated in a timely manner. Late preterm infants discharged home within the first week of life are especially at risk. Transcutaneous bilirubin screening should be performed prior to discharge or in the outpatient setting when there is concern. A thorough and comprehensive physical examination prior to discharge of the infant and documentation of findings are imperative. Documentation should include vital signs, evidence of adequate feeding and weight gain, evidence of normal voiding and stooling patterns, and adequate thermoregulation. A hearing screen should be obtained on all preterm and previously ill infants being discharged from the NICU. Risk factors, such as history of infection, ototoxic drug exposure, and severe jaundice, should be documented. Infants who fail a hearing screen should have the appropriate auditory follow-up in place prior to discharge. Late preterm infants should also have screening for congenital heart disease performed prior to discharge. Close neurodevelopmental follow-up is needed to identify any factors that would require timely interventions.

DISCHARGE OF THE PRETERM INFANT

Families of these infants experience an often overwhelming and stressful journey during their infant's stay in the NICU (Jeffries & Canadian Paediatric Society, Fetus and Newborn Committee, 2014). The NICU environment is often unfamiliar and highly technical causing parents to have a sense of fear and a lack of control over care of their infant interfering with the development of a trusting relationship.

After weeks or even months in the highly supportive environment of the NICU, discharge to home can be a challenge for many families and there is often growing concern for their ability to care for their infant. Discharge home of the preterm infant from the NICU requires comprehensive planning that will focus on health care maintenance and medical and neurodevelopmental follow-up. Preterm infants are at higher risk for adverse medical and neurodevelopmental outcomes, therefore their follow-up often requires a multidisciplinary approach sometimes involving multiple providers and therapists (Barkemyer, 2015).

Early intervention and high-risk clinics that offer in-depth neurodevelopmental follow-up are essential for optimal neurodevelopmental outcomes. Inclusion criteria for referral to these high-risk clinics should be available and referrals should be made prior to discharge. Early intervention is a prevention-focused program in the community with which the high-risk infants and their families become involved soon after discharge. Early intervention programs in the United States are federally funded and administered by states to provide timely evaluation and interventions for infants from birth through 2 years of age who are experiencing developmental delays or are at high risk for developmental delays (Barkemyer, 2015). Criteria for evaluation and services vary by state, but most high-risk graduates of the NICU meet these criteria (Barkemyer, 2015). Communication between the multidisciplinary care team and the parents after discharge is needed for optimal neurodevelopmental. Timing of the discharge depends on the stability of the infant and the ability of the caregivers to meet the needs of the infant in the home environment (Barkemyer, 2015). Adequate nutrition and acceptable growth is imperative for optimal brain growth of the preterm infant. Despite medical and pharmacologic advances in care for the premature and very low-birth-weight infant, nutritional care in the NICU is often unable to match growth rates achieved in utero (Barkemyer, 2015). Close monitoring of postdischarge weight and growth is essential for optimal brain growth. This can be done with regular plotting of weight, length, and head circumference against standardized curves for the preterm infant. Intraventricular hemorrhage occurs inversely with gestational age, with the highest rates in infants with gestational ages less than 28 weeks (Barkemyer, 2015). Grades III and IV (IVH) put the preterm infant at higher risk for poor neurodevelopmental outcomes that include intellectual disabilities, CP, or posthemorrhagic hydrocephalus (Barkemyer, 2015). Most often evolution of the IVH occurs after discharge and often necessitates the need for evaluation of serial imagining studies. According to Barkemyer (2015), assessment of head growth in all premature infants discharged is an important part of ongoing follow-up to recognize not only excessive head growth but also inadequate head growth, which is indicative of poor brain growth. Retinopathy of prematurity (ROP) is often a problem in infants born prematurely, usually seen more commonly in infants born before 28 weeks gestation. In most cases, ROP resolves without the need for intervention and without vision loss. When needed, treatment for ROP is essential because current interventions with cryotherapy and/or intraocular bevacizumab can significantly improve visual outcomes when offered in a timely manner (Barkemyer, 2015). Delays in screening and identification of infants who require intervention can result in unnecessary blindness.

Multiple studies have shown that families of premature infants graduating from the NICU experience levels of stress and anxiety at the time of discharge and need support during this process. Extra resources are especially needed for the families living in high-risk social environments. Involvement in the care of their infant from the time of initial hospitalization and throughout their infant's stay should be encouraged. Parents should be informed and educated regarding any and all of their infant's problems and medical interventions during their stay in the NICU. Besides community early- intervention programs and high-risk clinics, home health nursing, lactation specialists, and other available community supports should be put into place prior to discharge. The neonatal nurse practitioner should develop the skill to be able to summarize lengthy NICU stays in a document that is concise, understandable, and contains all the pertinent information for ongoing care.

After discharge, developmental care practices and interventions that include the parents are often complex. No longer is the infant the only "patient," instead the family requires support and sometimes interventions to keep them healthy to allow them to support their infant's continued medical and developmental growth. According to Benzies, Magill-Evens, Hayden, and Ballatyne (2013), several components were found to be important to a successful transition to home. These included psychosocial support for mothers and families to decrease stress, anxiety, and symptoms of depression, and increased self-efficacy and maternal sensitivity and responsiveness in interactions with their infant (Benzies et al., 2013). Ongoing parental educational programs can improve parental knowledge and increase parenting self-efficacy, thereby decreasing stress and anxiety (Benzies et al., 2013). This education may include information about neurological development and behavior that may be specific to their own infant (Benzies et al., 2013). Developmental interventions provided by the parents themselves may also improve self-efficacy and improve developmental outcomes for the infant. Interventions can include spending time talking or singing to their infant, spending face-to-face time, and providing bright interesting objects for them to look at. Giving their infant bells or rattles may improve the baby's tactile and sensory development, as will with hanging interesting mobiles above them while lying on a blanket. Smiling and making happy sounds is also important. Interventions that promote sensory neural development are important. Early intervention should be provided after discharge from the hospital.

Preterm infants develop significant nutritional deficits during their hospitalization in the NICU (Carver, 2005). Despite feeding interventions that attempt to promote and match intrauterine growth rates recommended by the AAP, preterm infants may continue to have growth restriction at the time of discharge (Nzegwu & Ehrenkranz, 2014). Growth failure in the immediate postdischarge period remains an extremely concerning and common problem for the premature and previously critically ill infant after discharge from NICU. Suboptimal postnatal growth in premature infants after discharge from the NICU is a common finding, especially in the very low birth weight and extremely low birth weight infants (Dusick et al., 2003). Suboptimal growth in these infants can put them at higher risk for impaired neurodevelopmental outcomes. Postdischarge nutritional practices vary widely and there are no widely accepted feeding recommendations that have elucidated any lasting effects on growth and neurodevelopment (Nzegwu & Ehrenkranz 2014). Practices range from breastfeeding to fortification of enteral feedings with nutrient-enriched products (Nzegwu & Ehrenkranz, 2014). Both the AAP and the World Health Organization endorse finding ways to support breastfeeding and lactation practices after discharge, which have been shown to increase the number of preterm infants receiving breast milk after discharge, which has been shown to be beneficial for growth and neurodevelopmental outcomes (Nzegwu & Ehrenkranz, 2014). An individualized approach is essential for each infant and family and close monitoring of growth parameters, such as weight, length, and head circumference and nutritional intake, should be assessed every 2 to 4 weeks after discharge (Nzegwu & Ehrenkranz, 2014). Lahood and Bryant (2007) describe developmental surveillance as a continuous process of skilled observation, eliciting and attending to parental needs and concerns, obtaining relevant history, and collaboration and open communication among all caregivers for that infant. A comprehensive, well-planned discharge of a medically stable infant will help ensure a safe and positive transition to home for both the parents and the infant.

REFERENCES

AAP Committee on Hospital Care and Institute for Family-Centered Care. (2003). Zero to three: Early experiences matter. Policy statement on family-centered care and the pediatrician's role. Retrieved from http://main.zerotothree.org

Als, H., & Brazelton, T. B. (1974). Comprehensive neonatal assessment (Brazelton neonatal behavior assessment). *Birth, 2,* 3–9.

Als, H., Tronick, E., Lester, B. M., & Brazelton, B. (1977). The Brazelton Neonatal Behavioral Assessment Scale (BNBAS). *Journal of Abnormal Child Psychology, 5*(3), 215–229.

Barfield, W. D., & Lee, K. G. (2016). Late preterm infants. In L. E. Weisman (Ed.), *UpToDate.* Waltham, MA: Wolters Kluwer.

Benzies, K. M., Magill-Evans, J. E., Hayden, K. A., & Ballatyne, M. (2013). Key components of early intervention programs for preterm infants and their parents: A systematic review and meta-analysis. *BMC Pregnancy and Childbirth, 13*(Suppl. 1), 510.

Barkemyer, B. M. (2015). Discharge planning. *Clinics in Perinatology, 64,* 545–556.

Blencowe, H., Cousens, S., Oestergaard, M., Chou, D., Moller, A. B., Narwal, R., . . . Say, L. (2015). National, regional, and worldwide estimates of preterm birth. *Lancet, 379,* 2162–2172.

Brazelton, T. B. (1974). Does the neonate shape his environment? *Birth Defects, 10*(2), 131–140.

Carver, J. D. (2005). Nutrition for preterm infants after hospital discharge. *Advances in Pediatrics, 52,* 23–47.

Clark, C. A., Woodward, L. I., Horwood, L. I., & Moor, S. (2008). Development of emotional and behavioral regulation in children born extremely preterm and very preterm biological and social influences. *Child Development, 79*(5), 1444–1462.

Correia, L. L. (2007). Maternal anxiety in the pre- and postnatal period: A literature review. *Revista Latino-Americana de Enfermagem, 15*(4), 677–683. doi:10.1590/S0104-11692007000400024

Coughlin, M. (2011). *Age-appropriate care of the premature and critically ill hospitalized infant: Guideline for practice.* Glenview, IL: National Association of Neonatal Nurses.

Coughlin, M. (2014). *Transformative Nursing in the NICU: Trauma- informed age-appropriate care.* New York, NY: Springer Publishing.

Coughlin, M., Gibbins, S., & Hoath, S. (2009). Core measures for developmentally supportive care in neonatal intensive care units: Theory, precedence, and practice. *Journal of Advanced Nursing, 65*(10), 2239–2248.

Doucette, J., & Pinelli, J. (2004). The effects of family resources, coping, and strains on family adjustment 18 to 24 months after NICU experience. *Advances in Neonatal Care, 4*(2), 92–104.

Dusick, A. M., Poindexter, B. B., Ehrenkranz, R. A., & Lemons, J. A. (2003). Growth failure in the preterm infant: Can we catch up? *Seminars in Perinatology, 27*(4), 302–310.

Esch, T., & Stefano, G. B. (2011). The neurological link between compassion and love. *Medical Science Monitor, 17*(3), RA65–RA75.

Finer, N. N., Robertson, C. M., Richards, R. T., Pinnell, L. E., & Peters, K. L. (1981). Hypoxic–ischemic encephalopathy in tern neonates: Perinatal factors and outcomes. *Journal of Pediatrics, 98*(1), 112–117.

Gibbins, S., Hoath, S. B., Coughlin, M. E., Gibbins, A., & Franck, L. (2008). The universe of developmental care: A new conceptual model for application in the neonatal intensive care unit. *Advances in Neonatal Care, 8*(3), 141–147.

Graven, S. (2011). Early visual development: Implications for the neonatal intensive care unit and care. *Clinics in Perinatology, 38*(4), 671–683.

Groopman, J. (2011, October). A child in time: New frontiers in treating premature babies. *The New Yorker: Medical Dispatcher.* Retrieved from http://www.newyorker.com/magazine/2011/10/24/a -child-in-time

Grunau, R. E., Holsti, L., & Peters, W. B. (2006). Long-term consequences of pain in human neonates. *Seminars in Fetal & Neonatal Medicine, 11*(4), 268–275.

Grunau, R. E., Porter, F. L., & Anand, K. J. S. (1999). Long-term effects of pain in infants. *Journal of Developmental and Behavioral Pediatrics, 20*(4), 19–29.

Grunau, R. E., Whitefield, M. F., & Petrie, J. (1998). Children's judgements about pain at age 8 to 10 years: Do extremely low birthweight (< or = 1000 grams) children differ from full birthweight peers? *Journal of Child Psychology and Psychiatry, 39*(4), 587–594.

Gudsnuck, K. M., & Champagne, F. A. (2011). Epigenetic effects of early developmental experiences. *Clinics of Perinatology, 38*(4), 703–717.

Hall, R. W. (2014). Pain management in newborns. *Clinics in Perinatology, 41*(4), 895–924.

Harris, D. D., Shepley, M. M., White, R. D., Kolberg, K. J. S., & Harrell, J. W. (2006). The impact of single family room design on patients and caregivers: Executive summary. *Journal of Perinatology, 26,* s38–s248.

Harrison, H. (1993). The principles for family-centered neonatal care. *Pediatrics, 92,* 643–650.

Jablonka, E., & Lamb, M. J. (2002). The changing concept of epigenetics. *Annals of the New York Academy of Science, 981,* 82–96.

Jain, L. (2011). The foundations of newborn brain development. *Clinics in Perinatology, 38*(4), xii–xiv.

Jeffries, A. L., & Canadian Paediatric Society, Fetus and Newborn Committee. (2014). Going home: Facilitating discharge of the preterm infant. *Paediatric Child Health, 19*(1), 31–36.

Judge, M. P., Chang, L., & Lammi-Keefe, C. J. (2015). Evidence of developmental continuity from birth to 1 year: Sleep temperament, problem solving, and recognition memory. *Advances in Neonatal Care, 15*(2), 125–133.

Kaaresen, P. I., Ronning, J. A., Ulvund, S. E., & Dahl, L. B. (2006). A randomized, controlled trial of the effectiveness of an early-intervention program in reducing parenting stress after preterm birth. *Pediatrics, 118*(1), e9–e19.

Kenner, C. (2012). Transition from hospital to home for parents of preterm infants. *Journal of Perinatal & Neonatal Nursing, 26*(1), 88–89.

Kugelman, A., & Colin, A. A. (2013). Late preterm infants: Near term but still in a critical developmental time period. *Pediatrics, 132*(4), 741–751.

Lahood, A., & Bryant, C. A. (2007). Outpatient care of the premature infant. *American Family Physician, 15*(8), 1159–1164.

Laudert, S., Liu, W. F., Blackington, S., Perkins, B., Martin, S., MacMillan-York, E., . . . Handyside, J. (2007). Implementing potentially better practices to support the neurodevelopment of infants in the NICU. *Journal of Perinatology, 27,* s75–s93.

Lester, B. M., Hawes, K., Abar, B., Sullivan, M., Miller, R., Bigsby, R., . . . Padbury, J. F. (2014). Single-family room care and neurobehavioral and medical outcomes in preterm infants. *Pediatrics, 134,* 754–760.

Loeser, J. D., & Treede, R.-D. (2008). The Kyoto protocol of IASP basic pain terminology. *Pain, 137*(3), 473–477.

Lopez, G. L., Hoehn Anderson, K., & Feutchinger, J. (2012). Transition of premature infants from hospital to home life. *Neonatal Network, 31*(4), 207–214.

Lowery, C. L., Hardman, M. P., Manning, N., Clancy, B., Whit Hall, R., & Anand, K. J. S. (2007). Neurodevelopmental changes of fetal pain. *Seminars in Perinatology, 33*(6), 275–282.

Lund, C. H., Brandon, D., Holden, A. C., Kuller, J., & Hill, C. M. (2013). *Evidence-based clinical practice guideline, neonatal skin care* (3rd ed.). Washington, DC: Association of Women's Health, Obstetric and Neonatal Nurses.

Lund, C. H., & Kuller, J. M. (2007). Integumentary system. In C. Kenner & J. W. Lotts (Eds.), *Comprehensive neonatal care: An interdisciplinary approach* (4th ed., pp. 65–91). St. Louis, MO: Elsevier Saunders.

MacDonald, M. G., & Seshia, M. M. K. (1997). *Avery's neonatology: Pathophysiology and management of the newborn* (7th ed.). Philadelphia, PA: Saunders.

Mahoney, A. D., Minter, B., Burch, K., & Stapel-Wax, J. (2013). Autism spectrum disorders and prematurity: A review across gestational age subgroups. *Advances in Neonatal Care, 13*(4), 247–251.

McAnulty, G. B., Butler, S. C., Bernstein, J. H., Als, H., Duffy, F. H., & Zurakowski, D. (2010). Effects of the newborn individualized developmental care and assessment program (NIDCAP) at age 8 years; preliminary data. *Clinical Pediatrics, 49*(3), 258–270.

McCain, G. C. (2003). An evidence-based guideline for introducing oral feeding to healthy preterm infants. *Neonatal Network, 22*(5), 45–50.

Monterosso, L., Kristjanson, L., & Cole, J. (2002). Neuromotor development and the physiologic effects of positioning in very low birth weight infants. *Journal of Obstetric, Gynecologic & Neonatal Nursing, 31*, 138–146.

Montirosso, R., Del Prete, A., Bellu, R., Tronick, E., Borgatti, R., . . . The Neonatal Adequate Care for Quality of Life (NEO-ACQUA) Study Group. (2012). Level of NICU quality of developmental care and neurobehavioral performance in very preterm infants. *Pediatrics, 129*(5), e1129–e1137.

Morse, S. B., Zheng, H. T., & Roth, J. (2009). Early school-age outcomes of late preterm infants. *Pediatrics, 123*(4), e622–e629.

Nightingale, F. (1860). *Nursing: What it is, and what it is not* (1st ed.). New York, NY: D. Appleton and Company.

Nzegwu, N. I., & Ehrenkranz, R. A. (2014). Post-discharge nutrition and the VLBW infant: To supplement or not supplement. *Clinics in Perinatology, 41*, 463–474.

Ohlinger, J., Brown, M. S., Laudert, S., Swanson, S., & Fofah, O. (2003). Development of potentially better practices for the neonatal intensive care unit as a culture of collaboration: Communication, accountability, respect and empowerment. *Pediatrics, 111*, e471–e481.

Pickler, R. H., McGrath, J. M., Reyna, B. A., McCain, N., Lewis, M., Cone, S., . . . Best, A. (2010). A model of neurodevelopmental: Risk and protection for preterm infants. *Journal of Perinatal & Neonatal Nursing, 24*(4), 356–365.

Pineda, R. G., Neil, J., Dierker, D., Smyser, C. D., Wallendorf, M., Kidokoro, H., . . . Inder, T. (2014). Alterations in brain structure and neurodevelopmental outcome in preterm infants hospitalized in different neonatal intensive care unit environments. *Journal of Pediatrics, 64*, 52–60.

Robertson, C., & Finer, N. (1985). Term infants with hypoxic-ischemic encephalopathy: Outcome at 3 to 5 years. *Developmental Medicine & Child Neurology, 27*(4), 473–484.

Rosier-van Dunne, F. M. F., van Wezel-Meijler, G., Groot, L. De., van Zyle, J. I., Odendaal, H. J., & de Vries, J. I. P. (2013). Echogenicity changes in the fetal brain, a 6-year follow-up study. *Journal of Maternal–Fetal & Neonatal Medicine, 26*(10), 1036–1041.

Santos de Carvalho Bonan, K. C., da Costa Pimentel Filho, J., Tristao, R. M., Lacerda de Jesus, J. A., & Junior, D. C. (2014). Sleep deprivation, pain and prematurity: A review study. *Arquivos de Neuro-Psiquiatria, 73*(2), 147–154.

Sarnat, H. B., & Sarnat, M. S. (1976). Neonatal encephalopathy following fetal distress: A clinical and electroencephalographic study. *Archives of Neurology, 33*, 696–705.

Schoenwolf, G. C., Bleyl, S. B., Brauer, P. R., Francis-West, P. H., & Philippa, H. (2015). *Larsen's human embryology* (5th ed.). New York; Edinburgh: Churchill Livingstone.

Shankaran, S., Pappas, A., McDonald, S. A., Vohr, B. R., Hintz, S. R., Yolton, K., . . . Higgins, R. D. (2012). Childhood outcomes after hypothermia for neonatal encephalopathy. *New England Journal of Medicine, 366*(22), 2085–2092.

Spittle, A. J., Thompson, D. K., Brown, N. C., Treyvaud, K., Cheong, J. L. Y., Lee, K. J., . . . Anderson, P. J. (2014). Neurobehavior between birth and 40 weeks' gestation in infants born <30 weeks' gestation and parental psychological wellbeing: Predictors of brain development and child outcomes. *BMC Pediatrics, 14,* 111. Retrieved from http://www.biomedcentral.com/1471-2431/14/111

Sullivan, R., Perry, R., Sloan, A., Kleinhaus, K., & Burtchen, N. (2011). Infant bonding and attachment to the caregiver: Insights from basic and clinical science. *Clinics of Perinatology, 38*(4), 643–655.

Velde, M. V., Jani, J., De Buck, F., & Deprest, J. (2006). Fetal pain perception and pain management. *Seminars in Fetal & Neonatal Medicine, 11*(4AQ115), 232–236.

Visscher, M., Odio, M., Taylor, T., White, T., Sargent, S., Sluder, L., . . . Bondurant, P. (2009). Skin care in the NICU patient: Effects of wipes versus cloth and water on stratum corneum integrity. *Neonatology, 96,* 226–234.

Vitaliti, S. M., Costantino, G., Puma, L., Re, M. P., Vergara, B., & Pinello, G. (2012). Painful procedures in the NICU. *Journal of Maternal-Fetal & Neonatal Medicine, 25*(54), 146–147.

Volpe, J. (Ed.). (1995). *Neurology of the newborn* (3rd ed., pp. 280–281). Philadelphia, PA: Saunders.

Volpe, J. J. (Ed.). (2008). *Neurology of newborn* (pp. 400–480). Philadelphia, PA: Elsevier Saunders.

Watson, A. (2010). Understanding neurodevelopmental outcomes of prematurity: Education priorities for NICU parents. *Advances in Neonatal Care, 13,* S21–S26.

Watson, A. (2013). Understanding neurodevelopmental outcomes of prematurity: Education priorities for NICU parents. *Advances in Neonatal Care, 13*(Suppl. 5), S21–S26.

Webb, A. R., Heller, H. T., Benson, C. B., & Lahav, A. (2015). Mother's voice and heartbeat sounds elicit auditory plasticity in the human brain before full gestation. Retrieved from www.pnas.org/cgi/doi/10.1073/pnas.1414924112

Woythaler, M. A., McCormick, M. C., & Smith, V. C. (2011). Late preterm infants have worse 24-month neurodevelopmental outcomes than term infants. *Pediatrics, 127*(3), e622–e629.

19

Complex Social Histories and Communicating With Parents: Critical Conversations for Sensitive Situations

Terri A. Cavaliere and Ana Arias-Oliveras

Chapter Objectives

1. Identify and apply four common ethical principles impacting neonatal care
2. Discuss recommendations for palliative and end-of-life care for infants
3. Define *moral distress*
4. Identify situations and conditions that create moral distress
5. Summarize research in palliative and end-of-life care for infants and moral distress
6. Analyze case presentations to identify the critical issues affecting the family and staff
7. Synthesize an approach to infants at the end of life, including care of families
8. Describe important aspects of critical discussions with parents in the neonatal intensive care unit (NICU)
9. Apply best practices for communicating with parents and professional care for high-risk infants

Advances in neonatology and perinatology have affected major improvements in mortality and morbidity of high-risk infants. This progress has resulted in changes in NICU patient characteristics over the past 30 years. The age of viability has been lowered dramatically as the complexity of diagnoses has expanded. Advanced practice nurses (APNs), neonatal nurse practitioners (NNPs), and clinical nurse specialists (CNS) are responsible for the care of patients who would not have survived several decades ago.

As is true in any medical specialty, progress comes with a price. Expansion in technology brings about heretofore-unknown ethical and moral dilemmas as well as the need to develop excellent communication skills in highly emotionally charged environments. Decision making regarding initiating or withholding treatments or relaying unpleasant information to families is a common event in the NICU.

Discussions about survival of an infant or the potential to survive with severe disabilities can be extremely difficult for families. Health care providers, particularly nurses, are vulnerable to moral distress while practicing in the NICU environment. Determining futility, quality of life, and when to initiate palliative care (PC) have been the core of much debate.

The ability of professionals to function in sensitive situations is generally not an innate talent but rather is a skill that must be taught and developed with continued practice. This is especially true in situations in which distressing news must be delivered to parents. Currently, education of APNs is complex and multifaceted. Each technological advance prompts additions to already crammed curricula. Priority is placed on pathophysiology, pharmacology, research, and clinical proficiency at the expense of seemingly less important, albeit critical, topics such as ethical decision making, palliative and end-of-life care, and communication skills. Little attention is paid to the issue of moral distress. As a result, with the exception of actual practical expertise, the majority of APNs enter the clinical arena unprepared to handle many of the difficult situations they face. This chapter covers a range of didactic information related to ethics, communication, and PC, followed by a series of case studies for practical applications. References are included to support the content and provide additional resources for the reader.

ETHICAL PRINCIPLES AND CONSIDERATION

Traditionally, decisions based on rule-based ethics depend on application of ethical principles such as autonomy, beneficence, nonmaleficence, and justice. These fundamental principles provide a framework employed in the approach to ethical dilemmas in the neonatal setting (Fanaroff, 2015). In this section, the learner will find definitions of these principles as well as information regarding futility as it pertains to ethical considerations and the distinction between withdrawal and withholding of care.

ETHICAL PRINCIPLES

The principle of *autonomy* recognizes the right of individuals to make their own medical decisions. When parents (or patients) consent to medical treatment, they are exercising their right of autonomy. These decisions should be made only after being fully informed. Parents or guardians act as surrogates in making medical decisions on behalf of the infant, in the *best interests of the infant*. Although it is not always easy to decide what are the best interests of others, it is accepted that the parents have the moral and legal authority to make decisions for their children. In an ideal situation, parents should have the time to consider details of decisions that will impact their child. Unfortunately for some parents, there may not be enough time prior to delivery for a thorough discussion on neonatal outcomes and decisions regarding neonatal resuscitation.

Neonatal health care providers strive to provide care that will promote the best interests of infants who are unable to make their own decisions. Beneficent acts result in a good outcome while avoiding harm to the patient. Thus, the principles of *beneficence* and *nonmaleficence* should be balanced. Some consider that the duty to avoid harm should be considered as the overarching principle (*primum non nocere*: first do no harm). Keep in mind that beneficence incorporates preventing and eliminating harm as much as possible, whereas the separate, distinct principle of nonmaleficence requires that we intentionally *act to avoid* harm. Together these principles remind us to be thoughtful and to proceed with care at all times. This requires consideration of the risks and benefits of treatments. Consider the use of postnatal steroids in babies with severe respiratory disease. In earlier years, prolonged courses of dexamethasone were used to assist in weaning babies from ventilator support. With the passage of time, data became available that linked poor neurodevelopment outcome in infants treated with high doses and long courses of steroids. Today, health care providers weigh the risks of poor neurodevelopmental outcome versus the benefits of using steroids in neonates. Parents are, or should be, counseled as to these risks and benefits prior to beginning steroid treatment.

There is one area in which parental wishes will not be honored. Certain religions have injunctions regarding what type of therapies may be refused (i.e., blood transfusions, removing life support, etc.). Adults have the right under any circumstances to refuse treatments. They are not, however, allowed to place their religious obligations on their children. Staff should, at all times, attempt to work with parents and avoid confrontations, but it is important to keep in mind that there are some situations that require administrative/legal consultation. Hospitals have ethics committees in place that provide assistance in situations of legal uncertainty. Despite the ethical correctness of an act, providers are not under obligation to carry out parental wishes if they are illegal. It is, therefore, important to be familiar with the laws regulating practice in jurisdictions in which care is provided. Following hospital policies that are contrary to laws will not provide protection for APNs.

We have collective data to predict outcomes such as gestational age, birth weight, use of antenatal steroids, neurodevelopmental outcomes, and so on. The decision to intervene at the limit of viability or to cease/withdraw life-sustaining measures should be collaborative. The health care provider will provide information to the family to enable and support its decision to pursue curative interventions.

As discussed previously, nonmaleficence obligates the health care provider to do no harm. The challenge arises when the health care provider and the family do not agree on what constitutes harm. For example, the family of a 23-week-gestation neonate requests that all interventions be provided. On the other hand, the health care team considers that aggressive care at the limit of viability may cause great harm, in terms of pain and suffering of the neonate, with very little positive benefit. Other illustrations are infants with grade IV intraventricular hemorrhage (IVH) and severe periventricular leukomalacia (PVL), or neonates born with conditions, such as anencephaly or bilateral renal agenesis and pulmonary hypoplasia, whose parents desire full resuscitation, including intubation and artificial ventilation to support continued existence.

The principle of justice pertains to social issues. Social benefits, such as medical care, should be distributed equally without regard to ethnicity, race, or ability to pay. Justice demands that (a) given similar situations, consumers have equal access to similar health care; and (b) the type of health care obtainable by one particular group of consumers takes into consideration the effects of such use of these resources on other groups (Fanaroff, 2015). In other words, health care should be allocated in an equitable manner.

Fanaroff (2015) provides a distinction between macroallocation and microallocation of resources. According to broad utilitarian philosophies, *macroallocation* entails distribution of resources to ensure the greatest good for the greatest number of people. This underlies government programs such as Medicaid and provisions of the Affordable Care Act. *Microallocation* has a more narrow focus and involves access opportunities for individual patients. Neonatal care is provided at enormous costs, especially in cases of extremely premature infants or those with complex medical conditions. Costs rise when other complications, such as necrotizing enterocolitis or sepsis, occur. Despite the concerns over the high cost of health care, it is rare for microallocation issues to be debated at the bedside (Fanaroff, 2015). However, it is critical for both micro- and macroallocation issues to be considerations for a just, efficient health care system.

ETHICS COMMITTEES

The Joint Commission for the Accreditation of Healthcare Organizations mandates that American hospitals establish a method for consideration and education on ethical issues in patient care (Caulfield, 2007). Most hospitals have complied with this directive through the creation of ethics committees that are both educational and advisory. Committee members are from diverse backgrounds to (a) provide clinical ethics consultation, (b) develop and/or revise policies pertaining to clinical ethics and hospital policy, and (c) facilitate education about topical issues in clinical ethics. Ethics committee members are often called upon to help in the resolution of ethical conflicts and in answering ethical questions through the provision of consultations. APNs should consider consulting ethics committees when they perceive that there is an ethical problem in the care of patients and they are unable to establish a resolution favorable to both the parents and the health care team.

LEGAL ISSUES

Consideration of the legal matters involved in neonatal care is beyond the scope of this chapter. The learner is referred to the many texts dealing with the subject. However, it bears mentioning that nurses have the individual responsibility to be aware of the legal statutes that impact their practice. Pleading ignorance is no excuse for engaging in illegal actions. There is usually an attorney who is a member of the ethics committee and consultation can be provided when the question of legality of a particular action arises.

FUTILITY

It is necessary to explore the concept of futility when considering treatment requests. The word *futile* is defined as serving no useful purpose, whereas *futility* is the quality of uselessness (Merriam-Webster, 2016). Futility from an ethical point of view infers that the treatment is nonbeneficial. There is a difference between a treatment having medical effect and whether it has medical benefit. Health care providers are under no ethical obligation to employ treatments that are not beneficial (Swaney, English, & Carter, 2016). For instance, cardiopulmonary resuscitation (CPR) for a neonate with the diagnosis of trisomy 13 with multiple congenital anomalies might restore effective cardiac rhythm (medically effective) but will the resuscitation provide a quality existence or change the underlying condition of the baby?

In addition to providing beneficial therapies while making decisions for infants, one must apply a best-interest standard as opposed to a "quality of life" standard. It is challenging to separate best interests from quality of life. Ethical decisions in neonatology are frequently difficult because of (a) uncertainty surrounding medical outcomes and prognoses, (b) lack of agreement over what treatments are beneficial for an infant, and (c) ambiguity in meaning of *best interests* and *quality-of-life standards*. These situations require collaboration between parents and providers to balance principles of beneficence, nonmaleficence, and justice.

Further details regarding ethics in neonatal care can be found in the works of Swaney, English, and Carter (2016) and Fanaroff (2015).

WITHHOLDING AND WITHDRAWING LIFE-SUSTAINING MEDICAL TREATMENT

The question of whether to withhold or withdraw treatment frequently arises during the course of caring for critically ill or extremely immature neonates. Withholding life-sustaining medical treatment (LSMT) consists of the option of excluding a treatment judged to be nonbeneficial. Withdrawing LSMT entails the decision to eliminate a treatment that has not achieved its intended beneficial effect (Fanaroff, 2015; Janvier, Barrington, & Farlow, 2014). From a personal point of view, it is frequently believed that there is a difference between these two actions, but from a moral/ethical viewpoint there is no difference. Fanaroff (2015) writes that, "If it is morally right (or wrong) to withhold treatment deemed to be ineffective, it is equally right (or wrong) to withdraw this same treatment after it is started, should it later become clear that the treatment is ineffective" (p. 33). Additional criteria for deciding whether to withhold or withdraw LSMT may include (a) the likelihood that death is inevitable and will occur despite the provision of intensive care, which proposes that the infant probably will not survive to be discharged from the NICU and is difficult to predict with certainty; (b) ineffective treatment that is not achieving its intended goal; and (c) poor quality of life. Despite the focus on the best-interest standard for treating infants, quality-of-life consideration, involving estimation of cognitive and neurodevelopmental outcome, is difficult to ignore (Fanaroff, 2015).

PERSONAL CONSIDERATIONS

Each of us is influenced by a multitude of personal values, morals, and attitudes that motivate every aspect of our lives. These deep-seated values have considerable power over our thoughts and behavior and often operate on an unconscious level. A key aspect of professional practice is the necessity for the provider to identify and examine the personal guidelines that motivate us. This exercise involves self-reflection and consideration of how our personal values "fit" the health care situations in which we practice. For example, if a neonatal advanced practice nurse's (NAPN's) beliefs deem drug addiction as sinful, this belief may influence the nurse to behave in a judgmental manner toward the mother of a neonate who is experiencing abstinence syndrome.

Although nurses must respect the beliefs of patients, there is no requirement that the nurses own beliefs must be violated during patient care. Therefore, it is important for nurses to investigate whether they can be replaced in situations that are contrary to their personal beliefs (e.g., participating in termination of pregnancies or removal of life support). If substitution of another nurse is not possible, the nurse may have to decide whether it will be tolerable to have personal values violated (see section "Understanding and Addressing Moral Distress").

PALLIATIVE CARE

PC is defined by the World Health Organization (WHO; 2015) as "an approach that improves the quality of life of patients and their families facing the problem associated with life-threatening illness, through the prevention and relief of suffering by means of early identification and impeccable assessment and treatment of pain and other problems, physical, psychosocial and spiritual." There are three general categories of newborns who benefit from PC: (a) those with congenital anomalies incompatible with life, (b) newborns at the limit of viability, and (c) infants with overwhelming illness not responding to life-sustaining interventions. Advances in technology have provided us the ability to sustain the lives of these infants beyond what was once considered unattainable. Determining futility, quality of life, and when to initiate PC has been the core of much debate. Who is best able to determine futility? Who is best able to determine what quality of life is? What is a good death? Who is ultimately making the decision to continue or forego medical interventions? (American Association of Pediatrics, 2013; Bidegain & Younge, 2015). Freibert and colleagues wrote that PC is concerned with optimal living in the face of a life-threatening condition; it is not merely about death and dying (Freibert, Bower, & Lookabaugh, 2012). The focus of PC should be to provide comfort to the patient and preserve quality of life (Catlin, 2011).

PC can be provided in other settings in addition to the immediate newborn period. For example, women whose fetuses have serious, life-threatening conditions and malformations who choosing to continue their pregnancies can be supported with PC services during their pregnancies (M. Conway-Orgell, personal communication, 2012; R. Spinazzola & B. Rochelson, personal communication, 2014). Determining the threshold of initiating PC is multifaceted and complex. Parents and health care professionals are faced with the burden of determining when to initiate withdrawal of life-sustaining interventions. Establishing goals related to end-of-life care with the family starts with an assessment of their understanding of the diagnosis and the infant's current status. You may ask the following: "What is your understanding of your baby's medical problems?" This will allow a baseline from which to continue your discussion. Investing the time to evaluate the parents' comprehension of the diagnosis will provide an opportunity to establish effective communication, build trust, and provide the family with the support needed (Catlin & Carter, 2002; Carter & Jones, 2013; Jellinek et al 1992; Mancini, Utahaya, Beardsley, Wood, & Modi, 2014).

LIMITS OF VIABILITY

The *limit of viability* is defined as the stage of fetal maturity that ensures a reasonable chance of extrauterine survival. Factors such as gender, birth weight, antenatal steroids, as well as single and multiple births, influence viability and affect outcome. However the major factor most responsible for viability is gestational age (Eherenkranz & Mercurio, 2016). The authors of the seventh edition of the *Textbook of Neonatal Resuscitation* (American Heart Association [AHA] & American Academy of Pediatrics [AAP], 2016), without actually using the term *limit of viability*, state that resuscitation need not be offered to neonates born at a *confirmed* gestational age of less than 22 weeks. Despite the recommendation of the AHA and AAP, resuscitation of extremely premature neonates in the delivery room is not regulated by professional associations of legal statutes. Health care providers retain the freedom to assess each situation on its own merits, considering parental wishes, the condition of the individual neonate, and their own judgments regarding medical futility (Arzuage & Meadow, 2014). Thus, the decision to provide or withhold aggressive medical management for those extremely premature neonates at 22 to 23 weeks gestation is complex and should embrace careful consideration of the factors previously mentioned as well as appraisal of prenatal data, assessment of family concerns prior to the delivery. Discussions with the family should include neonatal outcomes and options of intervening versus providing comfort care. In addition, parents should be asked what their understanding of the prognosis is and what they wish for their baby; if the medical team is to intervene, provide specific details; if comfort care is provided, what does that entail? Details for medical interventions should include assessment of respiratory effort, placement of an endotracheal tube, determination of when chest compressions are going to be initiated, when medications are going to be administered, and what determines ceasing all medical interventions.

Once resuscitative measures have been initiated, ongoing reassessments of the infant's response to the interventions are critical. The clinical course should dictate management. Parents expect a follow-up discussion about the infant's status, response to treatment, and what the next steps should be. Guidance during these difficult moments relies heavily on the medical team. Many factors influence end-of-life decision making. Parents are often faced with the pressures of family environment, societal expectations, and personal and religious beliefs (Gardner, & Carter, 2016; Stowkowski, 2012).

Perinatal PC

Prospective families who wish to continue their pregnancies have an opportunity to participate in the developing model of care called *perinatal PC* (Wool, 2011). Support is provided to help the transition from celebrating a life, to preparing for a goodbye. This multidisciplinary approach provides an extra layer of support, not only to the parents, but also to the siblings and other relatives who may also be affected. Once the diagnosis has been determined and shared with the family, there needs to be a holistic assessment in identifying their global needs. This will include, but is not limited to, the following: (a) Ask whether they have named the baby, if so, obtain the parent's permission to use the given name; (b) determine their understanding of the diagnosis and prognosis; (c) identify who will make the medical decisions regarding the baby (eldest male figure in the family, religious leader, etc.); (d) assess the family support system, this will guide the need for interhospital support groups versus community-based support groups or both; (e) assess how each family member is coping; identify individual needs of each parent/support person as well as collective needs of the family; (f) identify the goals and wishes for their baby; (g) assess how they feel about making memories with visuals such as photography and video; (h) determine preferences for the delivery (who will attend, religious rites [i.e., baptism, presence of clergy]); (i) determine preferences surrounding the funeral arrangements and an autopsy.

Special Considerations at End of Life in the NICU

End-of-life care refers to the process of providing supportive care and PC to the patient and families. The spectrum of time is variable from onset to bereavement. In the NICU, we need to create an environment that is conducive to the development of interdisciplinary collaboration at the end of life. This should include the medical team, nursing, pediatric subspecialist, chaplain, and social worker in addition to the family. Parents want to have the knowledge about the infant's condition and/or diagnosis so that they may prepare themselves for what may ultimately be their child's death. They want to feel supported and respected as they endure the journey of making difficult decisions while coping with the loss of the healthy baby whom they may not bring home (Kenner, 2014).

For the health care provider, once the decision is made to have a family meeting whether it is to divulge bad news or discuss end-of-life care, place and time of where to have the meeting should be a priority. Most NICUs do have a family room that is away from the bedside. This may help minimize the anxiety and tension surrounding the family. The next step will be to determine which of the interdisciplinary team members should attend this meeting. You want to create an environment of empathy and support. Having too many participants in the meeting may lead the family to feel overwhelmed. Begin the meeting by introducing the members of the interdisciplinary team, followed by asking the family to introduce family members to the team (this is if extended family members beyond parents are present). State the purpose of the meeting and then ask the family to share their understanding of the infant's condition and diagnosis. Provide detailed information minimizing the use of medical jargon. Allow intermittent moments of silence for the family to process the information discussed and allow them the opportunity to ask questions. The meeting should not exceed 30 minutes. If further discussions are needed, provide the family with the option of having multiple short meetings (Fanaroff, 2015; Gardner & Carter, 2016).

Cultural and Religious Considerations at End of Life

How does culture influence a physician–family relationship? How does culture influence a family's response to healing and suffering?

Culture fundamentally influences how individuals make meaning out of illness, suffering, and dying, and therefore influences how they make use of medical services at the end of life (Kagawa-Singer & Blackhall, 2001). *Acculturation* is considered to be the cultural modification of an individual, group, or people by adapting to or borrowing traits from another culture, also known as being "Americanized." Identifying the length of time a mother and/or the family unit has lived in the United States may help to minimize the risk of cross-cultural misunderstandings. With regard to end-of-life care, studies have shown cultural differences in truth telling, life-prolonging technology, and decision-making styles (Kagawa-Singer & Blackhall, 2001; Mancini et al., 2014). In the setting of the NICU, one must identify who makes the medical decisions for the patient, and who is the focal point of the family unit. This may or may not be the same person. In certain cultures, the eldest male figure is the only one who may volunteer information about the family, ask questions regarding the medical management, and ultimately make the medical decisions for the patient. In other cultures and religions, the spiritual leader of the community is the only one who may make the medical decisions and is present at the family meetings.

In summary, PC is based on a multidisciplinary framework that is beneficial to those infants with the following conditions: (a) congenital anomalies incompatible with life, (b) newborns at the limits of viability, and (c) infants with overwhelming illness who are not responding to life-sustaining interventions. Discussions with the family about medical management and when to withhold or withdraw treatment are multidimensional and complex. Special considerations, such as prenatal data, information received at consultation meetings, medical interventions, infant's response to those interventions (including laboratory test results and radiologic test results), are of utmost importance. Creating a collaborative team, which includes the family, will ensure effective communication, partnered goal-directed decision making, psychosocial care, comprehensive pain and symptom control, and provide grief support (Fribert et al., 2012).

ANALGESIA AND PAIN CONTROL AT THE END OF LIFE

Pain management is a critically important aspect of neonatal care that should not be overlooked at the end of life. Withdrawal or withholding treatment is *not* synonymous with withdrawing or withholding *care*. Therefore, attention must be given to alleviating infant suffering. Some may view providing analgesia as a form of euthanasia because it may hasten death of the patient by interfering with respiration. This leads to a discussion of the principle of double effect (PDE).

This principle is cited as a justification of administration of analgesia for pain relief despite the fact that it may lead to the predictable but unpremeditated, effect of producing respiratory depression that can accelerate death (Anderson, 2007). There is little evidence in the adult literature that opioid use at end of life hastens death (Anderson, 2007), yet a long-held belief that opioid use leads to death has resulted in undertreatment of patient suffering at the end of life.

APNs can apply the following four guidelines when assessing whether an action with both good (relief of suffering) and bad (degree of respiratory depression) outcomes is permissible: (a) The deed (pain administration) must itself be morally good or at least indifferent, (b) only the benefit (pain relief) must be intended even though the harmful (secondary) effect is predictable, (c) the beneficial effect must not be realized as a result of the harmful effect, and (d) the good result must outweigh the bad result (Anderson, 2007).

The American Nurses Association supported the promotion of comfort and pain relief in dying patients (American Nurses Association, 1991). It is an act of compassion, basic to nursing, to provide relief of pain and suffering for neonates and infants who are dying. Following the principles listed previously, analgesia is administered (a morally good act) with the intent of relief of suffering, *not* to cause respiratory depression and hasten death. The end result, relief of suffering, is not intentionally caused by the death of the patient, and the end result is death with peace and comfort, not death for the sake of ending a life.

UNDERSTANDING AND ADDRESSING MORAL DISTRESS

The advances in technology, which have led to great benefits for infants and their families, have at the same time created unforeseen problems for health care providers. Moral distress is pervasive and still largely unrecognized, yet it impedes the ability of professionals to deliver optimal care (Cavaliere, Daly, Dowling, & Montgomery, 2010). The first published reference to moral distress is credited to Jameton (1984), while observing nurses in practice settings. Jameton observed that nurses experienced anger and stress as they struggled to reconcile professional and personal values with the actualities of their work settings. Although this seminal work and majority of research have been in nursing, moral distress is not unique to nurses (Austin, Lemermeyer, Goldberg, Bergum, & Johnson, 2005; Chen, 2009; Hamric, & Blackhall, 2007; Hilliard, Harrison, & Madden, 2007; McCarthy & Gastmans, 2015; Sporrong, Hoglund, & Arnetz, 2006; Whitehead, Herbertson, Hamric, Epstein, & Fisher, 2015). Evidence in the literature documents moral distress in other health care professions. Since Jameton's original work was published, many others have added to the body of knowledge on the topic (Corley, 1995, 2002; Corley, Elswick, Gorman, & Clor, 2001; Corley & Minick, 2002; Corley, Minick, Elswick, & Jacobs, 2005; Elpern, Covert, & Kleinpell, 2005; Epstein & Delgado, 2010; Hamric, 2012; Hanna, 2004; Pauly, Varcoe, & Storch 2012; Rushton, 2006; Van Zuuren & van Manen, 2006; Wilkinson, 1987–1988; Woods, 2014; Zuzelo, 2007).

There are a variety of definitions proposed for moral distress (Cavaliere et al., 2010). For purposes of discussion in this chapter, moral distress is defined as physical and psychological pain and disrupted interpersonal relationships arising from patient care situations wherein the provider becomes cognizant of a moral problem, accepts moral responsibility, and makes a moral decision regarding a correct course of action. However, as a result of actual or perceived constraints, the nurse participates either by act or omission, in a manner he or she perceives to be morally wrong (Nathaniel, 2006). Note that moral distress is not the same as the confrontation of ethically troubling situations and does not occur independent of a nurse/provider–patient relationship. There are many events that cause distress in the health care setting but not every moral/ethical problem causes moral distress.

Table 19.1 summarizes potential causes of moral distress for nurses; these causes are substantiated by the many references regarding moral distress that are included in this chapter. Simply stated, anything that interferes with a nurse's ability to provide optimal patient care has the potential of causing moral distress (Cavaliere et al., 2010).

Moral distress exerts a heavy toll on nurses, impacting the quality, quantity, and cost of nursing care, and in some cases, on patient outcome (Corley et al., 2001; Pendry, 2007; Rushton, 2006; Wilkinson, 1987–1988). The literature confirms negative effects of moral distress on nurses (see Table 19.2 for specific consequences). As with the causes of moral distress, the references contained in this chapter provide support for data in the table.

Table 19.1 **Potential Causes of Moral Distress**

Issues surrounding end-of-life care

Futile, aggressive patient care without perceived patient benefit

Patient harm resulting from pain and suffering

Depersonalizing patients when meeting institutional requirements

Constraints caused by health policies and managed care directives

Inadequate staffing, floating

Working with incompetent colleagues

Effects of cost containment

Adapted from Cavaliere et al. (2010) and Corley (2002).

Table 19.2 **Impact of Moral Distress on Nurses**

Moral Distress
Contributes to feelings of frustration and powerlessness
Leads to loss of moral integrity
Creates dissatisfaction with the work environment
Produces stress-induced physical symptoms (headaches, sleeplessness, etc.), emotional and psychological pain (anxiety, withdrawal, depression)
Causes loss of capacity to care, failure to provide good care, avoidance of patient contact, emotional aloofness, cynicism, and sarcasm
When Ignored or Unaddressed Moral Distress
Progresses to burnout leading nurses to abandon the work setting, and at times, the profession

Webster and Bayliss (2000, p. 208) introduced the phenomenon of moral residue as a consequence of moral distress, describing it as an enduring, heart-rending reminder of times in which providers violated their own moral integrity in times of moral distress. They warn that it is "long-lasting, and powerfully integrated into one's thoughts and views of the self." Epstein and Delgado (2010) and Epstein and Hamric (2010) also discuss moral residue, stating that it is the moral residue that is detrimental to the individual and his or her career, especially when situations that cause moral distress continue unabated.

ADDRESSING MORAL DISTRESS

It may not be possible to completely eliminate moral distress from the practice setting. Hanna (2004) wrote that although moral distress has negative consequences, experiencing it may help to develop moral character. The author suggests that moral distress presents an opportunity for personal transformation and growth (McCarthy & Gastmans, 2015). Nevertheless, recognizing the consequences of moral distress, it is important that strategies exist to alleviate its impact. Several authors have proposed strategies to address moral distress (Austin et al., 2005; Beumer, 2008; Epstein & Delgado, 2010; Epstein & Hamric, 2009; Hamric, Davis, & Childress, 2006; Lilly et al., 2000; Puntillo & McAdam, 2006; Rushton, 2006). None of these has been accepted as best practice but many can be adapted for use in the clinical setting.

An approach to alleviating moral distress was created by the American Association of Critical-Care Nurses (AACN; Table 19.3). Other strategies that may be helpful in dealing with moral distress include (a) establishing support networks in the NICU and throughout the institution; assisting co-workers and colleagues who may be struggling with similar problems; (b) examining the work environment while keeping in mind that similar problems occur cyclically, representing an institutional problem not merely a patient or unit problem, necessitating identification of root causes; (c) seeking information about moral distress and locating educational material (literature searches), attending seminars and discussion groups, training staff to recognize moral distress, to identify barriers to change, and to create action plans; (d) creating interdisciplinary networks—to improve a system it is critical to have input from multiple professions, to collaborate in creation of policies, and to include discussion of moral distress in ethics consultations (Epstein & Delgado, 2010; Epstein & Hamric, 2009; Hamric, Davis, & Childress, 2006).

Table 19.3 Addressing Moral Distress

Stages	Actions/Activities	Goal/Rationale
Ask—Consider stage of self-awareness and reflection; provider experiences nonspecific suffering caused by threatened moral integrity and sense of self; symptoms may be physical, emotional, behavioral, or spiritual	1. Review the definition and symptoms of MD; ask whether you and/or other team members are experiencing MD. 2. Others (coworkers, friends, family) have noticed the signs/behaviors.	Identify presence of MD Identification is a prerequisite to addressing moral distress
Affirm—This stage identifies suffering as MD	1. Acknowledge presence of MD; commit to care for yourself 2. Validate your feelings and perceptions with others 3. Confirm professional responsibility to act 4. Search for resources: AACN, ANA, NANN, hospital policies 5. Gather the facts	Commit to addressing MD Prolonged/unrecognized MD may be harmful to personal and professional life; health care institutions have a moral responsibility to identify and relay their values to employees. Employees share the responsibility for creating a healthy work atmosphere

(continued)

Table 19.3 **Addressing Moral Distress (*continued*)**

Stages	Actions/Activities	Goal/Rationale

Assess—This stage identifies the source of MD	1. Continue gathering facts
	2. What is the source of MD?
	  a. In what situation do the signs and symptoms occur?
	  b. Do others experience similar reactions?
	3. What do you think is the correct action? To whom do you need to speak?
	4. What, if anything, is currently being done?
	5. Are you ready to take action?
	6. Identify risks and benefits involved in acting to eliminate the source of MD
		Establish readiness to act; create an action plan
		Greater details of this stage are available (AACN, n.d.; Rushton, 2006)

Act—During this stage, the plan of action is finalized and actions are taken	1. Prepare to act
	  a. Develop self-care plan
	  b. Identify possible sources of support: coworkers, managers, administrators, employee assistance programs, institutional ethics committee, chaplains
	  c. Locate outside sources for guidance: professional organizations, (e.g., ANA Code of Ethics, State Board of Nursing/ Nurse Practice Act, The Joint Commission)
	2. Act
	3. Maintain desired change
	  a. Anticipate and manage setbacks
	  b. Reevaluate—continue the 4 A's to identify and manage MD
		Preserve moral identity and authenticity
		Provide high-quality patient care and self-care

4 A's, ask, affirm, assess, act; AACN, American Association of Critical-Care Nurses; ANA, American Nurses Association; MD, moral distress; NANN, National Association of Neonatal Nurses.

Adapted from AACN (n.d.) and Rushton (2006).

COMMUNICATION WITH PARENTS

The one aspect of neonatal care that is applicable to every family is the need to communicate with parents. Parents deserve to be given complete, truthful, individualized, and consistent information by the medical and nursing team. Communication is a cornerstone of family-centered care and should be a priority, not an afterthought (Dupont-Thibodeau, Barrington, & Farlow, 2014; Hills, 2016; Yee & Ross, 2006).

Proficient communication skills are essential to providing optimal neonatal care. Like other skills taught in undergraduate nursing or APN courses, effective communication expertise must be incorporated into curricula. Although educational programs may encompass didactic content on professional patient-centered conversations, there is rarely opportunity to develop expertise in the clinical setting. There is a need for nursing faculty to assist students in developing competency in speaking to patients' families.

Although it has become a popular notion that decision making in the NICU should be a consensual process, shared by the parents and the health care team alike, parents need all the pertinent, complete information available about their child to be full participants in their care and in the decision-making process. In shared decision making, each member expresses his or her treatment preferences after discussing the relevant details and a final decision is reached. According to Fanaroff (2015), in the ideal situation, the burden and responsibility for the decision is shared by all members of the team, avoiding blame for a single person. Table 19.4 contains salient information in establishing effective communication with parents.

Table 19.4 **Communicating With Parents: Family-Centered Care**

Encourage parents' participation to enable them to be fully informed: integrate siblings and family members.

Remember basics of polite behavior: Introduce self and members of team, have seated conversations when possible, ask baby's first name; keep appointments is a timely manner, etc.

Know and understand your own beliefs and biases.

Strive to know the family: understand their situation, decision-making style, informational needs, communication preferences, religious/social/cultural background; their concerns; what is their understanding about infant's illness and prognosis; explore parental hopes and fears.

Customize information to the needs of parents—individualize for the infant and family situation; always be open and truthful, avoid giving false hope; provide balanced information; discuss quality of life, possibility of death and impairment.

Provide information accurately and with as much certainty about diagnosis and prognosis as possible. Identify areas of medical uncertainty.

Consider level of health literacy and language barriers; employ certified translators when needed.

Be proactive in situations in which a poor outcome is predicted or expected. Introduce end-of-life issue, palliative and hospice care, and family-supportive care; enlist aid of social worker, hospital chaplain or clergy, ethics committee, as needed. Inquire about spiritual or religious ceremonies. Explain what may occur regarding pain control and sedation. Assist in creating meaningful memories.

Identify and remove barriers that limit parents' ability to communicate.

(continued)

Table 19.4 Communicating With Parents: Family-Centered Care (*continued*)

Communicate frequently with parents, especially upon admission and at times of crisis, encourage parents to seek clarification of information as needed, and honor requests for meetings as much as possible.

Update parents frequently and as the condition changes; review goals of care; keep parents informed in a timely manner when special tests/investigations are planned.

Give parents time to process and absorb information.

Ensure consistency and continuity when communicating; considering staff rotation during shift changes and time off.

If an error occurs, be frank, candid, and timely in discussing the episode to parents.

Adapted from Fanaroff (2015) and Janvier et al. (2014).

CASE STUDIES

The following case studies are presented with a specific focus in mind (palliative and end-of-life care, communicating with parents when outcome is grim, and moral distress). Each one contains ethical issues that must be addressed. However, there is considerable overlap among the studies so the reader can apply more than one focus to each case study; for example, PC and difficult communication, and moral distress and ethical issues. Readers are encouraged to review the questions from all the case studies to examine whether they are applicable to the other studies. The answers to the following questions are influenced by many factors; in particular, personal values, professional experiences, state legislation, and institution-based policies. PC and ethics help to direct our interventions, discussions, and outcomes. The questions generate conversations regarding both PC and ethical situations that you may encounter. Please refer to the Bibliography to enhance the discussions and topics provided. The format of the answers differs from previous chapters due to the nature of the topics and the variability of the response to the question. We provide recommendations to lead the discussion; refer to specific sections of the chapter in addition to the References section.

Case 19.1

The neonatal nurse practitioner is called for an emergency cesarean section of a 35-year-old G5P1031 female at 27 weeks gestation. This pregnancy has been complicated by pregnancy-induced hypertension and a prenatal diagnosis of transposition of the great arteries (TGA). The mother has been an inpatient on the high-risk antepartum unit on two previous occasions for blood pressure control. Now the obstetrician (OB) informs you that the mother has developed HELLP (hemolysis, elevated liver enzymes, and low platelet count) syndrome so delivery is necessary. The parents do not want intervention and are requesting comfort care for the neonate because of prematurity and the heart defect.

(continued)

Case 19.1 (continued)

After speaking with the parent you understand that the family is considering palliative care (PC) and are enacting their right to parental autonomy. For them, the best interest of their child is to not intervene and allow a natural death.

Consider the following specific issues when answering the questions in Case Study 19.1: parental autonomy, beneficence/nonmaleficence, best interests of the child, withholding and withdrawing treatment, analgesia/pain control at end of life, PDE, ethics committees, limits of viability, futility, risks versus benefits of treatment, categories of candidates for PC, recommendations of professional societies, cultural and religious considerations at end of life.

1. *Is the health care provider obligated to honor the parents' request for nonintervention at 27 weeks gestation? What legal statutes impact the health care team's ability to honor the parent's wishes?*

   ANSWER: The answer to this question is dependent of the geographic location of your practice. You will not find the answer to this in the resources provided but it is advisable to research it for yourself.

2. *Considering the gestational age of the fetus and the comorbidity of TGA, is the prognosis bleak enough to warrant nonintervention? Does this represent a situation of futility?*

   The focus of discussion: Discuss long-term outcomes of TGA and survival at 27 weeks gestation. Definition of futility: Futility from an ethical point of view infers that the treatment is nonbeneficial. There is a difference between a treatment having medical effect and whether it has medical benefit. Refer to the chapter sections: Futility, Ethical Principles, and Special Considerations at End of Life.

3. *Who is best to determine futility?*

   ANSWER: If time permits, the neonatologist will be the person to counsel this family prenatally. The overall discussion will be based on the prognosis of a fetus born at 27 weeks gestation.

   The focus of discussion: Does the neonatologist have enough information to determine long-term outcomes of a fetus born at 27 weeks gestation with TGA? Should the neonatologist have a discussion with a pediatric cardiologist prior to the prenatal consult? Should the neonatologist have a discussion with the ethics committee prior to the prenatal consult? Refer to the chapter sections: Futility, Ethical Principles, and Special Considerations at End of Life.

4. *Who is best to determine what quality of life is?*

   The focus of discussion: Determine the factors that must be taken into consideration for the neonate's immediate and long-term prognosis. Does the family's perception of quality of life parallel the overall prognosis? Does the neonatologist and/or advanced

(continued)

Case 19.1 *(continued)*

practice nurse have a biased perception of quality of life? Refer to the chapter sections: Futility, Withholding and Withdrawing Life-Sustaining Medical Treatment, and Ethical Principles.

5. *Who should ultimately be involved in the decision to continue or forego medical interventions?*

   ANSWER: Variable upon the institution's policy. There may be limited participation from the multidisciplinary team in the discussion of curative efforts versus PC. Refer to the chapter sections: Futility, Ethical Principles, Palliative Care, and Special Considerations at End of Life.

6. *Differentiate between the parents' right to autonomy and the neonate's right to beneficence?*

   The focus of discussion: What is the overall prognosis of a fetus born at 27 weeks gestation? Does the diagnosis of TGA influence the parents' decision or is the aspect of prematurity the leading factor? Does the parents' autonomy supersede the neonate's right to beneficence or vice versa. Refer to the following section: Ethical Principles.

7. *Explore the difference, if any, between withholding and withdrawing care and the relationship between risks and benefits of treatment. What are some criteria to consider relative to decisions to withhold or withdraw life-sustaining medical treatment (LSMT), including the use of analgesia?*

   The focus of discussion: Fanaroff (2015) writes that, "If it is morally right (or wrong) to withhold treatment deemed to be ineffective, it is equally right (or wrong) to withdraw this same treatment after it is started, should it later become clear that the treatment is ineffective" (p. 33).

Criteria for LSMT to be considered: Infant's response to medical treatment, infant's current status, imminent death, and the presence of other comorbidities such as grade IV intraventricular hemorrhage. The use of analgesia is dependent on gestational age and unit-based policies. Refer to the chapter sections: Withholding and Withdrawing Life-Sustaining Medical Treatment, Palliative Care, and Special Considerations at End of Life.

8. *How are best interests of a neonate determined, and who should decide what these best interests are?*

   The focus of discussion: The neonatologist will provide information regarding long-term outcomes of a fetus born at 27 weeks gestation. There are limited data, if any, on the outcomes of a premature infant born with TGA at 27 weeks. Does this provide the neonatologist with enough data to present the family so that they may be able to consent to treatment or not?

(continued)

Case 19.1 (continued)

9. *Do you think it is possible to determine "best interests" without consideration of "quality of life"?*

   The focus of discussion: It is challenging to separate best interests from quality of life. Ethical decisions in neonatology are frequently difficult because of (a) uncertainty surrounding medical outcomes and prognoses, (b) lack of agreement over what treatments are beneficial for an infant, and (c) ambiguity in meaning of best interests and quality-of-life standards. Refer to the chapter section: Withholding and Withdrawing Life-Sustaining Medical Treatment.

10. *What are the categories of newborns who should be considered as candidates for PC?*

   ANSWER: There are three general categories of newborns who benefit from PC: (a) those with congenital anomalies incompatible with life, (b) newborns at the limit of viability, and (c) infants with overwhelming illness not responding to life-sustaining interventions.

11. *Is this patient a candidate?*

   The focus of discussion: Does the diagnosis of TGA compound the overall outcome of the fetus at 27 weeks gestation. Refer to the chapter sections: Palliative Care, and Perinatal Palliative Care.

12. *What standards and guidelines are available to assist families and staff in providing PC/hospice care to infants?*

   ANSWER: You should follow the policy and guidelines surrounding palliative care and hospice care both at the institution and state levels.

   The focus of discussion: What are the state provisions with hospice care in the community?

13. *Synthesize the procedure for initiating PC/hospice. Who should be involved? What resources are available to staff and parents?*

   Focus of discussion: Review the policy of PC/hospice at your institution. Once the parent(s) have made the decision to proceed with PC/hospice, create an environment that is conducive to the development of interdisciplinary collaboration at the end of life. This should include the medical team, nursing, pediatric subspecialist, chaplain, and social worker in addition to the family. Parents want to have the knowledge about the infant's condition and/or diagnosis so that they may prepare themselves for what may ultimately be their child's death. Local resources available to the staff and parents are specific to the area in addition to the national resources. Refer to the section Special Considerations at End of Life in the NICU. Compare and contrast these recommendations to the policies at your current institution. What improvements can be made?

Case 19.2

A 36-week gestational-age infant has been in the neonatal intensive care unit (NICU) for 6 months. Multiple congenital anomalies were present at birth and the baby has been ventilator dependent, with a tracheostomy, vesicostomy, and ileostomy in place. Other complications included pulmonary edema, as well as congestive heart failure as a result of cor pulmonale. Electroencephalogram revealed burst suppression and head ultrasound (HUS) showed cerebral atrophy, severe hydrocephalus ex vacuo with microcephaly occipitofrontal head circumference (OFC) was below the 5th percentile for age and weight). Peritoneal dialysis was initiated in light of renal failure. The infant experienced multiple episodes of sepsis because of the proximity of the ileostomy and peritoneal dialysis catheter. In the opinion of the neurodevelopmental pediatrician, there is profound delay and the outlook for productive life is bleak.

This family is not of American descent but has been legally in the United States for more than 20 years. Their religious and cultural backgrounds play a large role in their daily lives. There are five other siblings in the family, ranging in age from 16 to 26 years. Because of their religious beliefs, they were insisting that the baby receive maximum support and full resuscitation. They rarely visited but demanded that "everything be done" while awaiting a miracle, steadfastly insisting that the kidney failure be managed by dialysis until the oldest sibling could serve as a kidney donor.

In the opinion of the staff, the baby was not benefitting from any of the care that was provided and was, in fact, suffering from multiple interventions. There were several ethics committee consultations to discuss introducing palliative care (PC) and/or withdrawal of life-sustaining support.

Some of the nurses/staff expressed their frustration that caring for this baby in the face of the futility of the situation was a waste of health care resources, not only in terms of finances but also in allotting staff time in caring for the baby, who required cardiopulmonary resuscitation on an almost daily basis. The nurses expressed concern that they were actually hurting the baby and this violated their responsibility to protect the baby from harm. Thus, they experienced moral distress.

Consider the following specific issues when answering the questions in Case Study 19.2: parental autonomy, beneficence/nonmaleficence, quality of life versus best interests of the child, withholding and withdrawing treatment, role of ethics committees, futility, risks versus benefits of treatment, recommendations of professional societies, cultural and religious considerations when dealing with families. Also include subjects such as moral distress (causes, consequences, and approaches for relief) and guidelines for communication with parents.

1. *How far does the medical team go in honoring parental autonomy? Do parents' religious beliefs take precedence over the responsibility of the medical team to protect the baby from pain and suffering?*

   Focus of discussion: Discuss parental autonomy, futility, and the infant's right to beneficence and nonmaleficence. Refer to the chapter sections: Ethical Principles, Special Considerations at End of Life, Personal Considerations, Cultural Considerations at End of Life, Discussions With the Family, and Table 19.4.

(continued)

Case 19.2 (continued)

2. *What approach can the advanced practice nurse (APN) use when the parental autonomy and medical team conflict regarding beneficence and nonmaleficence toward baby?*

ANSWER: The APN can be a liaison between the family and medical team by the following:

Focus of discussion: Convey empathy and support to the family; validate their feelings; encourage expression of feelings, emotions, and desires; allow hope by offering truth and reality without denying hope; and provide frequent meetings to allow discussions surrounding their goals.

3. *Would this infant benefit from PC and withdrawal/withholding further care? Who should decide?*

Focus of discussion: There are three general categories of newborns who benefit from PC: (a) those with congenital anomalies incompatible with life, (b) newborns at the limit of viability, and (c) infants with overwhelming illness not responding to life-sustaining interventions. Does this infant meet the criteria? If so, who determines futility and what specific clinical data should be analyzed to determine futility? Refer to the chapter sections: Withholding and Withdrawing Life-Sustaining Medical Treatment, Palliative Care, and Futility.

4. *Synthesize the salient points to be included in conversations with the parents and siblings of the infant. Who should be included in the parent/staff conferences?*

ANSWER: Create an environment that is conducive to the development of interdisciplinary collaboration. This may include any of the following: the medical team, nursing, pediatric subspecialist, chaplain, and social worker in addition to the family.

5. *Is it ethical to consider issues of finances and allocation of resources at the bedside (ethical principle of justice)?*

ANSWER: These discussions should not occur at the bedside. As an APN, consider your role in this particular situation to facilitate a discussion away from the bedside. Consider offering a debriefing or similar setting to allow the nursing staff an opportunity to express their feelings. Refer to the chapter sections: Understanding and Addressing Moral Distress, and Tables 19.1, 19.2, and 19.3.

6. *Define moral distress. Explain why moral distress occurs. What are the causes of moral distress in neonatal nurses?*

Focus of discussion: Define moral distress as physical and psychological pain and disrupted interpersonal relationships arising from patient care situations wherein the provider becomes cognizant of a moral problem, accepts moral responsibility, and makes a moral decision regarding a correct course of action. Table 19.1 summarizes

(continued)

Case 19.2 *(continued)*

potential causes of moral distress for nurses; these causes are substantiated by the many references regarding moral distress that are included in this chapter. Simply stated, anything that interferes with a nurse's ability to provide optimal patient care has the potential of causing moral distress (Cavaliere et al., 2010). Discuss personal experiences. Refer to the chapter section: Understanding and Addressing Moral Distress, and Tables 19.1, 19.2 and 19.3.

7. *Analyze the situation relative to the moral distress of the nurses/staff in this case. What are the short- and long-term consequences of allowing moral distress to go unaddressed? Synthesize a plan for assisting the nurses/staff to deal with moral distress and achieve some degree of moral comfort while working with this infant and the family?*

   ANSWER: Refer to Tables 19.1, 19.2, and 19.3. Take into consideration personal experiences when synthesizing a plan.

8. *Who is best able to determine futility?*

   Focus of discussion: An ethics committee consult has been initiated. If the committee determines that parental autonomy supersedes the medical team's recommendation to withdraw support, should futility continue to be a topic of discussion? Refer to the chapter sections: Ethics Committee, Futility, and Ethical Principles.

9. *Who is best able to determine what quality of life is?*

   ANSWER: It is challenging to separate best interests from quality of life. Ethical decisions in neonatology are frequently difficult because of (a) uncertainty surrounding medical outcomes and prognoses, (b) lack of agreement over what treatments are beneficial for an infant, and (c) ambiguity in meaning of best interests and quality-of-life standards.

10. *What is a good death?*

    Focus of discussion: Personal considerations and professional experiences will influence this question. Refer to the chapter sections: Personal Considerations and Futility.

11. *Who is ultimately making the decision to continue or forego medical interventions?*

    ANSWER: Variable upon the institution's policy. There may be limited participation from the multidisciplinary team in the discussion of curative efforts versus palliative care. Refer to the chapter sections: Futility, Ethical Principles, Palliative Care, and Special Considerations at End of Life.

12. *How does culture influence a physician–family relationship? How does culture influence a family's response to healing and suffering?*

(continued)

Case 19.2 (*continued*)

The focus of discussion: Culture fundamentally influences how individuals make meaning out of illness, suffering, and dying, and therefore influences how they make use of medical services at the end of life. Define acculturation and how it impacts the physician–family relationship. Identify who makes the medical decisions for the patient, and who is the focal point of the family unit. This will impact the physician–family relationship tremendously. Refer to the chapter section: Cultural and Religious Considerations at End of Life.

Case 19.3

A 7-day-old full-term female neonate was admitted to the neonatal intensive care unit (NICU) from a pediatrician's office. The maternal, perinatal, and hospital courses were negative and noncontributory to the management of the case. The baby was discharged on day of life (DOL) 3 in stable condition and was breastfeeding well.

For the first few days there were no problems. The mother reported that the 3-year-old sibling came home from day care with a flu-like illness.

On DOL 6, the mother stated that the baby became fussy and did not nurse well. On the morning of admission, she became febrile (103.1°F/39.5°C) and was brought to the pediatrician's office in respiratory distress. The pediatrician observed a baby who was pale, tachypneic, hypotensive, bradycardic, and unresponsive. The family was sent directly to the NICU on the pediatrician's recommendation.

Stabilization of this baby included intubation, mechanical ventilation, intravenous (IV) fluids and inotropes, broad-spectrum IV antibiotics, and acyclovir. A chest radiograph showed complete bilateral consolidation. Right ventricular hypertrophy and myocardial dysfunction were evident on echocardiogram. Ultimately, a diagnosis of enteroviral sepsis was established. The medical staff was considering placing the baby on extracorporeal membrane oxygenation (ECMO). The parents disagree as to the proper course of treatment to select; the father wants "everything done," whereas the mother prefers a nonaggressive course and would like the baby to have a peaceful death. The neonatal advanced practice nurse (NAPN) assigned to the family is responsible for communication and support.

Consider the specific issue of communication with parents (in text and Table 19.3) when answering the questions in Case Study 19.3.

1. *Synthesize the salient points to be included in conversations with the parents and siblings of the infant. Who should be included in the parent/family/staff conferences? What information must be provided to the parents regarding the infant's diagnosis, current status, and long-term outcomes in order to equip them with sufficient data on which decisions can be made?*

(continued)

Case 19.3 *(continued)*

> **Focus of discussion:** The conversation with the family should reflect the following: Identify their needs collectively as a family and individually; allow the family to verbalize how they are coping; identify community support groups; identify in-hospital support groups/specialist; use child life specialists to support sibling(s).

Other considerations for family conferences: Schedule frequent meetings to minimize information overload. Identify the purpose of future meetings; for example, disclosure of lab results or radiographic imaging results. Assess the need for the participation of pediatric specialists.

Family conferences/meetings should have a purpose established prior to engaging in conversation. Core details about the current status, lab results, and long-term information should be presented with intervals of silence to allow the family to process the information. Refer to the chapter sections: Palliative Care, Perinatal Palliative Care, Special Considerations at the End of Life, Communication With the Family, and Table 19.4.

2. *Describe ways to support families when divulging "bad news."*

> **Focus of discussion:** Once the decision is made to have a family meeting whether it is to divulge bad news or discuss end-of-life care, place and time of where to have the meeting should be a priority. Describe what is the next step to support the family including members of the interdisciplinary team. Refer to the chapter sections: Palliative Care, Perinatal Palliative Care, Communicating With Parents, Table 19.4, and Special Considerations at End of Life in the NICU.

3. *What types of language could you use to facilitate parent–professional collaboration?*

> **Focus of discussion:** It is extremely important to minimize the use of medical jargon. What other terminology should be used to create a supportive dialogue and environment? Refer to the chapter sections: Perinatal Palliative Care, and Special Considerations at End of Life in the NICU.

4. *Is it appropriate to discuss palliative care (PC) for this newborn?*

> **Focus of discussion:** Prior to initiating the discussion of PC, the parents will need some time to establish congruency in their decision. Refer to Table 19.4.

Strive to know the family: Understand their situation, decision-making style, informational needs, communication preferences, religious/social/cultural background; their concerns; what is their understanding about infant's illness and prognosis; and explore parental hopes and fears.

5. *Why or why not?*

> **ANSWER:** Initiating PC discussion with a family who does not share the same goal(s) of treatment will hinder the relationship between the medical team and family.

(continued)

Case 19.3 (continued)

Supportive measures should be initiated to establish an assessment of the family needs and to create a plan of care. Refer to the chapter sections: Ethical Principles (parental autonomy), Palliative Care, Special Considerations at End of Life, Communication With Parents, and Table 19.4.

6. *Outline the approach for exploring the lack of congruency in parents' opinions regarding treatment options for the baby.*

   Focus of discussion: Create a table to establish the differences in opinion. Determine how to assess each parent's knowledge of the infant's condition, diagnosis, and futile interventions if applicable. Should this conversation happen collectively or on an individual basis? Discussions can be formatted as follows after the mentioned assessment has been completed: When discussing comfort care versus curative efforts, identify the options as follows:

   "If you were to choose comfort care, we can discuss how that would look like."
   "If you were to choose a trial of curative efforts, we can discuss how that would look like."

Refer to the chapter sections: Palliative Care, Special Considerations at End of Life, Communication With Parents, and Table 19.4.

7. *Explore the difference, if any, between withholding and withdrawing care and the relationship between risks and benefits of treatment. What are some criteria to consider relative to decisions to withhold or withdraw life-sustaining medical treatment (LSMT), include the use of analgesia?*

   The focus of discussion: Fanaroff (2015) writes that, "If it is morally right (or wrong) to withhold treatment deemed to be ineffective, it is equally right (or wrong) to withdraw this same treatment after it is started, should it later become clear that the treatment is ineffective" (p. 33).

Criteria for LSMT to be considered: Infant's response to medical treatment, infant's current status, imminent death, and the presence of other comorbidities such as grade IV intraventricular hemorrhage. The use of analgesia is dependent on gestational age and unit-based policies. Refer to the chapter sections: Withholding and Withdrawing Life-Sustaining Medical Treatment, Palliative Care, and Special Considerations at End of Life.

8. *Explore the ethical issues and principles relevant in this situation (i.e., autonomy, beneficence, nonmaleficence, etc.).*

   Focus of discussion: How will the medical team honor parental autonomy when there is not a congruent opinion? At this point, is there sufficient information to determine beneficence versus nonmaleficence? Refer to the chapter sections: Ethical Principles, and Personal Considerations.

REFERENCES

American Association of Critical-Care Nurses (AACN). (n.d.). 4As to rise against moral distress. Retrieved from http://www.aacn.org/wd/practice/docs/4as_to_rise_above_moral_distress.pdf

American Association of Pediatrics. (2013). Pediatric palliative care and hospice care commitments, guidelines and recommendations. *Pediatrics, 132,* 966–972.

American Heart Association, & American Academy of Pediatrics. (2016). *Textbook of neonatal resuscitation* (7th ed.), Elk Grove Village, IL: American Association of Pediatrics.

American Nurses Association. (1991). *Position statement on promotion of comfort and relief of pain in dying patients.* Washington, DC: Author.

Anderson, R. (2007). Boyle and the principle of double effect. *American Journal of Jurisprudence, 52*(1), 259–272. Retrieved from http://scholarship.law.nd.edu/ajj/vol52/iss1/9

Arzuaga, B. H., & Meadow, W. (2014). National variability in neonatal resuscitation practices at the limit of viability. *American Journal of Perinatology, 31*(6), 521–528. Retrieved from https://www.thieme-connect.com/products/ejournals/html/10.1055s-0033-1354566

Austin, W., Lemermeyer, G., Goldberg, L., Bergum, V., & Johnson, M. S. (2005). Moral distress in healthcare practice: The situation of nurses. *HEC Forum, 17*(1), 33–48.

Beumer, C. M. (2008). Innovative solutions: The effect of a workshop on reducing the experience of moral distress in an intensive care unit setting. *Dimensions of Critical Care Nursing, 27*(6), 263–267.

Bidegain, M., & Younge, N. (2015, June). Comfort care vs palliative care: Is there a difference in neonates? *NeoReviews, 16*(6). Retrieved October 4, 2015, from http://neoreviews.aappublications.org/content/16/6

Carter, B. S., & Jones, M. (2013). Evidence based comfort care for neonates towards the end of life. *Seminars in Fetal & Neonatal Medicine, 18,* 88–92.

Catlin, A. (2011). Transition from curative efforts to purely palliative care for neonates: Does physiology matter? *Advances in Neonatal Care, 11*(3), 216–222.

Catlin, A., & Carter, B. (2002). Creation of a neonatal end-of-life palliative care protocol. *Journal of Perinatology, 22*(3), 184–195.

Caulfield, S. E. (2007). Health care facility ethics committees: New issues in the age of transparency. *Human Rights, 34*(4). Retrieved from http://www.americanbar.org/publications/human_rights_magazine_home/human_rights_vol34_2007/fall2007/hr_fall07_caulfi.html

Cavaliere, T. A., Daly, B., Dowling, D., & Montgomery, K. (2010). Moral distress in neonatal intensive care unit registered nurses. *Advances in Neonatal Care, 10*(3), 145–156.

Chen, P. W. (2009). When doctors and nurses can't do the right thing. *The New York Times.* Retrieved from http:www.nytimes.com/2009/02/06/health/05chen.html

Corley, M. (1995). Moral distress of critical care nurses. *American Journal of Critical Care, 4*(4), 280–285.

Corley, M. (2002). Moral distress: A proposed theory and research agenda. *Nursing Ethics, 9,* 636–650.

Corley, M., Elswick, M., Gorman, M., & Clor, T. (2001). Development and evaluation of a moral distress scale. *Journal of Advanced Nursing, 33*(2), 250–256.

Corley, M., & Minick, P. (2002). Moral distress or moral comfort. *Bioethics Forum, 18,* 7–14.

Corley, M., Minick, P., Elswick, M., & Jacobs, M. (2005). Nurse moral distress and work ethical environment. *Nursing Ethics, 12,* 381–390.

Dupont-Thibodeau, A., Barrington, K. J., & Farlow, B. (2014). Communication with parents concerning withholding or withdrawing of life-sustaining interventions in neonatology. *Seminars in Perinatology, 38,* 38–46.

Ehrenkranz, R. A., & Mercurio, M. R. (2016). Limits of viability. *UptoDate.* Retrieved from htpps://www.uptodate.com/contents/limits of viability

Elpern, E. H., Covert, B., & Kleinpell, R. (2005). Moral distress of staff nurses in a medical intensive care unit. *American Journal of Critical Care, 14*(6), 523–530.

Engelder, S., Davies, K., Zeilinger, T., & Rutledge, D. (2012). A model program for perinatal palliative care services. *Advances in Neonatal Care, 12*(1), 28–36.

Epstein, E. G., & Delgado, S. (2010). Understanding and addressing moral distress. *Online Journal of Issues in Nursing, 15*(3), Manuscript 1. doi:10.3912/OJIN.Vol12No03Man01

Epstein, E. G., & Hamric, A. B. (2009). Moral distress, moral residue, and the crescendo effect. *Journal of Clinical Ethics, 20*(4), 330–342.

Fanaroff, J. M. (2015). Medical ethics in neonatal care. In R. J. Martin, A. A. Fanaroff, & M. C. Walsh (Eds.), *Fanaroff and Martin's neonatal-perinatal medicine: Diseases of the fetus and infant* (10th ed., pp. 24–40). Philadelphia, PA: Saunders.

Feudtner, C., Friebert, S., & Jewell, J. (2013). Pediatric palliative care and hospice care commitments, guidelines, and recommendations. *Pediatrics, 13*(5), 966–972.

Friebert, S., Bower, K. A., & Lookabaugh, B. (2012). *Caring for the pediatric patients* (4th ed.). Chicago, IL: American Academy of Hospice and Palliative Medicine.

Gardner, S. L., & Carter, B. S. (2016). Grief and perinatal loss. In S. L. Gardner, B. S. Carter, M. E. Hines, & J. A. Hernandez (Eds.), *Merenstein & Gardner's handbook of neonatal intensive care* (8th ed., pp. 865–902). St. Louis, MO: Elsevier.

Garten, L., Glockner, S., Siedentopf, J. P., & Buhrer, C. (2015). Primary palliative care in the delivery room: Patients' and medical personnel's perspectives. *Journal of Perinatology, 35*(12), 1000–1005.

Hamric, A. B., & Blackhall, L. I. (2007). Nurse–physician perspectives on the care of dying patients in intensive care units: Collaboration, moral distress, and ethical climate. *Critical Care Medicine, 35*, 422–429.

Hamric, A. B., Davis, W. S., & Childress, M. D. (2006). Moral distress in healthcare professionals. *Pharos, 69*(1), 16–23.

Hanna, D. R. (2004). Moral distress; the state of the science. *Research and Theory for Nursing Practice, 18*(1), 73–93.

Hilliard, R. I., Harrison, C., & Madden, S. (2007). Ethical conflicts and moral distress experienced by paediatric residents during their training. *Paediatrics & Child Health, 12*, 29–35.

Hills, P. (2016). Families in crisis. Theoretical and practical considerations. In S. L. Gardner, B. S. Carter, M. E. Hines, & J. A. Hernandez (Eds.), *Merenstein & Gardner's handbook of neonatal intensive care* (8th ed., pp. 821–864). St. Louis, MO: Elsevier.

Jameton, A. (1986). *Nursing practice: The ethical issues.* Englewood Cliffs, NJ: Prentice Hall.

Janvier, A., Barrington, K., & Farlow, B. (2014). Communication with parents concerning withholding and withdrawing of life-sustaining interventions in neonatology. *Seminars in Perinatology, 38*, 38–46.

Kagawa-Singer, M., & Blackhall, L. J. (2001). Negotiating cross-cultural issues at the end of life: "You got to go where he lives." *Journal of the American Medical Association, 286*(23), 2993–3001.

Kenner, C. (2014). Palliative and end-of-life care. In C. Kenner & J. W. Lott (Eds.), *Comprehensive neonatal nursing care* (5th ed., pp. 766–772). New York: Springer Publishing.

Lilly, C. M., De Meo, D. L., Sonna, L. A., Haley, K. J., Massaro, A. F., Wallace, R. F., & Cody, S. (2000). An intensive communication intervention for the critically ill. *American Journal of Medicine, 109*(6), 469–475.

Mancini, A., Utahaya, S. Beardsley, C., Wood, D., & Modi, N. (2014). *Practical guidance for the management of palliative care on neonatal units.* London, UK: Royal College of Pediatrics and Child Health.

McCarthy, J., & Gastmans, C. (2015). Moral distress: A review of the argument-based nursing ethics literature. *Nursing Ethics, 22*(1), 131–152.

Merriam-Webster. (2016). *The Merriam-Webster dictionary new edition.* Springfield, MA: Merriam-Webster.

Nathaniel, A. (2006). Moral reckoning in nursing. *Western Journal of Nursing Research, 28*(4), 419–438.

Pauly, B. M., Varcoe, C., & Storch, J. (2012). Framing the issue: Moral distress in health care. *HEC Forum, 24*, 1–12.

Pendry, P. S. (2007). Moral distress: Recognizing it to retain nurses. *Nursing Economics, 25*(4), 217–222.

Puntillo, K. A., & McAdam, J. L. (2006). Communications between physicians and nurses as a target for improving end-of-life care in the intensive care unit: Challenges and opportunities for moving forward. *Critical Care Medicine, 34*(11, Suppl.), S332–S340.

Raju, T. N., Mercer, B. M., Burchfield, D. J., & Joseph, G. F. (2014). Periviable birth: Executive summary of a joint workshop by the Eunice Kennedy Shriver National Institute of Child Health and Human Development, Society for Maternal–Fetal Medicine, American Academy of Pediatrics, and American College of Obstetricians and Gynecologists. *Obstetrics & Gynecology, 123*(5), 1083–1096. doi:10.1097/AOG.0000000000000243

Rushton, C. H. (2006). *The 4As to rise above moral distress.* Aliso Viejo, CA: American Association of Critical-Care Nurses.

Sporrong, S. K., Hoglund, A. T., & Arnetz, B. (2006). Measuring moral distress in pharmacy and clinical practice. *Nursing Ethics, 13,* 419–427.

Stowkowski, L. A. (2012). Dealing with death in the NICU—A conversation with neonatal palliative care expert. Retrieved from http://www.medscape.com.viewarticle/715963

Swaney, J. R., English, N., & Carter, B. S. (2016). Ethics, values, and palliative care in neonatal intensive care. In S. L. Gardner, B. S. Carter, M. E. Hines, & J. A. Hernandez (Eds.), *Merenstein & Gardner's handbook of neonatal intensive care* (8th ed., pp. 924–945). St. Louis, MO: Elsevier.

Van Zuuren, F. J., & van Manen, E. (2006). Moral dilemmas in neonatology as experienced by health care practitioners: A qualitative approach. *Medicine, Health Care and Philosophy, 9,* 339–347.

Webster, G. C., & Bayliss, F. E. (2000). Moral residue. In S. B. Rubin & L. Zoloth (Eds.), *Margin of error: The ethics of mistakes in the practice of medicine* (pp. 217–230). Hagerstown, MD: University Medical Group.

Whitehead, P. B., Herbertson, R. K., Hamric, A. B., Epstein, E. G., & Fisher, J. M. (2015). Moral distress among healthcare professionals: Report of an institution-wide survey. *Journal of Nursing Scholarship, 47,* 117–125.

Wilkinson, J. M. (1987–1988). Moral distress in nursing practice: Experience and effect. *Nursing Forum, 23*(1), 16–29.

Woods, M. (2014). Beyond moral integrity: Preserving the ethical integrity of nurses. *Nursing Ethics, 21*(2), 127–128.

Wool, C. (2011). Systematic review of the literature: Parental outcomes after diagnosis of fetal anomaly. *Advances in Neonatal Care, 11*(3), 182–192.

World Health Organization (WHO). (2015). Definition of palliative care. Retrieved from www.who .int/cancer/palliative/definition/en

Yee, W. & Ross, S. (2006). Communicating with parents of high-risk infants in neonatal intensive care. *Paediatrics & Child Health, 11*(5), 291–294.

Zuzelo, P. (2007). Exploring the moral distress of staff nurses in a medical intensive care unit. *Nursing Ethics, 16*(5), 344–359.

BIBLIOGRAPHY

Alelwani, S. M., & Ahmed, Y. A. (2014). Medical training for communication of bad news: A literature review. *Journal of Education and Health Promotion, 3,* 1–4.

Anderson-Fohr, S. (1998). The double effect of pain medication: Separating myth from reality. *Journal of Palliative Medicine, 1,* 315–328.

Atabay, G., Cangarli, B. G., & Penbek, S. (2015). Impact of ethical climate on moral distress revisited: Multidimensional view. *Nursing Ethics, 22*(1), 103–104.

Carter, B. S., & Leuthner, S. R. (2003). The ethics of withholding/withdrawing nutrition in the newborn. *Seminars in Perinatology, 27*(6), 480–487.

Catlin, A. (2011). Transition from curative efforts to purely palliative care for neonates: Does physiology matter? *Advances in Neonatal Care, 11*(3), 216–222.

Caulfield, S. E. (2007). Health care facility ethics committees: New issues in the age of transparency. *Human Rights, 34*(4). Retrieved from http://www.americanbar.org/publications/human_rights_ magazine_home/human_rights_vol34_2007/fall2007/hr_fall07_caulfi.html

Dupont-Thibodeau, A, Barrington, K. J., Farlow, B., & Janvier, A. (2014). End-of-life decisions for extremely low- gestational-age infants: Why simple rules for complicated decisions should be avoided. *Seminars in Perinatology, 38,* 31–37.

Epstein, E. G. (2008). End-of-life experiences of nurses and physicians in the newborn intensive care unit. *Journal of Perinatology, 28,* 771–778.

Epstein, E. G. (n.d.). *Ethics in medicine.* Seattle, WA: University of Washington School of Medicine, Seattle, Washington. Retrieved from https://depts.washington.edu/bioethx/topics/ethics.html

Ferrell, B. R. (2006). Understanding the moral distress of nurses witnessing medically futile care. *Oncology Nursing Forum, 33,* 922–930.

Gallagher, K., Marlow, N., Edgley, A., & Porock, D. (2012). The attitudes of neonatal nurses towards extremely preterm infants. *Journal of Advanced Nursing, 68*(8), 1768–1779. doi:10.10.1111/j.1365-2648.2011.05865.x

Gutierrez, K. (2012). Prognostic communication of critical care nurses and physicians at the end of life. *Dimensions of Critical Care Nursing, 35*(3), 170–182.

Hall, S. L., & Hynan, M. T. (Eds.). (2015). Interdisciplinary recommendations for the psychosocial support of NICU parents. *Journal of Perinatology, 35*(12, Suppl. 1).

Hamric, A. (2012). Empirical research on moral distress: Issues, challenges, and opportunities. *HEC Forum, 24,* 39–49.

Larcher, V. (2013). Ethical considerations in the neonatal end-of-life care. *Seminars in Fetal Neonatal Medicine, 18*(2013), 105–110.

Lorenz, J. M., & Hardart, G. E. (2014). Evolving medical and surgical management of infants with trisomy 18. *Current Opinion in Pediatrics, 26*(2), 169–176.

McGrath, J. (2014). Family: Essential partner in care. In C. Kenner & J. W. Lott (Eds.), *Comprehensive neonatal nursing care* (5th ed., pp. 739–765). New York, NY: Springer Publishing.

Mobley, M. J., Rady, M. Y., Verheijde, J. L. Patel, B., & Larson, J. S. (2007). The relationship between moral distress and the perception of futile care in the critical care unit. *Intensive and Critical Care Nursing, 23*(5), 256–263.

Moore, D., & Sheetz, J. (2014). Pediatric palliative care consultation. *Pediatric Clinics of North America, 2*(61), 735–747. doi:10.1016/j.pcl.2014.04.00

National Association of Neonatal Nurses. (2015, February). Palliative and end-of-life care for newborns and infants position statement #3063 NANN Board of Directors. Retrieved from http://www.nann.org/education/content/positionstatements.html

Parravicini, E., & Lorenz, J. M. (2014). Neonatal outcomes of fetuses diagnosed with life-limiting conditions when individualized comfort measures are proposed. *Journal of Perinatology, 34,* 483–487. doi:10.1038/jp.2014.40

Rosenzweig, M. Q. (2012). Breaking bad news: A guide for effective and empathetic communication. *Nurse Practitioner, 37*(2), 1–4. Retrieved from http://journals.lww.com/tnpj/Abstract/2012/02000/Breaking_bad_news_A_guide_for_effective_and.1.aspx

Samsel, C., & Lechner, B. E. (2015). End-of-life care in a regional level IV neonatal intensive care unit after implementation of a palliative care initiative. *Journal of Perinatology, 35,* 223–228.

Settle, P. D. (2014). Nurse activism in the newborn intensive care unit: Actions in response to an ethical dilemma. *Nursing Ethics, 21*(2), 198–209.

Webb, M. S., Passmore, D., Cline, G., & Maguire, D. (2014). Ethical issues related to caring for low birth weight infants. *Nursing Ethics, 21*(6), 731–741.

Weiner, J., Sharma, J., Lantos, J., & Kilbride, H. (2015, February). Does diagnosis influence end-of-life decisions in the neonatal intensive care unit? *Journal of Perinatology, 35*(2), 151–154.

Wilkinson, J. M. (1987–1988). Moral distress in nursing practice: experience and effect. *Nursing Forum, 23*(1), 16–29.

20

The Use of Simulation in Neonatal Advanced Practice Education: Case-Based Learning at Its Best

Desiree A. Diaz and Joan Esper Kuhnly

Chapter Objectives

1. Identify simulation best-practice methods
2. Identify simulation frameworks to create neonatal specific simulations
3. Identify ethical and practical risks related to simulation
4. Describe the methods for assessment, implementation and evaluation of simulation, and debriefing of students in simulation as it relates to best practice
5. Identify the level of simulations applicable to the advanced practice nurse at various points in the program

This chapter provides an overview of simulation pedagogy using evidence-based applications. Simulation in nursing has increased dramatically since the late 1990s (Hayden, Smiley, & Gross, 2014). The need for consistency in simulation standards has been echoed by many professional organizations that support simulation education (Chen, Grierson, & Norman, 2015; Jeffries, Dreifuerst, Kardong-Edgren, & Hayden, 2015). The creation of new teaching strategies requires increased continuing education to deliver best practice in educational standards.

The role of the advanced practice nurse within the clinical environment will require an understanding as well as a general comprehension of simulation best practice. The increased demand placed on health care providers to have adequate and competent staff at the bedside is reinforced by the Institute of Medicine's call for nurse educators who must not only engage in simulation to encourage practice at the full extent licensure allows, but are also expected to create and present interprofessionally within the work space. Practicing neonatal nurse practitioners are expected to teach, precept, and mentor neonatal nurses and future neonatal nurse practitioners in their role as an advanced practice nurse and educator in the clinical agency. Although simulation has frequently been used in neonatal resuscitation, the new neonatal nurse practitioner who has had positive experience with simulation in his or her academic program will embrace its use for more than resuscitation solely and realize the potential for teaching staff.

Simulation by definition is pretending to act in a manner as if the situation were real. A simulation typically consists of at least one participant and one observer. The observer can be the teacher or facilitator depending on the objectives of the activity. Group dynamics are usually presented in simulations in which there are a group of participants of three or more, while one participant acts as the nurse, the others are active observers (Jeffries, 2012).

The components of a simulation include all types of learning domains such as affective, cognitive, and kinesthetic (Adamson, Kardong-Edgren, & Willhaus, 2013). The learning domains also intersect with the knowledge, skills, and attitude encouraged by the quality standards (Sherwood & Zomorodi, 2014). The educator should take into account the identified domains (background, design, simulation experience, and outcomes [Jeffries, 2016]) when initiating a simulation activity. The beginning of that process is understanding best practice in simulation education.

STANDARDS OF BEST PRACTICE

Best practice in health care simulation begins with the understanding of basic terminology within the pedagogy. There is currently one set of health care simulation standards in the world and International Nursing Association of Simulation and Clinical Learning endorses them. The standards are renewed based on evidence in health science disciplines ("Standards of Best Practice: Simulation," 2013). Each standard requires a rigorous review of the literature to ensure the necessity of a standard and rationale for the expected outcomes. There are standards developed, including interprofessional education and research standards. In order to understand the development of neonatal simulations in relation to best practice, a review of each standard is presented.

TERMINOLOGY

A clear and consistent approach to educating participants is achieved through proper use of terms by each facilitator (Meakim et al., 2013). A full list of common and accepted terms can be found in the standards publication (Sittner, 2015). *Clinical reasoning, clinical scenario, assessment, guided reflection, fidelity, embedded participant, moulage, objectives,* and *prompt* are key terms that will be used throughout a standard simulation design. In an effort to standardize practice, the National League for Nursing (NLN) has developed a helpful simulation scenario template, which includes necessary components, including application to the test plan. Because simulation in nursing education initially focused on undergraduate education, the achievement of objectives has focused on application to components of the NCLEX (National Council Licensure Examination) test plan. However, as one develops simulation in graduate education, specifically the neonatal nurse practitioner (NNP) program, the objectives should be aligned with the NNP certification examination plan. Utilizing the NLN's template, the practicing NNP can then design simulation scenarios to teach neonatal nurses content that will align with the National Certification Corporation (NCC's) neonatal nurse certification exam on high-risk, low-incidence topics, such as exchange transfusion, or daily responsibilities such as communication with families.

PROFESSIONAL INTEGRITY OF PARTICIPANTS

Confidentiality within the simulation environment is crucial to a safe learning setting. Integrity within the environment relates to all aspects of the setting. Within the scenario performance, this includes specific content material presented as well as group dynamics (Gloe et al., 2013). Participants are more engaged and openly ask questions that expose performance gaps when they are comfortable and can reflect on practice (Jeffries, 2012).

The specific guidelines used for best practice in simulation were set forth by the International Nursing Association Clinical Simulation and Learning (INACSL) and endorsed by many medical simulation agencies around the world. This standard shapes the entire setting. Appropriate protection for participants is necessary to achieve meaningful cognitive and affective gains. The criteria in guideline one are essential for multiple scenarios that are run within any given day as well as repeated throughout the course (Gloe et al., 2013). Gloe and colleagues also specifically included the proviso that a breach in confidentiality relates to ethical misconduct. The specific citations for a breach in content security are dependent on facilitator and institutional policies. Participants should understand that when content is revealed, the next participant does not have the ability to respond as effectively as he or she would under the same stressors, thus limiting the value of the intended experience.

Feedback during and after the simulation is essential. Criterion two and three can be applied directly to this time in the learning activity. They are related to behaviors that occur during feedback. Civility is needed when a facilitator has to have a discussion of performance gaps. This is extremely important when critical elements were missed in the scenario performance. Specifics related to how to provide feedback are found in the debrief section of this chapter.

OBJECTIVES

The initial step in planning a simulation activity is determining your desired objectives. The objectives will guide the scenario. An objective should be measurable and have embedded opportunities within the scenario (Meakim et al., 2013). Creating objectives requires the instructor to prepare realistic goals. A guideline to follow is to include no more than three to four measureable objectives per simulation. Objectives should include assessments that are based in safety and are identified within the domains of active learning. When considering the objective, time management should be at the forefront. The question should be asked, "Does the participant have adequate time to complete this skill or task successfully in the allotted time?" This includes time to critically and clinically think within the simulation. An example of an appropriate objective would be: the nurse will call the NNP student or colleague in the neonatal intensive care unit (NICU) who will identify the rapid deterioration of a 25-week-gestation baby within 3 minutes. In this objective, can you identify the time elements needed for identification of deterioration? What are the expected signs that are being assessed? This objective is measurable and identifies the knowledge needed to physically act on the situation. The scenario would then need to have the props or moulage to facilitate the participant in meeting the objectives. A common pitfall by novice nurse educators is to include too many objectives in a given scenario. Maintaining a well-balanced simulation requires adequate attention to this concept. The idea is to simulate a realistic scenario that would include three to five obtainable objectives in the allotted time. The objectives should be discussed during the debriefing period to ensure all nurses present have the ability to engage in the process (Jeffries, 2012).

Objectives should be attainable for the participants who are engaging in the learning activity. Leveling of simulation scenarios via objectives may be beneficial to scaffold information that is expected of the participant. The same scenario may be used for multiple levels of students once the objectives appropriately reflect expected behaviors and are in alignment the curriculum (Lioce et al., 2013). It is imperative that the scenarios are planned appropriately for the different points in the NNP program. For example, beginning students may focus on history taking and physical examination skills. Second-year students may focus on critically evaluating a case and making management decisions based on their physical examination skills and then further communicating findings to interdisciplinary team members and/or the family. This is the same concept used for new graduates practicing on the unit. The initial simulation for staff nurses may be based on assessment of the neonate and notifying the provider of abnormal results, whereas additional simulations may include some psychosocial aspects of the family and interdisciplinary communication with social work, pharmacy, and potentially mental health services. Jeffries (2012) identified that effective use of simulation is best applied when the learner has the knowledge base and is aware of the objectives expected of him or her. Therefore, the scenarios should be a purposeful component of the course syllabus, intending to reinforce didactic knowledge that may or may not have been available for exposure in the clinical setting.

FACILITATION/FACILITATOR

The facilitator is essential in providing a well delivered simulation based education activity. The root of facilitation is the premise that learners can achieve expected outcomes and behaviors (Franklin et al., 2013). This standard requires the facilitator to be comfortable with different aspects of facilitation techniques. Techniques incorporated into the simulation are based in a constructivist and experiential learning method. The participants should be allowed to progress through the scenario without interruption, following a standard simulation design. Cues within the scenario allow guidance that is standardized among participants. A foundational element of simulation is that facilitating the learning process, rather than controlling it, is necessary for the process to be effective.

The facilitator is the educator guiding the learning experience, the NNP in the NICU, for example. According to the standard, a facilitator should have training in techniques to provide positive participant outcomes (Boese et al., 2013). This includes exploring performance gaps and promotes engaging discussions. The criteria outlined in the standard are based around clear communication, assessment, and professionalism.

Feedback is key for the facilitator. One must be able to maintain balance within the educational environment while providing honest feedback to all participants. The role is to actively engage the participants while allowing time for reflective pause and discussion.

DEBRIEFING

Debriefing is the most influential and important aspect of any simulation learning activity (Mariani, Cantrell, Meakim, Prieto, & Dreifuerst, 2013; McGaghie, Issenberg, Petrusa, & Scalese, 2010). Structured debriefing explores participants thought process and reinforces the cognitive aspect of learning. There are a variety of techniques that are used to discuss the scenarios (Raemer et al., 2011). Best practice is using a structured debriefing process in which a trained facilitator guides the participants, maintains a safe learning environment, and has viewed the scenario (Decker et al., 2013). A discussion among participants exposes the rationale behind individual participant responses within a debrief. The dialogue among peers as well as between facilitator and participant is crucial in experiential learning. There are multiple formats and styles used to elicit positive debriefing responses; however, here we will discuss two common types used.

Debriefing for Meaningful Learning

Debriefing for meaningful learning (DML) is a form of guided reflection that is based in education theory (Dreifuerst, 2012). Education theory is grounded in critical thinking and reasoning through reflection. DML is used to explore the thought process of the participants in a simulation while being guided by a trained facilitator. Participants and observers, as well as the hands-on person, engage within the scenario. The core principles are embedded in reflecting in, on, and beyond action. The debriefing method encourages participants to understand their own thought process. The elements of the guided reflection in DML are to engage, evaluate, explore, explain, elaborate, and extend one's thought process (Dreifuerst, 2012).

Plus/Delta

Plus/delta is an easy debriefing method to adopt. It is versatile in debriefing multiple groups within the clinical setting. A flip chart or white board is used to make a list of what was correct in the scenario and what could be changed for the better. The focus is on improvement of the outcome, not necessarily the rationale behind the thought process. The facilitator guides the discussion of performances and places them in the correct column on the chart or board.

PARTICIPANT ASSESSMENT AND EVALUATION

The seventh standard forms the basis for all evaluation methods (Sando et al., 2013). Evaluation is the purposeful outcome measure of simulation learning activities. It is important for participants to know which type of evaluation will be performed. A formative assessment forms or shapes the learning process. A summative assessment is a summary of a participant's learning, whereas a high-stakes assessment is a pass or fail test (Walters, 2014). Each type of evaluation should support the objectives of the simulation activity. The ideal scenario provides the opportunity for students to incorporate content and context through critical thoughts, which is accomplished by students being able to solve problems independently through progression without interruption of the simulation.

NLN JEFFRIES SIMULATION THEORY

A framework is needed when designing simulation activities. The NLN Jeffries Simulation Theory (Jeffries, 2016) takes into consideration all aspects of the simulation activity to ensure best practice and participant outcomes. The original framework (2012) has four components that include background, design, simulation experience, and outcomes (Jeffries, 2016). Each of the components is a cog in an interactive dynamic diagram. Each portion impacts the whole, causing a reaction within the learning activity; thus, consideration needs to be taken in each of the four components when creating simulation activities.

BACKGROUND AND DESIGN FEATURES

The objectives of the simulation must always be considered before creating the details of a simulation. Objectives guide the design and the props needed for participants to be successful. Simulating reality depends on how realistic the scenario that was created is. The realism creates the fidelity of the simulation activity (Jeffries, 2012). In the *Standard of Best Practice I: Terminology* (Meakim et al., 2013), *fidelity* is defined as the degree to which the simulation approaches reality, making it believable for the participants to act as they would in an actual clinical situation. Creating that realistic environment includes consideration of several factors, including the following:

> . . . . environment includes considering the physical factors such as the environment, equipment and tools; psychological factors such as potential emotional response or preconcieved beliefs; social factors such as participant motivation and goals; the group culture; and participant modes of thinking such as self awareness and trust. (Dieckmann et al., 2007; NLN-SIRC, 2013)

The standard further identifies high fidelity as a scenario that utilizes a full-scale computerized patient simulator or a standardized patient that provides a high level of interactivity and realism for the learner. It is imperative that designing the scenarios is dependent on the amount of fidelity that is appropriate to meet the goals while also using the resources available to the NNP faculty. For example, using a low- or medium-fidelity simulation manikin or model to practice intubation skills or line placement would be appropriate. If the goals of the scenario were to run a full-scale neonatal resuscitation, a high-fidelity simulator that has the ability to adjust cardiopulmonary, activity, and level of consciousness would be a more appropriate choice. In addition, one would require enough embedded participants (also known as a scenario guide, scenario role player, or confederate) who would simulate an interprofessional team to accomplish the simulation (Meakim et al., 2013). It is recommended that embedded participants who are students act only in roles with which they have experience.

Other simulation faculty or staff would act as other team members. For example, NNP students could act as an NICU nurse as they have experience being a NICU nurse, but it would not be appropriate to assign them a role as a respiratory therapist or attending neonatologist. It is also important to maintain fidelity by having staff or faculty who have the appropriate knowledge and/or scripts for their roles (Jeffries, 2012). If fellow students are to be used as the NICU nurse, for example, they should be prepared prior to running the scenario on what their role entails, whether they are supposed to provide any cues to the participants, and what resources they would have available if requested.

In order to facilitate participant success, there must be the proper equipment, setup, and props in the scene to enable the participant to become fully immersed in the environment. The fidelity does not require all the high-cost equipment, however, there must be props present to compensate for the altered equipment. Following is an example.

In a vented neonate, the endotracheal tube (ET) has been displaced. The object of the simulation is to discover the rapid decline in respiratory status and check placement of the tube. An actual ventilator is not needed as the skill associated with the simulation is not the ventilator setting, rather it is the need to assess placement of the ET tube. The inserted ET tube is needed because that is the outcome assessment for the simulation. A simple sign with ventilator settings on a cart with the proper tubing will illicit the same response (see Figure 20.1).

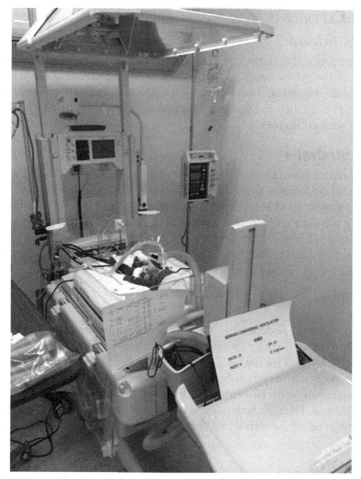

Figure 20.1 NICU Bedside Setup With Simulated Ventilator

Problem solving is noted within the complexity of the simulation scenario and based on the learning objectives. Reflective thinking within this component is supported by the standards of debriefing (Decker et al., 2013). Participant support and cues are the last aspect of the simulation design characteristics. Support for the participants is based on the environment and enhanced by facilitation standard (Franklin et al., 2013).

It is important not to underestimate the power of a cue in the simulation design. A cue is support to the participant that is planned (Jeffries, 2012). There are visual and verbal cues found within the scenario as well as unintentional cues provided by participants embedded in the scenario. A simple misplaced bottle of water can be misconstrued as an important aspect of the simulation and the participant begins an entirely different course of action based on the one misplaced prop. A visual cue provided by the manikins in the form of the baby turning blue alerts the NNP that there is respiratory distress. If there was no visual blue sign noted, there must be a cue in the form of monitor alarms sounding or the mother asking why it looks like her baby is not breathing. Careful consideration needs to be taken with everything that is found in the scene to facilitate participant success. If a cue is lacking or absent, the simulation designers must ask themselves how they would meet the objectives of the simulation.

SIMULATION EXPERIENCE

Facilitator/Participant

The interactive relationship between the facilitator and the participant is bidirectional. The characteristics of the relationship are dependent on each individual (Jeffries, 2016). This relationship is similar in all environments, such as the nurse educator in the hospital setting with the staff nurse, faculty and student in academia, as well as the charge nurse planning an onsite event with colleagues.

Educational Strategies

Educational practices take into account the diverse participant population and all learning styles. Jeffries (2012) identifies that educational strategies should incorporate active learning and diverse learning styles that are based on meeting expectations or objectives and provide feedback during and after the experience in order to promote the most optimal learning possible. The standards of best practice in simulation activities address all aspects of these two components (Borum, 2013). One must continually consider the objectives when creating a simulation while incorporating educational practices and outcomes into the design.

OUTCOMES

Outcome measurements are dependent on your primary objectives and audience. If the objective of the simulation is patient focused, the outcome measurement may be related to a patient-centered activity. Hospital-wide outcomes include measurements such as decreasing falls, infection rates, and system-wide measurements. Measurements should be concrete and clear. A participant objective can include behavior changes such as improving caring and empathy (Maruca, Díaz, Kuhnly, & Jeffries, 2015). The facilitator should have an understanding of what is being measured and the audience that is driving the simulation.

CONCLUSIONS

Simulation education and design are infused with theory and require consideration of best practices. The framework in which an educator chooses to design a simulation adheres to standards that often facilitate participant success. One must consider taking the time needed to create meaningful experiences that mimic reality. All participants should understand the use of simulation activities in their education and curriculum prior to participating in the activity. Increased fidelity suspends disbelief while participating in a scenario thereby creating the affective aspects of a live situation. The goal would be sustained knowledge, skills, and attitude gains that can be transferred into the live setting.

Case 20.1

Your nurse manager would like to have a simulation with the interdisciplinary team and has put you in charge of creating a learning activity to address the needs of the department.

(continued)

Case 20.1 (continued)

1. Prior to the actual design of a simulation for your interprofessional group, what factors should be taken into consideration?

A. Level of fidelity that is needed to meet objectives
B. The equipment and manikins that are available for use
C. The culture of the group involved in the activity
D. A and C
E. All of the above

ANSWER: E. *Jeffries (2012, 2016) explains the importance of taking into consideration the level of the learner, the culture within the organization related to interprofessional relationships, and the resources available to make the scenario real, thus creating a high level of fidelity. This includes the type of manikins that are available and appropriate props to meet the objectives of the simulation (Dieckmann et al., 2007). Each aspect of a simulation should facilitate learning.*

2. The standards of practice for simulation that were created by the International Nursing Association Clinical Simulation and Learning (INACSL) and promoted by Simulation in Healthcare include:

A. Standards of best practice in debriefing
B. Standards of best practice in interprofessional education
C. Standards of moulage
D. All of the above
E. A and B

ANSWER: E. *INACSL released standards in 2013 and added new standards in 2015 to include interprofessional education and simulation design. Moulage is part of creating realism. There is not a specific standard related to how to create realistic props.*

3. All of the following are the key steps in designing and implementing the simulation except?

A. Conduct a needs assessment to determine what potential learners would like to practice in the simulation setting or whether there is a need for improvement already identified.
B. Determine appropriate objectives for the learners in the learning activity but do not let learners know what the objectives are ahead of time so students can be surprised.
C. Design the simulation with team members who will be involved in simulation and debriefing.
D. The simulation should include all team members. The debriefing should also include all participants and they should be afforded an opportunity to evaluate the education activity.

ANSWER: B. *Interprofessional simulation is best conducted when appropriate team members are included in the planning (Raemer et al., 2011). Because the activity was designed as an interprofessional activity, one objective related to team communication would*

(continued)

Case 20.1 (*continued*)

be appropriate (Gosling, Sutherland, & Jones, 2012). However, learners should be aware of objectives prior to the simulation to promote the best learning and simulation experience (Jeffries, 2012). Debriefing must be included as the learning happens best when debriefing occurs after the simulation. Evaluation of the activity yields opportunities for future improvement (Deckers et al., 2013).

Case 20.2

Last year, the children's hospital adopted family-centered care as a core concept in their mission statement. You are a neonatal nurse practitioner (NNP) in a 24-bed Level III neonatal intensive care unit (NICU). In an effort to improve the patient satisfaction, the unit leadership team was given a directive by the agency's patient representative to address the deficit of families that feel they are not involved with discussion on their child's case.

1. ***The steps involved in addressing this gap between evidence-based care and current practice would include all of the following except:***
    A. Evaluation of current evidence to confirm the deficit identified by patient feedback does exist in relation to current practice.
    B. Key members of the interdisciplinary team should be involved in determining an action plan.
    C. Conduct constructive brainstorming discussions with current staff about the components of family-centered care identified in the literature.
    D. Disregard these discussions because you really don't see what this has to do with practicing as an NNP.

    ANSWER: D. *The case scenario refers to an educational need that should include evidence-based practice being consistent with family-centered care. The evidence should be gathered and evaluated and then presented to the key members of the interdisciplinary team, which could include medicine, nursing, advanced practice nursing, social services, dietitians, developmental therapists, and family support services (Melnyk et al., 2011). NNPs have positions of leadership and are integral members of the interprofessional teams and can impact practice changes (Gosling et al., 2012).*

2. ***The best suggestion on how one could improve the family's involvement in their child's case would be to suggest:***
    A. Parent attendance and participation in patient rounds and reports create a transparent environment that encourages parental involvement.
    B. Provide 24/7 visitation hours in the NICU for parents and any other significant people in their lives.

(continued)

Case 20.2 (continued)

C. Maintain an open NICU visitation policy for parents and significant family members with closure during 30-minute shift transitions twice a day and 1 hour for provider rounds once per day.

ANSWER: A. *Content should include the fact that addressing the knowledge deficit is the first step in solving this problem and through the process of presenting the content, root cause analysis can be conducted with the staff on how the patient rounding or reporting procedures could be done to include parents. An environment that promotes open, honest questions and concerns should be promoted to encourage staff to want to transform practice to align with current evidence. Offering 24/7 visitation is helpful in encouraging parental presence, but an invitation to participate in rounds and reports is much more deliberate an act of involvement for families (Gosling et al., 2012; Melnyk et al., 2011).*

3. ***Simulation may be utilized as a method for staff to become more comfortable with parent participation in rounds because:***
   A. Simulation is a safe environment for staff to practice a new skill.
   B. Staff should not need to practice patient-involved rounds in simulation because they should already be comfortable discussing the patient's case with the family.
   C. Simulation is a safe environment for staff to practice a new skill and additionally give the team an opportunity to debrief how the new policy went and determine any opportunities for improvement or challenges to overcome.

ANSWER: C. *Simulation of team communication and patient rounds with parents present could be used to breed familiarity with the process, allowing a safe environment for staff to express concerns about parents being present for discussions. The discussions may be more intense than anticipated during debriefing, due to challenges that need to be addressed (Jeffries, 2012).*

Case 20.3

As a neonatal nurse practitioner (NNP), you notice that when a call comes in from a pediatrician's office for a baby with significant hyperbilirubinemia, the nurses working on the unit have very little experience with exchange transfusions and express concern that they do not really know how to do one effectively.

1. ***As an NNP, your role in this process includes:***
   A. Ordering the appropriate lab tests, setting up potential exchange transfusion, and anticipating examination of the infant upon admission.

(continued)

Case 20.3 (*continued*)

B. Teaching the staff nurses how to set up the exchange transfusion and showing them where to find the written procedure for it.

C. Explaining the pathophysiology to the nurses so they understand the need for frequent lab draws during the transfusion.

D. A, B, and C

E. A and B

ANSWER: D. *Answers should include that the NNP should be a leader and take responsibility for safe patient care by nursing staff who may require education as well as referral to resources (Gosling et al., 2012).*

2. **After these patient needs are met, the NNP could proceed with which of the following plans?**

   A. Go home after working 24 hours and be thankful the baby's bilirubin came down adequately.

   B. Leave a note or send an e-mail for the leadership team to put potential options to maintain competency on high-risk, low-volume skills, such as exchange transfusions, on their next agenda.

   C. Volunteer to participate in the plan you suggest to the leadership team.

   D. B and C

   ANSWER: D. *It is necessary for all staff members to identify potential patient safety concerns; with simulation you can be part of the process to address this learning need to maintain skills competency with the nursing staff for such a high-risk, low-volume skill (Melnyk et al., 2011).*

3. **Skill attainment by staff can be best documented using:**

   A. A checklist of return demonstration

   B. Verification by return demonstration of appropriate setup of equipment and patient preparation after content is delivered to learners

   C. Learners take a pre- and posttest after an information session that covers applicable pathophysiology, implications for lab draws, patient indicators to be observed, assessment, and documentation requirements

   D. B and C

   ANSWER: D. *Completion of a checklist on return demonstration is appropriate but a response that is more specific is a better answer. Nurses would set up the equipment, conduct the assessments and procedure, understand the pathophysiology, and complete the documentation appropriately on an annual basis. If competency was not maintained, there should be communication about the error and the error should not impact the administrative evaluation of the employee. Leveled objectives for new NICU nurses versus experienced ones could be established or if the nurse actually conducted an exchange transfusion in practice, that competency could be checked off during the actual transfusion instead of in the simulation setting (Franklin et al., 2013; Gosling, 2012).*

ACKNOWLEDGMENTS

We would like to thank the University of Connecticut School of Nursing NNP/CRL for the collaboration and support. It is our honor to have worked with great providers such as Mary Whalen, Sandra Bellini, and Madge Buus Frank.

REFERENCES

Adamson, K. A., Kardong-Edgren, S., &Willhaus, J. (2013). An updated review of published simulation evaluation instruments. *Clinical Simulation in Nursing, 9*, e393–e400. doi:10.1016/j.ecns.2012.09.004

Boese, T., Cato, M., Gonzalez, L., Jones, A., Kennedy, K., Reese, C., . . . Borum, J. C. (2013). Standards of best practice: Simulation standard V: Facilitator. *Clinical Simulation in Nursing, 9*(6, Suppl.), S22–S25. doi:10.1016/j.ecns.2013.04.010

Borum, J. C. (2013). Introduction–Standard revisions. *Clinical Simulation in Nursing, 9*(6, Suppl.), S1. doi:10.1016/j.ecns.2013.05.009

Chen, R., Grierson, L. E., & Norman, G. R. (2015). Evaluating the impact of high- and low-fidelity instruction in the development of auscultation skills. *Medical Education, 49*(3), 276–285. doi:10.1111/medu.12653

Decker, S., Fey, M., Sideras, S., Caballero, S., Rockstraw, L., Boese, T., . . . Borum, J. C. (2013). Standards of best practice: Simulation standard VI: The debriefing process. *Clinical Simulation in Nursing, 9*(6, Suppl.), S26–S29. doi:10.1016/j.ecns.2013.04.008

Dieckmann, P., Gaba, D., & Rall, M., (2007). Deepening the theoretical foundations of patient simulation as social practice. *Simulation in Healthcare, 2*, 183–193.

Dreifuerst, K. T. (2012). Using debriefing for meaningful learning to foster development of clinical reasoning in simulation. *Journal of Nursing Education, 51*(6), 326–333. doi:10.3928/01484834-20120409-02

Franklin, A. E., Boese, T., Gloe, D., Lioce, L., Decker, S., Sando, C. R., . . . Borum, J. C. (2013). Standards of best practice: Simulation standard IV: Facilitation. *Clinical Simulation in Nursing, 9*(6, Suppl.), S19–S21. doi:10.1016/j.ecns.2013.04.011

Gloe, D., Sando, C. R., Franklin, A. E., Boese, T., Decker, S., Lioce, L., . . . Borum, J. C. (2013). Standards of best practice: Simulation standard II: Professional integrity of participant(s). *Clinical Simulation in Nursing, 9*, S12–S14. doi:10.1016/j.ecns.2013.04.004

Gosling, J., Sutherland, I., & Jones, S. (2012). *Key concepts in leadership*. Los Angeles, CA: Sage.

Hayden, J. K., Smiley, R. A., & Gross, L. (2014). Simulation in nursing education: Current regulations and practices. *Journal of Nursing Regulation, 5*(2), 25–27. Retrieved from http://ezproxy.lib.uconn.edu/login?url=http://search.ebscohost.com/login.aspx?direct=true&db=rzh&AN=2012637836&site=ehost-live

Institute of Medicine. (2011). *The future of nursing: Leading change, advancing health*. Washington, DC: National Academies Press. doi:10.17226/12956

Jeffries, P. R. (2012). *Simulation in nursing education: From conceptualization to evaluation*. Philadelphia, PA: National League for Nursing.

Jeffries, P. R. (2016). *The NLN/Jeffries simulation theory*. Philadelphia, PA: Wolters Kluwer.

Jeffries, P. R., Dreifuerst, K. T., Kardong-Edgren, S., & Hayden, J. (2015). Faculty development when initiating simulation programs: Lessons learned from the national simulation study. *Journal of Nursing Regulation, 5*(4), 17–23. Retrieved from http://ezproxy.lib.uconn.edu/login?url=http://search.ebscohost.com/login.aspx?direct=true&db=rzh&AN=2012860793&site=ehost-live

Lioce, L., Reed, C. C., Lemon, D., King, M. A., Martinez, P. A., Franklin, A. E., . . . Borum, J. C. (2013). Standards of best practice: Simulation standard III: Participant objectives. *Clinical Simulation in Nursing, 9*(6, Suppl.), S15–S18. doi:10.1016/j.ecns.2013.04.005

Mariani, B., Cantrell, M. A., Meakim, C., Prieto, P., & Dreifuerst, K. T. (2013). Structured debriefing and students' clinical judgment abilities in simulation. *Clinical Simulation in Nursing, 9*(5), e147–e155. doi:10.1016/j.ecns.2011.11.009

Maruca, A., Díaz, D. A., Kuhnly, J., & Jeffries, P. (2015). A content analysis of the simulated ostomy experience in undergraduate nurses. *Nursing Education Perspectives, 36*(6). doi:10.5480/15-1578

McGaghie, W. C., Issenberg, S. B., Petrusa, E. R., & Scalese, R. J. (2010). A critical review of simulation-based medical education research: 2003–2009. *Medical Education, 44*(1), 50–63. doi:10.1111/j.1365-2923.2009.03547.x

Meakim, C., Boese, T., Decker, S., Franklin, A., Gloe, D., Lioce, L., . . . Borum, J. C. (2013). Standards of best practice: Simulation standard I: Terminology. *Clinical Simulation in Nursing, 9*(6S), S3–S11. doi:10.1016/j.ecns.2013.04.001

Melnyk, B. M., & Fineout-Overholt, E. (2011). *Evidence-based practice in nursing & healthcare: A guide to best practice.* Philadelphia, PA: Wolters.

National League for Nursing Simulation Innovation Resource Center (NLN-SIRC). (2013). SIRC glossary. Retrieved from http://sirc.nln.org/mod/glossary/view.php?id¼183

Raemer, D., Anderson, M., Cheng, A., Fanning, R., Nadkarni, V., & Savoldelli, G. (2011). Research regarding debriefing as part of the learning process. *Simulation in Healthcare: Journal of the Society for Simulation in Healthcare, 6*(Suppl.), S52–S57. doi:10.1097/SIH.0b013e31822724d0

Sando, C. R., Coggins, R. M., Meakim, C., Franklin, A. E., Gloe, D., Boese, T., . . . Borum, J. C. (2013). Standards of best practice: Simulation standard VII: Participant assessment and evaluation. *Clinical Simulation in Nursing, 9*(6, Suppl.), S30–S32. doi:10.1016/j.ecns.2013.04.007

Sherwood, G., & Zomorodi, M. (2014). A new mindset for quality and safety: The QSEN competencies redefine nurses' roles in practice. *Nephrology Nursing Journal, 41*(1), 15–22, 72. Retrieved from http://www.prolibraries.com/anna/?select=session&sessionID=2965

Sittner, B. J. (2015). INACSL standards of best practice for simulation: Past, present, and future. *Nursing Education Perspectives, 36*(5), 294–298. doi:10.5480/15-1670

Standards of best practice: Simulation. (2013). *Clinical Simulation in Nursing, 9*, ii–iii. doi:10.1016/j.ecns.2013.05.008

Walters, L. (2014). *Simulation: The effects of simulation on high stakes testing in undergraduate nursing education.* Retrieved from http://ezproxy.lib.uconn.edu/login?url=http://search.ebscohost.com/login.aspx?direct=true&db=rzh&AN=2012683002&site=ehost-live

Afterword: Part One

Neonatal Nurse Practitioner Role Transition

Regina M. Cusson

This book uses a case study approach to examine maternal and neonatal social and physiological concepts to gain expertise in neonatal advanced practice nursing. There are other factors that influence expertise as the neonatal nurse transitions to the advanced practice role, such as role transition and the continuation of lifelong professional development. This epilogue addresses these crucial areas that must be considered when the neonatal nurse makes the decision to seek an advanced practice role. Successful development in the role is dependent on an understanding of and commitment to these important professional aspects of the neonatal advanced practice role.

ROLE TRANSITION

Life is full of role transitions and one's professional life is no exception. Although transitions are to be expected, they can bring about stress, even if the transitions are quite positive. When the neonatal nurse transitions to a role as advanced practice nurse, the transition can be overwhelming, even for experienced neonatal nurses. In fact, experienced neonatal nurses may be more prone to develop stress during role transition because they give up the security of being an experienced nurse for the uncertainty of functioning in the advance practice role. Previous research has demonstrated this expert-to-novice phenomenon (Cusson & Strange, 2008). Novice neonatal nurse practitioners (NNPs) with little clinical nursing experience also suffer from feelings of stress and inadequacy. The literature on role transition supports the universality of role transition as a time of stress, loss of confidence, and feelings of incompetence. Although role strain is a normal part of the transition process, strategies to enhance role transition are needed so that the novice NNP can fully actualize the new advanced practice role. Although most NNPs successfully transition after about a year in practice, it can take as long as 2 years before the new NNP develops the confidence and competence needed.

Meleis's (2010) transitions theory provides a helpful framework to use to consider this experience. Meleis indicates that *transition* is a central concept in nursing, from a patient, nurse, and organizational perspective. Particularly pertinent to role transition is Meleis's concept of situational transitions because the transition involves a personal and professional experience of moving to another level of practice. Barnes (2014, 2015) has described both successful and unsuccessful characterizations of role transition, providing additional support for the importance of a successful role transition in attainment of confidence, competence, and mature advanced practice.

There are several areas that can make a difference in preparing for the successful role transition from neonatal nurse to neonatal advanced practice nurse (Cusson & Viggiano, 2002). Simply being aware that the feelings of inadequacy and lack of confidence are normal and time-limited is the first step. Role strain is normal and needed for professional growth. Many successful nurses who seek upward mobility experience what is referred to as "the imposter syndrome." First described in nursing by Arena and Page in 1992, they detailed the experience of feeling like an imposter in the advanced practice role, fearing that others would find out their insecurities and inadequacies. Understanding that there are strategies that can be used to ameliorate the stresses of role transition can be enormously helpful.

Specific strategies can be utilized during the educational program to begin to prepare for role transition (Cusson & Viggiano, 2002). Participating in the choice of a preceptor can lead to feelings of empowerment, especially if the preceptor is someone known and respected. The importance of developing a mentoring relationship cannot be overemphasized. There is a difference between being a preceptor and being a mentor. A *mentor* is an experienced person who instructs, counsels, guides, and facilitates the development of others who are identified as protégés. The process of mentoring involves mutual respect, open communication, and trust. The mentoring relationship is guided by the mentor's belief in the protégé's ability to succeed. A mentor is someone who feels responsible for the success of the student. A mentor actively engages in finding experiences that will help to build the student's confidence and competence. Mentors remain a valuable source of support and guidance throughout one's professional career.

Making the most of the preceptorship means going above and beyond time limits and requirements. Sometimes the most valuable experiences occur after scheduled clinical hours, leading to extension of the clinical day. This often provides an opportunity to gain new skills. Being assertive in getting the experience needed in technical skills helps to decrease feelings of inadequacy and decreases the need to focus on technical skill development after completion of the program. There are also opportunities to explore all components of the advanced practice role during the preceptorship, not simply focusing on technical expertise. This is the absolute best time to gain experience in examining other aspects of the advanced practice role. Experience leads to feelings of confidence and to clinical competence in managing the high-risk infant's care. As the preceptorship develops, more autonomy should be expected. By the end of the preceptorship, the student should be able to handle all aspects of the beginning advanced practice nurse's role. Gaining proficiency in nonclinical aspects of the advanced practice role leads to increased role actualization. Seeking regular feedback from the preceptor can identify areas for growth. This provides the opportunity to develop a specific plan to strengthen competence in the areas identified as needing improvement. Developing strong communication skills is essential and will enhance developing relationships with new staff both during the preceptorship and throughout the professional career. Making the most of the clinical preceptorship and exploring opportunities for growth is invaluable in leading to a smooth transition.

Many of these strategies are also effective during the first advanced practice position. Being a good communicator aids in developing good relationships in the new position. Finding a mentor is key to success because the mentor can listen to areas of concern about perceived or real inadequacies in a nonjudgmental way, offering support and strategies for overcoming obstacles. Maintaining relationships begun during school also provides a source of support, as do friends and family members who can bolster flagging confidence. Many new advanced practice nurses are still recovering from the rigors of school and the process of securing needed certifications and licenses, while also relocating to a new agency or part of the country. Finding methods to decrease stress outside of work can also help during this period.

Acting like a professional, and not an hourly employee, who is willing to invest additional time and effort to become a valuable team member will go far in helping the NNP to become accepted in a new role and setting. Making your needs known is also important. Many novice practitioners are reluctant to admit to not knowing how to do something; this can lead to even more problems. Seeking guidance and searching out professional sources for the appropriate intervention helps to demonstrate that, although you may not know everything, you are willing to learn and know how to go about seeking the scientifically sound solution. This strategy also demonstrates a value on keeping knowledge up to date. Becoming active in a professional organization not only satisfies needed continuing-education requirements but also contributes to access to cutting-edge knowledge, which can be shared with colleagues. Becoming embedded in the nursing administrative structure also aids in sharing the advanced practice expertise outside of the neonatal intensive care unit and can make a major contribution to the institution. Facilitating role transition includes the strategies mentioned here and leads to integration into the practice setting, as well as to being a valued member of the health care team. With time and acceptance, feelings of inadequacy dissipate and the new advanced practice nurse begins to fulfill the multifaceted roles of the position.

REFERENCES

Arena, D., & Page, N. (1992). The imposter phenomenon in the clinical nurse specialist role. *Journal of Nursing Scholarship, 24,* 121–125.

Barnes, H. (2014). Nurse practitioner role transition: A concept analysis. *Nursing Forum, 50,* 137–146.

Barnes, H. (2015). Exploring the factors that influence nurse practitioner role transition. *Journal for Nurse Practitioners, 11,* 178–183.

Cusson, R. M., & Strange, S. N. (2008). Neonatal nurse practitioner role transition: The process of re-attaining expert status. *Journal of Perinatal & Neonatal Nursing, 22,* 329–337.

Cusson, R. M., & Viggiano, N. M. (2002). Transition to the neonatal nurse practitioner role: Making the change from the side to the head of the bed. *Neonatal Network, 21*(2), 21–27.

Meleis, A. (2010). *Transition theory.* New York: Springer Publishing.

Afterword: Part Two

Purposeful Plan for Lifelong Learning

Jacqueline M. McGrath

Providing excellent bedside caregiving can only be perpetuated through use of a purposeful plan for lifelong learning. Lifelong learning has been defined as an ongoing, almost continuous, voluntary, and self-motivated pursuit of knowledge for either professional or personal reasons (Davis, Taylor, & Reyes, 2014). Given the individual's attitude and personal motivations as well as a need for skill development (competence), approaches to lifelong learning must be flexible and diverse and occur during a variety of situations. The skill set needed for continued competence in a field of expertise includes taking responsibility for one's performance, with the awareness of when the needed skills are out of date or lacking; when this occurs the responsible practitioner seeks out experiences and knowledge to strengthen those skills. Furthermore, for those who respond better to external forces, specialty certification demands lifelong learning (Institute of Medicine, 2011).

A positive attitude about learning can be stimulated through an environment that fosters curiosity and inquisitiveness. Lifelong learning encourages creativity, imagination, resourcefulness, initiative, awareness, and responsiveness. These characteristics demonstrate the breadth of how lifelong learning might occur and how it can be purposefully sustained over the course of a life through several different strategies. Lifelong learning also enhances teamwork, engagement, active participation, and personal development, while at the same time increasing self-sustainability in the workplace, rather than competitiveness and employability. Lifelong learning is the foundation for how a novice neonatal nurse practitioner over time becomes an expert neonatal nurse practitioner (Benner, 1984).

Actively participating in lifelong learning enhances our ability to cope with and survive the burden of uncertainty. Lifelong learning includes awareness and reflection about everyday events such that knowledge is gained in the moment or in retrospect after an event occurs. It also provides the possibility of finding new and creative ways to handle a situation or negotiate conflict. More than 70% of adult learning is planned by the individual, such as choosing to attend a class or conference, or searching the literature for the latest article on a disease process (Gopee, 2005). Yet, for the learning to occur, the first step is taking the initiative to try something new.

Learning is not confined to the classroom or as the result of a testing situation; learning occurs daily throughout life because of the situations we encounter (Davis et al., 2014; Gopee, 2005). The learning we do is why we are different today from who we were yesterday.

Furthermore, learning can occur by becoming *more engaged* with the work. Engagement is the purposeful choice to become actively involved, be it with our health, workplace, or family life. Being fully engaged in the workplace supports the possibility of best outcomes no matter the situation because it demands thoughtful management of a multitude of tasks, setting priorities, managing time, solving problems, and improving skills. When engaging in each of these daily tasks, the expert practitioner is constantly learning and growing, using previous learning and experiences to be flexible in the moment but also taking in new knowledge at the same time such that "possibilities" are considered (Gopee, 2005). Informal learning is distinguishable by intent. It can occur almost anywhere and may, in some instances, be a by-product of other activities. It is often unplanned and occurs without explicit emphasis on learning, yet may still lead to the acquisition of valuable skills, knowledge, and attitudes (Davis et al., 2014). Learning can occur from communication and interaction with the environment; however, it is not just about being in the lecture hall or classroom—learning occurs when the learner is motivated to take in the information. The following strategies can be used to facilitate lifelong learning (Davis et al., 2014; Gopee, 2005).

Establishing a positive attitude about learning. A willingness to learn new things is playful and almost intuitive in a child but somehow is lost along the way in many adults. Yet, identifying problems and solutions as well as the opportunity to choose from a range of options can be part of the learning process. An attitude that learning is an aspect of excellent nursing practice fosters many transferrable skills that can be used throughout the workplace such as problem solving, project planning/management, independence, self-inquiry, self-discipline, and more important, self-confidence.

Questioning the status quo. It sometimes seems like it would be so much easier to go to work and provide care "the way we have always done it." But is that the best way? How many daily nursing care tasks are provided with no evidence? Have you ever asked, "Why do we do it this way?" A good example of questioning the status is quo is found in the work of Dr. Leslie Parker. Dr. Parker's current research examines the practice of gastric aspiration (Parker et al., 2015). Gastric aspirates are checked by neonatal nurses 8 to 12 times daily with no evidence that this assessment is making a difference in outcomes or that it is even safe for preterm infants. Yet, because we have always done it this way, the practice continues in most every neonatal intensive care unit (NICU). She asked why this was and has challenged us to consider whether this practice is in the best interest of the infant and even the nurse, given the time and cost involved in providing this assessment. This example of questioning the status quo could be applied to almost everything we do. Taking the time to be curious and responsible for why we do what we do is a great way to enhance learning and improve the caregiving environment.

Challenge your practice to use the most current evidence. Evidence-based practice is not just a trendy phrase; evidence-based practice facilitates best outcomes for patients. Yet, to truly be competent in the provision of evidence-based practice, the practitioner must develop and foster a number of strategies. First, he or she must learn skills to be able to search the literature using key words and terms to maneuver within at least two to three databases depending on the topic of interest. A really thorough search may require the assistance of a librarian, but beginning the process before getting the help of a librarian will save the practitioner and the librarian time. Second, the practitioner needs to be able to read research with a critical eye for the strengths and weaknesses of the study. Usually, developing this skill takes practice and can be facilitated by personal interactions or through journal club discussions. Lastly, the practitioner needs to synthesize the research findings. What do they mean in the context of how they were collected and what do they mean in the context of the care change you might be considering? Again, this skill can be facilitated with work-group discussions. No one is born being able to synthesize research; it takes time and practice but it is important in the provision of excellent evidence-based practice.

Consider the introduction of new technologies as an opportunity for learning. When new technologies are introduced in the clinical setting, learning about the technology can occur through several different avenues. As knowledge and skills become obsolete, individuals must continuously update their competencies using a process of continuous learning. This might include attending formal classes about the technology while also taking the time to explore the newest literature related to the technology. In addition, learning can be gained when working with others who have already gained this expertise with the technology.

Building on one's personal strengths and weaknesses. Lifelong learning empowers individuals to continue to grow and deepen their expertise. It can provide personal fulfillment; however, for this to occur, the practitioner must gain a personal awareness of his or her individual strengthens and weaknesses. Reflection about daily routines is a good place to begin. Considering what went well and what did not can provide a basis for developing a personal plan for growth. Some practitioners keep journals to record these reflections; writing down a plan actually increases the possibility that one will actually carry out the plan and thus increases the possibility of learning.

Mentorship. Challenging oneself to continue to grow comes easier for some than others. One strategy that can facilitate this possibility for growth is mentorship. Finding and working within a mentoring relationship is not just for when one is a novice in the clinical setting. Mentorship serves different purposes at different points in a lifetime. Mentors often challenge us to do things we would not consider doing without someone else pointing out the possibility of success. Mentors gently push their mentees to take risks, pursue ambitions, and to make positive changes that will propel their careers forward in ways the mentee might not have considered alone. Mentorship is a strategy for lifelong learning that is not always actively pursued; many believe mentoring relationships just happen but that is not the case; they are purposeful relationships that help us grow.

Use mobile technologies to support lifelong learning. One of my colleagues is an avid Google user. I have often sat with her during meetings or classes when she was using technology to find more information on the topic being discussed. It was amazing to me, at the time, how often what she found on the web quickly moved us along in our discussions and decision making. In today's increasingly fast-paced world of change, using mobile technologies to find information "in the moment" provides avenues that enhance our work. When used appropriately, this also can make the care we provide safer, more up to date, and evidence based. For example, checking medication dosing, looking up the right settings for ventilating an extremely preterm infant, or checking on the latest care for an infant with a rare disease that you have not dealt with for months can all make the care provided safer and more efficient in the moment.

Lastly, lifelong learning also includes personal growth that enhances a person's work–life balance. Work–life balance is a topic of concern for most practitioners. Yet, the evidence supports that a positive work–life balance actually enhances both the outcomes at work and in one's personal life. So do take the time to learn new things outside work. This can include such things as exploring a new hobby, taking a class in a foreign language, exploring the arts, taking the time to hike in a new park, or cooking a new dish for dinner. Not only do these activities provide balance and enjoyment, they also provide opportunities for continued learning.

REFERENCES

Benner, P. (1984). *From novice to expert: Excellence and power in clinical nursing practice.* Menlo Park, CA: Addison-Wesley .

Davis, L., Taylor, H., & Reyes, H. (2014). Lifelong learning in nursing: A Delphi study. *Nursing Education Today, 34*(3), 441–445.

Gopee, N. (2005). Facilitating the implementation of lifelong learning in nursing. *British Journal of Nursing, 14*(4), 761–767.

Institute of Medicine. (2011). *The future of nursing: Leading change, advancing health.* Washington, DC: National Academies Press.

Parker, L., Torrazza, R. M., Li, Y., Talaga, E., Shuster, J., & Neu, J. (2015). Aspiration and evaluation of gastric residuals in the neonatal intensive care unit: State of the science. *Journal of Perinatal and Neonatal Nursing, 29*(1), 51–59.

INDEX

Printed in the United States
by Baker & Taylor Publisher Services